2nd edition
surgery

The National Medical Series for Independent Study

2nd edition

surgery

Bruce E. Jarrell, M.D.

Professor and Chairman
Department of Surgery
University of Arizona
  College of Medicine
Tucson, Arizona

R. Anthony Carabasi, III, M.D.

Associate Professor of Surgery
Associate Professor of Radiology
Jefferson Medical College
Thomas Jefferson University
Director, Division of Vascular Surgery
Thomas Jefferson University Hospital
Philadelphia, Pennsylvania

Harwal Publishing

Philadelphia • Baltimore • Hong Kong • London • Munich • Sydney • Tokyo

A Waverly Company

Harwal

Editor: Jane Edwards
Editorial assistant: Joanne B. Crouch
Production coordinators: Keith LaSala, Judy Johnson,
  Laurie Forsyth
Illustrator: Wieslawa Langenfeld
Compositors: June Sangiorgio Mash, Richard Doyle,
  TeleComposition, Inc.

Library of Congress Cataloging in Publication Data

Surgery/[edited by] Bruce E. Jarrell, R. Anthony
Carabasi III.—2nd ed.
  p. 00 cm.—(The National medical series for
independent study)
(A Harwal publication)
  Includes index.
  ISBN 0-683-06270-0 (pbk. alk. paper): $23.00
  1. Surgery—Examinations, questions, etc.
2. Surgery—Outlines, syllabi, etc. I. Jarrell,
Bruce E. II. Carabasi, R. Anthony. III. Series.
IV. Series: A Williams & Wilkins medical
publication. [DNLM: 1. Surgery—examination
questions. 2. Surgery—outlines. WO 18 S9583]
RD37.2.S96 1990
617′.0076—dc20
DNLM/DLC
for Library of Congress   90-12980
                                              CIP

© 1991 Harwal Publishing

10 9 8 7 6 5

Dedication

We would like to dedicate this book to our wives, Leslie S. Robinson, M.D., and Jane Marko Carabasi, R.N., Ed.D. The many hours that we devoted were hours that obviously came from their time. Without their support and understanding, this effort would surely have failed.

Contents

Contributors

Frederick R. Armenti, M.D.
Instructor in Surgery
Jefferson Medical College
Thomas Jefferson University
Attending Cardiothoracic Surgeon
Thomas Jefferson University Hospital
Philadelphia, Pennsylvania

Vincent T. Armenti, M.D., Ph.D.
Assistant Professor of Surgery
Jefferson Medical College
Thomas Jefferson University
Attending Surgeon
Thomas Jefferson University Hospital
Philadelphia, Pennsylvania

Demetrius H. Bagley, M.D.
Professor of Urology
Associate Professor of Radiology
Jefferson Medical College
Thomas Jefferson University
Attending Urologic Surgeon
Thomas Jefferson University Hospital
Philadelphia, Pennsylvania

Bikash Bose, M.D.
Instructor in Neurosurgery
Jefferson Medical College
Thomas Jefferson University
Philadelphia, Pennsylvania
Consultant Neurosurgeon
Medical Center of Delaware
Alfred I. duPont Institute
St. Francis Hospital
Wilmington, Delaware

R. Anthony Carabasi, III, M.D.
Associate Professor of Surgery
Jefferson Medical College
Thomas Jefferson University
Attending Surgeon
Thomas Jefferson University Hospital
Philadelphia, Pennsylvania

Maryalice Cheney, M.D.
Assistant Professor of Surgery
Jefferson Medical College
Thomas Jefferson University
Attending Surgeon
Thomas Jefferson University Hospital
Philadelphia, Pennsylvania

Murray J. Cohen, M.D.
Assistant Professor of Surgery
Jefferson Medical College
Thomas Jefferson University
Associate Director, Trauma Program
Director, Surgical Intensive Care Unit
Thomas Jefferson University Hospital
Philadelphia, Pennsylvania

Herbert E. Cohn, M.D.
Professor of Surgery
Director, Graduate Medical Education
Vice Chairman, Department of Surgery
Jefferson Medical College
Thomas Jefferson University
Attending Surgeon
Thomas Jefferson University Hospital
Philadelphia, Pennsylvania

Anthony V. Coletta, M.D.

Instructor in Surgery
Jefferson Medical College
Thomas Jefferson University
Associate Director, Surgical Residency
  Program
Thomas Jefferson University Hospital
Philadelphia, Pennsylvania
Associate Attending Surgeon
Baltz Fellow for Surgical Education
Bryn Mawr Hospital
Bryn Mawr, Pennsylvania

Richard N. Edie, M.D.

Professor of Surgery
Jefferson Medical College
Thomas Jefferson University
Attending Surgeon
Thomas Jefferson University Hospital
Philadelphia, Pennsylvania

Diane Ruth Gillum, M.D.

Instructor in Surgery
Jefferson Medical College
Thomas Jefferson University
Attending Surgeon
Thomas Jefferson University Hospital
Philadelphia, Pennsylvania

Eric L. Hume, M.D.

Assistant Professor of Orthopedic Surgery
Jefferson Medical College
Thomas Jefferson University
Attending Orthopedic Surgeon
Thomas Jefferson University Hospital
Philadelphia, Pennsylvania

Bruce E. Jarrell, M.D.

Professor and Head
Department of Surgery
College of Medicine
University of Arizona
Health Sciences Center
Tucson, Arizona

Charles J. Lamb, M.D.

Attending Cardiothoracic Surgeon
Memorial Hospital of South Bend
St. Joseph's Medical Center
South Bend, Indiana

John H. Moore, Jr., M.D.

Assistant Professor of Surgery
Jefferson Medical College
Thomas Jefferson University
Attending Plastic Surgeon
Thomas Jefferson University Hospital
Consulting Surgeon
Magee Rehabilitation Hospital
Philadelphia, Pennsylvania

Michael J. Moritz, M.D.

Assistant Professor of Surgery
Jefferson Medical College
Thomas Jefferson University
Attending Surgeon
Thomas Jefferson University Hospital
Philadelphia, Pennsylvania

Pauline K. Park, M.D.

Assistant Professor of Surgery
Jefferson Medical College
Thomas Jefferson University
Attending Surgeon
Thomas Jefferson University Hospital
Philadelphia, Pennsylvania

D. Bruce Panasuk, M.D.

Instructor in Surgery
Jefferson Medical College
Thomas Jefferson University
Cardiothoracic Surgical Resident
Thomas Jefferson University Hospital
Philadelphia, Pennsylvania

John S. Radomski, M.D.

Assistant Professor of Surgery
Jefferson Medical College
Thomas Jefferson University
Attending Surgeon
Thomas Jefferson University Hospital
Philadelphia, Pennsylvania

Anne Louise Rosenberg, M.D.

Assistant Professor of Surgery
Jefferson Medical College
Thomas Jefferson University
Attending Surgeon
Thomas Jefferson University Hospital
Philadelphia, Pennsylvania

Francis E. Rosato, M.D.
Professor of Surgery
Chairman, Department of Surgery
Jefferson Medical College
Thomas Jefferson University
Attending Surgeon
Thomas Jefferson University Hospital
Philadelphia, Pennsylvania

Robert T. Sataloff, M.D.
Professor of Otolaryngology
Jefferson Medical College
Thomas Jefferson University
Attending Otolaryngologist
Thomas Jefferson University Hospital
Philadelphia, Pennsylvania

Joseph R. Spiegel, M.D.
Assistant Professor of Otolaryngology
Jefferson Medical College
Thomas Jefferson University
Attending Otolaryngologist
Thomas Jefferson University Hospital
Philadelphia, Pennsylvania

Jerome J. Vernick, M.D.
Clinical Professor of Surgery
Jefferson Medical College
Thomas Jefferson University
Director, Division of Trauma
Thomas Jefferson University Hospital
Philadelphia, Pennsylvania

Charles W. Wagner, M.D.
Associate Professor of Surgery and
  Pediatrics
University of Arkansas for Medical
  Sciences/Arkansas Children's Hospital
Medical Director, Arkansas Regional
  Organ Recovery Agency
Little Rock, Arkansas

Howard H. Weitz, M.D.
Clinical Associate Professor of Medicine
Jefferson Medical College
Thomas Jefferson University
Attending Physician
Thomas Jefferson University Hospital
Philadelphia, Pennsylvania

David A. Zwillenberg, M.D.
Clinical Associate Professor of
  Otolaryngology
Jefferson Medical College
Thomas Jefferson University
Attending Otolaryngologist
Thomas Jefferson University Hospital
Philadelphia, Pennsylvania

Preface

In keeping with the purpose of the *National Medical Series for Independent Study*, this book presents the core material of the specialty of surgery. The text is not meant to be all-inclusive and does not contain minutiae that we felt would be of little use to the reader. The authors have included not only didactic material but also facts that they find useful in clinical practice. Where controversy exists, we have attempted to present all sides fairly and to indicate factors that are essential in the decision-making process. We have also tried to stress situations in which surgeons and all others involved in patient care must work closely to make the most appropriate decisions regarding treatment.

In preparing the second edition of *Surgery*, we were able to focus on refining and updating the content and expanding the text when necessary. All of the chapters are now better organized in a more logical format. Certain chapters, such as Principles of Surgical Physiology and Liver, Portal Hypertension, and Biliary Tract, have been completely reorganized and expanded, and other chapters, such as Organ Transplantation, have been updated to reflect the rapid advances in the different fields of surgery. Two hundred study questions and explanations have also been added.

Surgery, 2nd edition, was written primarily for students and residents in general surgery, but practicing surgeons as well as physicians in other specialties will no doubt find it a useful reference. We hope that all readers will find *Surgery*, 2nd edition, represents a declaration of the state of surgical art in 1990.

Bruce E. Jarrell
R. Anthony Carabasi, III

Acknowledgments

The editors would first like to acknowledge Joseph S. Gonnella, M.D., Dean of Jefferson Medical College. Dr. Gonnella is nationally and internationally recognized as an expert in medical education, and his dedication to progress and excellence in this field has been our inspiration during the preparation of this book.

We would also like to express the admiration, appreciation, and affection that we feel for Francis E. Rosato, M.D., Samuel D. Gross Professor and Chairman of the Department of Surgery at Thomas Jefferson University. In our opinion, he is the ideal academic surgeon.

This work would not have been possible without the dedicated help of Mrs. Joanne Crouch. We gratefully acknowledge her assistance.

To the Reader

Since 1984, the *National Medical Series for Independent Study (NMS)* has been helping medical students meet the challenge of education and clinical training. In this climate of burgeoning knowledge and complex clinical issues, a medical career is more demanding than ever. Increasingly, medical training must prepare physicians to seek and synthesize necessary information and to apply that information successfully.

The *National Medical Series* is designed to provide a logical framework for organizing, learning, reviewing, and applying the conceptual and factual information covered in basic and clinical sciences. Each book includes a comprehensive outline of the essential content of a discipline, with up to 500 study questions. The combination of an outlined text and tools for self-evaluation allows easy retrieval of salient information.

All study questions are accompanied by the correct answer, a paragraph-length explanation, and specific reference to the text where the topic is discussed. Study questions that follow each chapter use current National Board format to reinforce the chapter content. Study questions appearing at the end of the text in the Challenge Exam vary in format depending on the book. Wherever possible, Challenge Exam questions are presented as a clinical case or scenario intended to simulate real-life application of medical knowledge. The goal of this exam is to challenge the student to draw from information presented throughout the book.

All of the books in the *National Medical Series* are constantly being updated and revised. The authors and editors devote considerable time and effort to ensure that the information required by all medical school curricula is included. Strict editorial attention is given to accuracy, organization, and consistency. Further shaping of the series occurs in response to biannual discussions held with a panel of medical student advisors drawn from schools throughout the United States. At these meetings, the editorial staff considers the needs of medical students to learn how the *National Medical Series* can better serve them. In this regard, the *National Medical Series* staff welcomes all comments and suggestions.

Part I
Introduction

1
Principles of Surgical Physiology

Michael J. Moritz

I. FLUID, ELECTROLYTE, AND ACID–BASE DISTURBANCES

A. Overview

1. Fluid and electrolyte **homeostasis** is determined by the individual's intake and output and is precisely regulated by the normal, healthy body.

2. The distribution of body water is shown in Table 1-1. The electrolyte composition and volume of various body fluids is shown in Tables 1-2 and 1-3. Table 1-4 shows the daily flux–losses and requirements—of water and electrolytes.

3. In disease states, regulatory mechanisms can become impaired and imbalances occur. The surgeon frequently encounters patients with these problems, which may be worsened by the additional stress of surgery, the use of tubes that drain fluids, which are not usually excreted, and the patient's inability to tolerate oral intake of fluids and nutrients.

B. Common acid–base disturbances

1. **Respiratory acidosis** is caused by carbon dioxide retention due to inadequate alveolar ventilation.
   a. Values. Arterial blood gases show increased P_{CO_2} and decreased pH.
   b. Compensation by renal bicarbonate (HCO_3^-) retention takes days.
   c. Treatment is improved ventilation.

2. **Respiratory alkalosis** is caused by an increased loss of carbon dioxide due to hyperventilation.
   a. Values. Arterial blood gases show decreased P_{CO_2} and increased pH.
   b. Treatment is decreased ventilation (e.g., sedatives) or rebreathing the same air to decrease carbon dioxide loss.

3. **Metabolic acidosis** is due to a loss of HCO_3^- or retention of some acids.
   a. Values. Serum electrolyte values reveal decreased HCO_3^- levels on an SMA6. A blood gas reveals a decreased pH.
   b. Compensation is by increased ventilation to lower carbon dioxide levels.
   c. A high anion gap defines conditions resulting from the accumulation of acids. Anion gap is defined as:

   $$\text{sodium } (Na^+) - [\text{chloride } (Cl^-) + HCO_3^-]$$

   with normal values equal to 15 or less.
   (1) Normal anion gap acidosis is due to HCO_3^- or Cl^- loss.
   (2) High anion gap acidosis is due to diabetic ketoacidosis, renal failure, overdose of methanol, ethanol, ethylene glycol (antifreeze), paraldehyde, or aspirin, and lactic acidosis.
   d. Treatment varies with the cause.
   (1) HCO_3^- loss due to diarrhea or pancreatic fistulas is treated with appropriate fluid and HCO_3^- replacement.
   (2) Acid retention requires specific therapy for each cause.
   (a) Diabetic ketoacidosis is treated with fluid replacement and insulin.
   (b) Renal acidosis is treated with HCO_3^- replacement and dialysis.
   (c) Lactic acidosis is managed with the treatment for shock (see Chapter 9 V).

Table 1-1. Distribution of Body Water

Compartment	Body Weight (%)*
Total body water	60
Extracellular fluid	20
Plasma	3–5
Interstitial fluid	15–18
Intracellular fluid	40

*Percentage decreases as body fat increases.

Table 1-2. Electrolyte Composition of Body Fluids

Fluid	Electrolyte Content (mEq/L)							
	Na^+	K^+	H^{+}*	Cl^-	HCO_3^-	Protein*	PO_4^-	SO_4^-
Plasma	142	4.5	. . .	100	25	16	2	1
Gastric juice								
High-acid	45	30	70	120	25	. . .	. . .	. . .
Low-acid	100	45	0.015	115	30	. . .	. . .	. . .
Intestinal juice	120	20	. . .	110	30	. . .	. . .	. . .
Bile	140	5	. . .	. . .	40	. . .	. . .	. . .
Pancreatic juice	130	15	. . .	. . .	80	. . .	. . .	. . .
Intracellular fluid	10	150	. . .	5	10	60	100	20

*Subject to wide variation in gastric and intestinal fluids.

Table 1-3. Volume of Gastrointestinal Tract Fluids

Fluid	Volume (ml) Produced per Day
Saliva	1500
Gastric secretions	2500
Bile	500–1500
Pancreatic juice	700
Small bowel secretions (succus entericus)	3000
Total	8200–9200

4. Metabolic alkalosis is due to loss of acid or loss of potassium (K^+). (Without adequate K^+, the kidney must exchange H^+ for Na^+, resulting in an acid loss in the urine.)

   a. Values. Serum electrolytes reveal elevated HCO_3^- and decreased K^+ levels.

   b. Compensation is by hypoventilation to increase carbon dioxide levels and renal HCO_3^- loss.

   c. Treatment varies with the cause. Loss of acid, usually from vomiting or nasogastric suctioning, requires fluid, K^+, and occasionally H^+ repletion. K^+ loss, usually due to diuretics, requires K^+ repletion.

C. Fluid and electrolyte imbalance in surgical patients

   1. Terms

      a. Volume

         (1) Too much water is defined as overhydration or **hypervolemia**.

         (2) Too little water is defined as dehydration or **hypovolemia**.

      b. Concentration is described in terms of Na^+, the principal extracellular cation (i.e., **hyper-** or **hyponatremia**).

Table 1-4. Normal Daily Fluid and Electrolyte Losses and Requirements

| Substance | Losses/24 hr | | | | | Requirements/24 hr/kg of body weight |
| | Urine | Insensible | | Feces | Total | |
		Skin	Lungs			
Water	1200–1500 ml†	200–400 ml†	500–700 ml‡	100–200 ml	2300–2600 ml	35 ml
Sodium	100 mEq§	40 mEq/L of sweat	...	...	80–100 mEq	1 mEq
Potassium	100 mEq‖	...	...	...	80–100 mEq	1 mEq
Chloride	150 mEq§	40 mEq/L of sweat	...	...	100–150 mEq	1.5 mEq
Bicarbonate	...	...	...	...	40 mEq*	0.5 mEq

*Lost in urine and lungs (as CO_2).
†25 ml/kg of body weight.
‡10 ml/kg of body weight.
§Varies with intake and with volume of urine and sweat. Autoregulated via renin–angiotensin–aldosterone system.
‖Aldosterone increases excretion.

(1) Note that there are three factitious causes of hyponatremia:
  (a) Dilutional hyponatremia (see I C 2 e)
  (b) Hyperlipidemia
  (c) Severe hyperglycemia
(2) With severe hyperglycemia, the serum Na^+ should be adjusted upward 3 mEq/L for every 100 mg/dl of glucose above normal [e.g., a serum glucose of 800 mg/dl (700 mg/dl above normal) will factitiously decrease serum Na^+ by about 21 mEq/L].

2. Types of imbalance. Any imbalance can be iatrogenic due to error or inattention.
  a. Isotonic dehydration is a proportionate loss of water and salt. This is the commonest imbalance in surgical patients. Common causes are:
  (1) Loss of blood (externally or internally)
  (2) Loss of gastrointestinal fluids from vomiting, nasogastric suction, fistula drainage, or diarrhea
  (3) Third-space losses. The third space, after intracellular and extracellular spaces, represents any soft tissue space. Injury or inflammation that leads to tissue swelling and fluid sequestration represents a third-space loss. Examples include burns, pancreatitis, peritonitis, bowel obstruction, retroperitoneal surgery, and cellulitis.
  b. Hypernatremic dehydration is the loss of water in excess of salt. It is caused by excessive loss of hypotonic fluid, for example, by perspiration, diabetes insipidus, osmotic diuresis (e.g., mannitol or hyperglycemia), and diarrhea.
  c. Hyponatremic dehydration is the loss of salt in excess of water. The commonest causes are renal salt wasting (e.g., diuretics or Addison's disease) and gastrointestinal losses.
  d. Hypernatremic overhydration is rare and due to the overzealous administration of hypernatremic fluids, such as fresh frozen plasma.
  e. Hyponatremic overhydration is common and generally is due to water overload with normal total body Na^+ (**dilutional hyponatremia**). It is usually **iatrogenic**, caused by the replacement of losses with inappropriately hypotonic fluids. It can also be due to the **syndrome of inappropriate antidiuretic hormone (SIADH) secretion**, which causes overconservation of free water. The treatment is **water restriction**.

3. Physiologic responses
  a. Dehydration causes activation of several neuroendocrine systems.
  (1) Renin is released by the juxtaglomerular apparatus, which senses the decreased circulatory volume. Renin, in turn, activates **angiotensin I**, which is then converted to angiotensin II.
  (2) Angiotensin II, a potent vasoconstrictor, also stimulates aldosterone and antidiuretic hormone (ADH) secretion.
  (3) Aldosterone acts on the renal tubules to conserve Na^+.
  (4) ADH, which is also secreted in response to an increase in plasma osmolarity, causes renal water conservation.
  b. ADH secretion is also increased by any significant stress, including trauma, burns, hemorrhage, sepsis, or major surgery. For example, increased ADH secretion persists for up to 5 days after surgery, accounting for the fluid retention that occurs postoperatively.
  c. Hypervolemia suppresses aldosterone and ADH secretion, allowing renal diuresis of salt and water. It also causes release of atrial natriuretic factor, which magnifies the diuresis.

D. Diagnosis of fluid–electrolyte disturbances

1. A history of fluid losses makes dehydration likely.
  a. External losses (e.g., bleeding, melena, vomiting, or diarrhea) are usually obvious.
  b. Internal losses (e.g., fluid lost into obstructed bowel, pancreatitis, or internal bleeding) may be subtle.

2. Physical examination must be attentive to:
  a. Vital signs. Orthostatic hypotension (pulse and blood pressure) must be checked.
  b. Changes in the patient's weight
  c. Skin turgor
  d. Moistness of mucous membranes
  e. Venous filling

3. Laboratory tests should always include:
  a. Hematocrit
  b. Serum Na^+, K^+, HCO_3^-, Cl^-, and glucose.

        c. Blood urea nitrogen (BUN) and creatinine

        d. Chest x-ray

        e. Other tests if needed

            (1) Serum osmolarity (normal: 285–295 mOsm/L). Serum osmolarity can be approximated by the formula:

$$\text{serum (mOsm/L)} = 2 \times Na^+ \text{ (mEq/L)} + \frac{\text{glucose (mg/dl)}}{18} + \frac{\text{BUN (mg/dl)}}{2.8}$$

            (2) Urine Na^+ and osmolarity

    4. Indirect measurements of circulating volume (i.e., central venous pressure and pulmonary arterial and wedge pressures) may be useful for diagnosis or for titrating treatment (rehydration).

E. Calculating the amount of the deficit

    1. A volume (water) deficit can be estimated clinically from the patient's body weight and appearance or can be calculated from the serum Na^+ level.

        a. Clinical estimates

            (1) In **mild dehydration**, the patient has lost 3% of total body water and complains of thirst.

            (2) In **moderate dehydration**, 6% of total body water is lost, and clinical signs of dehydration are evident:

                (a) Marked thirst and dry mucous membranes

                (b) Absent groin or axillary sweat

                (c) Loss of skin turgor

            (3) In **severe dehydration**, 10% of total body water is lost, clinical signs of dehydration are marked, orthostatic changes or hypotension may be present, and the patient may be confused or delirious.

        b. In hypernatremia, the water deficit can be calculated as follows: Given that normal serum Na^+ = 140 mEq/L and total body water = 0.6 × body weight (i.e., 60% of body weight), then

$$\text{water deficit} = \frac{\text{observed } Na^+ - 140}{140} \times 0.6 \times \text{body weight (kg)}$$

    2. Electrolyte deficits are calculated from laboratory tests.

        a. Na^+, Cl^-, and HCO_3^- deficits are calculated using the following equation:

$$\text{Deficit} = \begin{bmatrix}\text{normal value} - \\ \text{observed value (mEq/L)}\end{bmatrix} \times \begin{matrix}\text{electrolyte distribution in} \\ \text{body compartment (\%)}\end{matrix} \times \text{body weight (kg)}$$

        where the **Na^+ distribution = 60%**, the **Cl^- distribution = 20%**, and the **HCO_3^- distribution = 50%**. (Despite the fact that Na^+ is primarily an extracellular ion, the Na^+ space is considered to equal total body water because Na^+ controls total body osmolality. Therefore, 60% is used as the Na^+ distribution.)

        b. K^+ deficits are incalculable. **With a normal blood pH,** the estimate is:

            (1) For every 1.0 mEq/L decrease in the K^+ concentration between normal and 3.0 mEq/L, consider the total body deficit as 100–200 mEq.

            (2) For every 1.0 mEq/L decrease in the K^+ concentration below 3.0 mEq/L, consider the total body deficit as **another** 300–400 mEq/L.

F. Management of fluid, electrolyte, and acid–base imbalance

    1. Priorities

        a. Correct shock and restore blood volume to normal (see Chapter 9 V).

        b. Correct deficits.

            (1) Acid–base imbalance

            (2) Serum osmolarity

            (3) Electrolytes

        c. Define replacement therapy.

        d. Define maintenance requirements for fluids and electrolytes.

    2. Deficit correction is defined as the fluid and electrolyte therapy necessary to correct existing deficits. Deficit correction has **top priority** in fluid and electrolyte therapy.

    a. Examples of existing deficits include:

        (1) Blood volume deficit in acute or chronic blood loss

        (2) Extracellular or intracellular deficit in dehydration

    b. Replacement. In general, replace half of the calculated deficit quickly (over 12–24 hours), then re-examine the patient, recheck the laboratory studies, and reassess the need for further deficit correction.

3. Replacement therapy is defined as the fluid and electrolyte therapy necessary to replace abnormal (continuing) losses from or within the body (e.g., via drainage tubes). Replacement therapy has **second priority** in fluid and electrolyte therapy.

    a. Examples of continuing losses

        (1) Gastrointestinal losses (see Tables 1-2 and 1-5)

            (a) If these are purely gastric (succus gastricus), a solution providing 0.45% NaCl (½ normal saline) plus 20 or 30 mEq KCl/L is used for replacement.

            (b) If the fluid lost also contains intestinal juice (succus entericus), lactated Ringer's solution plus 10 mEq KCl/L is used for replacement.

        (2) Third-space loss

            (a) The amount of loss varies with the magnitude of the injury.

            (b) Lactated Ringer's or normal saline solution plus albumin is used for replacement.

    b. Replacement. Continuing losses require volume-for-volume replacement and must be added to maintenance requirements.

    c. Determining the electrolyte composition of continuing losses will aid in replacement therapy.

4. Maintenance therapy is defined as the fluid and electrolyte therapy necessary to maintain fluid and electrolyte balance in an individual.

    a. If inadequate calories are provided, maintenance therapy should be associated with a weight loss of approximately ¼ to ½ lb/day.

    b. Weight gain in the absence of adequate caloric intake implies excessive fluid intake.

5. Table 1-4 lists the daily maintenance requirements for fluid and electrolytes after existing deficits have been corrected. Table 1-5 lists commonly used electrolyte solutions and their principal uses.

G. Clinical examples

1. Maintenance therapy

    a. This provides the fluid and electrolytes necessary to satisfy the normal requirements in the absence of abnormal losses.

    b. Example. An average-sized (60-kg) woman has had an elective cholecystectomy. No nasogastric tube is placed, and there is no T tube.

        (1) Normal daily requirements for this patient would be calculated as follows:

            (a) Water: 35 ml/kg × 60 kg = 2100 ml.

            (b) Na^+: 1 mEq/kg × 60 kg = 60 mEq.

            (c) K^+: 1 mEq/kg × 60 kg = 60 mEq.

            (d) Cl^-: 1.5 mEq/kg × 60 kg = 90 mEq.

            (e) HCO_3^-: 0.5 mEq/kg × 60 kg = 30 mEq. (In a healthy individual, the bicarbonate buffer system is so efficient that small bicarbonate requirements can be ignored.)

        (2) Intravenous (IV) fluid orders would be:

            (a) 2000 ml 5% dextrose in ¼ normal saline with 30 mEq KCl/L

            (b) 500 ml 5% dextrose in ½ normal saline

        (3) This will provide:

            (a) 2500 ml of water

            (b) 84 mEq of Na^+

            (c) 60 mEq of K^+

            (d) 84 mEq of Cl^-

            (e) No HCO_3^-

        (4) In addition to the **type and quantity** of fluid ordered, the **rate of administration** should be stated (e.g., 100 ml/hr, 250 ml/hr, and so forth), depending on the volume of fluid required for a 24-hour period in a given patient.

2. Replacement therapy

    a. This provides the fluid and electrolytes necessary to replace abnormal losses from the body or within the body.

Table 1-5. Commonly Used Parenteral Solutions

Solutions	Na$^+$	K$^+$	Cl$^-$	HCO$_3$$^-$	Ca^{2+}	Principal Uses
	Electrolyte Content					
	(mEq/L)					
0.9% (isotonic) NaCl* (saline) [PSS or NS]	154	. . .	154	. . .	. . .	ECF replacement; correction of hyponatremia
0.45% (½ normal) NaCl* (½ PSS or ½ NS)	77	. . .	77	. . .	. . .	Na$^+$ maintenance; gastric fluid replacement
0.27% (¼ normal) NaCl* (¼ PSS or ¼ NS)	38	. . .	38	. . .	. . .	As for D5W below. Overuse will cause hyponatremia.
LR*	130	4	109	28	3	Best ECF replacement; correction of isotonic deficit
D5W	. . .	. . .	. . .	. . .	. . .	Correction or replacement of insensible water loss; correction of hyperosmolar dehydration. Overuse will cause hyponatremia.
	(mEq/dl)					
3% NaCl injection	51	. . .	51	. . .	. . .	Correction of symptomatic Na$^+$ deficit, 510 mEq/L
5% NaCl injection	85	. . .	85	. . .	. . .	Correction of symptomatic Na$^+$ deficit, 850 mEq/L
	(mEq/ampul)					
14.9% KCl (ampule)	. . .	40	40	. . .	. . .	Additive for K$^+$ maintenance; correction of K$^+$ and acid–base imbalance. Never add more than 40 mEq to each liter of fluid.
7.5% NaHCO$_3$$^-$ (ampule)	44.6	. . .	. . .	44.6	. . .	Additive for GI losses; correction of metabolic acidosis

PSS = physiologic strength saline; NS = normal saline; ECF = extracellular fluid; LR = lactated Ringer's solution; D5W = 5% dextrose in water; GI = gastrointestinal.
*With or without 5% dextrose.

   b. Example. The same patient as in I G 1 b develops an ileus after her cholecystectomy, requiring insertion of a nasogastric tube. Over the next 24 hours, there is 1600 ml of nasogastric drainage, which is bile-stained. Serum electrolytes are normal.
      (1) Requirements for this patient would be as follows:
         (a) For **replacement**, she would require 1600 ml as 5% dextrose in lactated Ringer's solution (D5LR) + 20 mEq KCl/L (from Table 1-2, gastric juice).
         (b) Her **maintenance** requirements would remain the same as in I G 1 b (1).
      (2) IV fluid orders would become:
         (a) 2000 ml 5% dextrose in ¼ normal saline + 30 mEq KCl/L
         (b) 2000 ml 5% dextrose in lactated Ringer's solution + 20 mEq KCl/L
         (c) Total volume is 4 L (1600 ml replacement plus 2400 ml maintenance) to run at a rate of 170 ml/hr (= 4 L/day)
         (d) Total Na$^+$ = 337 mEq; K$^+$ = 108 mEq; and Cl$^-$ = 295 mEq

   3. Hypernatremic dehydration
      a. In hypernatremic dehydration, the serum Na$^+$ concentration is elevated.
      b. Example. A 70-kg woman jogging on a hot day faints and is brought to the emergency room. Her vital signs are normal. She complains of thirst. Her serum Na$^+$ = 160 mEq/L.

Requirements for this woman would be calculated as follows:
(1) Water deficit:

$$= \frac{160 - 140}{140} \times (60\%) \, (70)$$

$$= \frac{20}{140} \times (0.6) \, (70)$$

$$= (0.14) \, (42)$$

$$= 5.9 \text{ L}$$

(2) Fluid requirement: 2.9 L + 2.4 L = 5.1 L of fluid in next 24 hours, containing 70 mEq Na^+.
   (a) The formula used here is ½ the water deficit (5.9 L/2) + normal daily fluid requirement (2.4 L).
   (b) To this is added the normal daily Na^+ requirement (70 mEq).

4. Isotonic dehydration
   a. In isotonic dehydration, the serum Na^+ concentration is normal.
   b. Example. A short, obese alcoholic patient presents with vomiting due to gastritis and with a fever of 100.6° F due to pneumonitis. He is complaining of thirst and a dry mouth and has no groin or axillary sweat. He is alert and normotensive. His weight is 100 kg; his serum Na^+ level is 140 mEq/L, and his serum K^+ level is 3.0 mEq/L. His requirements would be calculated as follows:
   (1) Fluid loss: 6% (based on clinical findings)
   (2) Isotonic fluid loss: 100 kg × 60% × 6% = 3.6 L.
   (3) Na^+ loss (in isotonic fluid): 140 mEq/L × 3.6 L = 504 mEq.
   (4) Twenty-four-hour Na^+ requirement: 504 mEq/2 + 100 mEq = 352 mEq.
   (5) Twenty-four-hour fluid requirement: 4.2 L/2 + 4.2 L = 6.3 L.
     (a) The daily fluid requirement is 4.2 L instead of 3.6 L because of the patient's fever: Each 1° rise in temperature increases the daily fluid requirement by about 10%.
     (b) The fluid and Na^+ replacement can be given as 5 L of 5% dextrose in ½ normal saline.
       (i) KCl should be added as indicated, at ½ of the deficit plus the daily requirement (100 mEq), provided that urine flow is adequate.
       (ii) Thus, since the patient has a K^+ deficit of 200 mEq (see I E 2 b), (½ × 200) + 100 mEq of KCl would be divided among all the solutions.

5. Hyponatremic dehydration
   a. In hyponatremic dehydration, the serum Na^+ concentration is decreased.
   b. Example. A muscular 50-year-old man with polycystic kidney disease presents with hypotension, weakness, confusion, oliguria, and no axillary sweat.
   (1) His past medical record shows that he has **polyuria,** he has been eating a low-salt diet because of mild hypertension, his BUN has been stable at 40 mg/dl, and his blood carbon dioxide content has been 20 mmol/L.
   (2) He now has a metabolic acidosis with a blood carbon dioxide content of 15 mmol/L and a serum Na^+ level of 120 mEq/L. His body weight is 90 kg, and his urine output is 1700 ml/day.
   (3) His requirements would be calculated as follows:
     (a) Fluid deficit = 10% dehydration × body weight (90 kg) × 60% = 5.4 L. This deficit is considered to be isotonic (i.e., Na^+ = 140 mEq/L).
     (b) Isotonic sodium deficit: 5.4 L × 140 mEq/L = 756 mEq.
     (c) Hypotonic sodium deficit: 54 L × 20 mEq/L = 1080 mEq.
       (i) The formula used here is Na^+ deficit × total body water [i.e., (normal Na^+ − observed Na^+) × body weight × Na^+ space]. See I E 2 a.
       (ii) For our patient, the figures used are: Na^+ deficit: 140 mEq/L − 120 mEq/L = 20 mEq/L. Total body water: 90 kg × 60% = 54 L.
     (d) Twenty-four-hour Na^+ requirement: ½ (1080 mEq + 756 mEq) + 75 mEq = 993 mEq.
     (e) HCO_3^- replacement is calculated as: 5 mEq/L deficit × 90 kg × 50% HCO_3^- space = 225 mEq.
   (4) The patient's 24-hour requirement can be given as 5 L of physiologic strength saline with one ampule of $NaHCO_3^-$ added to each liter at 200 ml/hr. Note that each liter is hypernatremic with 154 + 44 mEq Na^+.

II. NUTRITION IN THE SURGICAL PATIENT

A. Energy capacity of three sources of fuel

  1. Fat = 9 kcal/g.

  2. Carbohydrate = 3.4 kcal/g.

  3. Protein = 4 kcal/g.

B. Stored energy in a normal human

  1. Fat generally comprises 25% of body weight.

    a. A 70-kg man has about 17 kg of fat, equivalent to 160,000 kcal.

    b. There are three essential fatty acids: linoleic, linolenic, and arachidonic.

    c. During **fasting**, stored fat is metabolized to free fatty acids, ketone bodies, which are used for energy by most body tissues, and glycerol, a fuel for gluconeogenesis, which provides glucose for nerve cells and blood cells.

    d. Fat stores can last for up to 40 days of starvation.

  2. Carbohydrate is present in several forms in the body.

    a. Circulating **glucose** supplies about 80 kcal.

    b. **Liver glycogen** provides about 300 kcal of stored carbohydrate, which is released into the circulation as glucose.

    c. **Muscle glycogen** contains 600 kcal of carbohydrate, which is expended during muscle contraction.

    d. Total carbohydrate is approximately 290 g and is exhausted in 24 hours or less.

  3. Protein comprises about 12 kg of a 70-kg man for a caloric value of 48,000 kcal, most of which is *not* accessible as an energy source except during prolonged catabolism or starvation. Body protein is present in several forms:

    a. Muscle (skeletal, smooth, and cardiac)

    b. Other intracellular molecules, such as enzymes

    c. Circulating proteins, such as albumin and antibodies

    d. Structural proteins, such as collagen and elastin

C. Nutrient requirements

  1. Energy needs

    a. Basal caloric needs (e.g., for nonstressed persons at bed rest) are 25–35 kcal/kg/day.

    b. Most hospitalized patients require between 35 and 45 kcal/kg of body weight/day (1 kcal = 1 Cal = 1000 Cal).

    c. Patients with increased metabolism, such as those with multiple trauma, sepsis, extensive burns, or after surgery, may require 50–70 kcal/kg/day.

  2. Protein requirements

    a. The average 70-kg adult man uses about 70 g of protein a day.

      (1) This protein must be replaced to maintain protein equilibrium (or nitrogen equilibrium).

      (2) A total of 6.25 g of protein is equivalent to 1 g of body nitrogen.

    b. A daily intake of 1–1.5 g of protein per kg of body weight satisfies the requirements of most adult surgical patients.

    c. Protein intake may require restriction in diseases with impaired nitrogen excretion or metabolism, such as renal failure or hepatic cirrhosis.

    d. Increased protein intake is required in patients with conditions that cause excessive catabolism, such as sepsis, multiple fractures, or burns.

  3. A calorie-to-nitrogen ratio of 150–200 kcal/g of nitrogen is generally appropriate for surgical patients.

D. Malnutrition

  1. Causes of malnutrition in surgical patients are varied, and commonly, patients are malnourished for a combination of reasons.

    a. Increased catabolism, in excess of nutrient intake (e.g., a patient with sepsis may be unable to increase his oral intake to provide sufficient calories and protein)

  b. Nutrient losses (e.g., a patient with cirrhosis can lose albumin in ascitic fluid and become protein-depleted)

  c. Decreased intake, the commonest reason for malnutrition (e.g., impaired taste perception, a common occurrence in cancer patients, results in diminished oral intake)

  d. Decreased absorption (e.g., patients with malabsorption syndrome, intestinal fistulas, or short bowel syndrome may not absorb ingested nutrients)

  e. Multiple causes. A patient with pancreatic cancer may be malnourished because of decreased appetite, steatorrhea from pancreatic exocrine insufficiency, and increased nutritional requirements because of surgery; or a trauma patient may have a high expenditure of calories because of multiple injuries complicated by sepsis yet be unable to eat because of prolonged ileus.

 2. Protein–calorie malnutrition, the usual type of malnutrition in surgical patients, is characterized by diminished body stores of fat and protein. Marasmus, characterized by depletion of body fat but relative sparing of visceral protein, is uncommon in surgical patients.

 3. Protein malnutrition, which is similar to kwashiorkor, is characterized by depletion of body protein with relative sparing of body fat, as may occur in acutely ill, starved patients. Such patients may appear well nourished or even obese but are profoundly malnourished.

E. Evaluation of nutritional status. An accurate method to evaluate nutritional status is not available.

 1. The history and physical examination provide the best means of assessing the patient's nutritional status.

  a. A history of weight loss, change in appetite, or gastrointestinal symptoms is important.

  b. In the physical examination, malnutrition is suggested by muscle wasting, edema, or the loss of normal skin contours over bony prominences. **Anthropometric measurements**, such as the triceps skinfold thickness to estimate body fat and midarm muscle circumference to estimate skeletal muscle mass, are useful but imprecise.

  c. Indirect calorimetry is useful to measure the caloric requirements of acutely ill patients: Oxygen consumption and carbon dioxide production are measured and used to calculate caloric expenditure.

 2. Laboratory tests may be helpful.

  a. Serum albumin levels give an inexpensive measurement of visceral protein stores. Total iron-binding capacity and levels of serum transferrin, prealbumin, and retinol-binding protein can also be used.

  b. The total lymphocyte count may be decreased in malnutrition (less than 1500/mm^3 is abnormal).

  c. Delayed hypersensitivity to skin test antigens is correlated with nutritional status and with results of treatment, but the absence of delayed hypersensitivity is not specific for malnutrition.

 3. The patient's current nutrient intake is an important aspect of nutritional assessment that can be ascertained relatively easily.

F. Nutritional therapy

 1. Oral feeding is the most efficient, most pleasant, least expensive, and most widely used form of therapy.

  a. The patient's actual caloric and protein intake should be determined and compared to estimated requirements.

  b. For patients whose oral intake is insufficient for their estimated needs, a variety of oral supplements are available.

 2. Enteric feedings are useful for patients whose gastrointestinal tracts are functional but who are unable to take adequate nutrients by mouth.

  a. Routes available for administration

   (1) Feeding tubes are soft, small-diameter tubes passed via the nose into the stomach or duodenum.

   (2) Enterostomies are surgically created openings into the stomach (**gastrostomy**), small bowel (**jejunostomy**), or esophagus (**esophagostomy**). Enterostomies are appropriate for long-term enteric feedings.

   b. Nutrient solutions are available in a variety of formulas that provide the necessary nutrients in appropriate proportions.
   c. Complications of enteric feedings
      (1) Aspiration pneumonia can be avoided by eliminating large-volume, intermittent (bolus) feedings, and by feeding directly into the jejunum when patients are not alert.
      (2) Diarrhea is minimized by avoiding hyperosmolar or bolus feedings and by preventing bacterial overgrowth in the nutrient solutions.

   3. Parenteral nutrition (also called **intravenous hyperalimentation**) is used for patients who lack adequate intestinal function.
   a. Hypertonic nutrient solution is infused via a **central venous catheter** into the superior vena cava.
   b. Components include (see Table 1-5):
      (1) A source of **calories**, usually a combination of carbohydrate and fat
         (a) Carbohydrate calories are given as dextrose (glucose) at a concentration of up to 25%. Remember that 5% dextrose (D5W) contains 50 g/L equivalent to 200 kcal/L and has an osmolarity of 300 mOsm/L (normal serum: 290 mOsm/L).
         (b) Fat emulsions are available as 10% and 20% concentrations with a volume of 500 ml (50 g and 100 g a bottle equivalent to 450 and 900 kcal a bottle, respectively).
      (2) A protein source, available as a mixture of synthesized amino acids in concentrations of 3.5%–5%
      (3) Water
      (4) Vitamins, both water- and fat-soluble
      (5) Trace metals, needed primarily as enzyme cofactors—zinc, copper, manganese, and chromium
      (6) Minerals—K^+, Na^+, Cl^-, calcium, phosphate, and magnesium
   c. A typical prescription for **total parenteral nutrition (TPN)** is given in Table 1-6.
   d. Complications can be minimized by experience and by careful metabolic monitoring.
      (1) Complications related to central venous catheter insertion
         (a) Pneumothorax, arterial puncture, or malpositioning of the catheter can occur during attempts to insert the catheter. Complications are infrequent when the physician is experienced and the patient is cooperative, well hydrated, and has normal blood coagulation.
         (b) Great vein thrombosis can develop from a catheter that irritates the intima of the vena cava and subclavian vein. Thrombosis can be minimized by the use of soft catheters; some clinicians advocate adding small amounts of heparin to the infusion to minimize thrombosis.
         (c) Sepsis increases in incidence with faulty catheter maintenance techniques. The most frequent pathogens are *Staphylococcus* and *Candida*.
      (2) Metabolic complications can develop if either too much or too little of any nutrient is given and can be minimized by gradually increasing the volume and concentration of solutions and by judicious blood chemistry monitoring. The following complications are the commonest:
         (a) Water overload occurs when a patient receives excessive fluid (usually via a peripheral vein) in addition to parenteral feeding. Weight gain in excess of 3 lb/week is usually from overhydration. **Dilutional hyponatremia** is usually also present.
         (b) Hyperglycemia, most likely to develop in a diabetic patient or a stressed (i.e., septic) patient, occurs when glucose is administered more rapidly than the patient's pancreas can tolerate. When severe, hyperosmolar nonketotic hyperglycemia can occur and result in coma.
         (c) Hypoglycemia may occur if an infusion of hypertonic dextrose is stopped suddenly.
         (d) Metabolic acidosis occurs when excess Cl^- relative to acetate is given as the anion.
         (e) Essential fatty acid deficiency can occur if prolonged TPN is given without fat emulsions.
         (f) Hepatic cholestasis may develop in patients receiving high-caloric, high-carbohydrate, long-term TPN.

e. Special parenteral solutions
  (1) Patients with oliguric renal failure require:
    (a) A high dextrose concentration in a small daily volume
    (b) Essential amino acids instead of mixed essential and nonessential amino acids
    (c) High concentration (20%) fat emulsion
  (2) Patients with liver failure may be given a high percentage of branched-chain amino acids (leucine, isoleucine, valine) to reduce the risk of encephalopathy.

Table 1-6. Prescription for Daily Total Parenteral Nutrition

Calories
  10% fat emulsion* = 450 kcal given as 500 ml 10% fat
  Dextrose 500 g = 2000 kcal given as 1000 ml D50 (50% dextrose)

Protein
  8.5% amino acid solution = 85 g protein/L × 1 L

Minerals

Na$^+$	70 mEq
K$^+$	60 mEq
Total cations	130 mEq
Cl$^-$	50 mEq
Acetate†	65 mEq
Phosphate	15 mEq
Total anions	130 mEq
Ca^{2+} (gluconate)	10 mEq
Mg^{2+} (sulfate)	10 mEq

Trace Elements

Cu	1.0 mg
Cr	0.01 mg
Mn	0.5 mg
Zn	5.0 mg

Vitamins

Multivitamin solution	
Folic acid	0.4 mg
Cyanocobalamin (vitamin B$_{12}$)	5 mcg
Vitamin K	1.0 mg

    Totals
    Volume = 2500 ml
    Nonprotein calories = 2450 kcal
    Calorie:protein ratio = 180 kcal/g nitrogen

Schedule
  Continuous: 80 ml/hr for 24 hours plus fat solution, 500 ml over 8 hours‡
  Intermittent (nighttime feeding to allow daytime mobility): Infuse over 12 hours as follows:
    8:00 P.M. begin infusion at 50 ml/hr for 30 minutes
    8:30 P.M. increase rate to 170 ml/hr for 11 hours
    7:30 A.M. decrease rate to 50 ml/hr for 30 minutes
    8:00 A.M. stop infusion, flush central line with heparin (100 units/ml), and cap
  Concurrently run 10% fat emulsion over 8 hours

*Note that fat emulsions (10% and 20%) are isotonic with plasma and may be given by peripheral vein.

†Acetate is metabolized to bicarbonate in vivo.

‡Fat emulsions can be added to the total solution and infused as 2500 ml at 100 ml/hr over 24 hours.

(3) Formula modifications are also used in patients with sepsis, trauma, and congestive heart failure.

III. WOUND HEALING. Wound healing is the process by which injured tissue undergoes repair with restoration of tissue strength and resistance to infection and other external influences. It is a process critical to the practice of surgery.

A. **Three basic processes** are involved in wound repair.

1. **Collagen (connective tissue) is formed by fibroblasts** in a healing wound. Collagen is responsible for binding tissues together and, ultimately, is a major determinant of wound strength.
    a. Collagen is synthesized by fibroblasts. It is initially formed as protocollagen, a proline-rich collagen precursor, which is then hydroxylated to form collagen, a protein that contains glycine, proline, and hydroxyproline.
    b. Collagen is formed from three polypeptide chains that wind in a left-handed helix. The entire molecule is then twisted into a right-handed helix. Extensive cross-linking among molecules occurs and results in increased strength.
    c. Collagen synthesis requires ferrous iron, oxygen, ascorbic acid (vitamin C), and α-ketoglutarate. Vitamin C deficiency leads to incompletely synthesized and cross-linked collagen.

2. **Epithelial coverage of a wound occurs** as newly formed epithelial cells migrate onto the wound surface from the wound margin. Once covered (re-epithelialized), the wound has an intact barrier against infection from environmental organisms.
    a. **Fresh clean wounds have no resistance to infection** from surface contamination for the first 6 hours. By 5 days, the uncomplicated wound has the same resistance to infection as intact skin.
    b. Epithelium migrates slowly, and a **skin graft may be required** for complete wound healing of large open wounds.

3. **Contraction in the tissues of the wound** helps the wound to close by decreasing its surface area. Contraction occurs in open wounds and generally is not important in healing by first intention (see III C 1). The **myofibroblast** exerts a contractile force within the wound and is responsible for wound contraction.

B. **Three basic phases** occur in the healing process, which ultimately lead to the return of tissue strength.

1. **The lag phase** occurs during the first several days.
    a. There is an **acute inflammatory response** with cellular migration into the wound. Neutrophils predominate for the first 24–48 hours, and macrophages become active by the third day. In addition to other functions, these cells are responsible for removing devitalized tissue in preparation for capillary ingrowth.
    b. There is no increase in wound strength during this time.

2. **The proliferative phase** follows and is characterized by the migration of fibroblasts and capillaries into the wound. This phase lasts for 4–5 weeks.
    a. The fibroblasts begin to lay down collagen, which is detectable by the fourth day. Neutrophils and macrophages continue to be abundant in the wound.
    b. Capillary buds, originating in venules at the wound edges, grow across the wound to supply nutrients and oxygen to the cellular elements, particularly to the fibroblasts. Because of their rapid growth and immaturity, the capillaries remain highly permeable and susceptible to injury during this phase.
    c. **Wound strength** slowly increases during this phase and the next phase of healing.
        (1) After the first month, an uncomplicated wound has reached 50% of its final strength.
        (2) After the second month, the wound is at 75% of its final strength.
        (3) After the sixth month, the wound is at 95% of its final strength.

3. **The maturation phase** occurs when the cellular activity in the wound diminishes.
    a. Although the collagen content of the wound in this phase changes little, the wound continues to gain strength due to collagen cross-linking, remodeling, and contraction.
    b. Wounds rarely attain the same breaking strength that was present in the tissue prior to the injury. Some wounds do reach 80% of the original strength, but this may require years.

C. **Clinical management of wounds**

1. **First-intention healing.** When possible, the edges of a wound are immediately approximated after injury. This procedure, known as **primary wound closure**, allows the wound to heal by first intention. Epithelialization occurs within 48–72 hours, and wound healing proceeds as described in III B.

2. **Second-intention healing** occurs when the wound edges are left unopposed and open. This procedure, also known as **secondary closure**, allows necrotic and infected tissue to be readily accessible for surgical debridement. It is used primarily with grossly contaminated wounds.
   a. **Granulation tissue** forms on the wound surfaces when healing is by second intention.
      (1) Granulation tissue is beefy, red, moist tissue that contains high numbers of inflammatory cells and capillaries.
      (2) Granulation tissue is not sterile, but the large numbers of phagocytes act as a barrier to invasive infections.
      (3) When the bacterial counts fall as low as 10^4 organisms per mm³, usually the wound can either be closed, or a skin graft applied, or the tissue will support the ingrowth of epithelial cells.
   b. **Chronic granulation** is granulation tissue that is edematous with an associated exudate. This tissue is less vascular than healthy granulation tissue and will not support epithelialization. It must be surgically removed and new granulation tissue allowed to form.

3. **Third-intention healing** occurs with **delayed primary closure**, used to close wounds with low-grade bacterial contamination. In this procedure, the wound is left open and observed for several days. If the wound edges are healthy by the third or fourth day, they are approximated, and wound healing progresses with very little delay, similar to primary closure.

4. **Skin grafts** (see Chapter 26 I C) may be used to cover open wounds that are large and covered by healthy granulation tissue.
   a. The graft is a segment of epidermis and dermis, which has been surgically removed from another part of the body. When placed on a wound, the graft becomes vascularized from the underlying tissue. There are two thicknesses of grafts generally used.
      (1) A **split-thickness skin graft** is epidermis and a portion of the dermis and is usually 0.01–0.015 inch thick. A graft of this thickness allows the most rapid vascularization and is used on most wounds.
      (2) A **full-thickness skin graft** includes both epidermis and all of the dermis and is 0.02–0.025 inch thick. It is more often used in areas where cosmetic appearance is important.
   b. Movement between the graft and the wound disrupts the ingrowth of capillaries, making the graft fragile for weeks until firm adhesion occurs.

D. **Factors affecting wound healing**

1. **Age.** Young patients heal more rapidly than old patients.

2. **Severe malnutrition** impedes wound healing. In general, however, wounds get priority for biologic needs over other organ systems.

3. **Vascularity.** Highly vascular areas, such as the face, heal better than regions of poor vascularity, such as the pretibial area.

4. **Anti-inflammatory drugs,** such as steroids, delay wound healing if they are given during the first several days of healing but have little effect on healing if given after that time.

5. **Adequate levels of oxygen** are needed in the local wound area for unimpeded wound healing.
   a. Fibroblasts require oxygen to synthesize collagen, and phagocytes require oxygen to ingest and kill bacteria.
   b. Any process that interrupts the delivery of oxygen or other nutrients will impair healing; examples include hypoxemia, hypotension, vascular insufficiency, and local ischemia secondary to overtightened sutures.
   c. Radiation therapy causes obliteration of small vessels in the dermis, resulting in local ischemia and delayed wound healing.

6. Local sepsis is probably the commonest and most important cause of delayed wound healing or wound breakdown.

    a. The **usual source of bacterial contamination** is the patient's own bacteria. Environmental (i.e., exogenous) sources account for only about 5% of wound infections.

    b. Wounds may be **classified** by the **degree of bacterial contamination**; the risk of infection in each type is given in Chapter 2 II A 2.

        (1) A **clean wound** is one formed under relatively sterile conditions and in which the genitourinary, gastrointestinal, and tracheobronchial systems are not violated.

        (2) A **clean contaminated wound** occurs if one of these tracts is opened but minimal spillage has occurred. An example is a colectomy performed on bowel that has been mechanically cleaned. These wounds may usually be closed with healing by first intention.

        (3) A **contaminated wound** is one in which gross contamination has occurred. Wounds in direct contact with purulent material have a 50% or greater incidence of infection and, therefore, are usually left open to heal by second intention. Examples include surgery for an intra-abdominal abscess or perforated appendix.

    c. Prophylactic antibiotics (see Chapter 2 II A 4) may reduce the incidence of wound infections.

        (1) Antibiotics are probably of little benefit for clean wounds.

            (a) The only clean cases in which antibiotics are proven beneficial are those in which an infection would be life-threatening, such as when using a vascular prosthesis.

            (b) For grossly contaminated wounds, antibiotics are theraputic, not prophylactic. However, surgical debridement and irrigation are of prime importance in the management of this type of wound.

        (2) The **most appropriate use is for clean contaminated wounds**. The antibiotics should be given **before** or during the surgery. If they are given later than 3 hours after the wound is inoculated with bacteria, they have little effect.

        (3) The antibiotic used should be determined by the nature of the potential infecting organism. Bowel surgery patients should be treated with antibiotics effective against anaerobic and gram-negative organisms. Patients having upper torso surgery should be treated with antibiotics against gram-positive cocci.

E. Wound dehiscence, or **breakdown**, may occur in severely compromised wounds.

    1. Wound dehiscence generally occurs early postoperatively (usually 7–10 days after surgery) when the wound strength is low and wound stresses are high due to such conditions as abdominal distention, ileus, or respiratory difficulties.

    2. Dehiscence may be the result of any of the factors discussed in III D. In addition, during normal healing, collagenases are released at wound edges as part of collagen deposition and remodeling. In the compromised patient, this may weaken the tissue in which sutures are placed, resulting in tissue failure. Patients with systemic diseases, such as renal or hepatic failure, also have a high incidence of dehiscence.

    3. Wound dehiscence usually requires immediate surgery to repair the wound and prevent evisceration.

F. Scars from wounds vary greatly. Most wounds continue to remodel for more than 1 year. A wound that is unsightly several weeks following surgery may be cosmetically acceptable months or years later.

    1. Hypertrophic scars are composed of dense fibrous tissue in the dermis of the wound skin. They result from wounds that heal with excessive collagen synthesis, causing an unsightly scar with a raised surface. The etiology is unknown.

    a. The scar is tense, reddish in color, and associated with itching, hyperesthesia, and tenderness.

    b. These scars occur most commonly in blacks, Orientals, and dark-skinned white patients, and are commoner in young patients.

    c. The scars are classified into two general categories.

        (1) An **ordinary hypertrophic scar** lies entirely within the confines of the wound. Histologically, it shows an increased amount of normal-appearing collagen and numerous mature fibroblasts. There is scant ground substance. The scar usually stabilizes after 3 months and even regresses slightly and softens.

(2) A **keloid** is a scar that invades nearby normal tissue that was not previously involved in the wound. The scar continues to enlarge even after 6 months and does not usually regress or soften. Histologically, there are large swollen eosinophilic collagen bundles with abundant ground substance and scant fibroblasts.

2. **Treatment** of these scars is very difficult. Excision of the scar may result in its recurrence. Steroid injections into the scar or following excision may prevent recurrence, as may radiation therapy.

IV. HEMOSTASIS

A. **Components of hemostasis.** Hemostasis is the physiologic process by which bleeding—that is, blood leakage from an injured vessel—is controlled. Hemostasis consists of four components: the vessel response, platelet (thrombocyte) activities, the coagulation mechanism, and the fibrinolytic system.

1. **Vessel response**, namely **vasoconstriction**, is the first hemostatic response to occur after an injury to a blood vessel. Vasoconstriction is due primarily to smooth muscle contraction.

2. **Platelet activity.** Following the onset of vasoconstriction, the platelets begin to **adhere** and **aggregate**, eventually forming a **platelet plug**.
   a. **Adherence**
      (1) The platelets adhere chiefly to exposed subendothelial collagen, a process requiring **von Willebrand factor**. This platelet factor is produced by the endothelial cells and is related to factor VIII of the coagulation cascade (see IV A 3).
      (2) At the same time, platelet granules release adenosine diphosphate (ADP), which promotes a loose platelet aggregation.
   b. **Aggregation**
      (1) Arachidonic acid is then released from platelet phospholipids, and is converted by cyclooxygenase to the unstable cyclic endoperoxides prostaglandin G_2 (PGG$_2$) and prostaglandin H_2 (PGH$_2$).
      (2) Thromboxane synthetase converts PGH$_2$ to thromboxane A_2, which, in turn, induces further ADP release and, thus, enhances platelet aggregation.
      (3) **Aspirin** inhibits the cyclooxygenase-mediated formation of PGG$_2$ and PGH$_2$, thus interfering with platelet aggregation and subsequent plug formation. This defect lasts for the life of the platelet (7–10 days).
   c. **Platelet plug.** The aggregated platelets interact with thrombin and fibrin, fusing to form a plug.

3. **The coagulation mechanism** converts prothrombin to thrombin and leads to the formation of the **fibrin clot.** Two systems of interacting factors are involved, the intrinsic and the extrinsic pathways (Fig. 1-1).
   a. **The intrinsic pathway** involves only normal blood components.
      (1) **Factor XII (Hageman factor)** becomes bound to a damaged vessel and is activated (factor XIIa).
      (2) Factor XIIa (amplified by prekallikrein, and high-molecular-weight kininogen) activates **factor XI** (XIa).
      (3) Factor XIa, together with calcium, activates **factor IX**, which joins with **factor VIII**, calcium, and platelet factor 3 to activate **factor X** (Xa).
      (4) Factor Xa and **factor V** together convert **prothrombin (factor II)** to **thrombin.**
      (5) Small peptides are then split from **fibrinogen (factor I)** by thrombin to produce **fibrin monomers.** These are cross-linked by **factor XIIIa** (activated by thrombin) to form a stable **clot.**
   b. **The extrinsic pathway** requires the presence of a tissue phospholipid called thromboplastin.
      (1) **Factor VII** forms a complex with calcium and thromboplastin (also called factor III) to activate **factor X**. Platelet factor 3, released in the early stages of platelet adhesion, contributes to the factor IXa–VIIIa–calcium complex, which activates factor X.
      (2) The subsequent steps of the pathway are as described above. As Figure 1-1 shows, factors XII, XI, IX, and VIII are not involved.
   c. All of the soluble coagulation factors are manufactured by the liver except factor VIII (made by endothelium), calcium, thromboplastin, and platelet-derived factors.

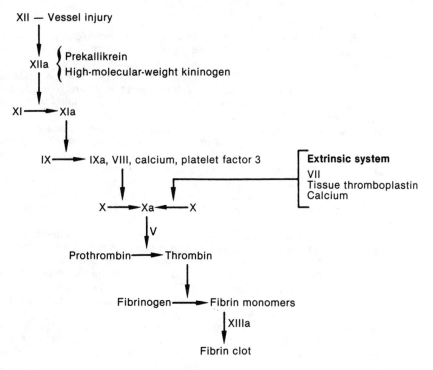

Figure 1-1. Coagulation cascade.

4. **Fibrinolytic system.** The vasculature must have a mechanism to balance the clotting process to terminate appropriately thrombus propagation and to maintain the circulating blood in a fluid state.

a. **Plasminogen**, an inactive protein, is converted to its active form, **plasmin**, by plasminogen activators.

b. The vascular endothelium, whose disruption initiates both platelet adherence and the coagulation cascade, is the primary source of plasminogen activators.

c. **Plasmin** digests fibrin, fibrinogen, and factors V and VIII.

d. **Homeostatic function.** Plasminogen becomes incorporated into a growing thrombus and eventually serves to eliminate the clot once its function is complete.

B. **Preoperative evaluation of hemostasis**

1. **The history** is important for identifying potential bleeding problems, particularly the personal medical history, the family history, and the medication history. Questions must be as direct as possible to obtain specific information.

a. **Personal medical history.** The patient must be asked specifically about bleeding that occurred after prior surgery, including circumcision, tonsillectomy, and dental extractions. Women should be asked about excessive menstrual flow.

b. **Family history.** Because many coagulation disorders are inherited, any history of spontaneous or postoperative bleeding in a relative warrants further investigation.

c. **Medication history.** Aspirin, nonsteroidal anti-inflammatory drugs, quinidine, cimetidine, tranquilizers, and certain antibiotics can all affect platelet production or performance. Patients should be asked what over-the-counter medications they are taking, since many preparations contain aspirin.

2. **Physical examination** should be thorough.

a. Petechiae, ecchymoses, and purpura are clues to possible coagulation disorders.

b. An enlarged spleen can sequester platelets and result in thrombocytopenia.

c. Jaundice, ascites, spider angiomas, hepatomegaly, or a small liver can indicate hepatic dysfunction. Because clotting factors are produced by the liver, hepatic disease can result in deficient clotting (i.e., coagulopathy).

3. Laboratory tests
   a. Peripheral blood smear, besides displaying red and white blood cell morphology, provides an estimate of the platelet count. Finding 15–20 platelets per oil immersion field indicates a normal platelet count; fewer than 5 is abnormally low.
   b. Platelet count is normally 200,000–400,000/mm^3. Counts below 100,000/mm^3 are regarded as thrombocytopenic, but 70,000 platelets/mm^3 are generally adequate for surgical hemostasis. Spontaneous bleeding is usually associated with counts below 20,000/mm^3.
   c. Bleeding time. The upper limit of normal is approximately 5 minutes.
      (1) Several standard tests are available, including the Duke and Ivy methods. Each requires familiarity with the technique if results are to be reproducible and meaningful.
      (2) A normal bleeding time implies an adequate number of platelets, normal platelet function, and a normal vascular response to an injury.
      (3) Thrombocytopenia, qualitative platelet defects (either intrinsic or related to drugs such as aspirin), and vascular wall abnormalities will cause a prolonged bleeding time.
   d. Tests of clotting factors
      (1) Prothrombin time (PT). The prothrombin time reflects the integrity of the **extrinsic coagulation system**. The control value is determined by each laboratory.
         (a) Deficiencies of factors I, II, V, VII, and X will be detected.
         (b) Abnormalities in factors VIII, IX, XI, and XII will not be detected.
      (2) Partial thromboplastin time (PTT). The partial thromboplastin time reflects the **intrinsic coagulation mechanism**—that is, all of the factors except factor VII. The normal value is usually less than 45 seconds.
      (3) Individual assays are also available for each of the clotting factors.
   e. Thrombin time (TT). This test measures the rate of conversion of fibrinogen to fibrin. The thrombin time will be prolonged by hypofibrinogenemia (< 100 mg fibrinogen/dl of plasma), by fibrin abnormalities, and by the presence of fibrin split products or heparin.
   f. Fibrin split products. These protein fragments are released from fibrinogen and fibrin by the action of plasmin. The normal range is 0–10 mg/ml of plasma. Fibrin split products will be increased in disseminated intravascular coagulation (DIC) and other fibrinolytic states.

4. Preoperative use of laboratory tests. There is disagreement among surgeons and hematologists on this topic.
   a. Some feel that a negative history and a normal-appearing blood smear or platelet count are adequate screens for most elective surgery. Others use the PT and PTT to screen preoperative patients further. In general, the PT and PTT will rarely be abnormal if the patient's bleeding history is negative and the peripheral smear is normal.
   b. Many hematologists feel that the bleeding time should be tested more frequently because the platelet count cannot detect qualitative platelet abnormalities.
   c. Ultimately, each physician must decide how much preoperative testing is warranted, based on the history and physical examination and the nature of the surgery that is planned.

C. Disorders of hemostasis

1. Platelet disorders
   a. Thrombocytopenia (platelet count below 100,000/mm^3) is the commonest cause of bleeding in the surgical patient. Surgical hemostasis requires a level of at least 70,000/mm^3. Thrombocytopenia has many causes.
      (1) Reduced production of platelets, caused by bone marrow failure, can be congenital, as in Fanconi's syndrome, or can be due to the toxic effects of radiation or of drugs, especially chemotherapeutic agents. The marrow may also be replaced with leukemic or other neoplastic cells, or involved in a fibrotic process (myelofibrosis). **Treatment** is to eliminate the effects of the underlying drug or the disease, if possible. If surgery is required, 6–8 units of platelets transfused just prior to the procedure should raise the count by 50,000–100,000/mm^3. Postoperatively, the count should be maintained above 50,000/mm^3.
      (2) Faulty platelet maturation can be secondary to megaloblastic anemia. **Treatment** is to replace the deficient vitamins—folate, B$_{12}$, or both.

(3) Abnormal platelet distribution occurs with splenomegaly, in which the spleen contains more than the usual 30% of the circulating platelets (see Chapter 22).

(4) Increased platelet destruction or loss can result from several causes:

(a) Autoimmune disorders [idiopathic thrombocytopenic purpura (ITP)

(b) Drug hypersensitivity reactions

(i) Some drugs (quinidine, sulfonamides), acting as haptens, can form an antigen–antibody complex that binds to the platelet membrane. Treatment is cessation of the drug.

(ii) Heparin is increasingly recognized as a cause of severe thrombocytopenia that appears to be antibody-related and can occur regardless of the duration, dose, route, or frequency of heparin administration. Platelet counts return to normal after the withdrawal of heparin. Patients receiving heparin should have platelet counts at least every other day.

(c) Disseminated intravascular coagulation [see IV C 3 c (1)]

(d) Hemorrhage, since platelets are lost, of course, along with all other blood components

(5) Dilutional thrombocytopenia can develop after large transfusions of banked blood, which contains few functional platelets.

b. Abnormal platelet function can produce hemostatic problems despite a normal platelet count.

(1) Causes of functional platelet abnormalities include:

(a) von Willebrand's disease [see IV C 3 a (1) (b)]

(b) Uremia. Both acute and chronic renal failure result in impaired platelet function with prolonged bleeding time.

(c) Idiopathic causes

(d) Drug effects

(i) Aspirin and other nonsteroidal anti-inflammatory drugs inhibit platelet aggregation by blocking the synthesis of the endoperoxides PGG_2 and PGH_2. Patients should stop aspirin use 1 week prior to surgery.

(ii) Penicillin G, carbenicillin, and ticarcillin can also impair platelet function.

(2) Treatment of disorders of platelet function is by **transfusion** of normal platelets preoperatively or by withdrawal of the offending drug if surgery can be delayed.

2. Blood vessel wall abnormalities, when serious, may prolong the bleeding time, although platelet count and function are usually normal.

a. Scurvy and Cushing's syndrome each cause a defect in the blood vessel connective tissue, leading to weakened vessel walls.

b. Henoch-Schönlein purpura, a hypersensitivity reaction, leads to inflammation of the capillaries with increased permeability.

c. Control of the disease process and awareness of the need for meticulous hemostasis in the operating room can minimize complications in these patients.

3. Disorders of blood coagulation

a. Congenital coagulation disorders

(1) Specific inherited deficiencies have been characterized. The first three disorders are uncommon; the latter eight are rare. Attention must be paid to which laboratory test is abnormal.

(a) Hemophilia A is a deficiency of the procoagulant activity of factor VIII; its antigenic activity is usually normal. The PT is normal, but the PTT is prolonged. A sex-linked recessive disorder, hemophilia A has an incidence of about 1 in 10,000 population.

(i) Severity depends on the degree of deficiency of factor VIII. Spontaneous bleeding can be avoided by plasma activity levels of at least 5%. Minor trauma may cause bleeding at levels between 5% and 25%, while surgical insult or major trauma is necessary to generate hemorrhage when levels are above 25%–30%.

(ii) Treatment consists of providing appropriate levels of factor VIII for the situation. A synthetic analogue of ADH, desmopressin (1-deamino-8-D-arginine vasopressin, or dDAVP), can elevate factor VIII levels threefold in hemophiliacs who have at least 1% factor VIII activity. Hemophiliacs may develop **inhibitors of factor VIII** for which surgical patients must be screened.

(b) Von Willebrand's disease (pseudohemophilia) can be transmitted as either an autosomal dominant or a recessive trait. It occurs as often as hemophilia A.

(i) The endothelium releases decreased amounts of factor VIII. This results in a defect in platelet adherence and **an abnormal bleeding time**. The antigenic activity of factor VIII is reduced as well as its procoagulant activity.

(ii) Unlike hemophilia, in which the factor VIII level remains constant, the level will vary in von Willebrand's disease.

(iii) The purified factor VIII used in classic hemophilia does not contain the **von Willebrand factor (factor VIII R:WF)** and is, therefore, ineffective for treatment. **Cryoprecipitate** provides both portions of the factor VIII complex and corrects the bleeding disorder. It should be started the day before surgery to correct the bleeding time.

(c) **Hemophilia B (Christmas disease)** is a sex-linked deficiency of factor IX. It occurs about one-tenth as often as hemophilia A. The manifestations, severity, and treatment are similar to those of hemophilia A. The **PTT is usually prolonged**.

(d) **Factor XI deficiency (Rosenthal's syndrome)** is a rare autosomal dominant disorder. The PTT is abnormal, and the PT is normal.

(e) **Factor XII deficiency** is usually asymptomatic.

(f) **Factor XIII deficiency** can be either autosomal dominant or sex-linked recessive. Fibrin monomers fail to cross-link, and the resulting weak clot will dissolve in 5 M urea. The PT, PTT, and TT are normal.

(g) **Factor V deficiency** is an autosomal recessive trait. Both the PT and PTT are prolonged.

(h) **Factor X deficiency** is an autosomal recessive disorder. The PT and PTT are prolonged.

(i) **Factor VII deficiency** is also inherited as an autosomal recessive trait. The PT is abnormal, and the PTT is normal.

(j) **Hypoprothrombinemia (factor II deficiency)**, a rare autosomal recessive disorder, prolongs both the PT and PTT.

(k) **Fibrinogen deficiency (afibrinogenemia)** is inherited in an autosomal recessive fashion; **qualitatively, abnormal fibrinogen (dysfibrinogenemia)** is autosomal dominant. In both types, the PT, PTT, and TT are all prolonged. A fibrinogen level of 100 mg/dl is needed for hemostasis.

(2) **Surgery in the patient with a congenital disorder of coagulation**

(a) **Prerequisites.** Before elective surgery, support must be available from a hematology consultant and from a coagulation laboratory capable of performing rapid factor assays. An adequate supply of the specific needed factor replacement must be on hand.

(i) Fresh frozen plasma, cryoprecipitate, and numerous factor concentrates are available in various strengths, so the strength must be known.

(ii) Levels of specific factors are expressed as a percent of normal activity. Levels above 30% are considered hemostatic and tests of coagulation are usually in the normal range. Factor concentrates are measured in units; 1 unit is the amount of factor present in 1 ml of plasma with 100% activity.

(b) **Plan for surgery.** The plasma level of the deficient factor should be brought to 100% of activity at the time of surgery, after which the level should be kept above 60% for 4 days, and then above 40% for 4 more days or until all sutures, clips, tubes, and drains are removed. The factor levels are monitored by assays, and replacement therapy is based on the factor's half-life.

b. **Acquired disorders of the coagulation system**

(1) **Disseminated intravascular coagulation (DIC)** results from the simultaneous activation of the coagulation and fibrinolytic systems. It occurs as a consequence of a severe underlying disorder, such as sepsis, malignancy, trauma, shock, or serious obstetric complications.

(a) **Presentation.** As the coagulation and fibrinolytic systems are activated, platelets and clotting factors are consumed and fibrin split products are released. Clinically, there is usually widespread hemorrhage. The PT and PTT are usually prolonged. The peripheral smear shows deformed red cells (schistocytes) from microangiopathic hemolysis. The presence of thrombocytopenia, decreased fibrinogen, and elevated fibrin split products help confirm the diagnosis.

(b) **Treatment.** It is most important to control the underlying disease process. Treatment beyond this is controversial.

(i) Some advocate the use of heparin to halt coagulation, believing that additional platelets and clotting factors would "fuel the fire."

(ii) However, in the face of diffuse hemorrhage, it would appear more prudent to provide maximum support, including platelets, fresh frozen plasma, and cryoprecipitate, while aggressively attacking the underlying disease process.

(2) Vitamin K deficiency. The liver requires vitamin K in order to synthesize factors II, VII, IX, and X. Vitamin K is produced by gut flora.

(a) A deficiency of vitamin K is common in surgical patients as a result of poor nutrition, antibiotic therapy that alters normal gut flora, obstructive jaundice with blockage of bile salts, or parenteral nutrition without vitamin K supplementation.

(b) Vitamin K in doses of 10–20 mg should begin to correct the defect in 8–12 hours. The dose is repeated, if possible, every 12 hours until the PT is corrected. For emergency surgery, the first dose is supplemented with fresh frozen plasma.

(3) Liver disease. All factors except factor VIII are reduced. Vitamin K will not be helpful if there is severe hepatocyte dysfunction.

(4) Exogenous anticoagulants (i.e., heparin or warfarin) will obviously cause clotting defects.

D. Bleeding during surgery. This can result from local factors or generalized disorders.

1. Local factors. If bleeding is from one site, such as the wound surface, it is most likely due to a **failure of local hemostasis** (e.g., an unligated vessel). The problem should be identified and corrected.

a. Direct pressure by finger or packs will usually control local bleeding until the source can be clearly identified. Once isolated, severed vessels can be clamped and then ligated, suture-ligated, or secured with metal clips, depending upon their size.

b. Electrocautery, although quicker than ligating, may cause more tissue necrosis if used improperly.

c. Chemical aids

(1) Epinephrine produces local vasoconstriction, but its use is limited by its systemic effects.

(2) Thrombin, applied topically, is effective because it induces the production of fibrin. Thrombin is frequently applied by means of gelatin foam (Gelfoam).

(3) Oxidized cellulose materials (Oxycel, Surgicel) serve as a scaffolding for clot formation. **Microfibrillar collagen (Avitene)** serves a similar function.

2. Generalized disorders

a. Underlying disorders. Bleeding during surgery may be the result of any of the previously described congenital or acquired disorders of platelets or of the coagulation system (e.g., hemophilia A, hypoprothrombinemia, or DIC).

b. Transfusion complications (see V C 2 c, 3)

V. TRANSFUSION THERAPY IN SURGERY (see Chapter 21 I C 3 d)

A. Blood components of several types are available for transfusion therapy.

1. Whole blood is collected in an anticoagulant–preservative solution and is stored at 4° C for up to 42 days. Two of the commoner solutions are citrate phosphate dextrose (CPD) and adenosine dextrose saline (AS-1).

a. Banked blood undergoes several **changes during storage.**

(1) Red blood cells progressively lose their viability. For example, if blood is transfused after it has been stored for 28 days, only 25% of its red cells will still be viable 60 days after the transfusion (the half-life of normal red blood cells is 120 days). Oxygen transport is also reduced because of a decrease in cellular 2,3-diphosphoglycerate (2,3-DPG); this shifts the oxygen–hemoglobin dissociation curve to the left.

(2) Clotting factors V and VIII rapidly deteriorate in banked blood, and **platelets** do not remain active past 24 hours.

(3) Changes in chemistry also take place: The **pH** of stored blood gradually decreases, reaching about 6.7 after 4 weeks of storage. The **potassium** concentration may be 25–30 mEq/L at this time. **Ammonia** also steadily rises.

b. Probably the only **indication for the transfusion of whole blood** is hypovolemia secondary to acute hemorrhage. **Fresh whole blood** (not more than 24 hours old) would be ideal for this purpose, since platelets and clotting factors would still be active and many of the adverse biochemical effects of stored blood would be avoided.

  c. Generally, whole blood is infrequently used. Transfusion is based on replacing the needed **components** of whole blood.

 2. Packed red blood cells are prepared by removing the plasma, leaving a hematocrit of 70%. Packed cells are indicated for most transfusions in which the goal is to increase the patient's oxygen-carrying capacity. Packed cells present less volume and a lower electrolyte load for the patient than whole blood.

 3. Fresh frozen plasma contains all of the coagulation factors lacking in banked whole blood, including factors V and VIII. It is used to replace clotting factors during massive transfusion of packed red cells or to correct the factor abnormalities found in conditions such as liver disease or DIC.

 4. Cryoprecipitate, a plasma derivative, contains high concentrations of factor VIII and fibrinogen, along with smaller amounts of other factors. It is used in factor VIII–deficient states, such as hemophilia and von Willebrand's disease, and in other states of uncontrolled bleeding such DIC.

 5. Specific factor concentrates provide replacement therapy for inherited deficiency states; several commercial products are available.

 6. Albumin is available in 5% and 25% concentrations. It is used as a volume expander. Unlike all of the above components, albumin is free from infectious risk.

B. Blood substitutes. Fluorocarbon emulsions possess oxygen-carrying capacity. They are being evaluated as blood substitutes. Since blood transfusion is associated with some risk of transmitted disease [e.g., hepatitis, acquired immune deficiency syndrome (AIDS)], a suitable blood substitute would be desirable.

C. Complications of transfusions

 1. Disease transmission
  a. Hepatitis is estimated to occur after about 2% of transfusions, although most cases are asymptomatic. The incidence is higher with pooled products, such as factor concentrates. It is also higher when paid donors are used as suppliers of blood. Effective screening can detect hepatitis B surface antigen; therefore, post-transfusion hepatitis is now due to non-A, non-B hepatitis. Approximately 70%–80% of post-transfusion hepatitis can now be identified with a new test for antibodies to hepatitis C. The risk of post-transfusion hepatitis should fall to less than 0.5%.
  b. Acquired immune deficiency syndrome (AIDS) is a severe defect in the immune system, which leaves its victim susceptible to opportunistic infections and rare neoplasms, such as Kaposi's sarcoma. This disease may be transmitted via blood obtained from affected individuals. Screening tests can detect the antibody response against the virus; however, there is a period of time early in the course of the infection when AIDS-contaminated blood can escape detection.
  c. Other diseases. Syphilis, brucellosis, malaria, and cytomegalovirus infection can also be transmitted in transfused blood.

 2. Immediate transfusion reactions
  a. Allergic reactions are the commonest type, occurring in up to 2% of transfusions.
   (1) Fever, chills, urticaria, and itching typically occur after at least half of a unit of blood or packed cells is transfused. Respiratory symptoms, such as wheezing or stridor, occur in severe cases.
   (2) An antihistamine, such as diphenhydramine, will control the minor symptoms; epinephrine and steroids are reserved for more serious cases.
   (3) If the reaction is typically allergic and responds to treatment, it is not necessary to stop the transfusion. However, if there is concern about a hemolytic reaction, the transfusion is stopped immediately.
  b. Febrile reactions are caused by antigens on white cells or platelets to which the patient is sensitive. They occur almost as frequently as allergic reactions. Fever, alone or with chills, occurs after half of a unit of blood has been transfused. Urticaria and respiratory symptoms do not occur. Antipyretics are given to reduce the fever.
  c. Hemolytic reactions are **fulminant reactions** usually due to the transfusion of **crossmatch incompatible** blood because of errors in crossmatching, typing, labeling, or patient identification.

(1) Typically, early reactions appear after only 50–100 ml of blood have been given. The patient may develop fever and chills with complaints of chest, back, or flank pain and dyspnea. Hypotension and shock may also occur.

(2) Intraoperative hemolytic reactions in anesthetized patients will not have symptoms. Instead unexplained, generalized bleeding is the first manifestation.

(3) Treatment of hemolytic reactions

    (a) This is an emergency due to the high mortality of DIC, acute renal failure (due to hemoglobinuria), and shock, which frequently occurs.

    (b) The transfusion is immediately stopped when any patient is suspected of having a hemolytic reaction.

    (c) The remaining transfusion blood and a fresh sample of the patient's blood are sent to the laboratory for retyping and crossmatching. Urine and serum samples should also be sent for free hemoglobin.

    (d) A Foley urinary catheter is inserted and diuresis is established rapidly by giving 25 g of mannitol and infusing lactated Ringer's solution at a rate that should ensure a urine output of at least 100 ml/hr. Sodium bicarbonate may also be given to alkalinize the urine and help prevent tubular damage.

(4) Delayed hemolytic reactions are considered to be anamnestic responses to prior transfusions or pregnancies. They cause hemolysis and jaundice that appear several days after the transfusion.

3. Complications of massive transfusions of banked blood. Rapid transfusion (within 12 hours) of an amount of stored blood equal to or greater than the patient's blood volume can lead to problems, due primarily to the changes that occur in stored blood (see V A 1 a).

a. Decreased oxygen-carrying capacity. Because the 2,3-DPG level gradually falls in stored blood, the hemoglobin affinity for oxygen increases, so that oxygen release to the tissues is less efficient.

b. Coagulation defects. These result from a dilutional effect, since whole blood stored longer than 24 hours has virtually no platelets and no factor V or factor VIII activity. Platelets and fresh frozen plasma must, therefore, be given in addition to banked blood.

c. Hypothermia. This rapidly develops if several units of blood are transfused without being warmed. Arrhythmias will commonly occur at body temperatures of 30° C. During a transfusion, the blood is warmed by immersing an in-line coil in a water bath that is near body temperature. The container of blood should *never* be warmed.

d. Metabolic effects

    (1) Hyperkalemia. Because the extracellular K^+ concentration rises in banked red cells, rapid administation of large amounts of old stored blood can cause transiently dangerous hyperkalemia. Therefore, when massive transfusions are required, blood less than 2–3 days old should be preferentially used or at least alternated with older blood to minimize this problem.

    (2) Acidosis and citrate toxicity

        (a) Normally, citric acid (from transfused blood) and lactic acid (from poorly perfused tissue) are rapidly metabolized. However, in the hypovolemic patient or the patient in shock with reduced hepatic blood flow, this will be slowed and severe acidosis can occur.

        (b) Some authorities advocate giving $NaHCO_3^-$ routinely with extensive transfusions in an attempt to minimize these changes in pH. One must proceed cautiously, however, since alkalosis acts synergistically with hypothermia and low 2,3-DPG levels to decrease the delivery of oxygen to the tissues. Also, alkalosis can lower the level of ionized calcium, which can cause serious cardiac arrhythmias.

        (c) For these reasons, **alkalinization** is probably **not routinely advisable** and should be used only if indicated by blood gas analysis.

    (3) Hypocalcemia

        (a) In citrate overload, the excess citrate binds ionized calcium. A low level of ionized calcium has a detrimental effect on myocardial performance. Thus, some authorities advocate routine administration of calcium in proportion to the number of units of blood transfused. However, the hypothermic patient's heart is very sensitive to the calcium ion.

        (b) Giving calcium gluconate 1 g/L of blood is probably safe, but, ideally, replacement should be guided by direct measurement of ionized calcium.

e. Respiratory insufficiency. Degenerating platelets and white cells in stored blood can microembolize and, when large amounts of banked blood are transfused, result in pulmonary damage and respiratory insufficiency. This complication is partially prevented by transfusing the blood through a micropore filter.

VI. SURGICAL ONCOLOGY

A. Overview. Cancer is a group of diseases caused by unregulated growth and spread of **neoplastic** cells. Neoplasias may be either **benign** (noninvasive growth, no metastases) or **malignant** (invasive growth, metastases).

1. Types
 a. Carcinomas are malignancies that arise from epithelium.
 b. Adenocarcinomas are malignancies that arise from epithelium and have a glandular component.
 c. Sarcomas are malignancies that arise from mesodermal tissues.

2. Neoplastic transformation. Neoplastic cells have "escaped" from the normal homeostatic inhibition (or regulation) of cell proliferation. **Causes of neoplastic transformation** are listed below with illustrative examples of human tumors. Because no single etiology is known for most human cancer, it is assumed that multiple factors lead to neoplastic transformation.
 a. Chemical carcinogens. Soot causes cancer of the scrotum of chimney sweeps (described by Pott in 1775); asbestos causes mesothelioma of the pleura; and smoking tobacco causes squamous cell carcinoma of the lung.
 b. Physical carcinogens. Ultraviolet light causes squamous carcinoma of the skin; ionizing radiation causes bone cancer in radium–dial workers, lung cancer in uranium miners, and leukemia in atomic bomb survivors (Hiroshima); and papillary thyroid cancer appears in individuals treated with neck irradiation.
 c. Hereditary factors are usually indirect (e.g., breast cancer is three times commoner in the daughters of women with premenopausal breast cancer). A few cancers have direct genetic links, such as retinoblastoma, colonic polyposis, and multiple endocrine neoplasia syndromes (e.g., pheochromocytoma, medullary carcinoma of the thyroid, and other endocrine tumors).
 d. Geographic factors are unexplained epidemiologic phenomena whereby a particular cancer is very common in certain locations (e.g., gastric cancer is common in Japan and esophageal cancer is common in southeastern China).
 e. Oncogenic viruses. Epstein-Barr virus is linked to Burkitt's lymphoma and nasopharyngeal carcinoma; herpes simplex virus-2 is linked to cervical cancer; human T-cell leukemia virus type 1 (HTLV-1) is linked to adult T-cell leukemia; and hepatitis B is linked to hepatocellular carcinoma.

B. Epidemiology. Cancer is the second leading cause of death in the United States (20% of all deaths). One in four persons living in the United States will develop cancer during his or her lifetime with an overall 5-year survival rate of 40%.

1. Mortality
 a. Overall, the highest number of deaths is caused by lung cancer (incidence rising), followed by colon and rectum cancer and breast cancer (incidence stable), and pancreatic cancer (incidence rising). Lung cancer is now the commonest cause of cancer death for both sexes (having exceeded breast cancer for women).
 b. A decreased number of deaths is found with gastric cancer and uterine/cervical cancer. For gastric cancer, the incidence is falling for unknown reasons. For uterine/cervical cancer, early diagnosis (Pap smear) and improved treatments are presumably responsible for the brighter outlook.

2. Incidence. Overall, the order is the same as for mortality. However, for women, the commonest form of cancer is breast cancer.

C. Biology of neoplastic cells

1. Characteristics
 a. Neoplastic cells proliferate more rapidly than normal cells.
 b. They tend to dedifferentiate into more "primitive" cells.
 c. They may have increased numbers of chromosomes (aneuploidy or polyploidy).

2. Growth rate
   a. If cancer begins from a single cell, then it takes 30 doublings to produce the one billion cells in a 1-cm nodule.
   b. Tumor doubling times of clinical cancers are usually in the range of 20–100 days.
   c. Most human tumors have been present for 1–10 years before they become clinically evident.

D. Clinical manifestations of cancer

   1. Seven classic symptoms of cancer are:
      a. Change in bowel or bladder habits
      b. A sore that does not heal
      c. Unusual bleeding or discharge
      d. Thickening or lump in the breast or elsewhere
      e. Indigestion or difficulty swallowing
      f. Obvious change in a wart or mole
      g. Nagging cough or hoarseness

   2. Other manifestations
      a. Growth, causing a mass, obstruction, or neurologic deficit
      b. Growth into neighboring tissues, causing pain, paralysis, fixation, or immobility of a palpable mass
      c. Tumor necrosis, causing bleeding or fever
      d. Systemic manifestation, such as thrombophlebitis, endocrine symptoms due to hormones secreted by the tumor, and cachexia
      e. Metastatic spread as the first symptom, such as enlarged lymph nodes, neurologic symptoms, or pathologic bone fractures

   3. Screening tests for cancer detection. Asymptomatic cancers detected by screening generally have a better prognosis than symptomatic cancers. Common screening tests and the current American Cancer Society recommendations for their use include:
      a. Mammography (annually after age 40–50)
      b. Stool for occult blood and digital rectal examination (annually after age 50)
      c. Pap smear of the cervix (every 3 years after two negative tests 1 year apart)

E. Staging of cancer. The standard staging of most cancers is based on the **tumor, nodes, and metastasis (TNM) system**. Various TNM classes are then grouped into stages. The staging of gastric cancer will be used to exemplify this system.

   1. T describes the primary tumor.
      a. T0: no evidence of primary tumor
      b. TIS (in situ): tumor limited to mucosa
      c. T1: tumor limited to mucosa or submucosa
      d. T2: tumor to but not through the serosa
      e. T3: tumor through the serosa but not into adjacent organs
      f. T4: tumor into adjacent organs (direct extension)

   2. N describes the involvement of lymph nodes with metastatic spread.
      a. N0: no metastases to lymph nodes
      b. N1: only perigastric lymph nodes within 3 cm of the primary tumor
      c. N2: only regional lymph nodes more than 3 cm from tumor but removeable at operation
      d. N3: other intra-abdominal lymph nodes involved

   3. M describes distant metastases.
      a. M0: no distant metastases
      b. M1: distant metastases

   4. Stage grouping. Staging is necessary to choose the appropriate therapy and to assess the prognosis. It also allows investigators to report their results in a standardized way so that conclusions regarding treatments and their outcomes are interpretable.
      a. Stage 0: TIS, N0, M0
      b. Stage 1: T1, N0, M0
      c. Stage 2: T2 or T3, N0, M0
      d. Stage 3: T1–3, N1 or N2, M0
      e. Stage 4: any T4, any T3, any N3, any M1

F. Diagnostic procedures

1. **Biopsy.** It is **mandatory** that tissue be obtained to prove microscopically that a malignancy is present. Therefore, a biopsy is always obtained in diagnosing and treating cancer. Several types of biopsy are described below.

   a. **Aspiration biopsy.** A narrow needle (e.g., 22-gauge needle) is inserted into the lesion, and **cells** are aspirated into the needle and deposited on slides. The specimen is very similar to that obtained by a Pap smear and is read by a **cytopathologist**.

   b. **Needle biopsy.** A large needle (e.g., 18-gauge) is inserted into the lesion and a core of tissue removed for histology. As a needle biopsy removes much more tissue than aspiration, complications (e.g., bleeding) are more likely, but the specimen is larger and the diagnosis obtained more precise.

   c. **Incisional biopsy** removes a superficial or accessible portion of the lesion. This is done for diagnosis as a prelude to appropriate therapies.

   d. **Excisional biopsy** removes completely a small discrete tumor without a wide margin of normal tissue and is not curative for malignancy. It is used when local removal will not interfere with the therapy to be used for definitive local control.

   e. **Staging laparotomy**, usually reserved for Hodgkin's disease, establishes the correct stage.

2. **Imaging studies**, such as computed tomography (CT scan), ultrasound, and magnetic resonance imaging (MRI) are useful for assessing the extent of spread when the study is **positive**. A negative imaging study does not exclude the possibility of microscopic disease spread.

G. Multimodality cancer therapy.
Most cancer patients are treated surgically with radiation, chemotherapy, and immunotherapy playing increasingly important roles. Choice of therapy is based on disease, stage, histologic grade, patient age, other concomitant diseases, and the intention of therapy (i.e., cure versus palliation).

1. **Surgery and radiation therapy** are both used for the treatment of the primary tumor and the regional lymph nodes. Neither has any effect on areas of distant spread.

2. **Chemotherapy and immunotherapy** are systemic therapies with the potential to affect distant areas of spread.

3. **Adjuvant therapy** is systemic therapy used for patients with local control (e.g., resection) who are at high risk of microscopic disease existing in lymph nodes or distant organs. A high proportion of these patients would develop recurrence at these sites, and adjuvant therapy attempts to destroy these distant, microscopic foci of cancer.

4. **Multimodality therapy** uses the advantages of each therapy to counteract the shortcomings of others. Examples follow:

   a. **Curable breast cancer.** Surgery is used for local control (mastectomy), or surgery (lumpectomy) plus radiation are used for local control. Surgery is used for staging of axillary lymph nodes, and postoperative chemotherapy is used for patients with positive malignancy in the nodes to decrease the chance of metastatic disease.

   b. **Pancoast tumor of the lung.** Preoperative radiation is used for regional spread into the brachial plexus to decrease the size and render the tumor surgically resectable.

   c. **Extremity sarcoma.** Incisional biopsy is used for diagnosis; preoperative radiation therapy is used to decrease tumor size; radical local resection is used for initial local control (see V1 H 2 b); postoperative adjuvant radiation is used for further regional control; and chemotherapy is used for systemic control.

H. Cancer surgery.
The principles of cancer surgery are based on removal of a tumor for cure. To prevent implantation of tumor cells at surgery, all dissection is done through uninvolved tissue, staying away from the tumor. To prevent vascular dissemination, tumors are minimally manipulated, and the vascular pedicle is ligated early. To prevent lymphatic spread, the same measures as above are performed, plus the lymph node draining area is removed **in continuity** with the tumor.

1. **Curative resection.** There are several types of curative resection, which vary with the tumor's size and biologic behavior.

   a. **Wide local resection.** For low-grade neoplasms that do not metastasize to regional lymph nodes or deeply invade surrounding tissue, wide local resection is adequate. Examples include basal cell carcinoma of the skin or mixed tumor of the parotid gland.

    b. Radical local resection. For neoplasms that deeply invade surrounding tissue, radical local resection is employed. Examples include extremity sarcoma where the resection includes the entire biopsy incision and the entire muscle compartment where the tumor lies.

    c. Radical resection with en bloc excision of lymphatic drainage is used for tumors that usually first metastasize to regional lymph nodes. Examples include colon cancer where the segment of colon plus regional mesentery and lymphatics are removed as one specimen.

    d. Super radical resections remove large portions of the body and are reserved for locally extensive disease with low likelihood of metastatic spread. Examples include pelvic exenteration [removal of rectum, bladder, uterus (in women), and all pelvic lymphatics and soft tissues] for locally advanced cancers of the rectum, cervix, uterus, or bladder.

2. Other surgical resections

    a. Resection of recurrent cancer is occasionally feasible with localized, low-grade recurrences. Examples include regional (lymph node) recurrence of colon cancer, local (anastomotic) recurrence of any gastrointestinal cancer, and local recurrence of skin cancer.

    b. Resection of metastases is feasible in several circumstances. The two commonest are isolated liver metastases from colon cancer and pulmonary metastases, especially from sarcomas sensitive to chemotherapy.

    c. Palliative surgery is used to relieve or prevent a specific symptom of a cancer patient without the intent to cure. An example is the removal of an obstructing or bleeding colon cancer in a patient with liver metastases.

    d. Debulking is the removal of the majority of a tumor, leaving residual disease. The rationale is that the remaining, smaller number of cancer cells will be more susceptible to chemotherapy or radiation therapy. Though not definitively proven, it appears to be useful for advanced ovarian cancers.

2

Problems in General Surgery

Michael J. Moritz

I. SURGICAL TUBES

A. Postoperative drainage tubes. Various types of tubes are used to drain either normal body fluid that cannot be handled by the body or abnormal material, such as pus. A tube can be mandatory, such as a chest tube for a tension pneumothorax, or optional.

1. Types of drains

a. **Closed drains** are tubes connecting a body cavity to a sealed reservoir.

   (1) **Gravity drainage** allows whatever material that collects to drain through the tube into a reservoir at a lower level.

   (2) **Underwater-seal drainage systems** prevent air and fluid from reentering the body. The end of the drainage tube is under water in a sealed drainage bottle at floor level. The water prevents air from reentering the tube, and the low level prevents fluid from siphoning back. This system is used for tubes in the pleural space.

   (3) **Suction drainage** applies a low level of suction to the drainage tube and can drain large volumes of fluid, such as the fluid that collects in the gastrointestinal tract. It also promotes closure of "dead space," allowing a better approximation of tissue surfaces.

b. **Open drains** are not sealed at either end. They allow bacteria and other materials access to the drained area and, as a result, carry a high risk of deep wound infection. Open drains have been used for many years, however, and are still part of the surgical routine in some centers.

c. **Sump drains** are double-lumen catheters that allow air or irrigation fluid to enter through one lumen while suction is applied to the other lumen. When air is allowed to enter, a filter should be used to prevent the entrance of microorganisms. Sump drains are used to evacuate particulate matter, such as debris from an abscess or as continuous irrigation catheters for closed spaces that are not otherwise accessible, such as deep abdominal abscesses.

2. Situations requiring drainage

a. Chest tube drainage of the pleural space is indicated to evacuate virtually all instances of **pneumothorax** (simple, tension).

b. A gastrointestinal tract that has been nonfunctioning for a prolonged period (more than 1 or 2 days) requires nasogastric drainage, usually with a sump tube.

   (1) The decompression lessens abdominal distention, intestinal dilation, nausea, and vomiting.

   (2) Drainage also allows a determination of the amount and type of fluid loss so that appropriate replacement can be made.

c. Areas where extensive dissection has been performed in a closed space may require drainage; for example, surgical procedures performed on solid organs, such as the liver or a kidney, where hemostasis is sometimes difficult and a postoperative hematoma is likely (see I A 4 c), or procedures, such as mastectomies or skin flaps, where there is a large raw area and little surrounding tissue to tamponade the bleeding.

d. Abscesses that do not communicate with the skin and, thus, do not provide direct access for local wound management require drainage. This usually involves a deep but well-walled-off abscess cavity, such as a subphrenic, subhepatic, or periappendiceal abscess. Drains should not be used to control a generalized infection, such as cellulitis or suppurative peritonitis.

3. Surgical procedures customarily requiring drainage
   a. In the gallbladder bed after cholecystectomy
   b. In the pancreatic region after pancreatic surgery
   c. Adjacent to or in the duodenal stump after gastrectomy with Billroth II reconstruction
   d. In the pelvis after low anterior resection of the colon
   e. In the splenic bed after splenectomy
   f. In the pleural space after thoracotomy (except for pneumonectomy)

4. Caveats and complications
   a. The presence of a drain does not guarantee that an abscess or other collection will not reform. The foreign body reaction can isolate a drain from adjacent tissues, preventing blood, pus, or other fluid from having access to the lumen.
   b. Drains and the tissues that they traverse can be colonized by microorganisms from exogenous sources. Drains, particularly open drains, increase the risk of infection. Avoiding bacterial colonization requires careful wound care at the drain's exit site.
   c. A drain should not be regarded as a substitute for hemostasis. Hematomas are likely to develop despite drainage if hemostasis is not adequate.
   d. A rigid drain may erode through the wall of a blood vessel or a hollow intestinal structure. This complication can be minimized by using soft drains and removing drains early.
   e. Excessive suction on a tube can also cause necrosis of nearby structures. Intermittent low-level suction is safer.
   f. A drain in direct contact with a fistula may perpetuate the fistula and delay its healing. The drain must be advanced beyond the fistula now and then if further healing is to occur.
   g. Drains may become detached from the skin and retract into the body, especially into the peritoneal cavity. Thus, they should always be firmly attached to the skin and should be marked with a radiopaque marker. A safety pin can also be used to keep drains outside the body.
   h. The free peritoneal space cannot be drained as tubes are quickly "walled off." Thus, diffuse peritonitis cannot be drained. Localized collections can be drained.

5. Removal. Drains should be removed when they have fulfilled their purpose.
   a. When the main risk of leakage has passed, the drain is removed.
      (1) After a cholecystectomy, if a leak from a bile duct injury is present, it should be evident in 1 or 2 days. Thus, drains are normally removed by the second day.
      (2) After urinary bladder procedures, a urinary leak will occur when the bladder catheter is removed. Thus, drains are removed a day after the catheter is removed.
   b. When a drain is used for postoperative fluid collections (i.e., blood, serum, or lymph), it is removed when no further drainage occurs.
   c. When the drain is used in a reconstructive procedure, it is removed once the repair is safe.
      (1) Following common duct exploration, a T tube is used to drain the bile duct until spasm of the sphincter of Oddi has resolved. The T tube is removed after a cholangiogram documents free flow of bile into the duodenum.
      (2) Following total gastrectomy or esophagectomy, the esophageal anastomosis is drained internally with a nasogastric tube. If an anastomotic leak is going to occur, it usually does so within the first week. Therefore, a "barium swallow" around the tube is performed to document that the anastomosis is intact and does not leak. The tube is removed if the anastomosis is intact.
      (3) Following gastrectomy and Billroth II reconstruction, a potential complication is disruption of the duodenal stump with formation of a duodenal fistula.
         (a) A tube may be placed within the duodenal lumen (duodenostomy) to prevent overdistention of the repaired duodenum, since this reduces the risk of disruption.
         (b) Once the patient has recovered from the surgical procedure, and if no signs of duodenal leakage have developed, the tube can be removed 2–4 weeks after surgery.

B. Gastrointestinal tubes

1. Cervical esophagostomy tubes are feeding tubes that are placed into the esophagus distally and exit the skin in the neck region proximally.

2. Gastrostomy tubes are large tubes inserted into the stomach through the skin and are usually used for feeding purposes but are also useful for prolonged gastric decompression.

    a. Once the tube is no longer necessary, it is removed. The tract formed between the skin and stomach will close over in 6–24 hours if a tube is not reinserted.

    b. They may be inserted surgically or via endoscopy [percutaneous endoscopic gastrostomy (PEG)].

3. Gastroesophageal balloon tamponade tubes (Sengstaken-Blakemore tube) are nasogastric tubes with inflatable balloons, which are used to compress and tamponade bleeding esophageal varices (see Chapter 14 II E 3 c).

4. Long intestinal tubes, particularly the double-lumen **Miller-Abbott tube** and the single-lumen **Cantor tube**, are introduced through the nose and allowed to pass into the small intestine.

    a. A weight or bag is at the leading tip, allowing peristalsis to carry the tube distally. In the absence of bowel motility, as with an ileus, the tube will generally not progress past the stomach.

    b. Long intestinal tubes can be useful for relieving small bowel obstruction.

        (1) They are used for recurrent obstructions. The tubes are not used for a first episode of small bowel obstruction; laparotomy and lysis of adhesions should be performed in such cases.

        (2) Multiple areas of partial obstruction, as with radiation enteritis, are treatable with a long tube.

        (3) Long intestinal tubes are less effective for late postoperative adhesions and for obstruction secondary to malignant disease.

5. Baker jejunostomy tubes. Long intestinal tubes may also be inserted directly into the intestine at the time of laparotomy. The tube most commonly used is the Baker jejunostomy tube, which is passed through a hole in the jejunum (jejunostomy) and then distally through the bowel. It is used either to splint the bowel in situations where adhesions are likely to recur or to decompress greatly distended bowel encountered at surgery.

6. Jejunostomy tubes are inserted into the jejunum as a surgical procedure. They exit on the abdominal wall and may be used for feeding purposes (see Chapter 1 II F 2).

7. Cecostomy tubes are large-caliber tubes that are surgically inserted into a distended cecum.

    a. Their commonest use is in colonic ileus, where marked colonic distention produces a cecum that is greater than 11 cm in diameter, so that cecal rupture is imminent.

    b. Colonic obstruction secondary to a malignant process is better treated with a proximal diverting colostomy than by cecostomy.

8. Rectal tubes are large-caliber tubes that are inserted into the rectum.

    a. The commonest use is to relieve colonic distention from a colonic ileus. It is the treatment of choice for sigmoid volvulus, where the tube is passed through the area of torsion under sigmoidoscopic visualization.

    b. Rectal tubes are best removed after several days because the thin-walled colon is prone to pressure necrosis.

C. Catheters and hemodialysis tubes

1. Tenckhoff peritoneal dialysis catheters are catheters inserted into the peritoneal cavity either for long-term dialysis therapy or for management of chronic ascites in patients with malignant disease. They may be inserted either percutaneously or surgically and can function for years if properly maintained with sterile technique.

    a. A Dacron cuff is glued to the Silastic catheter both where it enters the peritoneum and where it exits the skin.

    b. These cuffs become firmly incorporated into the surrounding tissue and function as mechanical barriers to organisms entering at the exit site in the skin.

2. Indwelling central venous catheters (Hickman-type catheters) maintain access to the veins for prolonged periods.

    a. They are typically used for:

        (1) Long-term hyperalimentation in patients with nutritional problems

        (2) Chemotherapy and phlebotomy in patients with malignant diseases

    b. The Hickman catheter has a Dacron cuff like that of the Tenckhoff catheter and, thus, may function for many years. Both single- and double-lumen styles are available; they can be inserted percutaneously or surgically.

3. **Arteriovenous shunts (Scribner shunts)** are external shunts still occasionally used for hemodialysis or plasmapheresis. It is a U-shaped cannula-and-tubing apparatus that is surgically inserted into an artery and a vein.
   a. The radial artery and a nearby vein are the usual vessels used.
   b. The patency of the ulnar artery should always be established before ligation and cannulation of the radial artery. This is done by means of the **Doppler test** or the **Allen test**.
      (1) The radial and ulnar arteries are occluded, and the patient then exercises the hand until the hand blanches.
      (2) The ulnar artery is released, and the patient is observed for blood flow into the hand.
      (3) If the hand blushes, then it has a dual blood supply.

II. **SURGICAL INFECTIONS.** Surgical infections are either infections that require surgical intervention to resolve completely or infections that develop as a complication of surgery. Some, of course, are in both categories.

A. **Overview**

1. **Characteristics of surgical infections** generally include the following:
   a. They usually involve either a penetrating injury (e.g., from trauma), a perforating injury (e.g., a perforated ulcer), or an operative site (e.g., the surgical wound).
   b. Often, multiple organisms are present.
   c. Treatment requires surgical drainage of the infection and debridement of necrotic or grossly contaminated tissue; **antibiotics alone will not resolve the infection**.

2. **Surgical wound infections** form the major type of surgical infections among hospitalized patients.
   a. **Incidence.** The incidence of wound infections is related directly to the nature of the surgical procedure performed. The classification of wounds by extent of contamination is described in Chapter 1 III D 6 b.
      (1) **Clean operative sites** from elective procedures (e.g., hernia repair) carry a 1%–2% risk of wound infection. Because the risk is low, the skin edges are closed primarily.
      (2) **Clean contaminated operative sites** (e.g., from a hysterectomy or cholecystectomy) have an infection rate of 5%–15%, and the skin edges are usually closed.
      (3) **Contaminated operative sites**, such as a colectomy, a gastrectomy for a bleeding ulcer, or a cholecystectomy in the presence of infected bile, have an infection rate of 10%–20% when the wound is closed; thus, it may be left open for delayed primary or secondary healing.
      (4) **Dirty operative sites** occur when an abscess or penetrating trauma has allowed bacteria to contaminate the region prior to surgical intervention. The incidence of wound infection is greater than 50%, and, therefore, the operative wound is usually left open to heal by second intention.
   b. **Clinical presentation.** Wound infection often presents as a spiking fever at about the fifth to eighth postoperative day. There may be localized wound tenderness, cellulitis, drainage from the wound, or dehiscence.
   c. **Treatment.** Simple incision and drainage will resolve most postoperative wound infections. Deeper wound infections, extensive necrosis, or wound breakdown may require open debridement.

3. **Prosthetic infections.** Prostheses are man-made implantable devices, including vascular grafts, heart valves, artificial joints, fascial replacements, metallic bone supports, and many others.
   a. **Clinical presentation.** An infected prosthesis usually causes either symptoms of local infection or generalized sepsis. The commonest organisms infecting prostheses are staphylococci. **These infections are life-threatening**.
   b. **Treatment.** Prophylactic antibiotics are always used when implanting a prosthesis; however, most prosthetic infections cannot be sterilized with antibiotics and, thus, require removal of the prosthesis.

4. **Prophylactic antibiotics** are antibiotics given shortly before, during, or shortly after surgery (i.e., during the perioperative period) to combat any bacterial contamination of tis-

sues that occurs during the operative procedure. The general rules for the use of prophylactic antibiotics are:

    a. The operation must carry a significant risk of a postoperative infection: A clean procedure would not require prophylactic antibiotics, but the following situations would:

        (1) Colon or rectal surgery (the patient is given oral nonabsorbable antibiotics plus intravenous antibiotics)

        (2) A procedure (e.g., vascular surgery) in which prosthetic material is to be used

        (3) A gynecologic procedure in which the vagina is opened

        (4) Gross contamination of the operative site

    b. The antibiotics used should be effective against the pathogens likely to be present in the operative site. Narrow-spectrum antibiotics should be used.

    c. The antibiotics must have reached an effective tissue level at the time of the incision. Thus, they should be given 1–2 hours prior to surgery.

    d. The antibiotics should be given for only 6–24 hours after surgery. Long-lasting regimens carry a high risk of superinfection and offer no additional protection.

    e. The benefits of the prophylactic antibiotic should outweigh its potential dangers, such as allergic reactions or the stimulation of bacterial or fungal superinfections from overgrowth of pathogens, such as gram-negative bacteria or *Candida*.

  5. Tetanus prophylaxis

    a. Active immunization with tetanus toxoid injections given in the recommended schedule results in a protective titer within 30 days. This is usually done in infancy (with DPT shots) or during military induction. A booster dose every 10 years is recommended by the American College of Surgeons.

    b. Prophylaxis at the time of injury

        (1) Any person with a penetrating injury must receive tetanus prophylaxis if previous immunization cannot be documented.

            (a) A previously immunized person should be given a booster dose if none has been given within the past 5 years.

            (b) A patient with a clean injury who has never been immunized may be given the first of three immunizing doses, but it is important that the patient receives the subsequent two doses.

            (c) A patient with a dirty wound who has never been immunized should be given **passive immunization** with human tetanus immune globulin intramuscularly.

                (i) The protection period has a half-life of 1 month.

                (ii) The first dose of tetanus toxoid may be given at the same time, but it should be given at a separate intramuscular site.

        (2) Adequate debridement of devitalized tissue and removal of all foreign debris are also essential.

        (3) The value of antibiotics, particularly penicillin, for the prophylaxis of tetanus-prone wounds is unproven. However, for patients who have a suspected *Clostridium tetani* infection or extensive necrosis, prophylactic penicillin should be given in high doses.

B. Abscesses

  1. Causative organisms

    a. Staphylococcal organisms (*S. epidermidis, S. aureus*) frequently infect cutaneous lesions (i.e., sebaceous cysts) or intracavitary locations (i.e., the pleural space) to form abscesses. They may also be blood-borne, resulting in multiple abscesses. Staphylococci usually produce **pus**, which must be drained to allow healing.

    b. Other organisms, including anaerobic and gram-negative organisms, can also cause both cutaneous and deep abscesses. Coliform organisms are often present in inguinal and perineal cutaneous abscesses.

  2. Cutaneous abscesses

    a. Types

        (1) Furuncles (boils) are cutaneous staphylococcal abscesses. They are frequently seen with acne and other skin disorders. The bacterial colonization begins in hair follicles and can cause both local cellulitis and abscess formation.

        (2) Carbuncles are cutaneous abscesses that spread through the dermis into the subcutaneous region. They may then spread over a large area, often with resultant sepsis. They are common in individuals with diabetes.

      (3) Hidradenitis suppurativa is an infection involving the apocrine sweat glands in the axillary, inguinal, and perineal regions. The infection results in chronic abscess formation and scarring, and often requires complete excision of the apocrine gland-bearing skin to prevent recurrence.

    b. Diagnosis. The microbiologic diagnosis is made by incising the abscess, then culturing and Gram-staining the pus, usually revealing gram-positive cocci. Subsequent culture reveals the bacterial type as well as its antibiotic sensitivity. Most staphylococcal organisms are resistant to penicillin; thus, one of the semisynthetic penicillins, erythromycin, or a cephalosporin should be used.

    c. Treatment

      (1) Drainage of pus

      (2) Appropriate antibiotic therapy

      (3) Wound care with irrigation and debridement when necessary

      (4) Excision of the involved area when it contains multiple small abscesses, sinus tracts, or necrotic tissue

  3. Intra-abdominal (peritoneal) abscesses

    a. Causes

      (1) Extrinsic causes include penetrating trauma and surgical procedures.

      (2) Intrinsic causes include perforation of a hollow viscus, such as the appendix, duodenum, or colon, seeding of bacteria from a source outside the abdomen, or ischemia and infarction of tissue within the abdomen, such as bowel ischemia.

    b. Sites. Multiple abscesses are present in up to 15% of cases. The commonest sites are the:

      (1) Subphrenic space

      (2) Subhepatic space

      (3) Lateral gutters along the posterior peritoneal cavity

      (4) Pelvis

      (5) Periappendiceal or pericolonic areas

    c. Signs and symptoms of infection, fever, pain, and leukocytosis are produced by abdominal abscesses.

      (1) These abscesses are frequently large and usually produce spiking fevers.

      (2) When there is a delay in seeking medical attention or a delay in diagnosis, patients may present with generalized sepsis with hypotension.

      (3) Postoperative abscesses usually produce fever during the second postoperative week.

      (4) Gastrointestinal bleeding or pulmonary, renal, or hepatic failure may occur.

    d. Diagnosis. The key to an expeditious diagnosis is a high index of suspicion.

      (1) The patient may have tenderness or an abdominal mass, particularly with a pelvic abscess, but often no physical findings are present.

      (2) Computed tomography (CT scan) and ultrasonography [and potentially magnetic resonance imaging (MRI)] are very useful and also can be used to guide the successful drainage of an abscess.

    e. Treatment

      (1) The mainstay of intra-abdominal abscess treatment is surgical intervention. This is particularly true when blood or debris is present in the abscess.

      (2) Deep infections usually require irrigation and drainage.

        (a) Classically, this has been performed as an open operative procedure.

        (b) More recently, ultrasound techniques and CT scanning have allowed precise localization of abscesses, and percutaneous drainage has been successful.

      (3) Ideally, drainage is performed without contaminating the general peritoneal cavity.

        (a) Pelvic abscesses may be drained transrectally or through the superior vagina.

        (b) Subphrenic abscesses may be drained posteriorly through a twelfth rib approach.

C. Cellulitis is an inflammation of the dermal and subcutaneous tissues secondary to **nonsuppurative** bacterial invasion. It may result from a puncture wound or any other type of skin break.

  1. Signs and symptoms

    a. Cellulitis produces redness, edema, and localized tenderness. Fever and leukocytosis are usually present.

    b. The cellulitis-causing bacteria may also infect the regional lymphatics, resulting in red, tender streaks on an extremity.

    c. A deep abscess can result in an overlying cellulitis and should be suspected when a patient does not rapidly respond to antibiotics.

2. **Treatment.** The usual organism is a *Streptococcus*, which is almost always sensitive to penicillin.

D. **Necrotizing fasciitis** is a rapidly progressive bacterial infection in which several different organisms invade the fascial planes. The infection travels rapidly along a fascial plane and causes vascular thrombosis as it progresses, resulting in necrosis of the tissue involved. The overlying skin may appear normal, leading the clinician to underestimate the severity of the infection. Necrotizing fasciitis may result from a small puncture wound, a surgical wound, or any open trauma.

1. **Signs and symptoms**
   a. Hemorrhagic bullae, edema, and redness may develop on the skin and crepitus may be present, although the skin may appear normal.
   b. The patient shows signs of progressive toxicity (fever, tachycardia) and may have localized wound pain.
   c. The necrotic wound or tissue involved usually has a foul serous discharge.

2. **Diagnosis. Gram-stain** reveals multiple organisms, which act synergistically, giving the fasciitis its rapidly progressive and destructive character, including:
   a. Microaerophilic streptococci
   b. Staphylococci
   c. Gram-negative aerobes and anaerobes

3. **Treatment** is surgical, and early diagnosis is extremely important.
   a. It is critical to remove all infected or devitalized tissue at the first debridement because any remaining necrotic tissue will continue the rapidly progressive necrosis.
   b. The removal of large amounts of skin and surrounding tissue and, occasionally, amputation of an extremity may be required.
   c. Daily debridement may be needed.
   d. Antibiotics, usually clindamycin and an aminoglycoside, in high doses are required.
   e. This infection is life-threatening, and prompt treatment is essential.

E. **Clostridial myositis and cellulitis (gas gangrene).** Gas gangrene is most commonly caused by *Clostridium perfringens* (*Clostridium welchii*).

1. **Characteristics of wounds likely to develop this condition**
   a. Extensive tissue destruction has occurred.
   b. There is marked impairment of the local blood supply, either from the injury itself, from complications of the injury (e.g., vascular thrombosis), or from iatrogenic causes (e.g., an overly tight orthopedic cast).
   c. The wound is grossly contaminated.
   d. There has been a delay in treatment (usually more than 6 hours).
   e. Surgical debridement has been inadequate.
   f. The patient has a preexisting condition that leads to immunologic incompetence, such as corticosteroid drug therapy.

2. **Clinical presentation**
   a. The onset of symptoms is usually 48 hours after injury but may occur as early as 6 hours after.
   b. The commonest complaint, severe pain at the site of injury, is due to the rapidly infiltrating infection. However, this pain may be missed because the patient is receiving narcotics. Any surgical patient who requires an increase in narcotics should be suspected of having a clostridial infection and should be examined before the narcotics dosage is changed.
   c. A rapid, weak pulse is usually present, and the patient appears diaphoretic, pale, and weak. There may be mental changes, including delirium or confusion. The temperature is often, but not always, elevated.
   d. The wound is more tender to the touch than is the usual postoperative wound. The skin may appear normal, but the wound usually drains a brownish serous fluid with a foul odor. Crepitus may appear around the wound edges but is often a late sign.
   e. Blood studies often reveal a falling hematocrit and a rising bilirubin due to hemolysis. The white blood count may be mildly elevated, but this is unreliable.
   f. Gram-stain of the wound discharge reveals large gram-positive bacilli. Numerous red blood cells are present but few white cells.
   g. A plain x-ray of the wound area may reveal air in the soft tissues.

3. Treatment. Adequate debridement at the time of initial injury is important for prophylaxis. Treatment for established clostridial infection includes extensive debridement within the tissue planes involved and antibiotics, especially penicillin. If extensive soft tissue necrosis is present in an extremity, amputation is performed.

a. Hyperbaric oxygen therapy is used, but its value is unproven.

b. Human tetanus immune globulin will not prevent or treat gas gangrene.

c. Delay in treatment to consider further diagnostic procedures or to observe the patient's course is usually catastrophic.

F. Infections after surgery

1. Gastrointestinal surgery

a. Upper gastrointestinal tract infections

(1) The rate of serious infections after operations on the upper gastrointestinal tract is 5%–15%.

(2) The **oral cavity** is colonized by large numbers of aerobic and anaerobic bacteria. These bacteria are generally killed in the low pH environment of the **stomach**, resulting in sterile cultures. Gastric cultures become positive when obstruction (or blood) is present.

(3) Prophylactic antibiotics are not necessary with elective gastric surgical procedures but should be used when obstruction, hemorrhage, or perforation is present.

(4) Patients with gastric malignancy or achlorhydria or who are taking anti-ulcer medications (H_2-blockers) should be given prophylactic antibiotics.

(5) The usual antibiotics employed are a cephalosporin or a penicillin–aminoglycoside combination to cover both aerobes and anaerobes.

b. Biliary tree infections

(1) The biliary tree is rarely colonized with bacteria in the normal individual. The colonization rate rises to 15%–30% for patients with chronic calculous cholecystitis and to over 80% in patients with common duct obstruction. Of those patients with positive cultures:

(a) *Escherichia coli* is present in over one-half of the cases, while other gram-negative organisms account for most of the remainder.

(b) *Streptococcus fecalis*, the aerobic gram-positive enterococcus, may also be present, and *Salmonella* strains are occasionally present. Anaerobic organisms, especially *C. perfringens*, are present in up to 20% of cases.

(2) No antibiotic prophylaxis is recommended for elective cholecystectomy.

(3) Therapeutic antibiotics are recommended in patients with cholangitis, with empyema or gangrene of the gallbladder, or with liver abscesses. A cephalosporin or aminoglycoside should be given for 5–7 days.

(4) Prophylactic antibiotics should be used in patients over 70 years of age and in those with common duct stones, a history of fever or chills, or a positive Gram stain of the bile.

c. Colonic and rectal infections

(1) Surgery performed on these segments of the bowel is frequently followed by wound and intraperitoneal infection (6%–60%).

(2) Normal human colonic flora is composed of both aerobes and anaerobes.

(a) **Aerobes** are present at levels of 10^8–10^9 bacteria per gram of stool. *E. coli*, the commonest aerobe, is the organism most often found in wound infections after colonic surgery.

(b) **Anaerobes** are present at levels of 10^{11} bacteria per gram of stool (1000-fold greater numbers than aerobes). Many types are present, but *Bacteroides fragilis* is the usual cause of anaerobic wound infection.

(c) Mixed aerobic and anaerobic infections are typical.

(3) An effective **preoperative regimen** combines the removal of gross feces (mechanical preparation of the bowel) with the use of oral nonabsorbable antibiotics.

(a) Mechanical removal of the feces is the most important factor in lowering the bacterial counts and the incidence of wound infections. Most regimens include aggressive purgation with potent oral agents, such as mannitol, polyethylene glycol, or magnesium sulfate, and with multiple enemas.

(b) Antibiotic prophylaxis will only reduce bacterial counts enough to lower the incidence of wound infection after adequate mechanical preparation. Single antibiotics or combinations of antibiotics are not effective unless they inhibit both aerobic and anaerobic organisms.

(i) Oral antibiotics, such as neomycin and erythromycin base, started 10–22 hours prior to surgery, result in maximal bacterial suppression at the time of surgery. Longer treatment periods allow resistant bacterial overgrowth.

(ii) Intravenous antibiotics may further lower the incidence of wound infection when given concomitantly with an oral antibiotic combination, but this is controversial.

(c) Preparation of the colon and rectum should be carried out before all elective operations unless a high-grade (complete) obstruction is present. The presence of obstruction calls for a preliminary colostomy to remove the feces mechanically. After adequate purgation, the elective procedure is performed under oral antibiotic "cover."

(d) In emergency procedures (e.g., after trauma) when no bowel preparation is possible, intravenous antibiotics should be given, and the wound should not be closed primarily. In these situations, colonic anastomoses are riskier than in elective situations.

2. Gynecologic surgery

a. The organisms involved usually colonize the vagina and include both aerobes and anaerobes.

b. Prophylactic antibiotics are useful for women undergoing hysterectomy.

3. Urologic surgery

a. Although the normal urinary tract is sterile, the commonest pathogen encountered is *E. coli*, followed by other gram-negative rods and enterococci.

b. The general principle that elective surgery should be postponed until any infection has been successfully treated is especially true for urologic surgery.

c. Chronic indwelling tubes (e.g., suprapubic bladder catheters and nephrostomies) are generally colonized with bacteria but do not require antibiotic therapy unless the patient has a symptomatic local infection, generalized sepsis, or catheter obstruction, or unless an urea-splitting organism, such as *Proteus*, is present.

d. When transurethral prostatectomy, cystourethroscopy (especially in males), or urethral surgery is planned, a urinary tract infection should be sought.

(1) If cultures are positive, the patient should be treated with an antibiotic specific for the infecting organism.

(2) The procedure should be postponed until cultures are negative.

(3) In the presence of urinary tract pathology, it may be impossible to sterilize the urine. Thus, antibiotics are used perioperatively both as treatment and prophylaxis.

4. Vascular surgery

a. The rate of infection when **vascular prosthetic grafts** are used varies between 1% and 6%. Infection may develop early (within months) or years later.

b. The source of infection may be direct contamination from the skin or surrounding tissues, or blood-borne organisms. The commonest infecting organism is *S. aureus*, followed by coagulase-negative *S. epidermidis*. Coliform infections are becoming commoner.

c. Perioperatively, prophylactic antibiotics will lower the incidence of graft infection from the high of 6% down to 1%. The recommended antibiotic is a cephalosporin.

d. Prophylactic antibiotics (penicillin) should also be used when a patient with a prosthetic graft undergoes a procedure associated with a transient bacteremia (such as dental extraction).

5. Cardiac surgery. The same sources of infection as for vascular surgery are present. Also, the extracorporeal circulation used for open heart surgery can be contaminated by *S. epidermidis* and *S. aureus*. Infections are severe and life-threatening and include sternal osteomyelitis and dehiscence and prosthetic valve endocarditis. The recommended antibiotic prophylaxis therapy is similar to that for vascular surgery.

6. Noncardiac thoracic surgery. Lung surgery has a high risk of infection when the lung is already infected or when a significant volume of lung is removed, as in a pneumonectomy, and a large dead space remains. For elective pulmonary resections, many surgeons use prophylactic antibiotics for the gram-positive cocci that colonize the upper respiratory tree, but it has not been definitively demonstrated that prophylactic antibiotics are useful.

7. Orthopedic surgery. Postoperative infections of bone or implanted prostheses are major life-threatening complications (similar to vascular and cardiac surgery). The commonest organisms are the staphylococci. Prophylactic antibiotics against these organisms are used routinely.

G. Infections after trauma

1. **Burns** (second- and third-degree) are prone to develop group A streptococcal infection during the first 5 days. Some burn centers recommend using penicillin G or a penicillinase-resistant synthetic penicillin during this time. To reduce the colonization of injured tissues, topical antibiotics should also be applied. These antibiotics should be effective against both gram-negative rods and gram-positive cocci. Purulent infection of intravenous catheter and cutdown sites is called suppurative thrombophlebitis and must be treated by excision of the vein.

2. **Penetrating abdominal trauma** should be treated with an antibiotic regimen that covers both anaerobic and aerobic organisms.

3. **Penetrating chest wounds** should be treated with antibiotics that are effective against organisms commonly found in the respiratory tract.

4. **Human bites** should be treated with penicillin because they are likely to contain mixed anaerobic and aerobic organisms. **Animal bites** warrant prophylactic antibiotics if there is extensive injury.

5. **Other soft tissue injuries** involving a large surface area should be treated with antibiotics effective against normal residents of the skin (gram-positive cocci). If extensive contamination from environmental pathogens is present, antibiotics providing coverage against anaerobic and gram-negative bacilli should be added.

III. POSTOPERATIVE COMPLICATIONS can be associated with any operation or can be related to a specific kind of surgery. The latter type are discussed in the relevant chapters, and only the general types of complications are discussed here. Thrombophlebitis and pulmonary embolus, which are common postoperative complications, are discussed in Chapter 8. Most surgical complications develop in relation to some event that occurs in the operating room, emphasizing the fact that **prevention** is the best form of management.

A. **Common postoperative problems** typically occur on certain postoperative days. Most of these problems produce **fever** and can be diagnosed by physical examination and simple laboratory tests.

1. **Pulmonary complications** are the commonest cause of fever during the first postoperative days. Most pulmonary problems develop because of prolonged mechanical ventilation or because of inadequate ventilation and a poor cough effort. They are made worse by oversedation, preexisting chronic pulmonary disease, or abdominal distention.
   a. **Atelectasis** is the usual problem. Nasotracheal aspiration or bronchoscopy will help to resolve atelectasis by removing secretions and inflating a collapsed lung.
   b. **Pneumonia** can supervene if the atelectasis is not quickly treated. Antibiotics should not be given unless evidence of infection is present.

2. **Urinary tract infection** typically causes the fever that develops on postoperative days 3–6.
   a. An indwelling catheter or preexisting bladder outlet obstruction is often the cause.
   b. Postoperative pain can cause patients to empty the bladder incompletely when voiding; the residual urine predisposes to infection.
   c. Urinary tract infection is best treated by:
      (1) Appropriate antibiotics
      (2) Relieving any obstruction that is present
      (3) Removing the catheter, if feasible

3. **Wound infections**, including intra-abdominal abscesses, are discussed in II.

4. **Dehydration** is common after surgery because of third-space sequestration of fluids in the operative site.
   a. Oliguria, tachycardia, and orthostatic hypotension may result.
   b. Treatment is rehydration.
   c. On the third or fourth postoperative day, the body begins to mobilize the third-space fluid, which increases the intravascular volume until the fluid is excreted by the kidneys.

5. **Overhydration** may occur in patients with impaired cardiac or renal function.

    a. Congestive heart failure or pulmonary congestion and impaired oxygenation may result.

    b. Attention to fluid balance and weighing the patient daily should prevent this problem.

    c. The intravascular volume increase that results from mobilization of third-space fluid should be anticipated.

B. General principles of management during the postoperative period are important both in preventing potential complications and in allowing early detection of problems that do develop. These principles include:

    1. Daily or more frequent examination of the patient, including the surgical wound

    2. Removal of all surgical tubes as soon as possible

    3. Early ambulation of the patient

    4. Close monitoring of fluid balance and electrolyte levels

    5. Adequate but not excessive pain medication

    6. Good nursing care

IV. GASTROINTESTINAL FISTULAS

A. Definitions

    1. Fistulas are abnormal communications between two or more hollow organs or between one hollow organ and a body surface. The variety of fistulas is almost limitless, due to the number of organs and sites that can be involved.

    2. Fistulas are **named** according to the sites that they join. Thus, a **bronchobiliary fistula** connects the bronchial tree with the biliary tree; a **gastrocutaneous fistula** communicates between the stomach and the skin.

B. Etiologies

    1. Congenital disorders. Distal tracheoesophageal fistula with esophageal atresia is the most important congenital fistula (see Chapter 29 IV).

    2. Trauma or operative injury. Traumatic or inadvertent operative injury or anastomotic breakdown can produce fistulization. Examples include a colocutaneous fistula from an anastomotic leak or a gastrocutaneous fistula complicating a splenectomy.

    3. Inflammation. Crohn's disease, for example, can cause many fistulas, including enterovesical and ileosigmoid.

    4. Malignancy. Fistulas can develop because of the destruction of organs by tumors. For example, a colovesical fistula might occur in a patient with a large sigmoid colon cancer that erodes into the urinary bladder.

    5. Radiation damage. An enterovaginal fistula can develop after pelvic irradiation for cervical carcinoma.

C. Complications

    1. Malnutrition can develop because of inadequate absorption of nutrients due to the short-circuiting of part of the bowel or due to external loss of ingested food (e.g., gastrocolic fistula and high-output enterocutaneous fistula, respectively) or because of increased caloric needs due to associated infection or stress.

    2. Fluid and electrolyte imbalances are frequent complications of fistulas, especially those involving the proximal bowel or pancreas. The electrolyte content of various gastrointestinal secretions is shown in Table 2-1. Electrolyte losses can be directly measured from a sample of the fistula drainage. For example, a pancreatic fistula developing after distal pancreatectomy, which drains 700 ml of bicarbonate-rich fluid a day, can produce dehydration and metabolic acidosis.

    3. Sepsis, a frequent accompaniment of fistulas, occurs because leakage of the organ's contents produces contamination of sterile spaces (e.g., peritoneum and pleura).

Table 2-1. Approximate Electrolyte Content of Gastrointestinal Secretions

Source	Electrolytes (mEq/L)			
	Na$^+$	K$^+$	Cl$^-$	HCO$_3$$^-$
Stomach	60	10	50–150	0–20
Duodenum	120	5	100	20
Bile duct	145	5	100	40
Pancreas	140	5	75	100
Ileum	100	5	65	30

    a. An abdominal abscess or wound infection can result.

    b. Distant infections, such as central venous catheter infections, can develop because of extensive skin contamination or bacteremia.

  4. Skin excoriation, often severe, can occur when intestinal secretions drain onto the abdominal skin. This skin disruption can be painful and can contribute to sepsis.

  5. Hemorrhage is an infrequent but potentially life-threatening complication of enteric fistulas. It occurs when the inflammation associated with a fistula erodes into a blood vessel, causing severe bleeding.

D. Evaluation. Management of the patient with an enteric fistula requires knowledge of the anatomy, etiology, and physiology of the defect.

  1. History and physical examination

    a. The history can provide useful etiologic information.

    b. Examining the patient provides information about the location of an external fistula and the character of its drainage. Dehydration and malnutrition can also be detected.

    c. The volume of drainage must be determined.

  2. Radiographic studies are vital in determining the dimensions of the fistula tract and organ involvement. Contrast material may be administered by mouth, by rectum, or directly into the fistula (**fistulogram** or **sinogram**).

    a. Ultrasonography, CT scan, and MRI can be useful in locating an undrained collection (e.g., an abscess), which may be associated with the fistula.

    b. Radiographs should also be used to **exclude the presence of intestinal obstruction** distal to the fistula (see IV E 6 a).

  3. Laboratory tests on the drainage are useful for determining the electrolyte content of the fistula, and bacteriologic cultures should be obtained in patients with suspected sepsis.

E. Management

  1. Hydration and correction of electrolyte disturbances require immediate attention.

  2. Control of infection also requires immediate attention. Antibiotics and operative drainage of abscesses may be required before patients improve: A fistula will not heal in the presence of an undrained collection.

  3. Control of external drainage helps to minimize further morbidity. Suction catheters, drains, collection bags, or operative diversion may be useful in protecting body surfaces from irritation. Bowel rest, provided by prolonged fasting, often diminishes gastrointestinal fluid losses.

  4. Therapy to inhibit organ-specific secretions is used when appropriate.

    a. For the stomach: H$_2$-blockers

    b. For the pancreas: octreotide

  5. Correction of malnutrition should begin as soon as the patient is stabilized. Most patients require parenteral nutrition. Occasionally, tube feedings of a low-residue diet, or even oral feedings, will be possible, especially with distal low-output fistulas.

  6. "Spontaneous closure" can occur in many patients with conservative therapy to minimize drainage and with appropriate nutrition. Closure with conservative measures may take from 2–8 weeks. However, spontaneous repair is unlikely, and operative repair is required when any of the following is present:

    a. Distal obstruction beyond the fistula site

b. Pus or foreign body at the fistula site
c. Severe bowel injury, such as radiation damage or extensive inflammatory bowel disease
d. Cancer at the fistula site
e. Epithelialization of the fistula tract

7. **Operative repair** should be performed electively, in a nonseptic, well-nourished patient. Operation typically involves:
   a. Identification of the fistula
   b. Resection of the fistula and damaged segments of bowel
   c. Anastomosis to restore bowel continuity

F. **Results.** Major improvements in fistula management have occurred in the past 2 decades with resultant increased survival rates.

1. **Mortality rates.** Until the mid-1960s, mortality rates were over 50% for gastric, duodenal, or small bowel fistulas.
   a. Management emphasized early attempts at operative repair before malnutrition developed.
   b. Major causes of death were electrolyte and fluid disturbances, malnutrition, and peritonitis.

2. **Present management** should lower the mortality rates to between 2% and 10%, depending on the etiology of the fistula.
   a. Sepsis and renal failure remain significant causes of death.
   b. Malnutrition and electrolyte disturbances have largely been eliminated as causes of death because of improved techniques of venous access, improved blood chemistry monitoring, and improvements in prolonged parenteral feeding.

V. HERNIA. A hernia is the abnormal protrusion of intra-abdominal tissue through a defect in the abdominal wall.

A. **Overview**

1. **Frequency of occurrence.** In both men and women, hernias occur most commonly in the inguinal region (75%–80% of all hernias). Incisional (ventral) hernias occur next in frequency (8%–10%), followed by umbilical hernias (3%–8%).

2. **Etiology.** Hernias can occur as a result of various factors.
   a. Congenital defects in the abdominal wall, such as in indirect inguinal hernia, are common.
   b. Enlarged foramen. A normal anatomic foramen that becomes pathologically enlarged can allow an organ to pass through the defect (e.g., the stomach passing into the chest through the esophageal hiatus is a **hiatal hernia**).
   c. Loss of tissue strength and elasticity, especially due to aging, may result in herniation, as in direct inguinal hernia.
   d. Trauma, especially **operative trauma** in which normal tissue strength is destroyed surgically, can lead to the development of hernia. Infection in the wound greatly increases the risk of hernia following surgery.
   e. Increased intra-abdominal pressure can result in hernia, such as:
      (1) Heavy lifting
      (2) Coughing, asthma, and chronic obstructive pulmonary disease (COPD)
      (3) Bladder outlet obstruction (e.g., benign prostatic hypertrophy)
      (4) Constipation or difficulty moving one's bowels, as occurs in carcinoma of the colon or rectum
      (5) Pregnancy
      (6) Ascites, intra-abdominal tumors, and abdominal distention
      (7) Obesity

3. **Descriptive terms.** Hernias may be described according to physical or operative findings.
   a. Complete. Both the hernia sac and its contents extend through the defect (e.g., in a complete inguinal hernia, both the sac and its contents extend into the scrotum).
   b. Incomplete. A defect is present but the sac and its contents do not yet pass through (e.g., in an incomplete inguinal hernia, the sac has not extended through the external inguinal ring).

     c. Reducible. The hernia contents can be pushed back into the abdomen.

     d. Irreducible (incarcerated). The hernia contents cannot be pushed back.

     e. Obstructing. The hernia contains a loop of bowel that is kinked and, therefore, obstructed.

     f. Strangulated. The tissue contained in the hernia is ischemic due to interruption of its blood supply.

     g. Sliding. The wall of the hernia sac, rather than being formed completely by peritoneum, is in part formed by the wall of another intra-abdominal structure, such as the colon or the bladder.

     h. Richter's hernia. One side of the bowel wall is trapped in the hernia rather than the entire loop of bowel.

   4. Complications. Hernias should be repaired electively to prevent the development of major complications.

     a. Intestinal obstruction may occur when a loop of bowel passes through the abdominal wall defect and becomes mechanically obstructed.

     b. Intestinal strangulation with **perforation** or **gangrene** may occur if the vascular pedicle to the herniated loop of bowel is also interrupted.

B. Inguinal hernias

   1. Anatomy of the inguinal region (Figures 2-1 and 2-2).

     a. The internal inguinal ring is an opening in the transversalis fascia lateral to the inferior epigastric vessels.

     b. The external inguinal ring is an opening in the external oblique aponeurosis.

     c. The inguinal canal is the communication between the internal and external rings.

       (1) The **anterior wall** of the canal is formed by the external oblique aponeurosis.

       (2) The **inferior wall** of the canal is formed by the inguinal ligament (**Poupart's ligament**) and its reflection.

       (3) The **roof** of the inguinal canal (**superior**) is made up of fibers of the internal oblique and transversus muscles, forming a structure termed the **conjoint tendon**.

       (4) The **posterior wall** or **floor** is formed by the transversalis fascia and aponeurosis.

         (a) Within the posterior wall of the inguinal canal is **Hesselbach's triangle**.

         (b) It is formed laterally by the inferior epigastric artery, inferiorly by the inguinal ligament, and superomedially by the lateral border of the rectus sheath.

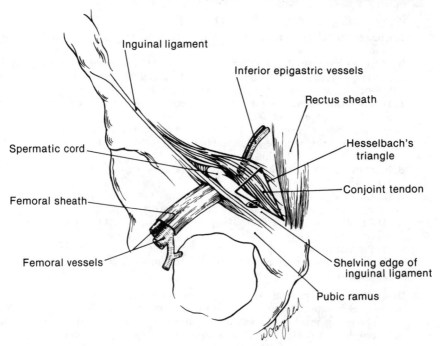

Figure 2-1. Anatomy of the inguinal region.

d. In men, the **spermatic cord structures** pass into the internal ring, traverse the inguinal canal, and pass through the external ring into the scrotum. In women, the **round ligament** traverses the inguinal canal. Structures within the spermatic cord include:

   (1) Arteries: testicular and cremasteric
   (2) Nerves: ilioinguinal, genital branch of the genitofemoral, and sympathetic nervous supply
   (3) Veins: pampiniform plexus
   (4) Vas deferens
   (5) Processus vaginalis: an evagination of peritoneum that accompanies the descent of the testicle and gubernaculum through the abdominal wall. Normally obliterated, it remains patent in an indirect hernia and forms the hernia sac.

2. Types of hernias
a. Indirect inguinal hernias

   (1) An indirect inguinal hernia passes through the internal inguinal ring and down the inguinal canal (see Figure 2-2). It may, on occasion, extend into the scrotum (complete hernia).
   (2) An indirect inguinal hernia, which occurs as a result of a congenitally patent processus vaginalis, allows free communication between the peritoneal cavity, inguinal canal, and scrotum. When incompletely obliterated, an indirect inguinal hernia or spermatic cord hydrocele may result.
   (3) Incidence
      (a) Indirect inguinal hernias are the commonest type of hernia in both men and women. They are five to ten times commoner in men than in women. Approximately 5% of men develop an inguinal hernia during their lifetime and require an operation.
      (b) Indirect inguinal hernias are five times commoner than direct hernias.
   (4) Indirect hernias may occur from infancy to old age but generally occur by the fifth decade of life.
   (5) A **pediatric inguinal hernia** (see Chapter 29 II) is almost always indirect and has a high risk of incarceration. It is commoner on the right (75%) and is often bilateral.

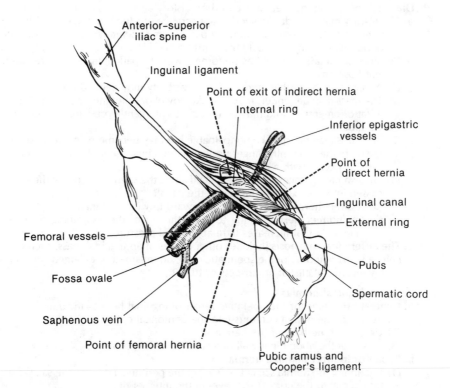

Figure 2-2. Sites of direct, indirect, and femoral hernias and their relationship to anatomic structures.

(6) Potential indirect hernias are associated with an undescended testis, a testis in the inguinal canal, and a testicular or spermatic cord hydrocele.

(7) Bilateral patent processus vaginalis occurs in up to 10% of patients with an indirect inguinal hernia.

b. Direct inguinal hernias. The inferior epigastric vessels are the anatomic landmarks that distinguish indirect and direct inguinal hernias.

(1) A direct inguinal hernia occurs in the floor of the inguinal canal, through Hesselbach's triangle (see Figure 2-1), due to an acquired weakness in the tissue.

(2) The hernia is a direct protrusion of abdominal structures into the floor of the canal posterior to the spermatic cord. It is not contained in the cord as the indirect hernia is, and it generally does not pass into the scrotum. The sac is a broadly based defect: It is much less often associated with strangulation than is an indirect inguinal hernia.

(3) Direct inguinal hernia increases in occurrence with age and is related to physical activity.

(4) A **recurrent inguinal hernia** usually occurs as a direct hernia. Generally the defect occurs in the most medial aspect of the repair of the floor of the inguinal canal.

c. Pantaloon hernias are combinations of direct and indirect hernias in which the hernia sac passes both medially and laterally to the epigastric vessels.

d. Femoral hernias

(1) A femoral hernia occurs when intra-abdominal contents protrude along the femoral sheath in the femoral canal (see Figure 2-2).

(2) The hernia contents protrude posteriorly to the inguinal ligament, anteriorly to the pubic ramus periosteum (i.e., **Cooper's ligament**), and medially to the femoral vessels.

(3) The hernia traverses the femoral canal and presents as a mass at the level of the foramen ovale. It may also turn cephalad once it has exited the foramen ovale and can cross anteriorly to the inguinal ligament.

(4) The sac frequently has a narrow neck, and 30%–40% of femoral hernias become incarcerated or strangulated.

(5) Femoral hernias are commoner in women than in men.

(6) Femoral hernias are related to physical exertion and to pregnancy.

3. Diagnosis of an inguinal hernia is based on history and physical examination.

a. The history may include the sudden appearance of a lump in the groin. The mass may be intermittently present and may be painful. Its appearance may be associated with strenuous activity. In some patients, it may extend into the scrotum (complete hernia).

b. Physical examination should be performed with the patient in both the recumbent and upright positions.

(1) A mass may be visible, and its size or visibility may depend on its position.

(2) The mass may be tender, may feel like bowel or other intra-abdominal tissue, such as fat or omentum, and may be reducible with gentle pressure. Bowel sounds may be audible.

(3) The mass may be small or nonpalpable but may become palpable as an impulse at the tip of the examining finger upon a sudden increase in the intra-abdominal pressure, as occurs with a cough.

(4) The examining finger should be placed along the spermatic cord at the scrotum and passed into the external ring along the canal.

(a) A **direct hernia** causes a bulge forward low in the canal.

(b) An **indirect hernia** lightly touches the tip of the examining finger during a maneuver that increases intra-abdominal pressure.

c. The differential diagnosis includes other causes of an inguinal mass, such as a hydrocele, a varix, a lipoma of the spermatic cord, an inflamed or enlarged lymph node, an undescended testicle, or an abscess or tumor.

4. Repair of inguinal hernias

a. General principles for the operative repair of inguinal hernias include:

(1) Return of the hernia contents into the peritoneal cavity

(2) Ligation of the base of the hernia sac

(3) Repair of the abdominal wall defect to prevent recurrence

b. Repair of indirect inguinal hernia involves:

(1) Ligation of the hernia sac at the level of the peritoneal cavity—the sac is usually anteromedial to the cord at the level of the internal ring

(2) Tightening of the internal ring in adults

(3) Repair of the inguinal canal floor in adults

c. Repair of direct inguinal hernia is based upon reinforcement of the inguinal canal floor after invaginating the hernia sac.

d. Repair of femoral hernia involves approaching the femoral sheath defect suprainguinally.

   (1) The space is closed by apposing Cooper's ligament and the posterior reflection of the inguinal ligament (Cooper's ligament repair) or by plugging the space with polypropylene mesh (Lichtenstein repair).

   (2) Often the floor of the inguinal canal is also reinforced, using the transversalis fascia.

e. Repair of the abdominal wall defect uses several techniques, which are discussed below.

   (1) Bassini repair

   (a) The transversalis fascia and conjoint tendon above are sutured to the reflection of the inguinal ligament (i.e., the shelving edge of Poupart's ligament) below.

   (b) The spermatic cord is returned to its normal anatomic location between the reinforced inguinal canal floor and the external oblique aponeurosis.

   (c) In women, the round ligament may be ligated and the internal ring closed.

   (2) Cooper's ligament repair (McVay's method)

   (a) This is similar to the Bassini repair except that the transversalis fascia is sutured to Cooper's ligament, which is the periosteum of the pubic ramus.

   (b) Because Cooper's ligament is more posterior than the inguinal ligament, a "relaxing" incision is often made in the anterior rectus sheath adjacent to the reflection of the external oblique aponeurosis. This allows the transversalis to be sutured to the ligament without undue tension.

   (3) Shouldice repair is also similar to the Bassini repair except that the transversalis fascia is divided longitudinally and imbricated upon itself in two layers. The internal oblique muscle and conjoint tendon are then sutured to the reflection of the inguinal ligament in two layers.

f. Recurrence rates after surgical repair vary, depending on the type of hernia, but hernias tend to recur in 3%–5% of cases.

g. Special situations

   (1) When **strangulation** or **necrosis of the incarcerated bowel** is suspected but the bowel returns to the peritoneal cavity spontaneously prior to visual examination by the surgeon, the abdomen should be opened and explored and any necrotic bowel should be resected.

   (2) Recurrent hernias or **hernias with large defects** may require the insertion of prosthetic material, such as polypropylene to repair the abdominal wall defect adequately.

   (3) Simple high ligation of the hernia sac is employed for hernias in the **pediatric agegroup**. No floor repair is needed.

   (4) A **truss** is a device that exerts external compression over the hernia defect, keeping the space obliterated. It is generally used only when surgery cannot be safely performed or when the patient refuses surgery.

C. Other types of abdominal wall hernias

1. **Umbilical hernias** occur at the umbilicus, usually in relation to the defect where the umbilical structures passed through the abdominal wall.

   a. Umbilical hernias occur ten times more often in women than in men.

   b. The defect is common in children but usually closes by age 2 years, and fewer than 5% of umbilical hernias persist into later childhood and adult life.

   c. In adults, umbilical hernias are often associated with increased intra-abdominal pressure, as with ascites or pregnancy.

   d. Repair of an umbilical hernia consists of a simple transverse repair of the fascial defect.

2. **Epigastric hernias** result from a defect in the linea alba above the umbilicus.

   a. They occur more commonly in men (in a 3:1 ratio).

   b. Some 20% of epigastric hernias are multiple at the time of repair.

   c. Repair (simple suturing) is associated with a recurrence rate as high as 10%.

3. **Ventral hernias** occur in the abdominal wall in areas other than the inguinal region.

   a. An incisional hernia, the commonest type of ventral hernia, results from poor wound healing in a previous surgical incision.

      (1) Common etiologic factors include wound infection or hematoma, advanced age, obesity, general debilitation or malnutrition, surgical technique, or a postoperative increase in abdominal pressure, as occurs with ileus, ascites, or pulmonary complications of surgery.

      (2) Incisional hernias are repaired after the patient has recovered from the surgical trauma.

   b. Spigelian hernias protrude through the abdominal wall along the semilunar line (the lateral edge of the rectus muscle) below the umbilicus at the semicircular line of Douglas (where the transversus abdominus and internal oblique aponeuroses change to pass anteriorly to the rectus muscle).

3
Medical Risk Factors in Surgical Patients

Pauline K. Park
Howard H. Weitz
Bruce E. Jarrell

I. INTRODUCTION. Even though the natural history of each medical disorder has a pattern of its own, certain considerations apply to most disease processes in evaluating and minimizing operative risk.

A. Overview. Operative risk is a function of many factors, including the baseline **general medical status** of the patient, the **natural history of the disease process** that precipitated the need for surgery, and any **alteration of the patient's baseline medical status** by the surgical process.

B. The history is the most helpful parameter in alerting the physician to certain risk factors, including:

1. Familial disorders, such as bleeding disorders or anesthetic complications

2. Prior difficulties with surgical procedures or anesthetics

3. Allergies or asthma

4. Current medications, such as steroids, diuretics, anticoagulants, or over-the-counter products, such as aspirin, that a patient might not consider a drug

C. Physiologic parameters. Attention to certain physiologic parameters in preoperative patients lowers the operative risk.

1. Electrolyte abnormalities (see Chapter 1 I) should be corrected.
   a. A history of nausea, vomiting, diarrhea, chronic anorexia, or bowel obstruction can be associated with dehydration and electrolyte shifts.
   b. In acute situations, serum electrolyte levels may not reflect the true fluid or metabolic status and should be interpreted with the clinical picture in mind.

2. Fluid status (see Chapter 1 I) should be assessed.
   a. Factors to consider include:
      (1) Past and current weight
      (2) Skin turgor, mucous membrane moistness, and axillary sweat
      (3) Jugular venous distention or pulmonary rales
      (4) Alterations in vital signs, such as blood pressure and heart rate
   b. In acute situations, volume status should be treated promptly.
      (1) Orthostatic blood pressure changes can be determined by a comparison of the supine and the upright blood pressures.
      (2) Hourly urine output should be determined, if time permits.
      (3) Even in urgent cases, such as perforated viscus, it may be beneficial to stabilize volume status preoperatively.

3. Red blood cell mass should be evaluated.
   a. A **hemoglobin level of 10 g/dl** of blood prior to major surgery is acceptable to most physicians; however, with the increased awareness of transfusion-related disease, this threshold has been questioned.
   b. Chronic anemia is usually well compensated by an increase in plasma volume. However, the **etiology** of the anemia should be determined as the underlying disease may affect the planned surgery. For example, cholelithiasis occurs frequently in patients with sickle cell anemia; thus, hydration and oxygenation should be carefully maintained in these patients during cholecystectomy to avoid precipitating a sickle crisis.

    c. Acute blood loss may not alter the peripheral blood hematocrit for up to 24 hours. Thus, the need for red cell replacement should be determined from other variables, such as obvious blood loss sites.

    d. Preoperative blood replacement should be considered in the following situations, though treatment should be individualized.

        (1) Hemoglobin $\leq$ 10 g/dl with anticipated operative blood loss

        (2) Clinical manifestations of hypovolemia due to blood loss within the last 12 hours

        (3) Suspected or demonstrated chronic contraction of blood volume

        (4) Patients with underlying cardiopulmonary disease and decreased oxygen delivery

  4. Malnutrition (see Chapter 1 II) can increase the operative risk; for example, absence of delayed-type hypersensitivity on skin testing and a nutritional deficit are both associated with increased septic-related deaths in elective surgical patients.

D. Infection (see Chapter 2 II) should be controlled prior to surgery.

  1. Elective procedures should be postponed until infections are under control; for example, urinary tract infection or a skin carbuncle should be treated prior to hernia repair.

  2. Prophylactic antibiotics (see Chapter 2 II A 4) may reduce the risk of infectious complications.

  3. In emergency situations that involve potential contamination, such as a perforated viscus or penetrating trauma, appropriate antibiotics should be given at the earliest possible time.

E. Prevention of complications. In acute conditions, such as acute appendicitis and small bowel obstruction, the prognosis depends on the prevention of complications that occur during the natural progression of the disease. It is important to establish the diagnosis and begin treatment *before* complications develop, even if a surgical procedure is required for diagnosis. For example, the overall mortality rate for simple appendicitis without rupture is less than 1% but increases to 3%–15% in patients whose appendix rupture.

F. Patient education. Making sure that the patient has a **realistic understanding of the prognosis and the expected outcome** of the operative procedure ensures the patient's cooperation postoperatively and, thus, improves the operative risk.

II. CARDIOVASCULAR DISEASE

A. Operative risk factors

  1. Goldman et al. (1977) devised a **risk factor index**, composed of risk factors that lead to an increased incidence of perioperative cardiac complications in patients over 40 years of age who undergo general surgery.

    a. Using multivariate analysis, each factor is assigned points (Table 3-1).

    b. Patients are classified into one of four risk groups based on a total point score (Table 3-2). Goldman's high-risk group was found recently to be at a lower risk than originally described.

  2. Other factors that increase the risk of perioperative cardiac complications are Canadian Cardiovascular Society class 3 and class 4 angina (see II B 3), unstable angina, and a history of pulmonary edema.

  3. Factors found **not** to increase cardiac risk are controlled diabetes mellitus, presence of a fourth heart sound, hypertension with a diastolic blood pressure less than 110 mm Hg, and hyperlipidemia.

  4. Anesthesia

    a. Inhalational anesthetic agents are myocardial depressants.

    b. Spinal and general anesthesias are associated with the **same cardiac morbidity and mortality**. Spinal anesthesia, because it may produce vasodilation with hypotension, is contraindicated in patients with a fixed cardiac output (i.e., severe aortic stenosis or severe left ventricular dysfunction).

Table 3-1. Cardiac Risk Index

Factor	Points
History	
Age > 70	5
Myocardial infarction within 6 months	10
Physical examination	
S_3 gallop or JVD	11
Valvular aortic stenosis	3
Electrocardiogram	
Rhythm on preoperative ECG other than sinus or PACs	7
More than 5 PVCs/min at any time prior to surgery	7
Poor general medical status	
$PO_2 < 60$ or $PCO_2 > 50$	3
$K^+ < 3.0$ or $HCO_3^- < 20$ mEq/L	
BUN > 50 or creatinine > 3 mg/dl	
Chronic liver disease, abnormal SGOT	
Bedridden due to noncardiac cause	
Surgical procedure	
Abdominal, thoracic, or aortic surgery	3
Emergency surgery	4

JVD = jugular venous distention; ECG = electrocardiogram; PAC = premature atrial contraction; PVC = premature ventricular contraction; K^+ = potassium; HCO_3^- = serum bicarbonate; BUN = blood urea nitrogen; and SGOT = serum glutamic oxalo-acetic transaminase. (Adapted from Goldman L, Caldera D, Nussbaum S, et al: Multifactorial index of cardiac risk in noncardiac surgical procedures. *N Engl J Med* 297:845, 1977.)

Table 3-2. Cardiac Perioperative Morbidity and Mortality

Class	Points	Cardiac Morbidity	Cardiac Mortality
I	0–5	0.7%	0.2%
II	6–12	5.0%	2.0%
III	13–25	11.0%	2.0%
IV	>25	4.0%	26.0%

(Adapted from Zeldin R: Assessing cardiac risk in patients who undergo noncardiac surgical procedures. *Can J Surg* 27:402, 1984.)

B. **Preexisting cardiovascular disease**

1. **Hypertension**
   a. Patients with hypertension have a 25% incidence of either hypotension or an exacerbation of hypertension during the perioperative period. The risk of **perioperative myocardial infarction** is increased if the blood pressure drops during surgery by 50% at any time or by 33% for 10 minutes or longer.
   b. **Diastolic blood pressure greater than or equal to 110 mm Hg** is a risk factor for development of perioperative cardiac complications.

2. **Myocardial infarction**
   a. Most perioperative myocardial infarctions occur during the first 4–5 postoperative days with a peak incidence on days 2 and 3. A mortality rate of up to 69% has been reported.
   b. Typical presentations of most postoperative myocardial infarctions are *not* associated with anginal pain but with new onset congestive heart failure, arrhythmias, and confusion.
   c. Myocardial infarction **within 6 months prior to surgery** increases the risk of perioperative reinfarction.
      (1) Initially, the reinfarction rate was found to be quite high: 35%, 0–3 months post–myocardial infarction, and 14%–18%, 4–6 months post–myocardial infarction.

(2) Modern cardiac medication and perioperative invasive hemodynamic monitoring have been shown to decrease this risk to 6%, 0–3 months post–myocardial infarction, and 4%, 4–6 months post-myocardial infarction.

d. Patients who survive coronary artery bypass surgery can usually undergo subsequent noncardiac surgery with low risk of perioperative myocardial reinfarction.

3. **Angina**
   a. Class 1 and 2 angina (chronic stable angina) is not a cardiac risk factor (Canadian Cardiovascular Society).
   b. Class 3 angina (angina walking up one flight of stairs or two blocks) is a cardiac risk factor and is similar in risk to having sustained a myocardial infarction during the 6 months prior to surgery.
   c. Class 4 angina (angina with any exertion) is double the risk of class 3 angina.
   d. For patients who are well maintained on an antianginal regimen, care must be taken to ensure effective antianginal therapy in the perioperative period.

4. **Congestive heart failure**
   a. Patients with a prior history but no preoperative clinical evidence of heart failure have a 6% incidence of perioperative pulmonary edema as contrasted with a 16% incidence of perioperative pulmonary edema in patients found to have clinical or radiographic evidence of heart failure preoperatively.
   b. Approximately 70% of patients who develop perioperative pulmonary edema do so in the first hour following surgery with the greatest onset during the first 30 minutes. Etiologies include:
      (1) Volume overload
      (2) Cessation of positive pressure ventilation with subsequent increase in preload
      (3) Anesthetic-induced myocardial depression
      (4) Postoperative hypertension

5. **Valvular heart disease**
   a. Significant aortic stenosis is a cardiac risk factor and is associated with an independent perioperative mortality of 13%.
   b. Aortic or mitral regurgitation. Operative risk is related to the status of **left ventricular function** rather than the degree of valvular regurgitation.
   c. Mitral stenosis. Volume status and heart rate are key factors in the perioperative period. Tachycardia decreases diastolic filling time and may result in pulmonary edema. Small fluid shifts may result in marked hemodynamic abnormalities.
   d. Prosthetic heart valves. Patients with prosthetic heart valves are at risk for **valvular thrombosis** and thromboembolic complications if anticoagulants are withheld for an excessive period perioperatively.
      (1) For most patients, anticoagulants can be discontinued up to 3 days before surgery and restarted 2–3 days following surgery without thromboembolic complications.
      (2) Patients with caged-disk prosthetic mitral valves are at high risk for valve thrombosis.
         (a) For these patients, warfarin (Coumadin) anticoagulation should be stopped 3 days prior to surgery and replaced with full-dose intravenous heparin, which is stopped 12 hours before surgery.
         (b) Once hemostasis is stable following surgery (usually at 12–24 hours postoperatively), heparin is resumed. Warfarin therapy is restarted once oral intake is resumed.

6. **Arrhythmias**
   a. Up to 84% of patients who undergo surgery develop cardiac arrhythmias, but less than 5% are clinically significant.
   b. The incidence of arrhythmia is highest when surgery lasts longer than 3 hours, during neurosurgical or thoracic surgery, and during endotracheal intubation.
   c. Metabolic abnormalities are the commonest cause of arrhythmia (i.e., hypoxia, hypercarbia, hypokalemia, and hyperkalemia). Therapy is aimed at reversal of these abnormalities.
   d. If antiarrhythmics are used during surgery, the following factors must be remembered:
      (1) The lidocaine half-life is increased during general anesthesia.
      (2) Procainamide excretion is delayed with renal dysfunction.
      (3) The use of type I antiarrhythmics (i.e., quinidine and procainamide) is associated with a worsening of ventricular arrhythmia in 10% of cases.

7. Bacterial endocarditis prophylaxis is indicated for procedures associated with **bacteremia** for patients with prosthetic heart valves, most congenital cardiac defects, surgically constructed systemic pulmonary shunts, rheumatic or other acquired valvular abnormalities, hypertrophic obstructive cardiomyopathy, prior history of bacterial endocarditis, and mitral valve prolapse with mitral regurgitation (see Table 3-3).

III. CHRONIC LUNG DISEASE is a common disorder, affecting surgical patients of all ages and diagnoses. It has multiple causes and, when severe, increases the risk of surgery. It may be symptomatic in the form of dyspnea or totally asymptomatic. There may be an acute infectious process superimposed upon a chronic disorder.

A. Preoperative evaluation

1. History. A history of lung disorders, including dyspnea, sputum production, recurrent bronchitis or pneumonia, emphysema, exposure to environmental toxins, systemic lung

Table 3-3. Infective Endocarditis Prophylaxis

Dental Respiratory Procedures	
Standard regimen	Penicillin V 2.0 g, orally, 1 hour before, **and** Penicillin V 1.0 g, orally, 6 hours after, **or** Penicillin G, 2 million units, intravenously or intramuscularly, 30–60 minutes before, **and** Penicillin G, 1 million units, intravenously or intramuscularly, 6 hours later
Maximal protection (e.g., prosthetic valve)	Ampicillin 1.0–2.0 g, intravenously or intramuscularly, **and** Gentamicin 1.5 mg/kg, intramuscularly or intravenously ½ hour before procedure, **and** 6 hours later, penicillin V, 1.0 g, orally, **or** Repeat parenteral regimen 8 hours after procedure
Penicillin-allergic oral regimen	Erythromycin 1.0 g, orally, 1 hour before, **and** Erythromycin, 500 mg, 6 hours later
Penicillin-allergic parenteral regimen	Vancomycin 1.0 g, intravenously, **slowly** over 1 hour, beginning 1 hour before
Gastrointestinal Genitourinary Procedures	
Standard regimen	Ampicillin 2.0 g, intramuscularly or intravenously, **and** Gentamicin 1.5 mg/kg, intramuscularly or intravenously, ½ to 1 hour before procedure; one follow-up dose may be given 8 hours later
Oral regimen, minor/repetitive procedure; low-risk point	Amoxicillin 3.0 g, orally, 1 hour before procedure, **and** Amoxicillin 1.5 g, orally, 6 hours later
Penicillin-allergic regimen	Vancomycin 1.0 g, intravenously, **slowly** over 1 hour, **and** Gentamicin 1.5 mg/kg, intramuscularly or intravenously, 1 hour before procedure; may be repeated once 8–12 hours later

(Adapted from Shulman ST, et al: *Circulation* 70:1123A, 1984 with permission of the American Heart Association, Dallas, Texas.)

diseases, or previous lung surgery, should alert the physician to the possibility of chronic lung disease. **Cigarette smoking**, the commonest cause of chronic lung disease, is toxic to respiratory epithelium and celia and results in impaired mucus transport with consequent impaired resistance to infection.

2. **Physical examination.** Abnormal findings include:
   a. Anatomic abnormalities, such as scoliosis or chest wall abnormalities (e.g., from obesity)
   b. Findings on auscultation of the chest, including decreased breath sounds, wheezing, and rhonchi or rales
   c. Signs of inadequate oxygenation, such as cyanosis, finger clubbing, and the use of accessory muscles for breathing

3. **Chest x-ray.** Abnormal findings include blebs, pneumonitis, and flattening of the diaphragm.

4. **Laboratory studies.** Arterial blood gases provide information on adequacy of ventilation and oxygenation. Abnormal laboratory values include hypoxemia and hypercarbia on arterial blood gases and secondary polycythemia.

B. **Pulmonary function studies.** The correlation of the preoperative pulmonary function tests with postoperative complication rates is controversial.

1. **Spirometry and arterial blood gases** should be performed in patients with the following:
   a. Productive cough and dyspnea
   b. History and physical findings suggestive of pulmonary disease
   c. Age greater than 60
   d. Greater than 20 pack-year history of cigarette smoking
   e. Morbid obesity
   f. Abnormal chest x-ray findings
   g. Planned thoracic procedures with or without pulmonary resection
   h. Planned upper abdominal procedures, especially abdominal aortic aneurysmectomy

2. **Guidelines to identify patients at high risk for nonthoracic surgery**
   a. Forced expiratory volume in 1 second (FEV_1) < 1.0 L
   b. Forced vital capacity (FVC) < 70%–75% predicted
   c. FEV_1/FVC < 70% expected
   d. End tidal CO_2 > 45
   e. Maximum voluntary ventilation (MVV) < 50% predicted
   f. Maximal expiratory flow rate (MEFR) < 200 L/min

3. After **bronchodilator therapy**, pulmonary function tests may be repeated to assess improvement after treatment. Failure to improve after therapy may be an indication of high risk.

4. **Ventilation perfusion scans, quantitation of CO_2 diffusion capacity**, and **determinations of pulmonary artery pressures** may be necessary, if indicated. **Split lung pulmonary function** tests may be required in pulmonary resections, because the segment to be resected may be considerably diseased and may not contribute significantly to pulmonary function.

C. **Operative risk factors**

1. **Preexisting lung disease**
   a. **Chronic obstructive pulmonary disease (COPD).** Patients with obstructive lung disease are at the highest risk for pulmonary complications.
   b. **History of 20 pack-years** or consumption of **more than 20 cigarettes a day** increases the risk of postoperative pulmonary complications.
   c. **Asthma.** Patients with asthma are at risk for bronchospasm.
   d. **Bronchitis.** Patients with active bronchitis should be stabilized with antibiotics prior to operation.
   e. **Restrictive lung disease, neuromuscular disorders, or chest wall abnormalities.** These patients have an impaired ventilatory reserve as a result of weak muscles or abnormal mechanics of ventilation.
   f. **Pulmonary vascular disease**
   g. **Obesity** increases the work of ventilation and impairs the function of the chest wall, leading to decreased functional residual capacity. Postoperative atelectasis is common.
   h. **Age.** There is a slight decrease in pulmonary function with increasing age, although advanced age in itself is not necessarily a risk factor for pulmonary complications.

2. Operative variables
   a. Type of surgery influences the pulmonary risk.
   (1) Thoracotomy and upper abdominal surgery are associated with the most marked changes in postoperative lung volumes and up to 70% risk for postoperative pulmonary complications.
   (a) Chest wall and diaphragmatic excursion mechanics are altered, leading to decreased total lung capacity (TLC), functional residual capacity (FRC), and tidal volume (TV).
   (b) Postoperative pain causes hypoventilation and a poor cough reflex, leading to retention of secretions and ventilation–perfusion shunting.
   (2) Lower abdominal surgery is associated with fewer pulmonary complications than thoracic and upper abdominal surgery.
   (3) Extremity surgery rarely affects postoperative pulmonary function.
   b. Vertical midline incisions are more prone to respiratory complications as compared to transverse, muscle-splitting incisions.
   c. Length of surgery. Surgery that takes over 3.5 hours is associated with increased pulmonary complications.
   d. Anesthesia
   (1) **Mechanical ventilation** impairs many protective mechanisms, such as ciliary function and mucus transport. It also increases the risk of pneumothorax from ruptured pulmonary alveoli.
   (2) **General anesthesia** may decrease FRC for up to 1 week postoperatively.
   (3) **Spinal anesthesia** has been shown to have no difference in pulmonary morbidity than general anesthesia
   (4) **Regional anesthesia** is not associated with postoperative changes in FRC as compared to general anesthesia.
   (5) **Inhalational anesthetics** may exacerbate bronchospasm.

D. Postoperative complications occur in up to 50% of patients with chronic lung disease and up to 70% of patients with abnormal pulmonary function tests. Pulmonary secretions tend to accumulate after the hypoventilation secondary to decreases in FRC and splinting from pain.

   1. Atelectasis is the commonest complication, followed by **pulmonary infection**, both of which may lead to pulmonary failure. These are usually due to retained tracheobronchial secretions.

   2. Other significant complications include:
   a. Bronchospasm
   b. Pulmonary edema
   c. Aspiration of gastric contents
   d. Pneumothorax

E. Pre- and postoperative management may improve pulmonary function and reduce the number of postoperative complications in high-risk patients.

   1. Preoperative management
   a. Cessation of cigarette smoking at least **8 weeks** preceding elective surgery has been shown to decrease postoperative pulmonary complications.
   b. Incentive spirometry may improve impaired function and reduce postoperative atelectasis.
   c. Chest physiotherapy may help to mobilize secretions, but it should be reserved for patients with lobar collapse or high sputum production because it may exacerbate bronchospasm.
   d. Bronchodilators, such as aminophylline, may improve function in patients with asthma or COPD.
   e. Aerosol B_2 agonists and mucolytic drugs (such as acetylcysteine) may help to liquefy and mobilize retained secretions. Postural drainage also expedites this.
   f. Antibiotics should be used in patients with acute bronchitis or purulent sputum production prior to surgery. Elective procedures should be delayed until after treatment.
   g. Steroids should not be used routinely but should be used preoperatively only when absolutely necessary, because of their adverse effects on wound healing and response to infection.

h. Preoperative patient education on the methods of coughing and deep breathing, incentive spirometry, and other pulmonary therapy, as well as postoperative expectations, is important.

2. Postoperative management
   a. Extubation should be performed only after the patient is awake and has full respiratory muscle strength.
   (1) Parameters for extubation include:
      (a) Negative inspiratory force (NIF) $\geq$ 20 cm H_2O
      (b) Vital capacity (VC) $\geq$ 15 ml/kg body weight
      (c) TV $\geq$ 5 ml/kg body weight
      (d) Respiratory rate $\leq$ 30/minute
   (2) After extubation, respiratory sufficiency should be carefully observed and evaluated. Arterial blood gases should be measured, and chest x-ray should be performed, but a physical examination should be done first.
   b. Oxygen should be administered, if necessary, but should be given cautiously in patients with COPD. It should be heated and humidified.
   c. Early mobilization. Patients should be out of bed and upright as much as possible, as this simple maneuver improves FRC 10%–20%. This allows gravity to assist more in respiration and also helps to minimize secretion retention.
   d. Nasogastric tube. If an ileus is present, pulmonary aspiration of gastric contents should be prevented by the use of a nasogastric tube. Once gastric emptying is satisfactory, the nasogastric tube should be removed promptly to allow the patient to cough more effectively.
   e. Preoperative aminophylline should be continued through the postoperative period, particularly if the patient is undergoing abdominal surgery, as it has been shown to improve **diaphragmatic function** immediately postoperatively.
   f. Narcotics should be used judiciously to avoid oversedation and respiratory depression while still allowing adequate analgesia for effective coughing. **Epidural narcotics** may be useful in maintaining postoperative analgesia while minimizing sedation.
   g. Pneumothorax should always be suspected if sudden respiratory insufficiency occurs.

IV. CHRONIC RENAL DISEASE

A. Preoperative evaluation. Preoperative condition of patients with chronic renal disease is strongly dependent upon the residual **glomerular filtration rate (GFR)** and the presence of other major disease processes.

1. GFR 25% of normal. The kidney loses its ability to correct many different abnormalities.
   a. Fluid and electrolyte homeostasis is altered.
   (1) This results in:
      (a) Hypertension
      (b) Peripheral edema
      (c) Hyponatremia as a result of fluid retention
      (d) Salt retention
      (e) Metabolic acidosis as a result of failure to excrete organic acids, such as phosphates and sulfates
      (f) Hyperkalemia
   (2) Certain renal diseases, such as chronic pyelonephritis, medullary cystic disease and other interstitial disease, may result in salt wasting and subsequent dehydration.
   b. Nutritional status is impaired.
   (1) Proteinuria may be as high as 25 g/day.
   (2) Decreased body stores of nitrogen are catabolized more often as uremia progresses.
   (3) Decreased dietary intake may result from anorexia, nausea, malabsorption, or dietary restrictions placed by the physician.
   c. Metabolism or excretion of medications, especially many antibiotics and radiopaque iodinated angiographic dye, is impaired.
   d. Immune function is affected.
   (1) This results in:
      (a) Increased urinary tract infections as a result of oliguria

           (b) Impaired mucocutaneous barriers, which may be secondary to pruritus or epidermal atrophy

           (c) Increased pulmonary infections, which are related in part to decreased pulmonary clearance mechanisms

           (d) Increased incidence of malignancies

           (e) Impaired phagocytosis

        (2) The response to vaccines may be normal or mildly impaired.

        (3) The elimination of certain viruses, such as hepatitis B virus, is impaired. This is a major problem in dialysis patients because as many as 60% of patients become chronic antigen carriers once they contract the infection.

    e. Hematologic functions are altered.

        (1) Anemia occurs as the GFR drops and becomes profound as the GFR approaches zero.

        (2) Coagulation defects occur as a result of altered platelet adhesion and aggregation and abnormalities in the coagulation cascade, especially with a creatinine greater than 6 mg/dl (see Chapter 1 IV A).

    f. Cardiac and other vascular abnormalities develop, including:

        (1) Increased incidence of atherosclerosis

        (2) Pericarditis and pericardial effusions

    g. Altered calcium metabolism and parathyroid hormone metabolism result in secondary hyperparathyroidism and bone disease with hypocalcemia and hyperphosphatemia.

2. GFR less than 5% of normal. Dialysis is required for maintenance of bodily functions.

    a. Dialysis corrects or improves many of the uremic symptoms and abnormalities, such as fluid and electrolyte problems, hypertension, and nutritional problems related to dietary intake.

    b. Complications related to dialysis

        (1) **Peritoneal dialysis** is associated with an increased risk of peritonitis.

        (2) **Hemodialysis** requires systemic heparin levels that may worsen the coagulopathy of chronic renal failure. In addition, the vascular access necessary for dialysis is associated with blood-borne infections, especially staphylococcal infections.

3. Renal failure. Patients are susceptible to appendicitis, cholecystitis, diverticulitis, and peptic ulcer disease. In addition, they may require surgery for problems related specifically to their disease, such as vascular access procedures and urologic procedures.

B. Perioperative management

1. Residual renal function, which may be adversely affected by a surgical procedure, is best protected by the following maneuvers:

    a. Correction of overhydration or dehydration and any accompanying electrolyte disorder, either by medical management or by the use of dialysis

    b. Proper treatment of infections, especially urinary tract infections

    c. Avoidance of nephrotoxic drugs

2. Dialysis patients with no preservable renal function should be treated similarly.

    a. Nephrotoxic drugs may be used safely if blood levels are followed and if other side effects, such as ototoxicity, are monitored.

    b. Urinary bladder catheters should not be used in patients with no preservable renal function or with oliguria.

3. General medical preparation

    a. Anemia is well tolerated by patients with renal failure.

        (1) A hematocrit of 20%–25% (i.e., 7–8 g/dl) is adequate for most major surgical procedures.

        (2) Preoperative transfusions should be given during dialysis to minimize hyperkalemia.

    b. Routine dialysis should be undertaken 24 hours prior to elective surgery to minimize the effects of the intravenous heparin given with dialysis and to allow the patient to stabilize post-treatment. The following conditions should be addressed specifically:

        (1) **Hyperkalemia** must be treated expeditiously. A reading of the potassium level must be obtained immediately preceding surgery, and treatment must be instituted if the level is greater than 5.0 mEq/L. Exchange resins, such as sodium polystyrene sulfonate (Kayexalate) can control potassium levels and may be given as an enema, but dialysis may also be required.

      (2) Acidosis should be corrected by either bicarbonate administration or dialysis therapy.

      (3) Coagulopathy of chronic renal failure is best controlled preoperatively by adequate dialysis. Bleeding tendencies during or after surgery may also be controlled by the administration of cryoprecipitated plasma.

      (4) Pericarditis and pericardial effusion should be resolved prior to the administration of a general anesthetic because of impaired cardiac output and the risk of pericardial tamponade.

      (5) Uremic signs and symptoms, such as asterixis, hemorrhagic disorders, and seizures, should be treated with dialysis prior to surgery.

   c. Steroids should be given in the perioperative period to patients on long-term steroid therapy.

   d. Malnutrition

      (1) Elective surgery should be postponed for patients with malnutrition until the nutritional status improves.

      (2) In emergency surgery, the nutritional requirements should be supplied intravenously postoperatively until adequate oral intake is possible.

   e. Systemic disorders, such as diabetes mellitus or a thyroid disorder, should be controlled.

C. Operative management follows the same basic principles as those for any surgical patient. However, patients with uremia or gastrointestinal pathology require special consideration as patients with chronic renal disease have delayed healing of serosal surfaces and a higher anastomotic disruption rate.

   1. Fluid management must be closely monitored.

   2. Anesthesia. The altered metabolism and excretion in chronic renal disease must be taken into consideration when using anesthesia, particularly muscle relaxants, since prolonged drug action may lead to hyperkalemia and postoperative recurarization (recurrent paralysis) with catastrophic results.

   3. Maintenance of diuresis with osmotic or diuretic agents in patients with preservable renal function may protect against further renal insult.

D. Postoperative complications are commoner in patients with chronic renal disease. Overall mortality ranges from 0%–6% for major surgery.

   1. Hyperkalemia occurs in up to 38% of patients and is due to blood transfusions, operative trauma, hematomas, and the patient's catabolic state.

   2. Labile blood pressures, with hypertension or hypotension are common, and may be difficult to manage, given the fluid restrictions imposed by renal failure.

   3. Wound healing is impaired and results in complications in up to 40% of cases. Wound infections are very common (occurring in up to 33% of cases) when the gastrointestinal tract is opened.

   4. Postoperative hematomas in the operative site are common (occurring in up to 15% of cases) and frequently become secondarily infected.

   5. Gastrointestinal complications postoperatively are also common and may result in nausea, vomiting, anorexia, hiccups, or prolonged ileus. Upper gastrointestinal bleeding, esophagitis, and stomatitis may also occur.

   6. Shunt thrombosis may occur postoperatively, especially in the presence of hypotension.

   7. Postoperative dialysis

      a. Dialysis should be withheld for 24 hours postoperatively, if possible, as it requires the use of heparin, acutely lowers the platelet count, and causes transient hypotension and hypoxia during treatment.

      b. It should be performed **emergently** for the following:

         (1) Severe volume overload

         (2) Acidosis with the inability to give sodium bicarbonate secondary to volume overload

         (3) Hyperkalemia unresponsive to medications

         (4) Signs of uremia (i.e., pericarditis, mental status changes, or asterixis)

V. LIVER DISEASE. Hepatic insufficiency increases the risk of complications and death in the postoperative period. Recognition and management of liver disease preoperatively can minimize the postoperative problems.

A. Preoperative evaluation. Liver disease should be suspected, based on the history and physical examination.

1. History

a. Jaundice, pancreatitis, hepatitis, biliary stone disease, malignancy (e.g., gastrointestinal or breast cancer), or enzyme deficiencies (e.g., α_1-antitrypsin deficiency)

b. Hemolytic or parasitic disease

c. Drug or alcohol abuse

d. Upper gastrointestinal bleeding, delirium tremens, or encephalopathy

e. Possible contact with infectious hepatitis agents (e.g., via tattoos or blood transfusions)

f. Environmental or other exposure to hepatotoxins, particularly hepatotoxic anesthetic agents

2. Physical examination

a. Jaundice, ascites, peripheral edema, muscle wasting, testicular atrophy, palmar erythema, or gynecomastia

b. Evidence of portal hypertension, including caput medusae (dilated periumbilical vessels) or splenomegaly

c. Evidence of bleeding disorders, encephalopathy, asterixis, or spider angiomas

d. Hepatomegaly or a shrunken liver, especially with a rounded edge or with palpable nodules upon its surface; also, hepatic tenderness to percussion.

3. Laboratory tests may confirm the diagnosis but can be normal in some cases, even in the presence of moderate liver disease.

a. Most useful are the serum bilirubin, glutamic oxaloacetic and glutamic pyruvic transaminases (GOT and GPT), alkaline phosphatase, albumin, and prothrombin time.

b. Hepatitis B surface antigen should be sought if its presence is suspected, particularly since the hospital staff may be exposed.

4. Liver biopsy may be necessary preoperatively if an acute hepatitis, particularly acute alcoholic hepatitis, is suspected.

B. Operative risk factors and their management in patients with preexisting liver disease have not been fully defined, but several generalizations are useful.

1. Acute hepatitis. It is advisable to delay elective surgery in patients with acute hepatitis until the hepatitis is resolved.

a. Acute alcoholic hepatitis

(1) General anesthesia is associated with an operative mortality of 50% or more when portal decompressive surgery is performed.

(2) Abstinence from alcohol for 6–12 weeks to normalize bilirubin levels prior to elective surgery is recommended.

b. Acute drug-induced hepatitis. The results of studies have ranged from no increase in risk to as high as a 20% morbidity and mortality rate.

c. Acute viral hepatitis. It is recommended that elective surgery be deferred for more than 1 month or more after the acute illness.

2. Chronic liver failure from cirrhosis. Patients will tolerate most surgical procedures well if they are in a relatively compensated state preoperatively. The risk appears to be similar to that of patients undergoing portal decompressive procedures (see Child classification, Chapter 14 Table 14-1).

3. Obstructive jaundice is associated with postoperative renal failure, coagulation disorders, gastrointestinal hemorrhage, and delayed wound healing. It has been postulated that these complications may be the result of endotoxemia secondary to infection in the biliary tree. Management should include careful preoperative hydration, correction of coagulopathy, and attention to postoperative renal function.

4. Coagulopathy, especially if secondary to vitamin K deficiency or thrombocytopenia, should be corrected.

5. **Malnutrition**, with its attendant increased risks of infection and wound complications, should be improved by adequate nutrition and treatment of current infections.

6. **Narcotics and sedatives** that may precipitate hepatic encephalopathy must be avoided.

7. **Fluid and electrolyte balance.** Hypokalemia and alkalosis must be corrected.

8. **Anesthetics.** All inhalational anesthetics reduce hepatic blood flow to some extent. Isoflurane is associated with minimal hepatic metabolism and, therefore, may be the inhalational anesthetic of choice.

VI. DIABETES MELLITUS affects 2%–5% of the general population. As many as one-half of these patients have no symptoms until a stressful situation, such as sepsis or surgery, results in overt manifestations of hyperglycemia.

A. **Overview.** The diabetic patient frequently requires surgery for **complications of the diabetes** as well as for nondiabetic surgical problems.

1. **Age.** The diabetic patient is generally **older physiologically** than the chronologic age would suggest and, thus, should be treated as an older patient.

2. **Mortality rates**
   a. **The mortality rate for surgery** in diabetics is approximately 2%.
      (1) Close to 30% of deaths result from **cardiovascular complications**.
      (2) Close to 16% of deaths are related to **sepsis**, particularly from staphylococcal infections.
   b. **The mortality rate for emergency surgery** in diabetics is several times higher than that for elective procedures. For example, in diabetics, mortality for emergency cholecystectomy for acute cholecystitis is as high as 22%, as compared to a less than 1% mortality for elective cholecystectomy.

B. **Preoperative evaluation.** The patient history should emphasize the diabetes and its management, and the physical examination should include an assessment of the preoperative risk.

1. **History**
   a. The **type of diabetic control** used, **dosage schedule**, and the **adequacy of control** should be determined.
   b. The propensity to develop ketosis, ketoacidosis, and hyper- or hypoglycemia and a history of **"brittleness"** (unpredictable wide swings in blood glucose level) should be assessed.

2. **Physical examination.** Specific questions related to the **complications of diabetes**, such as nephropathy, neuropathy, peripheral vascular and coronary artery disease, and retinopathy, should be answered.
   a. **Retinopathy** is associated with nephropathy and diffuse microvasular disease.
   b. **Autonomic neuropathy** occurs as a result of diabetic degeneration of the autonomic nervous system. This may be manifested as:
      (1) Postural hypotension
      (2) Bladder emptying problems
      (3) Impaired intestinal motility
      (4) Gastroparesis
      (5) Impotence
      (6) Cardiac autonomic dysfunction
   c. **Somatic neuropathy,** with "stocking–glove" loss of sensation increases the risks of injury (of which the patient may not be aware) to an insensate foot.
   d. Patients with uncontrolled diabetes are prone to **infections**, and the presence of ongoing infection should be investigated.
   e. **Cardiovascular disease** and **hyperlipoproteinemias** may be present.

3. **Laboratory studies.** The patient's **fluid** and **electrolyte** status should be assessed, especially in relation to the acuteness of the disease requiring surgery and associated vomiting and diarrhea.

C. Preoperative management of the diabetic patient depends upon the severity of the diabetes and the severity of the acute disease.

    1. The serum glucose level should be monitored. If possible, glucose levels should be stable and less than **250 mg/dl**.

    2. The anion gap should be followed, and if it is elevated, arterial blood gases should be tested. The usual finding is low serum bicarbonate and a decreased pH. This may be due to:
        a. Diabetic ketoacidosis
        b. Lactic acidosis
        c. Retained organic acids containing phosphates and sulfates secondary to chronic renal disease

    3. Radiopaque dye studies performed on diabetics increase the risk of acute renal failure. This is especially true in patients over 40 years of age or with a creatinine level greater than 2 mg/dl.

D. Perioperative management

    1. Drug therapy
        a. Orally administered hypoglycemic agents should be discontinued on the day of surgery.
        b. Sulfonylurea drugs have a prolonged half-life (e.g., the half-life of chlorpropamide is 38 hours) and should be withheld at least 1 day prior to surgery.

    2. Insulin therapy is usually given in **one-half to two-thirds of the daily dose as NPH insulin** on the morning of surgery; an intravenous drip of glucose-containing solution should be administered to maintain glucose metabolism and prevent ketoacidosis.

E. Postoperative management. Intermittent doses of regular insulin titrated to frequently determined blood glucose levels until patients tolerate regular diets and resume their previous stable regimens comprises the postoperative diabetic management.

F. Emergency management

    1. Hyperglycemia. Diabetic patients with emergent surgical conditions, such as perforated viscus or acute cholecystitis, may develop extremely high glucose levels secondary to stress or ongoing infection. These patients require **correction of the acute disease process** before the diabetes can be completely controlled.

    2. Diabetic ketoacidosis. Patients with diabetic ketoacidosis are hyperglycemic, ketotic, and acidotic. They are also dehydrated with decreased body stores of potassium and sodium and may have Kussmaul's respirations (rapid deep breaths).
        a. There is a drop in serum sodium levels of 1.7 mEq/dl for each 100 mg/dl that the glucose is elevated.
        b. Massive free water deficits may occur secondarily to osmotic diuresis from glucosuria.
        c. Ketoacidosis is best corrected by administration of intravenous fluids, insulin, bicarbonate, and potassium.
        d. Surgery should be postponed until the ketoacidosis is at least partially resolved, as measured by improvement in pH, hydration, and correction of electrolye abnormalities and serum glucose levels.

    3. Hyperosmolar nonketotic states. The stress of surgery, infection, or the high glucose load of hyperalimentation may induce a nonketotic, hyperglycemic, hyperosmolar coma in patients with adult-onset diabetes.
        a. This condition is not associated with acidosis but is otherwise very similar to diabetic ketoacidosis.
        b. Management principles include intravenous fluids, insulin and potassium supplementation as necessary.

Part I Introduction

Directions: Each question below contains five suggested answers. Choose the **one best** response to each question.

1. A 70-kg, 60-year-old man with normal renal function underwent a vagotomy and hemigastrectomy for an obstructing duodenal ulcer. Intraoperative fluid losses were appropriately replaced, and he was considered normovolemic. On the first postoperative day, his nasogastric tube drained 5000 ml of bile-stained fluid. What volume of parenteral fluids should be ordered for this patient over the next 24 hours?

(A) 2500 ml

(B) 5000 ml

(C) 7500 ml

(D) 10,000 ml

(E) 12,000 ml

2. Which of the following statements best describes human nutrient requirements?

(A) The average healthy human requires approximately 1 g protein/kg body weight

(B) Approximately 1 g protein is equivalent to 6.25 g body nitrogen

(C) Most hospitalized patients require about 20 kcal/kg body weight/day

(D) Oleic acid is an essential fatty acid, which must be supplied enterally or parenterally

(E) If essential fatty acids are not given, essential fatty acid deficiency will develop within 5 days

3. Important components of collagen synthesis and wound strength and contraction include all of the following EXCEPT

(A) fibroblasts

(B) myofibroblasts

(C) vitamin C

(D) vitamin D

(E) arterial Po_2

4. The most important aspect in treating disseminated intravascular coagulation (DIC) is to

(A) administer heparin

(B) administer platelets

(C) treat the underlying disease process

(D) achieve normal levels of fibrinogen

(E) transfuse with fresh frozen plasma and cryoprecipitate

5. Citrate overload can complicate massive transfusion. Which of the following statements is true regarding citrate overload?

(A) Citrate binds calcium, and hypocalcemia has detrimental effects on myocardial function

(B) Citrate, as citric acid, results in profound metabolic acidosis

(C) Citrate is directly nephrotoxic

(D) Citrate overload causes seizures

(E) Citrate binds potassium, causing profound hypokalemia

6. All of the following components or qualities of stored whole blood tend to decrease over time EXCEPT

(A) red blood cell viability

(B) potassium concentration

(C) pH

(D) platelet activity

(E) oxygen-carrying capacity

7. In women, the leading cause of death by cancer is

(A) lung cancer

(B) uterine cancer

(C) cervical cancer

(D) breast cancer

(E) pancreatic cancer

8. Appropriate circumstances for the insertion of drains at the time of appendectomy surgery include which of the following?

(A) Unruptured appendicitis with cloudy fluid in the peritoneal space

(B) Ruptured appendicitis with diffuse bacterial peritonitis

(C) Uncomplicated appendicitis in a patient with hemophilia A

(D) Ruptured appendicitis with a localized abscess

(E) Gangrenous appendicitis without an abscess

9. Following active immunization with tetanus toxoid injection, how often should a tetanus toxoid booster be given?

(A) Every year
(B) Every 2 years
(C) Every 5 years
(D) Every 10 years
(E) Never

10. Which of the following statements best characterizes a cutaneous abscess?

(A) Hidradenitis suppurativa is an infection of the exocrine glands
(B) *Streptococcus* is the commonest infecting organism in an upper extremity furuncle
(C) Gram-negative cocci are the likely pathogens in an abscess in the inguinal area
(D) The most effective treatment for a cutaneous abscess is penicillin
(E) A carbuncle is a cutaneous abscess that burrows through the dermis into subcutaneous tissue

11. All of the following statements concerning intra-abdominal abscesses are correct EXCEPT

(A) a common cause is perforation of a hollow viscus
(B) treatment usually includes surgical exploration with drainage of the abscess
(C) a high index of suspicion is essential for the diagnosis because there may be no physical signs of infection
(D) ultrasonography, CT scan, or MRI can be used to direct surgical drainage
(E) these infections are usually due to staphylococcal organisms

12. All of the following statements characterize necrotizing fasciitis or its treatment EXCEPT

(A) surgical debridement is essential
(B) high doses of antibiotics are required for treatment
(C) adequate tetanus immunization prevents this infection
(D) the skin overlying the infection site often appears normal
(E) the organisms likely to be involved are staphylococci, microaerophilic streptococci, and gram-negative anaerobes

13. A hollow viscus forms part of the wall of the hernia sac in

(A) sliding hernia
(B) Richter's hernia
(C) incarcerated hernia
(D) direct inguinal hernia
(E) pantaloon hernia

14. The hernia most frequently seen in women is the

(A) femoral hernia
(B) indirect inguinal hernia
(C) epigastric hernia
(D) direct inguinal hernia
(E) pantaloon hernia

15. Which of the following studies is most helpful in evaluating a patient's risk for a routine operative procedure?

(A) History
(B) Physical examination
(C) Chest x-ray
(D) Electrocardiogram
(E) Liver function profile

16. Elective surgery is contraindicated in patients with

(A) serum creatinine levels above 2.5 mg/dl
(B) atrial fibrillation
(C) chronic obstructive lung disease with a P_{CO_2} of 45 mm Hg
(D) a history of a subendocardial myocardial infarction (4 weeks ago)
(E) a history of a stroke (6 months ago)

17. Alveolar hypoventilation in an overweight patient is caused principally by

(A) retention of carbon dioxide
(B) impaired chest wall expansion and contraction
(C) bronchospasm
(D) increased pulmonary dead space
(E) increased pulmonary arterial resistance

18. The quickest method to determine the effectiveness of pulmonary ventilation preoperatively and postoperatively is by

(A) arterial blood gas analysis
(B) serial spirometry
(C) pH determination
(D) chest x-ray
(E) pulmonary dead space

19. The commonest cause of pulmonary insufficiency in the early postoperative period following major abdominal surgery is

(A) aspiration of gastric contents
(B) bronchospasm
(C) atelectasis
(D) pneumothorax
(E) pulmonary edema

20. Patients with chronic renal failure are likely to present with all of the following clinical manifestations EXCEPT

(A) overhydration and overnourishment, resulting in an increased weight gain
(B) impaired immune function, resulting in an increased incidence of infection
(C) altered platelet function, resulting in an increased incidence of wound hematomas
(D) anemia with the ability to tolerate a hematocrit of 27%
(E) pericarditis, resulting in pericardial effusion

21. Postoperative dialysis should be performed emergently for all of the following conditions EXCEPT

(A) congestive heart failure secondary to volume overload
(B) uncorrectable acidosis
(C) hyperkalemia unresponsive to medication
(D) uremic pericarditis
(E) serum creatinine greater than 10 mg/dl

Directions: Each question below contains four suggested answers of which **one or more** is correct. Choose the answer

    A if **1, 2, and 3** are correct
    B if **1 and 3** are correct
    C if **2 and 4** are correct
    D if **4** is correct
    E if **1, 2, 3, and 4** are correct

22. A 45-year-old insulin-dependent, diabetic woman presents with a 3-day history of anorexia, nausea, and severe right upper quadrant pain. She has a history of postprandial colicky right upper quadrant pain dating back 10 years. On examination, she has a temperature of 101° F, right upper quadrant tenderness, and peritoneal signs. Other vital signs are all entirely normal. The patient is not orthostatic. Her admission serum electrolytes (in mEq/L) reveal the following: sodium, 130; potassium, 3.1; carbon dioxide, 15; chloride, 95; and blood glucose, 327. Correct statements regarding this woman's condition include which of the following?

(1) She has a metabolic acidosis
(2) She has diabetic ketoacidosis
(3) She has a high anion gap
(4) She requires immediate surgery

23. A 30-year-old man with severe hyperlipidemia presents with acute pancreatitis characterized by severe epigastric pain and three episodes of vomiting. The duration of symptoms prior to this visit to the emergency room is 6 hours. The patient is in shock with a blood pressure of 100 and a pulse of 120 supine. The important causes of this patient's shock include

(1) decreased extracellular fluid volume
(2) external losses of isotonic fluids secondary to vomiting
(3) third-space losses
(4) sepsis

24. A 45-year-old man undergoes a hemigastrectomy and Billroth II reconstruction for an antral gastric cancer. Postoperatively, for the first 3 days, the patient's nasogastric tube drained between 500–1000 ml of bile-tinged fluid daily. This fluid loss is replaced with the appropriate volume of 5% dextrose in ¼ normal saline with 20 mEq/L potassium chloride (KCl). Maintenance fluids during this time were given as 5% dextrose in ¼ normal saline with 10 mEq/L KCl. On the third postoperative day, the patient has a seizure, and his electrolytes are (in mEq/L): sodium, 118; potassium, 3.3; carbon dioxide, 22; and chloride, 95. Correct statements regarding this man's condition include which of the following?

(1) The patient has had inadequate replacement of sodium
(2) The patient has a profound metabolic alkalosis from extensive nasogastric drainage
(3) The primary problem is hypochloremia
(4) The total body sodium is normal

25. Replacement of electrolyte deficits are determined by calculating the deficit in mEq and multiplying that by the electrolyte distribution in the body. True statements regarding electrolyte distribution include which of the following?

(1) Bicarbonate distribution equals 50% of body weight
(2) Chloride distribution equals 20% of body weight
(3) Sodium distribution equals 60% of body weight
(4) Potassium distribution equals 40% of body weight

SUMMARY OF DIRECTIONS

A	B	C	D	E
1, 2, 3 only	1, 3 only	2, 4 only	4 only	All are correct

---

26. Common metabolic complications of total parenteral nutrition include which of the following?

(1) Nonketotic hyperosmolar coma
(2) Hypoglycemia
(3) Metabolic acidosis
(4) Azotemia

27. Protein intake should be reduced in patients with which of the following conditions?

(1) Uremia
(2) Sepsis
(3) Hepatic encephalopathy
(4) Multiple long bone fractures

28. Recommended nutrients for long-term parenteral nutrition include which of the following?

(1) Fat solution
(2) Amino acids
(3) Magnesium
(4) Plasma proteins

29. Correct statements concerning lactated Ringer's solution include which of the following?

(1) It can correct body water deficits in isotonic dehydration
(2) It is isotonic with extracellular fluid
(3) It contains 130 mEq sodium/L solution
(4) It contains 2.5 g albumin/dl solution

30. The rate of wound healing may be influenced by multiple factors, including

(1) malnutrition
(2) previous radiation treatment
(3) vascularity
(4) aspirin

31. Correct statements concerning hypertrophic scar formation include which of the following?

(1) Most of these scars have completed remodeling by 3 months
(2) These scars are commoner in black and Oriental patients than in white patients
(3) Treatment is by early excision and injection of bupivacaine, a long-acting local anesthetic
(4) Histologically, these scars appear as large, swollen, eosinophilic collagen bundles

32. Causes of vitamin K deficiency include

(1) malnutrition
(2) total parenteral nutrition
(3) obstructive jaundice
(4) antibiotic therapy

33. Many postoperative problems can be anticipated, provided that the physician knows that

(1) urinary tract infections frequently cause fever on postoperative days 3 through 6
(2) wound infections frequently cause fever on postoperative days 5 through 8
(3) pulmonary complications are the commonest cause of fever in the first few postoperative days
(4) the body accumulates third-space fluid for the first 4 postoperative days, making fluid supplementation necessary

34. Correct statements regarding infections of prosthetic devices include which of the following?

(1) Because the prosthesis is insensate, it is frequently asymptomatic
(2) Prophylactic antibiotics are always used when implanting a prothesis
(3) Proper treatment of an infected prothesis is high-dose antibiotics to sterilize the prothesis, and if that is ineffective, then surgery is an option
(4) Prosthetic infections are life-threatening

35. Clinical manifestations of gas gangrene include

(1) confusion
(2) mildly increased leukocyte count
(3) foul odor of the wound
(4) onset 48 hours after injury

36. One week after a venous cutdown on the saphenous vein at the ankle, a patient develops fever, chills, and a red streak over the saphenous vein, beginning at the site of the intravenous catheter. Pus can be expressed from the venous cutdown site. Proper management of this patient's infection includes

(1) removal of the intravenous catheter
(2) excision of the involved segment of the saphenous vein
(3) intravenous administration of antibiotics after culturing and Gram-staining the pus
(4) intravenous administration of heparin to prevent venous thrombosis

37. Gastrointestinal fistulas may develop as a result of

(1) penetrating abdominal trauma
(2) congenital anomaly
(3) inflammation
(4) malignancy

38. A patient who has undergone surgical repair of a pyloric ulcer has developed an enterocutaneous fistula that is draining 300 ml of succus entericus daily. Management of this patient should include

(1) contrast radiography of the gut
(2) prompt operative repair of the fistula
(3) control of external drainage
(4) increase in the oral fluid and nutrient intake

39. Persistent patent processus vaginalis may result in

(1) a femoral hernia
(2) an indirect inguinal hernia
(3) a direct inguinal hernia
(4) a spermatic cord hydrocele

40. Proper repair of an adult indirect inguinal hernia applies which of the following principles?

(1) The abdominal wall defect is repaired
(2) The external oblique aponeurosis contributes significantly to the strength of the repair
(3) The hernia sac is ligated at its base
(4) The spermatic cord is placed deep to the transversalis fascia to eliminate the internal ring

41. Correct statements concerning cigarette smoking include which of the following?

(1) It is probably the commonest cause of preventable chronic lung disease
(2) It directly affects respiratory epithelium and cilia
(3) A history of 20 pack-years is associated with increased operative risk
(4) It can be stopped 2 weeks prior to elective surgery to reduce the operative risk

42. General endotracheal anesthesia results in which of the following alterations in pulmonary function?

(1) Impaired ciliary function
(2) Respiratory alkalosis
(3) Altered chest wall mechanical properties
(4) Increased functional residual capacity

43. Which of the following medications can reduce postoperative pulmonary complications?

(1) Aminophylline
(2) Ampicillin
(3) Prednisone
(4) Terbutaline

44. Patients with chronic liver disease and acute alcoholic hepatitis undergoing surgery can develop which of the following difficulties?

(1) Lethargy and hepatic coma due to regular doses of narcotics
(2) Acute liver failure and death
(3) Coagulopathy due to thrombocytopenia or impaired absorption of vitamin K
(4) Postoperative delirium tremens

45. A 65-year-old woman with known insulin-dependent diabetes presents in the emergency room in diabetic ketoacidosis and free air on abdominal x-rays. Her management should include

(1) intravenous fluid resuscitation
(2) potassium replacement
(3) broad-spectrum intravenous antibiotics
(4) exploratory laparotomy once her diabetes is well controlled

ANSWERS AND EXPLANATIONS

1. The answer is C. [*Chapter 1 I F 1 a–d, G 1 b (1), 2*] In a patient who is normovolemic, the first priority of fluid therapy is volume-for-volume replacement. Since the patient described in the question lost 5000 ml of fluid through nasogastric drainage, then 5000 ml of water and electrolyte therapy is necessary to replace this loss. The second priority is maintenance therapy—that is, administration of the fluid and electrolytes necessary to satisfy normal requirements; normal daily requirements are calculated according to weight. In this case, the patient will require 2500 ml of fluids for maintenance. Thus, the total fluid requirement for a 24-hour period is 7500 ml.

2. The answer is A. [*Chapter 1 II C 1, 2*] Protein requirement for a normal, healthy adult is 1 g/kg/day. Stressed, hospitalized patients may require up to 1.5 g/kg/day. A total of 6.25 g protein contain 1 g body nitrogen. Basal caloric needs for nonstressed adults are 25–35 kcal/kg/day, and this increases to 35–45 kcal/kg/day for stressed, hospitalized patients. Linoleic, linolenic, and arachidonic acids are the essential fatty acids. Absence of intake of essential fatty acids will cause symptoms of essential fatty acid deficiency but only after a prolonged period of time (generally longer than 4 weeks).

3. The answer is D. [*Chapter 1 III A 1, 3*] Collagen, which is formed by fibroblasts, is responsible for binding tissues together and ultimately is a major determinant of wound strength. Proline, hydroxyproline, and glycine are very important in collagen synthesis as are adequate tissue oxygen, ferrous iron, α-ketoglutarate, and ascorbic acid. Myofibroblasts are responsible for wound contraction, which occurs in a wound and helps it to close by decreasing its surface area.

4. The answer is C. [*Chapter 1 IV C 3 b (1)*] Disseminated intravascular coagulation (DIC) results from the simultaneous activation of the coagulation and fibrinolytic systems as a consequence of a severe underlying disorder, such as sepsis, malignancy, trauma, shock, or serious obstetric complications. Platelets and clotting factors are consumed, and fibrin split products are released. Clinically, there is widespread hemorrhage. The consumptive coagulopathy of DIC cannot be interrupted until the underlying pathologic process that precipitated the disorder has been controlled. Until this is accomplished, administration of platelets, fresh frozen plasma, and cryoprecipitate are helpful adjuncts. Heparin administration, although advocated by some, probably is inadvisable in the profusely bleeding patient with DIC.

5. The answer is A. [*Chapter 1 V A 1, C 3 d (3)*] Citrate is the commonest anticoagulant used in blood storage solutions. Its anticoagulant properties are due to its abilities to bind calcium, an essential component of the coagulation cascade. In citrate overload, citrate binds ionized calcium, resulting in hypocalcemia. This has profound effects on myocardial function and the clotting cascade. Citrate is given as the salt, not the acid, and does not cause metabolic acidosis. Citrate is not directly nephrotoxic, nor does it cause seizures. Citrate does not bind potassium.

6. The answer is B. [*Chapter 1 V A 1, 2*] There is a progressive increase in the potassium concentration of stored blood, which may reach 30 mEq/L after 3–4 weeks. This is an important consideration when massive transfusions are required and in patients with renal disease. Red blood cells gradually lose their ability to survive. For example, if blood is transfused after storage for 28 days, only 25% of the red cells will be viable 60 days after the transfusion. Oxygen transport is also reduced because of a decrease in cellular 2,3-diphosphoglycerate. The pH of stored blood gradually decreases, reaching about 6.7 after 4 weeks of storage. Platelets become inactive after only 24 hours of storage.

7. The answer is A. [*Chapter 1 VI B 2*] Lung cancer has passed breast cancer to become the commonest cause of death from cancer in women. It has long been the commonest cause of death from cancer in men. Increased smoking by women is suspected as the cause of this increase.

8. The answer is D. [*Chapter 2 I A 2 d*] Drains are necessary where a deep abscess cavity exists, as with a periappendiceal abscess. Drains are not appropriate where diffuse peritonitis exists or where postoperative bleeding in the large peritoneal space is anticipated.

9. The answer is D. [*Chapter 2 II A 5 a*] Active immunization results when tetanus toxoid injections are given on the recommended schedule, usually in infancy (with DPT shots) or during military induction. A follow-up booster every 10 years is recommended by the American College of Surgeons. However, any person with a penetrating injury must receive tetanus prophylaxis if previous immunization cannot be documented or if more than 5 years have passed since the last immunization.

10. The answer is E. [*Chapter 2 II B 2 a–c*] Cutaneous abscesses are of three types: furuncles, carbuncles, and hidradenitis suppurativa. Furuncles are cutaneous staphylococcal abscesses that are frequently seen with acne. Carbuncles are cutaneous abscesses that spread through the dermis into the subcutaneous region. Hidradenitis suppurativa is an infection involving the apocrine sweat glands. Staphylococci are the most likely causative organisms.

11. The answer is E. [*Chapter 2 II B 3 a, d, e*] Intra-abdominal abscesses can result from penetrating trauma, surgical procedures, perforation of a hollow viscus, seeding of bacteria from outside the abdomen, or ischemia and infarction of tissue within the abdomen. Although abscesses in the abdominal region produce the signs and symptoms of any abscess—fever, pain, and leukocytosis—a high index of suspicion is essential as there may be no physical signs of infection. The mainstay of treatment is surgical intervention with drainage and debridement of the abscess. Ultrasonography, CT scan, and MRI are useful in localizing the abscess and guiding the drainage procedure. The usual flora are enteric—aerobic and anaerobic.

12. The answer is C. [*Chapter 2 II D 1–3*] Necrotizing fasciitis is a rapidly progressive bacterial infection in which several different organisms—staphylococci, microaerophilic streptococci, and gram-negative anaerobes—invade the fascial planes. The infection results in necrosis of the tissue involved; however, the overlying skin may appear normal, leading the physician to underestimate the severity of the infection. On the other hand, the patient with necrotizing fasciitis often is critically ill with a high fever, leukocytosis, and severe pain in the affected area. Treatment is largely surgical: It is critical to remove all infected or devitalized tissue at the first debridement so that the rapidly progressive necrosis does not continue. Daily debridement may be needed, and antibiotics in high doses are required. This is not a clostridial infection, and tetanus immunization against the toxin produced by *C. tetani* is not protective.

13. The answer is B. [*Chapter 2 V A 3 g, h, B 2 b, c*] Hernias may be described according to physical or operative findings. In a sliding hernia, the wall of the hernia sac, rather than being formed completely by peritoneum, is formed by the wall of another intra-abdominal structure, such as the colon or the bladder. In a Richter's hernia, one side of the bowel wall is trapped in the hernia rather than the entire loop of bowel. In incarcerated hernia, the contents of the hernia sac are trapped within the sac. A direct inguinal hernia is a protrusion of abdominal structures directly through the floor of the canal behind the spermatic cord. A pantaloon hernia is a combination of a direct and indirect hernia in which the hernia sac passes around the inferior epigastric vessels both medially and laterally.

14. The answer is B. [*Chapter 2 V B 2 a (3) (a)*] Although indirect inguinal hernias are five to ten times commoner in men than in women, they are still the commonest type of hernias seen in women. They may occur from infancy to old age but generally occur by the fifth decade of life. An indirect inguinal hernia passes through the internal inguinal ring and down the inguinal canal. It occurs as a result of a congenitally patent processus vaginalis, which allows free communication between the peritoneal cavity and inguinal canal.

15. The answer is A. [*Chapter 3 I B*] The history is the most helpful study in evaluating a patient's operative risk because it gives a complete profile of the patient and how he or she has reacted to stress and to other adverse conditions in the past. A history of familial disorders, prior illnesses, prior difficulties with surgical procedures or anesthetics, the presence of allergies or asthma, and the effects of medications, including over-the-counter products, should be included. Physical examination, chest x-ray, electrocardiogram, and a liver function profile are useful, but an alert physician will suspect problems from the history alone.

16. The answer is D. [*Chapter 3 II B 2 c*] A myocardial infarction within 3–6 months of surgery carries a much higher operative mortality due to the risk of perioperative recurrence. Perioperative myocardial infarctions occur in the first postoperative week and have a mortality as high as 50%. There is little difference in the risk of recurrence between a subendocardial and a transmural myocardial infarction. Emergency procedures that cannot be avoided require careful operative management.

17. The answer is B. [*Chapter 3 III C 1 g*] Because obesity markedly increases the work of respiration and impairs the bellows function of the chest wall, the obese surgical patient is at increased risk for respiratory failure postanesthesia as a result of alveolar hypoventilation. As a result of the failure to move enough air in and out of the lungs, carbon dioxide retention and inadequate oxygenation of blood occur. Brochospasm and increased pulmonary dead space and pulmonary resistance have no particular association with obesity.

18. The answer is A. [*Chapter 3 III A 4*] Arterial blood gas analysis is the fastest and simplest method to determine effective ventilation. If the Po_2 is low, there is inadequate alveolar gas exchange. If the Pco_2 is high in the absence of primary metabolic alkalosis, then there is CO_2 retention and inadequate ventilation. In the presence of a low Pco_2 without a primary metabolic acidosis, there is hyperventilation.

19. The answer is C. [*Chapter 3 III D 1*] The commonest complication in the postoperative period after abdominal surgery is atelectasis (i.e., alveolar and segmental collapse), which causes fever and can lead to pulmonary insufficiency. Aspiration of gastric contents, pulmonary embolism, bronchospasm, pneumothorax, and pulmonary edema are significant, albeit less common, pulmonary complications of the postoperative course and, thus, should be suspected and excluded.

20. The answer is A. [*Chapter 3 IV A 1 b (3), d, e, f (2), B 3 a*] Although patients with chronic renal disease are often overhydrated and as a result overweight, the weight gain is due to peripheral edema, not to an increased food intake. Patients with renal failure have decreased body stores of protein, which is catabolized more as uremia progresses. There is usually decreased dietary intake as a result of anorexia, nausea, malabsorption, or perhaps dietary restriction by the physician. Immune function is affected, resulting in more infections; hematologic functions are impaired, resulting in anemia and altered platelet adhesion and aggregation, and cardiac and vascular abnormalities develop, including pericarditis and atherosclerosis.

21. The answer is E. [*Chapter 3 IV D 7 b*] Postoperative dialysis should be performed emergently to treat the following conditions: hyperkalemia unresponsive to exchange resins, uncorrectable acidosis because sodium bicarbonate is contraindicated secondary to volume overload, signs of uremia (i.e., pericarditis), and congestive heart failure secondary to volume overload. The decision to perform emergent dialysis would not ever be based solely on serum creatinine levels. Dialysis should be postponed for 24 hours postoperatively, if possible, as it requires the use of heparin, acutely lowers the platelet count, and can cause transient hypotension and hypoxia during treatment.

22. The answer is A (1, 2, 3). [*Chapter 1 I B 3*] Insulin-dependent diabetics who develop infectious problems are notoriously susceptible to ketoacidosis. Thus, the patient described in the question has diabetic ketoacidosis with a modestly elevated blood sugar of 327 mg/dl. There is a metabolic acidosis as noted by the decreased serum carbon dioxide of 15 mEq/L (normal: 20–24 mEq/L). The anion gap measures $130 - (15 + 95) = 20$, which is high (normal is less than 15). Note that diabetic ketoacidosis is frequently accompanied by hypokalemia. This patient does require surgery for acute cholecystitis but not immediately. Correction of fluid deficits, acidosis, and hyperglycemia takes priority. After these are corrected, the patient should undergo surgery expeditiously.

23. The answer is B (1, 3). [*Chapter 1 I C 2 a (3)*] Acute pancreatitis is similar to a chemical burn of the retroperitoneum and peritoneal space, which results in a massive "third-space loss" of isotonic fluid into the retroperitoneal and intraperitoneal spaces. This causes a decrease in circulating volume and in extracellular fluid volume, which can culminate in shock. The patient has vomited three times within 6 hours, which does not represent a large enough volume loss to account for his shock. Sepsis can be a very late complication of pancreatitis, appearing several days after the initial onset, but it would not account for shock at the time of presentation with such a short duration of symptoms.

24. The answer is D (4). [*Chapter 1 I C 2 e, 3 b*] Postoperative dilutional hyponatremia is a common occurrence when fluid deficits are replaced with hyponatremic solutions. High antidiuretic hormone levels postoperatively lead to retention of free water and dilutional hyponatremia. When this becomes severe, seizures can result. The patient's sodium replacement is probably appropriate. The patient's serum carbon dioxide (bicarbonate) is normal, and he does not have a metabolic alkalosis. The patient's chloride is slightly decreased, which is also dilutional.

25. The answer is A (1, 2, 3). [*Chapter 1 I E 2*] Potassium (K^+) is primarily an intracellular cation, and its deficit cannot be determined in the method described in the question as the serum electrolyte determination does not reflect intracellular events accurately. For K^+, a concentration between normal and 3 mEq/L is equivalent to a body deficit of 100–200 mEq. For each mEq below 3 mEq/L, another 300–400 mEq of deficit is allotted.

26. The answer is A (1, 2, 3). [*Chapter 1 II F 3 d (2)*] Metabolic complications are common with total parenteral nutrition and require close monitoring of the patient's physical examination and blood chemistries, particularly after the initiation of therapy. Hyperosmolar nonketotic hyperglycemia, which results in coma, occurs from excessive glucose administration above the body's ability to handle it. Hypoglycemia can occur if the infusion of hypertonic glucose is suddenly stopped. Metabolic acidosis occurs when excess chloride relative to acetate (the form in which bicarbonate is given) is administered as the anion. Azotemia due to dehydration or the excessive administration of amino acids is not a common occurrence with total parenteral nutrition.

27. The answer is B (1, 3). [*Chapter 1 II C 2*] Patients with impaired ability to excrete or tolerate the nitrogenous wastes of amino acid metabolism, particularly those with uremia and hepatic encephalopathy, do not tolerate intravenous protein administration well and should receive a reduced amount of amino acids. Patients with sepsis and multiple injuries are often highly catabolic and require increased amounts of calories and protein.

28. The answer is A (1, 2, 3). [*Chapter 1 II F 3 a, b; Table 1-6*] Parenteral nutrition can be used to provide all or part of a patient's nutrients for an indefinite period of time. Because it completely bypasses the gastrointestinal tract, parenteral nutrition is useful for patients who lack intestinal function. Parenteral nutrient solutions should include a fat solution as a source of calories and to prevent essential fatty acid deficiency; amino acids as a protein source; and a variety of minerals, including magnesium. Plasma proteins, on the other hand, are not considered nutrients.

29. The answer is B (1, 3). [*Chapter 1 Table 1-5*] Lactated Ringer's solution is a balanced electrolyte solution that contains 274 mOsm/L. It is slightly hypo-osmolar to extracellular body fluid, which contains about 310 mOsm/L. However, lactated Ringer's solution is an excellent fluid for correction of isosmolar body water deficits. The solution contains 130 mEq sodium, 4 mEq potassium, and 3 mEq calcium/L with 109 mEq chloride and 28 mEq bicarbonate/L. It is a crystalloid solution and contains no albumin. It can also be used as a replacement solution for some gastrointestinal losses because of their similar electrolyte compositions.

30. The answer is A (1, 2, 3). [*Chapter 1 III D 1–5*] Wound healing may be influenced by a variety of factors. Young patients heal more rapidly than old patients, and malnutrition can impede wound healing even though the biologic needs of wounds take priority over those of the organ systems. Highly vascular regions, such as the face, heal more rapidly than regions of poor vascularity, such as the pretibial area. Aspirin irreversibly inhibits platelet function but has no direct effect on wound healing.

31. The answer is C (2, 4). [*Chapter 1 III F 1*] Most scars continue to remodel for more than 1 year. Hypertrophic scars, which result from wounds that heal with excessive collagen synthesis, are unsightly and have a raised surface. They occur most commonly in black, Oriental, and dark-skinned white patients, and in relatively young patients. An ordinary hypertrophic scar lies entirely within the confines of the wound, but a keloid invades nearby normal tissue that was not previously involved in the wound. Histologically, these scars are large, swollen, eosinophilic collagen bundles. The treatment of these scars is very difficult as excision often results in recurrence. Thus, any excision is done late, allowing maximal time for the scar to remodel and regress. As part of treatment, steroids are frequently injected into the scar and surrounding tissues.

32. The answer is E (all). [*Chapter 1 IV C 3 b (2)*] Vitamin K, a fat-soluble vitamin, is acquired both from diet and as a product of metabolism of the gastrointestinal bacterial flora. Malnutrition and total parenteral nutrition without vitamin K supplements will lead to deficiency. Obstructive jaundice will block the passage of bile salts to the gut; these are necessary for the absorption of fat-soluble vitamin K. Antibiotic therapy can alter the normal flora of the gut, resulting in a deficiency. Thus, a deficiency of vitamin K is common in surgical patients for all of the above reasons.

33. The answer is A (1, 2, 3). [*Chapter 2 II A 2 b; III A 1–5*] Common postoperative problems typically occur on certain postoperative days. Urinary tract infection, triggered by an indwelling catheter or preexisting vesical outlet obstruction, is the typical cause of fever that develops on postoperative days 3 through 6. Wound infection often presents as a spiking fever on postoperative days 5 through 8. Pulmonary complications, the commonest cause of fever in the first few postoperative days, develop as a result of prolonged mechanical ventilation or because of inadequate ventilation and a poor cough effort. Dehydration is common after surgery because of third-space sequestration of fluids in the operative site; however, by the third or fourth postoperative day, the body begins to mobilize third-space fluid, making fluid restriction or diuresis necessary.

34. The answer is C (2, 4). [*Chapter 2 II A 3*] Due to the risks of prosthetic infection, prophylactic antibiotics are mandatory when implanting a prosthetic device. Although the prosthesis itself is insensate, the surrounding tissues are not, and these infections come to medical attention quickly. Infected prostheses cannot generally be sterilized with antibiotics, and removal of the prosthesis is almost always required. Because prostheses are frequently placed in direct contact with the blood and because resulting infections are difficult to eradicate, prosthetic infections are considered life-threatening.

35. The answer is E (all). [*Chapter 2 II E 1, 2*] Gas gangrene is caused by *Clostridium perfringens*. Wounds that are susceptible include those with extensive tissue destruction, marked impairment of blood supply, or gross contamination, particularly when surgical wound treatment has been delayed or debridement inadequate. The onset of symptoms is usually 48 hours after injury. The commonest complaint is severe pain at the site of injury. The skin may appear normal, but the wound usually drains a serous fluid with a brownish color and a foul odor. The white blood cell count may be mildly elevated, and the patient may become confused or delirious.

36. The answer is A (1, 2, 3). [*Chapter 2 II G 1*] The patient described in the question has the classic signs and symptoms of suppurative thrombophlebitis. Proper management of this infection includes removal of the intravenous catheter, excision and drainage of the infected vein site, and administration of appropriate antibiotics.

37. The answer is E (all). [*Chapter 2 IV B 1–5*] The causes of gastrointestinal fistulas are many. Fistula-forming abdominal trauma may be accidental or an inadvertent surgical injury (e.g., a gastrocutaneous fistula after splenectomy). The most important fistulous congenital anomaly is a distal tracheoesophageal fistula with esophageal atresia. Crohn's disease is an inflammatory bowel disease that usually affects the ileum; a fistula connecting the ileum to another site is a common complication. Fistulas can develop because of the destruction of organs by tumors; for example, a colovesical fistula may occur in a patient with a large sigmoid colon cancer.

38. The answer is B (1, 3). [*Chapter 2 IV D 2, E 3*] Radiography with contrast medium given either by mouth, rectum, or fistula, is important in defining the location and dimensions of the fistula. The use of suction catheters or various bags as collection devices to control the drainage from fistulas is important to prevent skin excoriation and further morbidity. Prompt operative intervention to repair the fistula is usually not indicated, although early surgery to drain an abscess may be necessary. With the availability of long-term parenteral nutrition, the intravenous route is usually preferred for fluid and nutritional maintenance in patients with high-output fistulas. With the proximal fistula described above, increased oral intake will likely increase the fistula output and make dehydration and malnutrition worse, not better.

39. The answer is C (2, 4). [*Chapter 2 V B 1 d (5), 2 a (2)*] The processus vaginalis is an evagination of peritoneum that accompanies the descent of the testicle and gubernaculum through the abdominal wall. Normally obliterated, it remains patent in an indirect hernia and forms the hernia sac. Thus, a patent or incompletely obliterated processus vaginalis allows communication between the peritoneal cavity and the scrotum, resulting in an indirect inguinal hernia or a spermatic cord hydrocele.

40. The answer is B (1, 3). [*Chapter 2 V B 4 a, b*] Operative repair of inguinal hernias includes a return of the hernia contents into the peritoneal cavity, ligation of the base of the hernia sac, and repair of the abdominal wall defect to prevent recurrence (about 3% recur). To repair the abdominal wall defect, the transversalis fascia and conjoint tendon are sutured to either the inguinal ligament or Cooper's ligament, which is responsible for the strength of the repair. The spermatic cord is returned to its normal anatomic location within the inguinal canal in almost all repairs.

41. The answer is A (1, 2, 3). [*Chapter 3 III A 1, C 1 b, E 1 a*] Cigarette smoking is the commonest cause of chronic lung disease. It is toxic to respiratory epithelium and cilia and results in impaired mucus transport with consequent impaired resistance to infection. A history of 20 pack-years or more than 20 cigarettes a day increases the risk of postoperative pulmonary complications. Cessation of smoking at least 8 weeks prior to elective surgery is associated with a decreased incidence of pulmonary complications.

42. The answer is B (1, 3). [*Chapter 3 III C 2 d (1)*] Both the anesthetic and the technique employed in its use can have adverse effects on postoperative function. Anesthesia markedly interferes with the normal clearing mechanisms of the tracheobronchial tree by impairing ciliary action, mucus function, cough reflexes, sighs, and other reflex actions. The chest wall dynamics are altered due to muscle relaxation and impaired diaphragmatic excursion, and the risk of pneumothorax is increased by positive pressure ventilation. Anesthesia may decrease functional residual capacity, resulting in hypoxemia.

43. The answer is E (all). [*Chapter 3 III E 1 a–h*] Bronchodilators, such as aminophylline or terbutaline, may improve pulmonary function in patients with asthma or chronic obstructive pulmonary disease. Antibiotics, such as ampicillin, should be used in patients with acute bronchitis or purulent sputum production prior to surgery; elective surgery should be delayed until after treatment. Steroids may improve pulmonary function for patients with bronchospasm, but should be given cautiously because they have adverse effects on wound healing and response to infection.

44. The answer is E (all). [*Chapter 3 V B 1–8*] Management of surgical patients with preexisting liver disease and alcoholic hepatitis has not been fully defined, but several important generalizations should be considered. It is advisable to delay elective surgery in patients with acute alcoholic hepatitis until the hepatitis has resolved, as use of a general anesthetic in these patients is associated with an operative mortality rate of 50% or more. Coagulopathy, especially if due to a vitamin K deficiency or thrombocytopenia, should be corrected with transfusion of blood products. Any central nervous system depressant should be avoided in patients with liver failure as it may precipitate hepatic encephalopathy. Postoperative delirium tremens from alcohol withdrawal has a very high mortality.

45. The answer is A (1, 2, 3). [*Chapter 3 I D 3; VI B 2 a (4), F 2*] Initial management of a patient presenting with a surgical abdomen and diabetic ketoacidosis includes intravenous fluid resuscitation, electrolyte replacement, intravenous antibiotics, and surgical exploration to correct the cause of the exacerbated diabetes. Surgery should be undertaken as soon as the patient is stabilized as the mortality increases with delay and the diabetes cannot be well-controlled in the presence of severe infections.

Part II
Thoracic Disorders

4

Principles of
Thoracic Surgery

D. Bruce Panasuk
Richard N. Edie

I. GENERAL PRINCIPLES OF THORACIC SURGERY

A. Anatomy of the thoracic cavity

1. **The chest wall** (Figure 4-1) is formed by the sternum, ribs, vertebral column, intercostal muscles, vessels (which run on the undersurface of the ribs), and nerves. Its inferior border is the diaphragm. It is lined internally by the parietal pleura.

2. **The mediastinum** (Figure 4-2) forms the compartment between the pleural cavities for the length of the thorax.
   a. **Superior mediastinum.** Superiorly, the fascial planes communicate with the neck, thus allowing neck infection to extend into the mediastinum.
   b. **The anterior mediastinum** comprises the thymus gland, lymph nodes, ascending and transverse aorta, and great veins. It is bordered anteriorly by the sternum, posteriorly by the upper dorsal spine, and inferiorly by the anterior border of the heart.
   c. **The middle mediastinum** comprises the pericardium, heart, trachea, hilar structures of the lung, phrenic nerves, and lymph nodes. It is bordered superiorly by the anterior border of the heart, inferiorly by the diaphragmatic surface, and posteriorly by the anterior border of the dorsal spine.
   d. **The posterior mediastinum** comprises the sympathetic chains, vagus nerves, esophagus, and descending thoracic aorta.

3. **Lungs and tracheobronchial tree** (Figure 4-3)
   a. **The right lung** has three lobes—the upper, middle, and lower—separated by two **fissures**.
      (1) The **major (oblique) fissure** separates the lower lobe from the upper and middle lobes.
      (2) The **minor (horizontal) fissure** separates the upper lobe from the middle lobe.
   b. **The left lung** has two lobes—the upper and the lower. The **lingula** is a portion of the upper lobe. The lobes are separated by a **single oblique fissure**.
   c. **Bronchopulmonary segments** are intact sections of each lobe that have a separate blood supply, allowing segmental resection. There are 10 bronchopulmonary segments on the right and 8 broncopulmonary segments on the left.
   d. **The tracheobronchial tree** (see Chapter 5 IX A) is formed from respiratory epithelium with reinforcing cartilaginous rings; the branching **bronchial tubes** are progressively smaller, down to a diameter of 1–2 mm.
   e. **The blood supply** is dual.
      (1) **Pulmonary artery** blood is **unoxygenated**.
      (2) **Bronchial artery** blood is **oxygenated**.
   f. **Lymphatic vessels** are present throughout the parenchyma and toward the hilar areas of the lungs.
      (1) Lymphatic flow in the pleural space is from parietal pleura to visceral pleura.
      (2) Lymphatic drainage within the mediastinum is cephalad, flowing toward the scalene nodal areas along the paratracheal areas.
      (3) Generally, lymphatic drainage affects ipsilateral nodes, but contralateral flow often occurs from the left lower lobe.

B. General thoracic procedures

1. **Radiologic diagnostic procedures.** The standard procedures are **chest x-ray** and **tomography** of a lesion. **Computed tomography (CT scan)** has been shown to be extremely useful

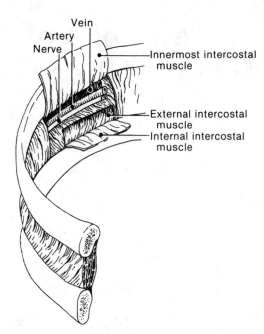

Vein
Artery
Nerve
Innermost intercostal muscle
External intercostal muscle
Internal intercostal muscle

Figure 4-1. Chest wall. (Adapted from Way L: Thoracic wall, pleura, lung, and mediastinum. In *Current Surgical Diagnosis and Treatment*, 6th ed. Los Altos, CA, Lange, 1983, p 268.)

in localizing a process anatomically as well as in delineating cavitation, calcification, lymphadenopathy, or multiple lesions. **Magnetic resonance imaging (MRI)** may be used when a vascular lesion is suspected or if vascular involvement is anticipated.

2. Endoscopy

a. Laryngoscopy is occasionally an important procedure when carcinoma of the lung is suspected. Tumor involvement of the left or both recurrent laryngeal nerves (signifying inoperability) can be diagnosed via laryngoscopy when suspicion is raised by vocal cord paralysis with resultant hoarseness.

b. Bronchoscopy is useful in many diseases of the tracheobronchial tree for both diagnostic and therapeutic purposes.

(1) Diagnostic uses

(a) To confirm a lung or tracheobronchial tumor suggested by history, physical examination, or chest x-ray

(b) To identify the source of hemoptysis

(c) To obtain specimens for culture and cytologic examination from an area of persistent pulmonary atelectasis or pneumonitis

(2) Therapeutic uses

(a) To remove a foreign body

(b) To remove retained secretions (e.g., after administration of general anesthesia or from aspiration of gastric contents)

(c) To drain lung infections, such as abscesses

(3) Types

(a) Rigid bronchoscopy allows visualization of the trachea and main bronchi to the individual lobes.

(i) It is excellent for biopsies of endobronchial lesions and for clearing of thick secretions and blood.

(ii) The performance of rigid bronchoscopy under local anesthesia requires considerable skill.

(b) Flexible fiberoptic bronchoscopy is used more frequently.

(i) It is particularly helpful for visualizing lobar bronchi and small bronchopulmonary segments and for the biopsy of lesions in that area.

(ii) Although not as effective as rigid bronchoscopy, it may also be used for clearing secretions.

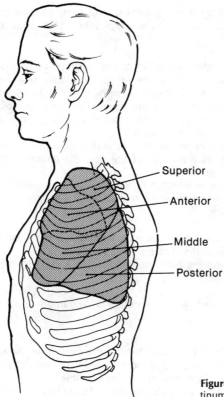

Figure 4-2. The anatomic compartments of the mediastinum.

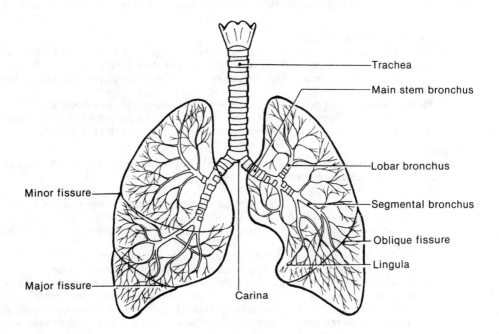

Figure 4-3. Lungs and tracheobronchial tree. (Courtesy of Thomas C. King and Craig R. Smith, Columbia Presbyterian Hospital, New York.)

      (iii) It is especially useful when the patient is intubated, allowing the broncho-scope to be introduced through the endotracheal tube, thus retaining the airway.

    (4) Specific advantages

      (a) Biopsy for suspicion of endobronchial or parenchymal tumor may be performed transbronchially via the bronchoscope in approximately one-third of cases. Pneumothorax is a rare complication, occurring in less than 1% of cases.

      (b) Parenchymal biopsies are useful for suspicion of infection as well. Infections, such as those due to *Pneumocystis carinii*, can only be diagnosed with fixed-tis-sue specimens and so require biopsy.

      (c) Widening of the tracheal carina in patients with lung tumors can be seen on bronchoscopy. It suggests distortion of the tracheal anatomy by subcarinal nodes and is a poor prognostic sign.

  c. Mediastinoscopy is a procedure in which a lighted hollow instrument is inserted be-hind the sternum at the tracheal notch and directed along the anterior surface of the trachea in the pretracheal space.

    (1) Diagnostic uses

      (a) Direct biopsy of paratracheal and subcarinal lymph nodes. Positive nodes in this area usually (but not always) indicate unresectability.

      (b) It is also useful for diagnosing other pulmonary problems, such as sarcoidosis, lymphoma, and infections.

    (2) Mortality rate is about 0.1%.

    (3) Complications include hemorrhage, pneumothorax, and injury to the recurrent la-ryngeal nerves.

3. Scalene node biopsy

  a. The scalene node–bearing fat pad is located behind the clavicle in the region of the sternocleidomastoid muscle. This area should be palpated in patients suspected of hav-ing lung tumors and should be biopsied if nodes are palpable.

  b. Tumor is found in 85% of patients with palpable nodes but in less than 5% of patients with nonpalpable nodes.

  c. The scalene nodes are surrounded by important structures, including the pleura, sub-clavian vessels, the thoracic and other large lymph ducts, and the phrenic and vagus nerves. The principal **complications** of scalene node biopsy result from injury to these structures.

4. Diagnostic pleural procedures

  a. Thoracentesis. Pleural effusions are examined for organisms in suspected infections and are examined cytologically in suspected malignancies. Positive cytologic findings prove a tumor to be inoperable. Pneumothorax is the principal complication of this procedure.

  b. Pleural biopsy. Either percutaneous or open pleural biopsy yields a positive diagnosis in 60%–80% of patients with tuberculosis or cancer when a pleural effusion or pleural-based mass is present. Pneumothorax is the principal complication of this procedure.

5. Lung biopsy

  a. Diagnostic uses. Percutaneous lung biopsy may be used for either a localized peripher-al lesion or a diffuse parenchymal process.

  b. Types

    (1) Needle biopsy is an excellent means for obtaining tissue for tumor diagnosis. How-ever, sampling errors do exist, and a biopsy negative for tumor does not rule out the existence of a tumor. Needle biopsy is also useful for the diagnosis of infections and inflammatory processes.

      (a) The needle can be guided by ultrasonography, fluoroscopy, or CT.

      (b) Complications of needle biopsy are pneumothorax and hemorrhage.

    (2) Open lung biopsy is necessary if needle biopsy fails to diagnose the problem. Open biopsies or resections are ultimately necessary for many lesions of the chest. To ex-pose different areas in the chest, different **thoracic incisions** are necessary, including:

      (a) Median sternotomy (Figure 4-4) for exposure of the heart, pericardium, and structures in the anterior mediastinum

      (b) Posterolateral thoracotomy (Figure 4-5) for exposure of the lung, esophagus, and posterior mediastinum

      (c) Axillary thoracotomy (Figure 4-6) for limited exposure of the upper thorax dur-ing such procedures as upper lobe biopsy or sympathectomy

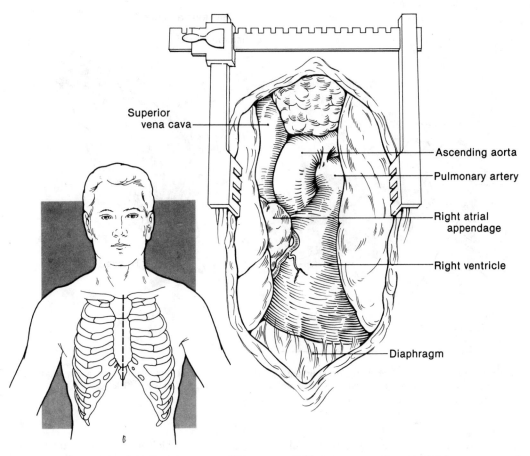

Figure 4-4. Median sternotomy. (Adapted from Kirklin JW, Barratt-Boyes BG: Hypothermia, circulatory arrest, and cardiopulmonary bypass. In *Cardiac Surgery*, New York, Wiley, 1986, p 62.)

(d) Anterolateral thoracotomy (Figure 4-7) for rapid exposure in patients with thoracic trauma or in patients with a very unstable cardiovascular status who cannot tolerate a lateral incision. This type of procedure also allows for excellent control of the airway during the incision.

(e) Anterior parasternal mediastinotomy (Chamberlain procedure), a 2–3-cm parasternal incision that allows insertion of a mediastinoscope into the mediastinum or, more commonly, direct visualization and biopsy of mediastinal lymph nodes.

II. THORACIC TRAUMA. Most thoracic trauma can be managed nonoperatively, using expeditious control of the airway and thoracostomy tube drainage of the pleural space. Less than 25% of chest injuries require surgical intervention. Thoracic trauma can be divided into immediately life-threatening injuries and potentially life-threatening injuries, according to the designation by the American College of Surgeons Committee on Trauma.

A. Immediately life-threatening injuries are those which can cause death in a matter of minutes and, therefore, must be rapidly identified and treated during the initial evaluation and resuscitation.

1. Airway obstruction quickly leads to hypoxia, hypercapnia, acidosis, and cardiac arrest. The highest priority is rapid evaluation and securing the upper airway by clearing out secretions, blood, or foreign bodies; endotracheal intubation; or cricothyroidotomy.

2. Tension pneumothorax implies that the pleural air collection is under significant positive pressure so as to cause a marked mediastinal shift.

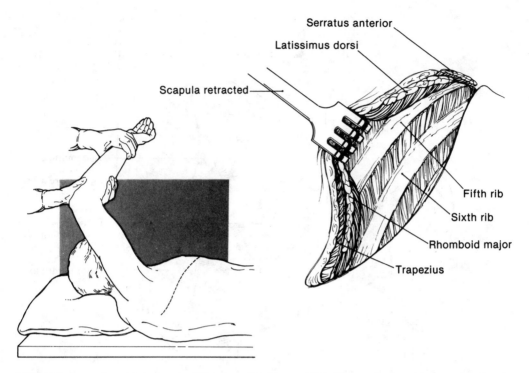

Figure 4-5. Posterolateral thoracotomy. (After Bryant LR, Morgan CV Jr: Chest wall, pleura, lung, and mediastinum. In *Principles of Surgery*, 5th ed. Edited by Schwartz SI, et al. New York, McGraw-Hill, 1989, p 634.)

    a. Causes. It is caused by a check-valve mechanism in which air can escape from the lung into the pleural space but cannot be vented. It is a cause of **sudden death**.

    b. Clinical presentation. The collapsed lung results in chest pain, shortness of breath, and decreased or absent breath sounds on the affected side. Hypotension results from vena caval distortion, which decreases the venous return to the heart.

    c. Treatment. The thorax must be decompressed with a needle, which is replaced by an intercostal tube with underwater seal and suction.

3. Open pneumothorax describes an injury in which an open wound in the chest wall has exposed the pleural space to the atmosphere.

    a. Clinical presentation. The open wound allows air movement through the defect during spontaneous respiration, causing ineffective alveolar ventilation.

    b. Treatment involves covering the wound and inserting a thoracostomy tube. Later, debridement and closure of the wound may be necessary.

4. Massive hemothorax occurs with the rapid accumulation of blood in the pleural space, which causes both compromised ventilation as well as hypovolemic shock.

    a. Treatment entails securing intravenous access and beginning volume restoration followed immediately by placement of a thoracostomy tube.

    b. Complications

        (1) If the hemothorax is inadequately drained, the patient may develop an empyema or fibrothorax, both of which would require subsequent thoracotomy and decortication.

        (2) Initial drainage of 1000 ml or more or continued hemorrhage at the rate of 200 ml an hour for 4 hours are indications for prompt surgical exploration.

5. Cardiac tamponade occurs with the rapid accumulation of blood in the pericardial sac, which causes compression of the cardiac chambers, decreased diastolic filling, and hence, decreased cardiac output.

    a. Clinical presentation includes hypotension with neck vein distention.

    b. Treatment is prompt pericardial decompression either by pericardiocentesis (if in extremis) or via median sternotomy or left anterior thoracotomy (if more stable).

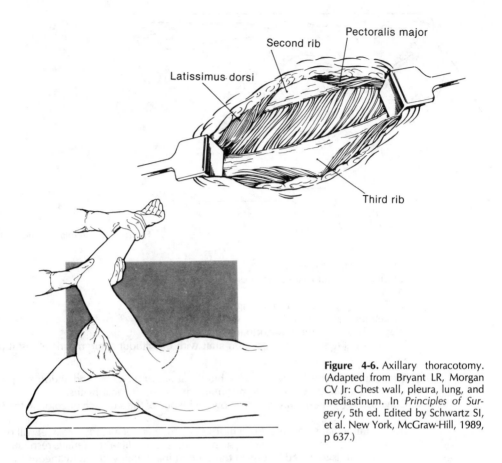

Figure 4-6. Axillary thoracotomy. (Adapted from Bryant LR, Morgan CV Jr: Chest wall, pleura, lung, and mediastinum. In *Principles of Surgery*, 5th ed. Edited by Schwartz SI, et al. New York, McGraw-Hill, 1989, p 637.)

  6. Flail chest. Blunt chest trauma, causing extensive anterior and posterior rib fractures or sternocostal disconnection, results in paradoxical chest wall movement.
   a. Clinical presentation. Paradoxical chest wall movement interferes with the mechanics of respiration and if severe, causes acute alveolar hypoventilation. Morbidity is also related to underlying lung injury.
   b. Treatment includes adequate pain control (intercostal blocks or epidural narcotics) and aggressive pulmonary toilet. Mechanical ventilation may be required in severe cases.

 B. Potentially life-threatening injuries are those which, left untreated, would likely result in death, but which usually allow several hours to establish a definitive diagnosis and institute appropriate treatment.

  1. Tracheobronchial disruption usually occurs within 2 cm of carina.
   a. Diagnosis is made by bronchoscopy and is suspected when a:
    (1) Collapsed lung fails to expand, following placement of a thoracostomy tube
    (2) Massive air leak persists
    (3) Massive progressive subcutaneous emphysema is present
   b. Treatment is by primary repair.

  2. Aortic disruption is the result of a deceleration injury in which the mobile ascending aorta and arch move forward while the descending thoracic aorta remains fixed in position by the mediastinal pleura and intercostal vessels. This movement causes a tear at the aortic isthmus, just distal to the takeoff of the left subclavian artery.
   a. Clinical presentation. The aortic injury usually results in **fracture** of the **intima** and **media** with the adventitia remaining mostly intact. However, complete disruption of all layers can occur with the hematoma contained only by the intact mediastinal pleura.
   b. Chest x-ray findings include:
    (1) Widened mediastinum

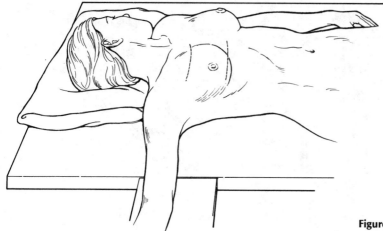

Figure 4-7. Anterolateral thoracotomy.

    (2) Indistinct aortic knob
    (3) Depressed left main stem bronchus
    (4) Apical cap
    (5) Deviation of trachea to the right
    (6) Left pleural effusion
  c. Diagnosis is confirmed by aortogram.
  d. Treatment is repair by interposition graft with or without some means of distal perfusion.

3. Diaphragmatic disruption results from blunt trauma to the chest and abdomen, producing a radial tear in the diaphragm, beginning at the esophageal hiatus.
  a. Diagnosis is by chest x-ray, which shows evidence of the stomach or colon in the chest.
  b. Treatment
    (1) The immediate placement of a nasogastric tube (if not already in place) will prevent acute gastric dilation, which can produce severe, life-threatening respiratory distress. This is followed by urgent transabdominal repair with simultaneous treatment of any associated intra-abdominal injuries.
    (2) If rupture is not diagnosed until 7–10 days later, transthoracic repair is recommended to free any adhesions to the lung that might exist.

4. Esophageal disruption usually results from penetrating rather than blunt trauma.
  a. Clinical presentation. It causes rapidly progressive mediastinitis.
  b. Treatment is wide mediastinal drainage and primary closure with tissue reinforcement (pleura, intercostal muscle, or stomach).

5. Cardiac contusion results from direct sternal impact. It ranges in severity from subendocardial or subepicardial petechiae to full-thickness injury.
  a. Functional complications
    (1) Arrhythmias (i.e., premature ventricular contractions, supraventricular tachycardia, and atrial fibrillation)
    (2) Myocardial rupture
    (3) Ventricular septal rupture
    (4) Left ventricular failure
  b. Diagnosis is made by electrocardiogram, isoenzymes, and 2-D echocardiogram.
  c. Treatment includes cardiac and hemodynamic monitoring, appropriate pharmacologic control of arrhythmias, inotropic support if cardiogenic shock develops.

6. Pulmonary contusion is the commonest injury seen in association with thoracic trauma (30%–75% of all patients suffering major chest injury).
  a. Causes. It is caused by blunt trauma, which produces capillary disruption with subsequent intra-alveolar hemorrhage, edema, and small airway obstruction.
  b. Diagnosis is by chest x-ray, arterial blood gas, and clinical symptoms of respiratory distress.
  c. Treatment includes fluid restriction, supplemental oxygen, vigorous chest physiotherapy, adequate analgesia (epidural narcotics), and prompt chest tube drainage of any associated pleural space complication.

5
Chest Wall, Lung, and Mediastinum

D. Bruce Panasuk
Richard N. Edie

I. DISORDERS OF THE CHEST WALL

A. Chest wall deformities

1. **Pectus excavatum (funnel chest).** An exceedingly depressed sternum is the **commonest chest wall deformity.** It is usually asymptomatic, but it may cause some functional impairment. **Surgery** is indicated for moderate to severe deformities and is performed at 4–5 years of age. The operation involves:
   a. Excision of all involved costal cartilages
   b. An osteotomy of the sternum
   c. Overcorrection of the sternal defect with a bone wedge
   d. Use of a supporting bar behind the sternum (optional)

2. **Pectus carinatum (pigeon breast).** An overly prominent sternum is less likely to cause functional impairment than a depressed sternum. The repair is similar to that for pectus excavatum.

3. **A distal sternal defect** occurs as part of the **pentalogy of Cantrell** (see Chapter 29 III A 2 d).

4. **Poland's syndrome** is a unilateral absence of costal cartilages, pectoralis muscle, and breast. **Surgery** is indicated for protection of the underlying thoracic structures and for cosmetic reasons.

5. **Thoracic outlet syndrome**
   a. Clinical presentation. Compression of the neurovascular structures at the thoracic outlet by bony structures causes arm and neck pain.
      (1) The cause may be a cervical rib or arm or neck trauma.
      (2) The pain usually involves the ulnar aspect of the arm, but it may also involve the back of the neck and the interscapular area.
      (3) Arterial or venous involvement is less common.
   b. Diagnosis is based on the history and physical examination. Ulnar nerve conduction studies are helpful in confirming the diagnosis.
   c. Treatment is to decompress the thoracic outlet, usually by resecting the first rib and the cervical rib, if present, via an axillary or posterior approach. Surgery also involves releasing the nerve bundles from surrounding scar tissue usually via a supraclavicular approach.

B. Chest wall tumors

1. **Benign tumors**
   a. Fibrous dysplasia of the rib occurs posteriorly or on the lateral portion of the rib. It is not painful and is slow-growing. It may occur as part of Albright's syndrome.
   b. Chondroma is the commonest benign tumor of the chest wall. It occurs at the costochondral junction.
   c. Osteochondroma occurs on any portion of the rib.

2. **Malignant tumors** include fibrosarcoma, chondrosarcoma, osteogenic sarcoma, myeloma, and Ewing's sarcoma.

3. **Treatment** of chest wall tumors involves wide excision and reconstruction, using autologous or prosthetic grafts, or both.

II. DISORDERS OF THE PLEURA AND PLEURAL SPACE

A. **Spontaneous pneumothorax** occurs when a **subpleural bleb** ruptures into the pleural space with resultant loss of negative intrapleural pressure, allowing the **lung** to **collapse**.

1. **Incidence.** Young adults 18–25 years of age are most commonly affected, although older persons with asthma or chronic obstructive pulmonary disease are also susceptible.

2. **Symptoms** include chest pain, cough, and dyspnea and range from mild to severe.

3. **Diagnosis** is made by physical examination and chest x-ray.

4. **Treatment** is by chest tube drainage of the pleural space.
   a. **Indications for surgery**
      (1) Recurrent pneumothorax (ipsilateral or contralateral)
      (2) Persistent air leak for 7–10 days
      (3) Incomplete lung expansion
   b. **Procedure** is stapling of apical blebs and pleural abrasion.

B. **Pleural effusions**

1. **Etiology.** Causes of pleural effusions are congestive heart failure, infection, and malignant neoplasm.

2. **Treatment** is aimed at the underlying cause and includes thoracentesis (for either diagnostic or therapeutic purposes) and pleural drainage.

C. **Pleural empyema.** Pus in the pleural space usually accumulates secondary to pulmonary infection.

1. **Pathophysiology** of empyema evolves in three stages.
   a. **Acute or serous phase** (onset to 7 days) during which pleural fluid is initially produced
   b. **Transitional or fibrinopurulent phase** (7–21 days) during which fluid gravitates to dependent areas and undergoes septation and loculation
   c. **Chronic or organized phase** (> 21 days) in which fibrin and pleura fuse and thicken around the periphery of the fluid, resulting in frank abscess formation

2. **Diagnosis** is made by thoracentesis in a patient with pleural effusion and fever.
   a. The aspirated fluid is sent for laboratory studies: If organisms are seen on Gram stain, if organisms are cultured out, or if the pH is below 7.4, the diagnosis is probably an empyema.
   b. On gross examination, if the fluid is very cloudy or is foul-smelling, an empyema is quite likely.

3. **Treatment**
   a. **Early empyemas** associated with pneumococcal pneumonia may be treated with repeated aspiration and antibiotics.
   b. **Established empyemas**, which usually have thicker fluid, need continuous closed drainage. If the empyema is loculated and, therefore, not completely drained by the intercostal tube, then thoracotomy, debridement, and decortication are necessary.
   c. **Small dependent empyemas** that do not respond to chest tube drainage need open drainage via localized rib resection, especially in poor-risk patients.

D. **Pleural tumors. Mesothelioma** is related to asbestos exposure.

1. **Localized mesotheliomas** usually arise from the visceral pleura and are treated by local excision.

2. **Malignant mesothelioma** presents with a pleural effusion, and it is almost always a fatal disease. Patients may require palliative decortication for control of pain and to improve pulmonary function. Use of intrapleural chemotherapy following surgical resection may improve survival.

III. PULMONARY INFECTIONS

A. **Lung abscess**

1. **Etiology.** Abscess of the lung usually occurs secondary to aspiration. It occurs in the de-

pendent segments of the lung (i.e., the posterior segment of the upper lobe or the superior segment of the lower lobe). These are most often anaerobic infections.

2. Treatment
   a. Intravenous antibiotics are the usual treatment; over 90% of acute lung abscesses resolve with antibiotic therapy, **penicillin** being the most effective. There is no proven efficacy of intracavitary antibiotic instillation.
   b. Transbronchial drainage via a rigid or flexible bronchoscope is occasionally successful.
   c. Indications for surgery
      (1) Failure of the abscess to resolve with adequate antibiotic therapy
      (2) Hemorrhage
      (3) Inability to rule out carcinoma
      (4) Giant abscess (> 6 cm in diameter)
      (5) Rupture with resulting empyema. This can be treated initially by chest tube drainage of the pleural space but may require open drainage and decortication with or without actual resection.

B. Bronchiectasis is a complication of repeated pulmonary infections, which causes bronchial dilatation. The disease usually affects the lower lobes. It occurs in adults and children who present with a chronic illness accompanied by excessive sputum production.

   1. Diagnosis. Bronchography is the definitive diagnostic study. **Bronchoscopy** may also be helpful to determine the specific segmental location of secretions and to identify foreign bodies, bronchial stenosis, or neoplasms.

   2. Treatment
      a. Medical treatment resolves most cases.
      b. Surgical treatment involves segmental resection of the affected area, and best results are obtained in patients with localized disease.

C. Tuberculosis

   1. Incidence. Approximately 25,000 new cases of tuberculosis are diagnosed each year in the United States.

   2. Treatment
      a. Chemotherapeutic agents are now used to treat this disease. Fewer than 5% of patients require pulmonary resection as part of their therapeutic regimen, and this is usually performed after a course of chemotherapy.
      b. Indications for surgery
         (1) Bronchopleural fistula with empyema
         (2) Destroyed lobe or lung
         (3) Persistent open cavities with positive sputum
         (4) Post-tubercular bronchial stenosis
         (5) Pulmonary hemorrhage
         (6) Suspected carcinoma
         (7) Aspergilloma
         (8) Bronchiectasis

IV. SOLITARY PULMONARY NODULES (COIN LESIONS) are well-circumscribed, peripheral nodules, which are manifestations of neoplastic disease (e.g., bronchogenic carcinoma) or of granulomatous or infectious processes (e.g., tuberculosis).

A. General characteristics

   1. Solitary pulmonary nodules are usually asymptomatic.

   2. They occur more often in men than in women.

B. Benign versus malignant etiology

   1. When no other tumor is known to be present, the solitary pulmonary nodule is rarely a sign of metastatic disease.

   2. If the patient is younger than 40 years of age, there is a two-thirds chance that the lesion is benign.

3. The likelihood of cancer is higher in men than in women.

4. The **risk of carcinoma** in solitary pulmonary nodules is age-related. In patients who undergo surgery, the probability of cancer is about 33%, the probability of granuloma is about 33%, and the probability of tuberculoma is about 20%. The lesions of the remaining surgical patients are due to other causes.

5. X-ray evidence of a benign lesion includes the following:
   a. Calcification is present, particularly concentric, heavy, or popcorn-like calcification. If the calcification appears as small flecks, a malignant lesion should be suspected.
   b. X-rays taken 1 year or more apart show no growth in the size of the lesion.
   c. The lesion size is less than 1 cm in diameter. The larger the lesion, the greater the chance of malignancy.
   d. Computed tomography (CT) scan demonstrates a well-circumscribed lesion. Multiple lesions that are demonstrated on CT but are not seen on plain film suggest either metastatic disease or satellite lesions from carcinoma or granulomas. [There is no advantage of magnetic resonance imaging (MRI) over CT scan for imaging of solitary pulmonary nodules.]

V. BRONCHOGENIC CARCINOMA

A. Overview

1. Incidence
   a. Bronchogenic carcinoma is the **leading cause of cancer death in the United States**.
   b. Approximately 130,000 new cases are diagnosed each year in this country.
   c. About 95% of lung cancers occur in patients who are over 40 years of age.

2. Etiology
   a. Seventy-five percent of all lung carcinomas are **related to smoking;** affected individuals usually have a history of smoking one or more packs of cigarettes daily for 20 years.
   b. There is no known environmental cause. However, chronic exposure to various substances may play a role; nickel, asbestos, arsenic, radioactive materials, and petroleum products have all been implicated.

B. Pathology

1. Adenocarcinoma is now the **commonest lung carcinoma**, representing 30%–45% of all malignant lung cancers. It is less strongly associated with smoking and occurs more commonly in women.
   a. Histology reveals distinct acinar formation of cells, which arise from the subsegmental airways in the periphery of the lung.
   b. Characteristics
      (1) Many of these tumors are formed in conjunction with lung scars, representing a response to chronic irritation.
      (2) Growth may be slow, but the cancer metastasizes readily by a vascular route. It may spread diffusely throughout the lung via the tracheobronchial tree.
   c. Variants. Bronchoalveolar carcinoma is a variant of adenocarcinoma, which represents a highly differentiated form that spreads along alveolar walls.
      (1) It occurs in three forms: solitary nodule, multinodular, and diffuse/pneumonic types.
      (2) It has the best prognosis of all the cell types.

2. Squamous cell carcinoma is the second commonest carcinoma of the lung, representing 25%–40% of all malignant lung tumors. It is associated with smoking.
   a. Histology reveals intercellular bridge formation and cell keratinization. It is thought to arise from squamous metaplasia of the tracheobronchial tree.
   b. Characteristics
      (1) Approximately two-thirds of squamous cell carcinomas occur centrally in the lung fields.
      (2) The tumor is bulky and is associated with bronchial obstruction.
      (3) It is characterized by slow growth and late metastasis.
      (4) It undergoes central necrosis and cavitation.

3. Small cell anaplastic (oat cell) carcinoma, which is highly malignant, represents approximately 15%–25% of all malignant lung tumors.

   a. Histology reveals clusters, nests, or sheets of small, round, oval or spindle-shaped cells with dark round nuclei and scanty cytoplasm.

     (1) Electron microscopy reveals the presence of neurosecretory cytoplasmic granules.

     (2) This, together with observed production of biologically active substances, has led to their classification as neuroendocrine tumor of the amine precursor uptake and decarboxylation (APUD) system.

   b. Characteristics

     (1) It is usually centrally located.

     (2) It metastasizes early by the lymphatic and vascular routes.

     (3) It may be curable (small peripheral stage I) if it is resected at an early stage. If unresectable, it usually responds to combination chemotherapy.

   c. Prognosis is quite poor.

4. Undifferentiated large cell carcinoma is the rarest of the major cell types of lung cancer.

   a. Histology reveals anaplastic, large cells with abundant cytoplasm and no apparent evidence of differentiation.

   b. Characteristics

     (1) It may be located either centrally or peripherally.

     (2) It is a highly malignant lesion, which spreads early.

   c. Prognosis. It has a poorer prognosis than the more differentiated non–small cell carcinomas.

5. Other tumors, such as bronchial adenoma, papilloma, and sarcomas, are rare.

C. Clinical presentation

1. Pulmonary symptoms include cough, dyspnea, chest pain, fever, sputum production, and wheezing. Patients may be **asymptomatic**, the only clue to the cancer being an abnormal chest x-ray.

2. Extrapulmonary symptoms

   a. Metastatic extrapulmonary manifestations include weight loss, malaise, symptoms referable to the central nervous system, and bone pain.

   b. Nonmetastatic extrapulmonary manifestations (paraneoplastic syndromes) are secondary to hormone-like substances that are elaborated by the tumor. These include Cushing's syndrome, hypercalcemia, myasthenic neuropathies, hypertrophic osteoarthropathies, and gynecomastia.

3. A Pancoast tumor involving the superior sulcus may produce symptoms related to brachial plexus involvement, sympathetic ganglia involvement, or vertebral collapse secondary to local invasion. This may result in pain or weakness of the arm, edema, or **Horner's syndrome** (i.e., ptosis, miosis, enophthalmos, and anhidrosis).

D. Diagnosis

1. Abnormal chest x-ray is the commonest finding.

   a. The tumor may present as a nodule, an infiltrate, or atelectasis.

   b. An abnormal chest x-ray is more likely to represent carcinoma in patients over age 40.

2. CT scan assesses the extension of the tumor and evaluates the possibility of mediastinal metastasis.

3. Bronchoscopy assesses the bronchial involvement and the resectability and obtains tissue for cytologic examination.

4. Mediastinoscopy or mediastinotomy obtains mediastinal lymph nodes for pathologic examination and aids in the staging of the disease. Positive findings may or may not preclude a curative resection, depending on the pathologic cell type, the extent of nodal involvement, and the condition of the patient.

5. Percutaneous needle biopsy may be used to obtain tissue for cytologic examination.

E. Staging of lung carcinoma is fundamental for the evaluation of treatment protocols (Table 5-1). It is based on information obtained during preoperative evaluation, findings at mediastinoscopy (above), thoracotomy, and pathologic findings of the surgical specimens. Definitions of tumor size (T), lymph node metastasis (N), and distant metastasis (M) comprise the **TNM classification of carcinoma of the lung** by the revised International Clinical Staging System.

Table 5-1. Stage Grouping in Cancer of the Lung

Stage Grouping	Tumor	Nodal Involvement	Distant Metastasis
Occult carcinoma	TX	N0	M0
Stage 0	TIS	Carcinoma in situ	. . .
Stage I	T1	N0	M0
	T2	N0	M0
Stage II	T1	N1	M0
	T2	N1	M0
Stage IIIa	T3	N0	M0
	T3	N1	M0
	T1–3	N2	M0
Stage IIIb	Any T	N3	M0
	T4	Any N	M0
Stage IV	Any T	Any N	M1

1. **T (primary tumors)**
    a. **TX:** Tumor proven by the presence of malignant cells in bronchopulmonary secretions but not visualized by x-ray or by bronchoscopy, or any tumor that cannot be assessed, as one in a retreatment staging
    b. **TO:** No evidence of primary tumor
    c. **TIS:** Carcinoma in situ
    d. **T1:** A tumor that is 3.0 cm or less in greatest dimension, surrounded by lung or visceral pleura and without evidence of invasion proximal to a lobar bronchus at bronchoscopy
    e. **T2:** A tumor more than 3.0 cm in greatest dimension or a tumor of any size that either invades the visceral pleura or has associated atelectasis or obstructive pneumonitis that extends to the hilar region. At bronchoscopy, the proximal extent of demonstrable tumor must be within a lobar bronchus or at least 2.0 cm distal to the carina. Any associated atelectasis or obstructive pneumonitis must involve less than an entire lung.
    f. **T3:** A tumor of any size with direct extension into the chest wall (including superior sulcus tumors), diaphragm, or the mediastinal pleura or pericardium without involving the heart, great vessels, trachea, esophagus, or vertebral body, or a tumor in the main bronchus within 2 cm of the carina without involving the carina
    g. **T4:** A tumor of any size with invasion of the mediastinum or involving the heart, great vessels, trachea, esophagus, vertebral body, or carina or the presence of malignant pleural effusion

2. **N (nodal involvement)**
    a. **N0:** No demonstrable metastasis to regional lymph nodes
    b. **N1:** Metastasis to lymph nodes in the peribronchial or the ipsilateral hilar region, or both, including direct extension
    c. **N2:** Metastasis to ipsilateral mediastinal lymph nodes and subcarinal lymph nodes
    d. **N3:** Metastasis to contralateral mediastinal lymph nodes, contralateral hilar lymph nodes, ipsilateral or contralateral scalene or supraclavicular lymph nodes

3. **M (distant metastasis)**
    a. **M0:** No (known) distant metastasis
    b. **M1:** Distant metastasis present

F. **Treatment**
    1. **Surgical treatment**
        a. **Pulmonary resection** (i.e., lobectomy, extended lobectomy, or pneumonectomy) is the only potential cure for bronchogenic carcinoma. The surgical approach is to resect the involved lung, regional lymph nodes, and involved contiguous structures, if necessary.
            (1) Lobectomy is used in disease localized to one lobe.
            (2) Extended resections and pneumonectomy are used when the tumor involves a fissure or is close to the pulmonary hilus.
            (3) Wedge resections or bronchial segmentectomy may be used in localized disease in high-risk patients.
        b. **Contraindications for thoracotomy.** One-half of all patients with lung carcinomas are not candidates for thoracotomy at the time of diagnosis.
            (1) Extensive ipsilateral mediastinal lymph node involvement (N2 disease), particularly high paratracheal and subcarinal

(2) Any contralateral mediastinal lymph node involvement (N3 disease)
(3) Distant metastases
(4) Malignant pleural effusion
(5) Superior vena cava syndrome
(6) Recurrent laryngeal nerve involvement
(7) Phrenic nerve paralysis
(8) Poor pulmonary function (relative contraindication)

2. **Adjuvant therapy.** Further treatment using radiotherapy, chemotherapy, or both is indicated for some advanced-stage tumors.

a. **Radiotherapy** is particularly helpful in patients with Pancoast's tumors. It has been helpful in the treatment of other tumors, but it is generally indicated in postoperative treatment of patients with positive mediastinal metastasis.

b. **Chemotherapy**, in general, has not helped to prolong survival or to provide palliation in patients with lung carcinoma, whether combined with surgery or used alone. Chemotherapy with multiple agents has shown some success in controlling oat cell carcinoma, particularly when combined with radiation therapy.

c. Preoperative chemotherapy (with or without radiation therapy) in patients with stage IIIa disease, particularly those with known N2 involvement, has recently been used in attempts to convert advanced local disease into a resectable lesion. However, the efficacy of this therapy has yet to be determined, although early results appear promising.

G. **Prognosis** depends primarily on cell types and stage of disease at the time of diagnosis.

1. Five-year survival based on **cell type**
a. Bronchoalveolar carcinoma, 30%–35%
b. Squamous cell carcinoma, 8%–16%
c. Adenocarcinoma, 5%–10%
d. Small cell carcinoma, < 3%

2. Five-year survival based on **postoperative pathologic stage**
a. Stage I, 60%–80%
b. Stage II, 40%–55%
c. Stage IIIa, 10%–35%

VI. **BRONCHIAL ADENOMAS.** The term **adenoma** is an unfortunate misnomer since these lesions are all **malignant neoplasms,** albeit relatively low grade in character. They arise from the epithelium, ducts, and glands of the tracheobronchial tree and include the carcinoid tumor, adenoid cystic carcinoma (cylindroma), and mucoepidermoid carcinoma.

A. **Carcinoid tumors**, which comprise 80%–90% of bronchial adenomas, occur mainly in the **proximal bronchi** (20% main stem bronchi, 60% lobar or segmental bronchi, 20% peripheral parenchyma).

1. **Characteristics**
a. They arise from **Kulchitsky-type cells** and are seen most commonly in the fifth decade of life.
b. They are slow growing and protrude endobronchially, often causing some degree of bronchial obstruction.
c. Regional lymph node metastases occur in 10% of patients, mostly those with the **atypical variant** of carcinoid tumors, which is characterized by pleomorphism, increased mitotic activity, disorganized architecture, and tumor necrosis. Of these patients, 70% present with metastases.

2. **Signs and symptoms** include cough (47%), recurrent infection (45%), hemoptysis (39%), pain (19%), and wheezing (17%). Approximately 21% are asymptomatic.

3. **Chest x-ray** may reveal evidence of atelectasis or pulmonary nodule.

4. **Treatment** for carcinoid tumor is surgical excision.
a. **Lobectomy** is the most commonly performed procedure.
b. **Wedge excision** or **segmentectomy** can occasionally be used for peripheral typical carcinoids.
c. **Pneumonectomy** should rarely be required, especially since the introduction of **bronchoplastic techniques**, which allow **sleeve resection** of lesions involving the main stem bronchi or bronchus intermedius.

      d. Prognosis should be more than 90% 5-year survival for typical carcinoid tumors, decreasing to less than 50% for the atypical variant.

B. Adenoid cystic carcinoma (cylindroma) comprises approximately 10% of bronchial adenomas.

    1. Characteristics
      a. They **occur more centrally** in the lower trachea/carina area and in the orifices of the main stem bronchi.
      b. Although considered a low-grade malignancy, the adenoid cystic carcinoma is more aggressive than is the carcinoid tumor.
      c. Metastases tend to occur late, but about one-third of patients present with metastases, commonly along perineural lymphatics to regional lymph nodes but also distantly to liver, bone, and kidneys.

    2. Treatment is by generous en bloc excision of the tumor, including peribronchial tissue and regional lymph nodes. This may require lobectomy, sleeve resection, or both. **Radiation therapy** should be considered in all inoperable patients, and in those in whom residual tumor remains after resection.

    3. Prognosis is less favorable than in carcinoid tumor, 5-year survival being approximately 50%.

C. Mucoepidermoid carcinoma accounts for less than 1% of bronchial adenomas.

    1. Characteristics
      a. Location and distribution in the tracheobronchial tree is similar to carcinoid tumors.
      b. High-grade and low-grade variants exist, although the latter type predominates.

    2. Treatment principles as outlined for carcinoid tumors apply to low-grade mucoepidermoid carcinoma. High-grade variants should be approached and managed like other bronchial carcinomas.

VII. HAMARTOMAS

A. Pathology. These are benign pulmonary tumors and histologically are classified as adenochondromas. They occur within the substance of the lung and usually present as solitary pulmonary nodules.

B. Treatment involves removal during a diagnostic thoracotomy for evaluation of the solitary nodule.

VIII. METASTATIC TUMORS

A. Metastatic tumors are common to the lung, which may be the only site of metastases from a nonpulmonary primary tumor.

B. Treatment

    1. Single or multiple metastatic tumors can be removed from the lung as part of the treatment protocol.

    2. The best treatment results are obtained with tumors for which there is effective chemotherapy. This combination approach has been used frequently in patients with pulmonary metastases from osteogenic sarcoma and in some patients with metastases from colon carcinoma.

IX. DISORDERS OF THE TRACHEA

A. Anatomy

    1. Structure
      a. The trachea is 11 cm from the cricoid to the carina with a range in the adult of about 10–13 cm in length and 2.3–1.8 cm in diameter.
      b. The trachea is encircled by 18–22 cartilaginous rings. The **cricoid cartilage** is the only

complete tracheal ring. The remaining rings are incomplete with a membranous portion posteriorly.

c. The trachea is vertically mobile. When the neck is extended, one-half of the trachea is in the neck, and when the neck is flexed, all of the trachea is behind the sternum.

2. Relationship to other organs
a. The thyroid isthmus is at the second or third tracheal ring.
b. The innominate artery crosses the trachea in its midportion.
c. The aorta arches over the trachea in its distal portion.
d. The esophagus is posterior to the trachea throughout its course.

3. Blood supply is segmental and is shared with the esophagus. Blood is supplied by the inferior thyroid artery, the subclavian artery, the supreme intercostal artery, the internal mammary artery, the innominate artery, and the bronchial circulation.

B. Congenital lesions

1. Types
a. Stenosis. There are three types of tracheal stenosis—generalized, funnel, and segmental. The bronchi may be small in congenital tracheal stenosis, and an associated pulmonary artery sling, in which the artery tethers the trachea, may be present. **Webs** may also be present.
b. Congenital tracheomalacia. Cartilaginous softening is due to compression of the trachea by vascular rings, which are anomalies of the aortic arch. These anomalies include double aortic arch, right arch with left ligamentum arteriosum, aberrant subclavian artery, or aberrant innominate artery. The diameter of the trachea is normal, but the wall is collapsible.

2. Diagnosis
a. Signs and symptoms
(1) Inspiratory and expiratory wheezing, which may be paroxysmal
(2) Feeding problems
(3) Frequent infections
b. Diagnostic studies
(1) Air tracheography (tomography)
(2) Bronchoscopy
(3) Angiography to assess vascular anomalies

3. Treatment
a. Stenosis and webs are usually **treated conservatively** because of the difficulty in performing tracheal reconstruction in infants.
(1) A web may be removed endoscopically.
(2) Tracheostomy may be helpful and should be performed in a narrow area to avoid injury to normal areas of the trachea.
b. Chondromalacia is treated by **aortopexy,** performed under bronchoscopic guidance to maximize the tracheal lumen. The patient may still have some airway problems for a period of time postoperatively.

C. Neoplasms of the trachea

1. Types
a. Primary neoplasms are rare.
(1) Squamous cell carcinomas are the commonest neoplasms of the trachea. They may be exophytic, may cause superficial ulceration, or may be multiple lesions with interposed areas of normal trachea. The tumor spreads through the regional lymph nodes and by direct extension to mediastinal structures.
(2) Adenoid carcinoma is slow-growing with a prolonged course. It infiltrates airways beyond the gross tumor, and it spreads paratracheally.
(3) Other primary tracheal neoplasms include carcinosarcomas, pseudosarcomas, mucoepidermoid carcinomas, squamous papillomas, chondromas, and chondrosarcomas.
b. Secondary tumors to the trachea are usually from the lung, the esophagus, or the thyroid gland.

2. **Diagnosis**
   a. **Radiographic studies** include chest x-ray, tracheal tomogram, and fluoroscopy for evaluation of the larynx. Instillation of contrast medium is rarely necessary for the evaluation of tracheal tumors.
   b. **Bronchoscopy** is deferred until the final operation because the biopsy may be hazardous due to bleeding or obstruction of the airway. Frozen section examination is adequate for assessment of the tracheal tumor.
   c. **Pulmonary function testing** is mandatory if carinal or pulmonary resection is contemplated.

3. **Treatment** is by tracheal resection.
   a. **Overview**
      (1) **Preoperative antibiotics** are selected on the basis of preoperative tracheal cultures.
      (2) When there is airway obstruction, **anesthesia** should be induced with halothane.
      (3) High-frequency **ventilation** may be helpful, and it may be possible to pass a small tube beside the tumor.
      (4) In the **resection procedure**, up to one-half of the trachea may be removed.
         (a) Adequate mobilization can usually be obtained by simply flexing the patient's neck, although laryngeal or hilar release techniques are occasionally necessary.
         (b) An end-to-end anastomosis is performed.
   b. **Incisions used**
      (1) A cervical incision is used for resection of the upper half of the trachea.
      (2) A posterolateral thoracotomy is used for the lower portion of the trachea.
      (3) The entire trachea can be exposed via a combined cervical incision and median sternotomy.

4. **Prognosis** is similar to that for resectable carcinoma of the lung (see V G 2).

X. LESIONS OF THE MEDIASTINUM (see Chapter 4 I A 2)

A. **Anterior mediastinal lesions**

1. **Thymoma** (see Chapter 16 IV B 1)

2. **Teratomas**
   a. **Incidence.** Teratomas occur most frequently in adolescents, and 80% of these tumors are benign.
   b. **Etiology.** They originate from the branchial cleft pouch in association with the thymus gland. All tissue types are present in these tumors, including ectodermal, endodermal, and mesodermal elements.
   c. **Diagnosis.** Teratomas are diagnosed radiographically and may appear as smooth-walled cystic lesions or as lobulated solid lesions. Calcification is often present.
   d. **Treatment** is total surgical excision.

3. **Lymphoma.** Fifty percent of patients with lymphomas (including those with Hodgkin's disease) have mediastinal lymph node involvement; however, only 5% of patients with lymphomas have *only* mediastinal disease.
   a. **Symptoms** of mediastinal lymphoma include cough, chest pain, fever, and weight loss.
   b. **Diagnosis** is by chest x-ray and lymph node biopsy, using either mediastinoscopy or anterior mediastinotomy.
   c. **Treatment** is nonsurgical.

4. **Germ cell tumors.** These tumors are very rare, occurring as less than 1% of all mediastinal tumors. They metastasize to pleural lymph nodes, the liver, bone, and retroperitoneum.
   a. **Histologic types**
      (1) Seminoma
      (2) Embryonal cell carcinoma
      (3) Teratocarcinoma
      (4) Choriocarcinoma
      (5) Endodermal sinus tumor
   b. **Symptoms** include chest pain, cough, and hoarseness due to invasion of the vagus nerves.
   c. **Diagnosis.** They are diagnosed radiographically.
   d. **Treatment** is by as complete surgical excision as possible.
   e. **Adjuvant therapy.** Seminomas are very radiosensitive, and the other cell types may benefit from chemotherapeutic agents.

B. Middle mediastinal lesions are usually cystic in nature. The two commonest are pericardial cysts and bronchogenic cysts.

1. **Pericardial cysts** are usually asymptomatic and are found on chest x-ray. They are smooth-walled and most commonly occur in the cardiodiaphragmatic angle. Surgery is usually performed as a diagnostic procedure to identify the lesion.

2. **Bronchogenic cysts** generally arise posteriorly to the carina. They may be asymptomatic, or they may cause pulmonary compression, which can be life-threatening, particularly in infancy. The usual **treatment** is surgical excision.

3. **Ascending aortic aneurysms** are also included as middle mediastinal masses due to the location of the great vessels in this compartment.

C. Posterior mediastinal lesions are neurogenic tumors located in the paravertebral gutter. About 10%–20% are malignant.

1. **Incidence.** Seventy-five percent of these neurogenic tumors occur in children under 4 years of age. Malignancy is most likely to occur if the tumor arises in childhood.

2. **Histologic types**
   a. Neurilemomas, which arise from the Schwann cells of the nerve sheath
   b. Neurofibromas, which can degenerate into neurosarcomas
   c. Neurosarcomas
   d. Ganglioneuromas, which originate from sympathetic ganglia
   e. Neuroblastomas, which also arise from the sympathetic chain. Neuroblastomas may have **metastasized** to bone, liver, and regional lymph nodes by the time diagnosis is made. Also, direct extension to the spinal cord may occur.

3. **Pheochromocytomas** occur in the mediastinum, although rarely; they behave similarly to the usual intra-adrenal pheochromocytomas.

4. **Symptoms**
   a. Symptoms include chest pain secondary to compression of an intercostal nerve. If the tumor grows intraspinally, it may cause symptoms of spinal cord compression. Rarely, these tumors have an endocrine function and can secrete catecholamines.
   b. The symptoms of neuroblastoma include fever, vomiting, diarrhea, and cough.

5. **Diagnosis** is by chest x-ray and CT scan.

6. **Treatment** is by surgical excision. Postoperative radiation is helpful in the treatment of malignant tumors.

6
Heart

D. Bruce Panasuk
Charles J. Lamb
Richard N. Edie

I. ACQUIRED HEART DISEASE

A. Overview

1. **Epidemiology**
   a. Approximately 3 million myocardial infarctions are recorded annually in the United States with an accompanying mortality rate of 10%–15%.
   b. Acquired valvular disease is less frequent than coronary artery disease but still accounts for significant morbidity and mortality.

2. **Signs and symptoms**
   a. **Dyspnea** is due to pulmonary congestion, which is the result of increased left atrial pressure.
   b. **Peripheral edema** may be the result of significant right-sided congestive heart failure.
   c. **Chest pain** may be caused by angina pectoris, myocardial infarction, pericarditis, aortic dissection, pulmonary infarction, or aortic stenosis.
   d. **Palpitations** may indicate a serious cardiac arrhythmia.
   e. **Hemoptysis** may be associated with mitral stenosis or pulmonary infarction.
   f. **Syncope** may result from mitral stenosis, aortic stenosis, or heart block.
   g. **Fatigue** is the result of decreased cardiac output.

3. **Physical examination** should include:
   a. **Blood pressure**, which should be measured in both arms and legs
   b. **Peripheral pulses.** The quality and regularity of pulses are important.
      (1) Pulsus alternans is a sign of left ventricular failure.
      (2) Pulsus parvus et tardus may be seen with aortic stenosis.
      (3) A wide pulse pressure with a "water-hammer pulse" is seen with increased cardiac output or decreased peripheral vascular resistance, as in aortic insufficiency or patent ductus arteriosus.
   c. **Neck veins.** Central venous pressure may be indirectly inferred from the height of the internal jugular vein filling.
   d. **Heart**
      (1) **Inspection and palpation of the precordium**
         (a) Normally, the apical impulse is appreciated at the midclavicular line, fifth intercostal space. In left ventricular hypertrophy, the apical impulse is increased and displaced laterally.
         (b) With right ventricular hypertrophy, a parasternal heave is appreciated.
         (c) Thrills from valvular disease may be felt.
      (2) **Auscultation.** The quality of heart tones, type of rhythm, murmurs, rales, and gallops are all important.

4. **Preoperative management**
   a. **Laboratory studies** should include the following: complete blood count (CBC), sequential multiple analyzer series 6 (SMA6), prothrombin time (PT), partial thromboplastin time (PTT), platelet count, serum creatinine, and serum bilirubin.
   b. **Chest x-ray** and **electrocardiogram**
   c. **Cardiac catheterization** is the definitive preoperative study.
   d. **Pulmonary function studies** are important in patients with known pulmonary disease.
   e. **Psychological preparation** of the patient is an important aspect and should include familiarizing the patient with the postoperative procedures in the intensive care unit.
   f. **Perioperative antibiotics** play an important role in the prevention of sepsis.

5. Postoperative management is critical to the success of any cardiac operation.
   a. Intensive care units must be equipped and staffed to handle cardiac surgery patients.
   b. Drugs used postoperatively include those administered to improve myocardial contractility, to maintain urine output, or to abolish or control cardiac arrhythmias. In addition, patients may require blood products to treat anemia or to help correct coagulopathies.

6. Cardiac arrest
   a. Causes of cardiac arrest include:
      (1) Anoxia
      (2) Coronary thrombosis
      (3) Electrolyte disturbances
      (4) Myocardial depressants: anesthetic agents, antiarrhythmic drugs, or digitalis
      (5) Conduction disturbances
      (6) Vagotonic maneuvers
   b. Immediate cardiopulmonary resuscitation is critical, as brain injury results after 3–4 minutes of diminished perfusion.
   c. Treatment should include:
      (1) Establishing an **airway** and giving **ventilatory support**. These are best accomplished by endotracheal intubation and controlled ventilation.
      (2) Cardiac massage. Closed-chest cardiac massage is usually appropriate. In the patient with cardiac tamponade, acute volume loss, an unstable sternum, or an open pericardium, open-chest cardiac massage usually is required.
      (3) Electrical defibrillation, if cardiac arrest is the result of ventricular fibrillation
      (4) Drug therapy. Commonly used agents include:
         (a) Epinephrine, for its cardiotonic effect
         (b) Calcium, also for its cardiotonic effect
         (c) Sodium bicarbonate, to treat associated acidosis
         (d) Vasopressor agents, to support blood pressure
         (e) Atropine, to reverse bradycardia
      (5) Replacement of **blood volume**, if necessary

7. Extracorporeal circulation. The rationale for using extracorporeal circulation is to provide the operating team with a motionless heart and a bloodless field in which to work while simultaneously perfusing the different organ systems with oxygenated blood.
   a. Hypothermia is employed during the procedure to improve the tolerance of the myocardium to ischemia. This is complemented by the use of cardioplegic solution to protect the myocardium.
   b. Pathophysiologic effects of extracorporeal circulation include:
      (1) Widespread total body inflammatory response with initiation of humoral amplification systems, including:
         (a) Coagulation cascade
         (b) Fibrinolytic system
         (c) Complement activation
         (d) Kallikrein-kinin system
      (2) Release of vasoactive substances
         (a) Epinephrine
         (b) Norepinephrine
         (c) Histamine
         (d) Bradykinin
      (3) Retention of both sodium and free water, causing diffuse edema
      (4) Trauma to blood elements, resulting in hemolysis of red cells and destruction of platelets
      (5) Respiratory insufficiency, which is usually self-limited

8. Prosthetic valves. These fall into three general categories: tissue valves, mechanical valves, and human allograft valves.
   a. Tissue valves consist primarily of porcine heterografts. These valves usually do not require anticoagulation postoperatively; however, they lack long-term durability with a 10%–30% failure rate at 10 years.
   b. Mechanical valves are durable for long periods of time, but they require permanent anticoagulation therapy.
   c. Human allograft (cryo preserved) valves do not require anticoagulation and at the present time, have demonstrated long-term durability. Wider use of this valve is anticipated, especially in the aortic position.

B. Aortic valvular disease

1. Aortic stenosis
 a. Etiology
  (1) Congenital stenosis. Bicuspid valves usually develop calcific changes in the fourth decade and symptoms by the sixth decade.
  (2) Acquired stenosis results from progressive degeneration and calcification of the valve leaflets.
  (3) Patients with a history of rheumatic fever rarely have isolated stenosis but usually have a mixed lesion of stenosis and insufficiency.
 b. Pathology
  (1) Thickening and calcification of the leaflets result in a decreased cross-sectional area of the valve, which may be as narrow as 0.5–0.7 cm² in severe aortic stenosis (the normal aortic valve is 2.5–3.5 cm²).
  (2) Critical aortic stenosis imposes a significant **pressure load** on the left ventricle, which increases left ventricular work, resulting in concentric left ventricular hypertrophy (without associated dilation). Eventually, myocardial decompensation occurs.
 c. Clinical presentation
  (1) Classic symptoms are angina, syncope, and dyspnea.
  (2) Symptoms usually occur late in the course of the disease and represent myocardial decompensation. Sudden death is a frequent occurrence in untreated patients at this stage.
  (3) Life expectancy averages 4 years after the onset of symptoms.
 d. Diagnosis
  (1) Physical examination reveals the classic systolic crescendo-decrescendo murmur, heard best in the second right intercostal space. Radiation of the murmur to the carotids is common.
   (a) Often, an associated thrill is appreciated.
   (b) A narrowed pulse pressure along with pulsus parvus et tardus is frequently found.
  (2) Chest x-ray usually shows a heart of normal size. Calcification of the aortic valve may be seen.
  (3) Electrocardiogram demonstrates left ventricular hypertrophy.
  (4) Cardiac catheterization is important to measure the pressure gradient across the aortic valve, to calculate its cross-sectional area, and to identify any associated mitral valve or coronary artery disease, which occurs in 25% of the patients.
 e. Treatment
  (1) Surgical correction is recommended for patients with symptoms of syncope, angina, or dyspnea or with a peak systolic gradient across the aortic valve greater than 50 mm Hg or with a valve area less than 0.7 cm².
  (2) Surgery consists of **excision** of the diseased valve and replacement with one of the prosthetic valves.

2. Aortic insufficiency
 a. Etiology. Myxomatous degeneration, aortic dissection, Marfan's syndrome, bacterial endocarditis, rheumatic fever, and annuloaortic ectasia are common causes.
 b. Pathology
  (1) The underlying pathologic process may be a fibrosis and shortening of the valve leaflets (as occurs in rheumatic fever), a dilatation of the aortic annulus (as occurs in Marfan's syndrome), or myxomatous degeneration of the leaflets.
  (2) Aortic insufficiency imposes a significant **volume load** on the left ventricle in accordance with Starling's law of the heart. This leads to early left ventricular dilatation. If uncorrected, this may lead to left ventricular failure with pulmonary congestion. Secondary mitral insufficiency may occur at this stage.
 c. Clinical presentation
  (1) There is a greater variability in time between the onset of aortic insufficiency and the appearance of symptoms than occurs with aortic stenosis.
  (2) Early symptoms include palpitations secondary to ventricular arrhythmias, and dyspnea on exertion.
  (3) Later, severe congestive heart failure is seen. Death results from progressive cardiac failure.

d. Diagnosis
   (1) Physical examination
      (a) The characteristic diastolic murmur is heard along the left sternal border. The duration of the murmur during diastole often correlates with the severity of the aortic insufficiency. The murmur radiates to the left axilla.
      (b) The pulse pressure is often widened. Short, intense peripheral pulses ("**water-hammer pulses**") are characteristic.
   (2) Chest x-ray shows left ventricular dilatation.
   (3) Cardiac catheterization with aortography is used to quantitate the degree of aortic insufficiency.
e. Treatment
   (1) Surgery is recommended whenever ventricular decompensation is demonstrated. Patients at this stage may or may not have significant symptoms.
   (2) Valve replacement with a prosthesis is the indicated therapy.

C. Mitral valve disease

1. Mitral stenosis
   a. Etiology. Although only 50% of patients report a history of rheumatic fever, this is thought to be the cause of mitral stenosis in virtually all cases. **Congenital defects** causing adult mitral stenosis are very rare.
   b. Pathology
      (1) The time interval between the episode of rheumatic fever and the manifestation of mitral stenosis averages between 10 and 25 years.
      (2) The underlying pathologic changes are fusion of the commissures and thickening of the leaflets with or without shortening of the chordae tendineae.
      (3) The normal **cross-sectional area** of the mitral valve is 4–6 cm². In mild mitral stenosis, the area is reduced to 2–2.5 cm²; in moderately severe stenosis, to 1.5–2 cm²; and in severe stenosis, to 1–1.5 cm².
      (4) Pathophysiologic changes include:
         (a) Increased left atrial pressure
         (b) Pulmonary hypertension
         (c) Atrial fibrillation
         (d) Decreased cardiac output
         (e) Increased pulmonary vascular resistance
   c. Clinical presentation
      (1) Dyspnea is the most significant symptom. It indicates pulmonary congestion secondary to increased left atrial pressure.
      (2) Other manifestations include:
         (a) Paroxysmal nocturnal dyspnea and orthopnea
         (b) Chronic cough and hemoptysis
         (c) Pulmonary edema
         (d) Systemic arterial embolization, usually from a left atrial thrombus
      (3) Long-standing pulmonary hypertension may result in right ventricular failure and secondary tricuspid regurgitation.
   d. Diagnosis
      (1) Physical examination. The typical patient is thin and cachectic. Auscultation reveals the **classic triad** of an apical diastolic rumble, opening snap, and loud first heart sound.
      (2) Chest x-ray typically shows a prominent pulmonary vasculature in the upper lung fields. The cardiac silhouette may be normal or may show a double density of the right heart border. A lateral chest x-ray with a barium swallow may detect left atrial enlargement.
      (3) Electrocardiogram may be normal or may show P-wave abnormalities, signs of right ventricular hypertrophy, and right axis deviation.
      (4) Cardiac catheterization is used to calculate the mitral valve cross-sectional area, the mitral valve end diastole pressure gradient, pulmonary artery pressure, and any associated valvular or coronary artery disease.
      (5) M-mode, 2-D, and Doppler echocardiography may complement cardiac catheterization in the diagnosis of mitral stenosis.
   e. Treatment. Surgery is recommended for all patients with symptomatic mitral stenosis. The choice of operative approach depends on the extent of these changes.

(1) Closed or **open mitral valve commissurotomy** should be attempted for a patient with simple fusion of the commissures and minimal calcification, although a later prosthetic valve replacement may be necessary.

(2) Mitral valve replacement is required for patients with severe disease of the chordae tendineae and papillary muscles.

(3) Permanent anticoagulant therapy is especially important for mechanical prosthetic valves in the mitral position to prevent thromboembolization.

2. Mitral insufficiency

a. Etiology. Mitral insufficiency is usually due to rheumatic fever. Other causes include:

(1) Myxomatous degeneration

(2) Papillary muscle dysfunction or rupture secondary to coronary artery disease

(3) Bacterial endocarditis

b. Pathology

(1) The pathogenesis in mitral insufficiency secondary to rheumatic fever is similar to that in mitral stenosis. Why insufficiency predominates in some patients and stenosis in others is not understood.

(2) Pathophysiologic changes include:

(a) Increased left atrial pressure during systole

(b) Late-appearing pulmonary vascular changes, including increased pulmonary vascular resistance

(c) Increased left ventricular stroke volume

c. Clinical presentation

(1) Many years may elapse between the first evidence of mitral insufficiency and the development of symptoms.

(2) In general, symptoms occur late in the course of cardiac decompensation, and include dyspnea on exertion, fatigue, and palpitations.

d. Diagnosis

(1) Physical examination reveals a holosystolic blowing murmur at the apex that radiates to the axilla, accompanied by an accentuated apical impulse. The duration of the murmur in systole correlates with the severity of the disease. Atrial fibrillation may be present.

(2) Chest x-ray demonstrates an enlarged left ventricle and atrium.

(3) Electrocardiogram shows evidence of left ventricular hypertrophy in 50% of cases.

(4) Cardiac catheterization is important to determine left ventricular function, the degree of the mitral valve insufficiency, the pulmonary artery pressure, and any associated valvular or coronary artery disease.

e. Treatment

(1) Medical treatment with digitalis, diuretics, and vasodilator agents, has a significant place in the treatment of stable mitral insufficiency and in preparation for surgery.

(2) Surgical indications include:

(a) Progressive congestive heart failure

(b) Progressive cardiac enlargement

(c) Mitral insufficiency of acute onset, as from ruptured chordae tendineae

(d) Disease in more than one valve

(3) Mitral valve repair with annuloplasty has gained popularity recently, but **mitral valve replacement** remains the preferred treatment.

D. Tricuspid valve, pulmonic valve, and multiple valvular disease

1. Tricuspid stenosis and insufficiency

a. Etiology

(1) Organic tricuspid stenosis is almost always due to rheumatic fever and is most commonly found in association with mitral valve disease. Isolated tricuspid disease is rare.

(2) Functional tricuspid insufficiency is the result of right ventricular dilatation secondary to pulmonary hypertension and right ventricular failure. Functional insufficiency is commoner than organic tricuspid valve disease.

(3) Tricuspid insufficiency is sometimes seen in the carcinoid syndrome, secondary to blunt trauma or secondary to bacterial endocarditis in drug addicts.

b. Pathology

(1) The pathogenesis in tricuspid stenosis secondary to rheumatic fever is similar to that in mitral valve disease.

(2) Elevation of right atrial pressure secondary to tricuspid stenosis leads to peripheral edema, jugular venous distention, hepatomegaly, and ascites.

c. Clinical presentation

(1) Moderate isolated tricuspid insufficiency is usually well tolerated.

(2) When right-sided heart failure occurs, symptoms (edema, hepatomegaly, ascites) develop.

d. Diagnosis

(1) Physical examination

(a) Tricuspid insufficiency produces a systolic murmur at the lower end of the sternum.

(b) Tricuspid stenosis produces a diastolic murmur in the same region.

(c) A prominent jugular venous pulse may be observed.

(d) The liver may be pulsatile in tricuspid insufficiency.

(2) Chest x-ray shows enlargement of the right heart, which may also be reflected on the electrocardiogram.

(3) Cardiac catheterization is the most accurate guide to diagnosing tricuspid disease. It should include evaluation of any associated aortic or mitral valve lesions.

e. Treatment

(1) Isolated tricuspid disease, especially tricuspid insufficiency, may be well tolerated without surgical intervention.

(2) In mild to moderate tricuspid insufficiency associated with mitral valve disease, opinion varies concerning the need for tricuspid surgery.

(3) In the case of extensive tricuspid insufficiency associated with mitral valve disease, the consensus is that either **tricuspid repair** or **tricuspid valve replacement** is appropriate.

(4) Tricuspid stenosis, when significant, is remedied by **commissurotomy** or **valve replacement**.

(5) Valve excision alone may be indicated in certain cases of tricuspid insufficiency secondary to endocarditis, especially in intravenous drug abusers.

2. Pulmonic valve disease

a. Pathology. Acquired lesions of the pulmonic valve are uncommon. The carcinoid syndrome, however, may produce pulmonic stenosis.

b. Treatment. Surgical **repair** or **replacement of the valve** is carried out when warranted by the degree of dysfunction.

3. Multiple valvular disease

a. Pathology. More than one valve may be involved in rheumatic fever as indicated in the foregoing discussions. Abnormal physiologic responses to multivalvular disease may be additive but usually reflect the most severely affected valve.

b. Treatment involves **repair** or **replacement of all valves** with significant dysfunction.

E. Coronary artery disease

1. Etiology and epidemiology

a. Atherosclerosis is the predominant pathogenetic mechanism underlying obstructive disease of the coronary arteries. Uncommon causes of coronary artery disease include vasculitis (occurring with collagen vascular disorders), radiation injury, and trauma.

b. Atherosclerotic heart disease represents the commonest cause of death in the United States and most other developed nations.

c. Coronary artery disease is four times more prevalent in men than in women, although the incidence in women is rapidly increasing.

d. Risk factors for coronary artery disease that have been identified by epidemiologic studies include:

(1) Hypertension

(2) Smoking

(3) Hypercholesterolemia

(4) Family history of heart disease

(5) Diabetes

(6) Obesity

2. Pathophysiologic effects of ischemic coronary artery disease on the myocardium include:

a. Decreased ventricular compliance

b. Decreased cardiac contractility

c. Myocardial necrosis

3. **Clinical presentation.** Coronary artery disease may take the form of:
   a. **Angina pectoris**
      (1) Angina pectoris typically presents as substernal chest pain lasting 5–10 minutes. The pain may be precipitated by emotional stress, exertion, or cold weather and is relieved by rest.
      (2) Angina may be characterized by its patterns of occurrence:
         (a) Stable angina: angina that is unchanged for a prolonged period
         (b) Unstable angina: angina that shows a recent change from a previously stable pattern, including new-onset angina
         (c) Angina at rest
         (d) Postinfarction angina
   b. **Myocardial infarction**
   c. **Congestive heart failure**
   d. **Sudden death**

4. **Diagnosis**
   a. **History.** The diagnosis of angina pectoris due to coronary artery disease is most often made from the patient's history.
   b. **Electrocardiogram**
      (1) The electrocardiogram is normal in up to 75% of patients when they are at rest without pain.
      (2) ST-segment changes and T-wave changes may be seen.
      (3) Evidence of a previous infarction may be apparent.
   c. **Exercise stress testing** will induce angina in approximately 80% of patients.
   d. **A radiothallium scan** of the heart may be helpful.
   e. **Cardiac catheterization and coronary angiography** provide the most accurate means of determining the extent of coronary artery disease. Obstruction is considered physiologically significant when the diameter of the vessel on angiography is narrowed by 50%. In addition, left ventricular function may be assessed by the ventriculogram and hemodynamic measurements.

5. **Treatment**
   a. **Medical treatment.** Management of coronary artery disease is initiated with medical therapy in patients with stable angina and with no evidence of congestive heart failure.
      (1) Drugs used include nitrates, β-blockers, digitalis derivatives, and calcium channel blockers.
      (2) In addition, the patient is encouraged to adopt a low-fat diet, stop smoking, and begin a graded exercise program.
   b. **Surgical treatment**
      (1) Coronary artery bypass. Coronary artery obstructive disease is treated surgically by providing a bypass around physiologically significant lesions, using a reversed autogenous saphenous vein or internal mammary artery (IMA).
      (2) Percutaneous transluminal coronary angioplasty (PTCA) is an increasingly more frequent alternative to coronary artery bypass in select "morphologically" favorable lesions.
         (a) Indications for coronary artery bypass include:
            (i) Intractable or unstable angina pectoris
            (ii) Angina pectoris with left main coronary artery obstruction, obstruction of the three main coronary arteries (**"triple-vessel disease"**) with depressed ventricular function, or proximal obstruction of the left anterior descending artery
         (b) Relative contraindications for coronary artery bypass include:
            (i) Stable angina pectoris with single-vessel right coronary artery or circumflex coronary artery disease is not usually considered an indication for surgery.
            (ii) Congestive heart failure may be an anginal equivalent and respond favorably to coronary artery bypass. However, severe congestive heart failure *without* angina is a relative contraindication to bypass surgery.
            (iii) Acute myocardial infarction that presents in less than 6 hours is generally treated with thrombolytic therapy and percutaneous transluminal coronary angioplasty, although some centers continue to advocate emergency bypass surgery.

c. Prognosis after bypass surgery
  (1) The results of coronary artery revascularization depend on the patient's preoperative left ventricular function. A left ventricular systolic ejection fraction of less than 0.3 constitutes an increased but acceptable operative risk.
  (2) In patients with stable angina, the accepted operative mortality rate is around 1%. About 85%–95% of patients are helped significantly with 85% having complete freedom from angina.
  (3) Surgery increases survival in patients with "left main disease" and triple-vessel disease with depressed ventricular function.
  (4) Ten-year patency rates for IMA grafts are more than 90%, whereas vein graft patency is only 50% at 10 years. Therefore, the IMA is the conduit of choice for coronary artery bypass. There has been recent work using the gastroepiploic artery as a bypass conduit with early favorable results. Definitive recommendation must await long-term follow-up.

6. Surgical treatment of myocardial infarction complications. Myocardial infarction and many of its complications are treated medically, but some complications warrant surgery. These include the following:
  a. Ventricular aneurysms. The scarred myocardium may produce either akinesia or dyskinesia of ventricular wall motion, decreasing the ejection fraction.
    (1) This may result in congestive heart failure, ventricular arrhythmias, or, rarely, systemic thromboembolization.
    (2) Surgical correction of the aneurysm is undertaken when these problems occur.
    (3) Coronary revascularization may also be warranted at the same time.
  b. Ruptured ventricle is rare, and the mortality rate approaches 100% without surgery.
  c. Rupture of the interventricular septum carries a high mortality rate. Again, early operative repair is important.
  d. Mitral valve papillary muscle dysfunction or rupture
    (1) Usually the posterior papillary muscle is involved.
    (2) Treatment is by mitral valve replacement or repair.
    (3) Long-term survival is dependent on the extent of myocardial damage.

F. Cardiac tumors

1. Types of tumors
  a. Benign tumors
    (1) **Myxomas**, which account for 75%–80% of benign cardiac tumors, may be either pedunculated or sessile. Most are pedunculated and are found in the left atrium attached to the septum.
    (2) Other benign tumors include rhabdomyomas (commonest in childhood), fibromas, and lipomas.
  b. Malignant tumors. Overall, primary malignant tumors account for 20%–25% of all primary cardiac tumors. The various types of sarcomas are the commonest.
  c. Metastatic tumors occur more frequently than primary cardiac tumors (benign or malignant).
    (1) Autopsy studies show cardiac involvement by metastatic disease in about 10% of patients who have died of malignancy.
    (2) Melanoma, lymphoma, and leukemia are the tumors that most often metastasize to the heart.

2. Clinical presentation. Cardiac neoplasms may be manifested by pericardial effusion, resulting in cardiac tamponade; or by congestive heart failure, arrhythmias, peripheral embolization (especially with myxomas), or other constitutional signs and symptoms.

3. Treatment is by **surgical excision** if possible.

G. Cardiac trauma. Injuries to the heart may be divided into several categories.

1. Penetrating injury may involve any area of the heart, although the anterior position of the right ventricle makes it the most commonly involved chamber.
  a. Penetrating wounds may result from gunshots, knives, and so forth. In addition, penetrating injury may be iatrogenic, as results from catheters or pacing wires.
  b. Bleeding into the pericardium is a common consequence. **Pericardial tamponade** may result, manifested by:
    (1) Distended neck veins

(2) Hypotension

(3) Pulsus paradoxus

(4) Distant heart sounds

  c. Small wounds may spontaneously seal, in which case pericardiocentesis may suffice; however, open thoracotomy may be required.

  2. Blunt trauma may be more extensive than is usually appreciated.

    a. History of a significant blow to the chest, with or without fractured ribs or sternum, should create a high index of suspicion of a cardiac contusion or infarction. A patient with such a history should be observed and monitored in a manner similar to a patient suffering from myocardial infarction, because the trauma is likely to cause a similar myocardial injury.

      (1) Serial electrocardiograms and cardiac enzyme studies should be obtained.

      (2) Echocardiography may be helpful in determining myocardial injury.

      (3) The appearance of new murmurs should be investigated and may call for cardiac catheterization.

    b. Treatment. Blunt trauma may cause rupture of a tricuspid, mitral, or aortic valve, requiring treatment by valve replacement or repair.

H. Pericardial disorders

  1. Pericardial effusion

    a. The pericardium responds to noxious stimuli by an increased production of fluid.

    b. A pericardial effusion volume as small as 100 ml may produce symptomatic tamponade if the fluid accumulates rapidly, while larger amounts may be tolerated if it accumulates slowly.

    c. Pericardial effusion is treated by pericardiocentesis or by tube pericardiostomy via a subxyphoid approach.

    d. Chronic effusions, such as those that occur with malignant involvement of the pericardium, may require pericardiectomy via left thoracotomy or sternotomy.

  2. Pericarditis may be acute or chronic.

    a. Acute pericarditis

      (1) Causes of acute pericarditis include:

        (a) Bacterial infection, as from staphylococci or streptococci. Acute pyogenic pericarditis is uncommon and is usually associated with a systemic illness.

        (b) Viral infection

        (c) Uremia

        (d) Traumatic hemopericardium

        (e) Malignant disease

        (f) Connective tissue disorders

      (2) Treatment consists of managing the underlying cause. Open pericardial drainage may be required. Most cases of acute pericarditis resolve without serious sequelae.

    b. Chronic pericarditis may represent recurrent episodes of an acute process or undiagnosed long-standing viral pericarditis. The etiology is often impossible to establish. It may go unnoticed until it results in the chronic constrictive form, causing chronic tamponade.

    c. Chronic constrictive pericarditis presents with dyspnea on exertion, easy fatigability, marked jugular venous distention, ascites, hepatomegaly, and peripheral edema.

      (1) Chest x-ray may show pericardial calcification.

      (2) Cardiac catheterization may be needed to confirm the diagnosis.

      (3) Once the diagnosis has been established in the symptomatic patient, **pericardiectomy** should be undertaken with or without the use of cardiopulmonary bypass.

II. CONGENITAL HEART DISEASE

A. Overview

  1. The incidence of congenital heart disease is approximately 3/1000 births.

  2. Etiology. In most cases the etiology is unknown.

    a. Rubella occurring in the first trimester of pregnancy is known to cause congenital heart disease (e.g., patent ductus arteriosus).

    b. Down's syndrome is associated with endocardial cushion defects.

3. Types. The commonest forms of congenital heart disease are in decreasing order:
   a. Ventricular septal defect
   b. Transposition of the great vessels
   c. Tetralogy of Fallot
   d. Hypoplastic left heart syndrome
   e. Atrial septal defect
   f. Patent ductus arteriosus
   g. Coarctation of the aorta
   h. Endocardial cushion defects

4. History
   a. The mother should be questioned about difficulties during the pregnancy, especially in the first trimester.
   b. The mother often states that the child shows the following symptoms, which indicate pulmonary overcirculation and congestive heart failure.
      (1) Easy fatigability and decreased exercise tolerance
      (2) Poor feeding habits and poor weight gain
      (3) Frequent pulmonary infections
   c. A history of cyanosis should be sought, as this indicates a right-to-left shunt.

5. Physical examination
   a. Abnormalities in growth and development should be identified.
   b. Cyanosis and clubbing of the fingers may be noted.
   c. Examination of the heart should proceed in the same manner as in the adult.
      (1) Systolic murmurs are frequently found in infants and small children and may not be of clinical significance.
      (2) A gallop rhythm is of great clinical importance.
      (3) Congestive heart failure in children is frequently manifested by hepatic enlargement.

B. Patent ductus arteriosus

1. Pathophysiology
   a. In the normal infant born at term, the ductus arteriosus closes within the first few days of life.
   b. Hypoxia and certain prostaglandins may act to keep the ductus open.
   c. The natural history in patent ductus arteriosus is variable.
      (1) A small percentage of patients will experience heart failure within the first year of life, while others will suffer later from pulmonary vascular disease if undiagnosed.
      (2) Many patients will remain asymptomatic and will be diagnosed later upon routine examination.
      (3) Patent ductus arteriosus may be seen in combination with other defects, such as ventricular septal defect and coarctation of the aorta.

2. Clinical presentation. Common presenting complaints are dyspnea, fatigue, and palpitations, signifying congestive heart failure.

3. Diagnosis is based primarily on the physical findings.
   a. Physical examination
      (1) The classic continuous "machinery-like" murmur is usually heard, but it may be absent until age 1 year.
      (2) Other signs include a widened pulse pressure and bounding peripheral pulses.
      (3) Cyanosis may be seen in patent ductus arteriosus that is associated with other anomalies or in right-to-left shunt from pulmonary vascular disease.
   b. Cardiac catheterization is useful in determining the existence of other associated lesions.

4. Treatment
   a. Surgical management consists of **ligation of the ductus**. This is reserved for:
      (1) Premature infants with severe pulmonary dysfunction
      (2) Infants who suffer from congestive heart failure within the first year of life
      (3) Asymptomatic children with a patent ductus that persists until the age of 2 or 3 years
   b. Indomethacin, a prostaglandin inhibitor, has been used in attempts to close the ductus in premature infants with symptomatic simple patent ductus arteriosus.

C. Coarctation of the aorta

   1. Overview. Coarctation is found twice as often in male as in female children.

      a. It is commonly located adjacently to the ductus arteriosus.

      b. Coarctation may be fatal in the first few months of life if not treated.

      c. Associated intracardiac defects, present in up to 60% of patients, include patent ductus arteriosus and ventricular septal defect.

   2. Clinical presentation

      a. Some children are asymptomatic for varying periods of time.

      b. In others, symptoms suggesting congestive heart failure are present shortly after birth.

      c. Headaches, epistaxis, lower extremity weakness, and dizziness may be seen in the child with symptomatic coarctation.

   3. Diagnosis

      a. Physical findings include:

         (1) Upper extremity hypertension

         (2) Absent or diminished pulses in the lower extremities

         (3) A systolic murmur

      b. Chest x-ray may reveal ''rib-notching'' in older children, representing collateral pathways via intercostal arteries.

      c. Cardiac catheterization is usually recommended to define the location of the coarctation and any associated cardiac defects.

   4. Treatment

      a. Surgical correction of the coarctation is indicated for all patients and may be delayed until age 5 or 6 years in asymptomatic patients.

      b. Operative procedures include:

         (1) Resection and **end-to-end anastomosis**

         (2) Prosthetic patch graft

         (3) A **subclavian flap procedure**

      c. Any associated defects must also be corrected.

   5. Complications

      a. Residual hypertension may be a problem postoperatively.

      b. Spinal cord injury due to ischemia during surgery may manifest itself postoperatively.

      c. Postoperative mesenteric ischemia is seen in a small but significant number of cases and is related to postoperative hypertension.

D. Atrial septal defects

   1. Classification. Atrial septal defects occur twice as frequently in female as in male children. Three types are commonly seen:

      a. Ostium secundum defects, which account for most atrial septal defects, are found in the midportion of the atrial septum.

      b. Sinus venosus defects are located high up on the atrial septum and are often associated with anomalies of pulmonary venous drainage.

      c. Ostium primum defects are components of atrioventricular septal defects and are located on the atrial side of the mitral and tricuspid valves.

      d. A **patent foramen ovale** is **not** considered an atrial septal defect.

   2. Pathophysiology

      a. Atrial pressures are equal on both sides of a large atrial septal defect.

      b. Since atrial emptying occurs during ventricular diastole, the direction of shunt at the **atrial level** is determined by the relative compliances of the **right** and **left ventricles** (diastolic phenomena). Since the right ventricle is more compliant than the left, **flow is left to right across an atrial septal defect**.

      c. This results in a modest increase in pulmonary blood flow, which causes mild growth retardation.

      d. If uncorrected, pulmonary vascular disease may develop, resulting in cor pulmonale.

   3. Clinical presentation. Mild dyspnea and easy fatigability are seen in infancy and early childhood. Such symptoms increase in severity with age and may manifest in adulthood as congestive heart failure, often brought on by the onset of atrial fibrillation.

4. Diagnosis

a. **Physical examination** reveals a systolic murmur in the left second or third intercostal space and a fixed, split, second heart sound.

b. **Chest x-ray** reveals moderate enlargement of the right ventricle and prominence of the pulmonary vasculature.

c. **Electrocardiogram** reveals right ventricular hypertrophy.

d. **Cardiac catheterization** can make the diagnosis from the "step-up" in oxygen saturation in the right atrium. The amount of left-to-right shunt may be calculated.

5. Treatment is based on the size of the left-to-right shunt.

a. Spontaneous closure is extremely rare after age 2.

b. Surgical closure of the defect is indicated if the pulmonary blood flow is one and one-half to two times greater than the systemic blood flow.

c. Surgery carries a mortality risk of less than 1%.

d. Ideal time for closure is age 4 or 5, prior to beginning school.

E. Ventricular septal defects

1. Classification. Ventricular septal defects are the commonest congenital heart defects. Associated anomalies, such as coarctation of the aorta, are common. They may be classified according to their location in the ventricular septum:

a. Infracristal (membranous), the commonest type

b. Supracristal

c. Atrioventricular canal type

d. Muscular

2. Pathophysiology

a. Ventricular **pressures** are **equal** on either side of a large ventricular septal defect.

b. Since ventricular emptying occurs during systole, the direction of the shunt at the ventricular level is determined by the **relative resistances** of the **pulmonary** and **systemic circuits** (systolic phenomena).

(1) Since the pulmonary vascular resistance is much less than the systemic vascular resistance, **flow is left to right across a ventricular septal defect**.

(2) This causes markedly increased pulmonary blood flow, which imposes a volume load on the left ventricle and may lead to early congestive heart failure.

c. Other adverse effects of pulmonary overcirculation include:

(1) Poor feeding

(2) Failure to thrive

(3) Frequent respiratory tract infections

(4) Increased pulmonary vascular resistance

(5) Development of irreversible pulmonary vascular occlusive disease if untreated

(a) This results in a higher pulmonary vascular resistance than systemic resistance, and reversal of flow occurs (Eisenmenger's syndrome).

(b) At this point, the patient is inoperable

3. Clinical presentation

a. Small ventricular septal defects rarely cause significant symptoms in infancy or early childhood and may undergo spontaneous closure before they are recognized.

b. Symptoms are usually seen with ventricular septal defects, which approach the diameter of the aortic root.

(1) Children with large defects usually have dyspnea on exertion, easy fatigability, and an increased incidence of pulmonary infections.

(2) Severe cardiac failure may be seen in infants but is less common in children.

4. Diagnosis

a. **Physical examination** reveals a harsh pansystolic murmur.

b. **Chest x-ray and electrocardiogram**, especially in large ventricular septal defects, show evidence of biventricular hypertrophy.

c. **Cardiac catheterization** is essential for delineating the severity of the left-to-right shunt, pulmonary vascular resistance, and the location of the defects.

5. Treatment

a. Surgical closure of the defect should be performed in:

(1) Infants with significant cardiac failure or increased pulmonary vascular resistance

(2) Asymptomatic children with significant shunts who have not had spontaneous closure by age 2 years

      (3) Patients with pulmonary blood flow one and one-half to two times greater than systemic flow

    b. Operative mortality risk (< 5%) is related to the degree of preoperative pulmonary vascular disease.

F. Tetralogy of Fallot

1. Pathophysiology

    a. The tetralogy of Fallot, one of the commonest **cyanotic congenital heart disorders**, consists of:

      (1) Obstruction to right ventricular outflow

      (2) A ventricular septal defect

      (3) Hypertrophy of the right ventricle

      (4) An overriding aorta

    b. The addition of an atrial septal defect (which is of little further physiologic significance) turns the condition into the **pentalogy of Fallot**.

    c. Since resistance to right ventricular outflow exceeds the systemic vascular resistance, the shunt is right to left, resulting in desaturation of the blood and cyanosis.

    d. Exercise tolerance is limited because of the inability to increase pulmonary blood flow.

2. Clinical presentation

    a. Cyanosis and dyspnea on exertion are routinely seen in patients with tetralogy of Fallot. Children soon learn that by squatting they can temporarily alleviate these symptoms.

      (1) Squatting increases the systemic vascular resistance, which decreases the magnitude of right-to-left shunt and causes an increase in pulmonary blood flow.

      (2) The cyanosis is seen at birth in 30% of the cases, by the first year in 30%, and later in childhood in the remainder. Polycythemia and clubbing accompany the cyanosis.

    b. Cerebrovascular accidents and brain sepsis constitute the major threats to life, as cardiac failure is rare.

3. Diagnosis

    a. **Physical examination** reveals clubbing of the digits and cyanosis. A harsh systolic murmur of pulmonary stenosis is often heard.

    b. **Cardiac catheterization** is important for determining the level of pulmonic outflow obstruction and the size of the main and branch pulmonary arteries.

4. Treatment depends on many variables, including the anatomy of the defect and the age of the child.

    a. Total correction is undertaken after the age of 2 years.

    b. Controversy exists over whether the defect should be corrected before this age. Many feel that a palliative **systemic-to-pulmonary** (Blalock-Taussig) **shunt** should be done initially, followed by definitive correction at a later date.

    c. The risk of surgery depends on the age of the patient and the degree of cyanosis.

    d. After correction, a dramatic improvement is usually seen.

G. Transposition of the great arteries

1. Pathophysiology

    a. Transposition of the great arteries (TGA) occurs when the **aorta** arises from the morphologic **right ventricle**, and the **pulmonary artery** arises from the morphologic **left ventricle**. This results in two independent parallel circuits.

    b. Survival is dependent on a **communication** between the right and left sides of the heart to allow mixing of oxygenated and unoxygenated blood. This usually occurs across an atrial septal defect, although a patent ductus arteriosus or ventricular septal defect could also be present.

2. Diagnosis is based on arterial blood gas, chest x-ray, and echocardiogram

3. Treatment

    a. Initial **balloon atrial septostomy** is performed to increase the size of the interatrial communication and facilitate mixing of blood.

    b. This is followed by definitive surgical correction.

    c. Operative procedures include:

      (1) Atrial inversion (Senning or Mustard procedures)

      (2) Arterial switch (Jatene operation)

Part II Thoracic Disorders

STUDY QUESTIONS

Directions: Each question below contains five suggested answers. Choose the **one best** response to each question.

1. Hoarseness secondary to bronchogenic carcinoma is usually due to extension of the tumor into what structure?

(A) Vocal cord
(B) Superior laryngeal nerve
(C) Left recurrent laryngeal nerve
(D) Right vagus nerve
(E) Larynx

2. Which of the following findings indicates incurability of a lung cancer?

(A) Recurrent pneumonia
(B) Sputum cytology positive for cancer
(C) Shortness of breath
(D) Left vocal cord paralysis
(E) Clubbing of the digits

3. A patient undergoes a left scalene node biopsy to rule out carcinoma of the lung. One hour later the patient is cyanotic, dyspneic, and has a marked tachycardia with decreased breath sounds on the left. What is the maneuver that is most likely to improve the patient's condition?

(A) Blood transfusion
(B) Insertion of a right subclavian catheter and administration of intravenous fluids
(C) Endotracheal intubation
(D) Insertion of a left chest tube
(E) Re-exploration of the wound

4. All of the following symptoms and signs are indicative of a tension pneumothorax EXCEPT

(A) chest pain
(B) shortness of breath
(C) absent breath sounds unilaterally
(D) shifting of the trachea toward the pneumothorax
(E) hypotension

5. A 24-year-old man involved in a motor vehicle accident presents with blood pressure 80/60, heart rate 135, and respirations 45 and labored. Physical examination reveals agitation, sternal flail, and absent breath sounds in the left hemithorax, which is crepitant to palpation and resonant to percussion. The initial maneuver should be to

(A) obtain a chest x-ray
(B) intubate the patient
(C) place a left chest tube
(D) begin two large-bore intravenous needles
(E) place antishock garment

Questions 6 and 7

Chest x-ray of a 55-year-old man involved in a high-speed motor vehicle accident shows a widened mediastinum and pneumomediastinum, and electrocardiogram shows sinus tachycardia with frequent premature ventricular contractions.

6. All of the following maneuvers are appropriate at this time EXCEPT

(A) aortogram
(B) bronchoscopy
(C) continuous cardiac monitoring
(D) left thoracotomy
(E) endotracheal intubation

7. Expected physiologic changes due to blunt chest trauma include all of the following EXCEPT

(A) elevated P_{CO_2}
(B) increased compliance
(C) elevated A gradient
(D) decreased ventricular contractions
(E) elevated shunt fractions

(end of group question)

8. Management of a lung abscess refractory to prolonged antibiotic treatment include all of the following EXCEPT

(A) lobectomy
(B) open drainage
(C) tube drainage
(D) intracavitary antibiotic instillation
(E) bronchoscopic endobronchial drainage

9. Indications for resection in patients with pulmonary tuberculosis include all of the following EXCEPT

(A) destroyed lung or lobe
(B) residual cavity with positive sputum
(C) residual cavity with negative sputum
(D) hemoptysis
(E) suspected carcinoma

10. All of the following diagnoses in a 60-year-old man with a peripheral solitary pulmonary nodule (coin lesion) are likely EXCEPT

(A) bronchogenic carcinoma
(B) tuberculosis
(C) metastatic colon cancer
(D) hamartoma
(E) sarcoidosis

11. Unfavorable prognostic findings in a patient with non–small cell carcinoma include all of the following EXCEPT

(A) pulmonary osteoarthropathy
(B) chest wall invasion
(C) adenocarcinoma cell type
(D) hoarseness
(E) pleural effusion

12. The most acceptable measure in the management of a patient with a suspected carcinoma of the lung and with no evidence of spread is

(A) surgical resection of the lesion
(B) intense radiation therapy
(C) chemotherapy
(D) chemotherapy followed by resection
(E) re-evaluation in 2 months to determine if the lesion is larger or has spread

13. Middle mediastinal masses include all of the following EXCEPT

(A) bronchogenic cyst
(B) ascending aortic aneurysm
(C) pericardial cyst
(D) ganglioneuroma
(E) lymphoma

14. The usual management of cardiac arrest should include all of the following protocols EXCEPT

(A) immediate resuscitation, as irreversible brain damage will result after 3–4 minutes of diminished perfusion
(B) establishment of an airway and ventilatory support
(C) open-chest cardiac massage
(D) defibrillation, if cardiac arrest is due to ventricular fibrillation
(E) administration of cardiotonic agents

15. All of the following complications of myocardial infarction are indications for surgical correction EXCEPT

(A) ventricular premature beats
(B) a ventricular aneurysm
(C) a ruptured ventricle
(D) a ruptured intraventricular septum
(E) papillary muscle dysfunction

16. True statements concerning pericardial disease include all of the following EXCEPT

(A) the pericardium responds to noxious stimuli by an increased production of fluid
(B) a rapidly accumulating pericardial effusion must have a volume of at least 250 ml before symptoms will occur
(C) pericardial effusion is treated by tube pericardiostomy
(D) chronically occurring effusions (e.g., from malignant involvement of the pericardium) are best treated by creation of a pericardial window
(E) constrictive pericarditis most likely follows an occult viral infection

17. In the normal term infant, the ductus arteriosus closes within the first few days of life. If the ductus remains patent, the clinical features likely to result include

(A) a classic "machinery-like" murmur
(B) right-to-left shunt
(C) clubbing of the fingers
(D) coarctation of the aorta
(E) cyanosis

18. Coarctation of the aorta is best characterized by which of the following statements?

(A) It is found twice as often in female as in male children
(B) Physical findings include decreased pulsations in the upper and lower extremities
(C) Surgical correction is indicated in all patients, ideally when the child is 1–2 years old
(D) Hypotension is a frequent postoperative problem
(E) Headaches, lower extremity weakness, and dizziness are seen in the child with symptomatic coarctation

Directions: The groups of questions below consist of lettered choices followed by several numbered items. For each numbered item select the **one** lettered choice with which it is **most** closely associated. Each lettered choice may be used once, more than once, or not at all.

Questions 19–23

Match the following.

(A) Mechanical cardiac valve prosthesis
(B) Tissue valve cardiac prosthesis
(C) Both
(D) Neither

19. Higher incidence of thromboembolism

20. Usually fails gradually rather than abruptly

21. Requires anticoagulation indefinitely

22. Frequent cure of acute bacterial endocarditis by antibiotics alone

23. Has a low incidence of valve-induced hemolysis

Questions 24–27

For each clinical presentation listed below, select the cyst or tumor that is most likely to be associated with it.

(A) Neuroblastoma
(B) Bronchogenic cyst
(C) Thymoma
(D) Pericardial cyst
(E) Teratoma

24. Cardiophrenic angle

25. Myasthenia gravis

26. Posterior mediastinum

27. Calcification

Questions 28–31

Echocardiographic examination of the left-sided cardiac chamber reveals the morphology listed below. Match each set of morphologic data with the most appropriate anatomic valvular lesion.

(A) Left atrium: normal
   Left ventricle: hypertrophy
   Aorta: normal
(B) Left atrium: dilatation/hypertrophy
   Left ventricle: normal
   Aorta: normal
(C) Left atrium: normal
   Left ventricle: dilatation
   Aorta: dilatation
(D) Left atrium: dilatation
   Left ventricle: dilatation
   Aorta: normal

28. Aortic regurgitation

29. Aortic stenosis

30. Mitral regurgitation

31. Mitral stenosis

ANSWERS AND EXPLANATIONS

1. The answer is C. [*Chapter 4 I B 2 a*] Bronchogenic carcinoma invades the left recurrent laryngeal nerve as it passes around the aortic arch; when this happens, hoarseness results. This finding indicates nonresectability of the tumor.

2. The answer is D. [*Chapter 4 I B 2 a*] Vocal cord paralysis is evidence of invasion of the recurrent laryngeal nerve by the cancer. Recurrent pneumonia, a positive sputum cytology, shortness of breath, and clubbing of the digits are general symptoms and signs that can be present in the absence of tumor extension or metastasis.

3. The answer is D. [*Chapter 4 I B 3 c*] The pleura of the lung lies immediately adjacent to the scalene fat pad. If the pleura is injured during scalene node biopsy, a pneumothorax can result, causing the symptoms that developed in the patient described in the question. Other nearby structures include the lymph duct structures, the brachial plexus, the vagus and phrenic nerves, and the subclavian vessels. Any of these structures can also be injured during scalene node biopsy with corresponding symptoms.

4. The answer is D. [*Chapter 4 II A 2*] Tension pneumothorax results from the trapping of air within the pleural space of the affected lung. The resultant total-volume (air and lung) increase on the affected side shifts the mediastinum away from that side. Hypotension results from impaired venous return, which is due to distortion of the vena cava by the mediastinal shift.

5. The answer is C. [*Chapter 4 II A 2 a–c*] While all of the maneuvers described in the question are appropriate in the evaluation and resuscitation of the multiply injured patient, the findings listed are indicative of a left tension pneumothorax. Immediate treatment is to decompress the pleural space by chest tube insertion.

6. The answer is D. [*Chapter 4 II A 5, 6, B 1, 2, 5, 6*] Causes for the chest x-ray and electrocardiographic findings described in the question are multiple and include aortic rupture, cardiac tamponade, tracheobronchial disruption, hypoxia, and cardiac contusion. A more precise diagnosis would be mandatory prior to undertaking thoracotomy, since operative strategy would vary greatly, depending on which of these injuries is present.

7. The answer is B. [*Chapter 4 II A 6*] Blunt thoracic trauma with or without flail chest results in chest wall muscle damage and pain with resultant splinting and loss of chest wall elasticity. Intra-alveolar hemorrhage and interstitial edema cause a reduction of pulmonary parenchymal elasticity. Therefore, both lung and chest wall compliance are decreased. All of the remaining features would be expected on the basis of the same pathophysiology.

8. The answer is D. [*Chapter 5 III A 2 a*] Acute lung abcesses usually respond to intravenous antibiotic therapy; however, scarring can occur, preventing resolution and mandating surgical intervention. Choice of procedure is determined largely by the patient's general status. Low-risk patients tolerate lobectomy well, whereas high-risk patients can be treated by either open or closed drainage techniques. Endobronchial drainage facilitated by the rigid or fiberoptic bronchoscope is occasionally successful.

9. The answer is C. [*Chapter 5 III C 2 b*] An open cavity with negative sputum is not generally felt to be an indication for resection. These patients usually do well on long-term follow-up. Complications of tuberculosis that require resectional therapy include lung destruction with or without secondary bacterial infection, hemoptysis when the site of bleeding can be accurately identified, and residual cavities with persistent positive sputum, which do not respond to continued chemotherapy. If carcinoma is suspected, then surgery is necessary to rule this out.

10. The answer is E. [*Chapter 5 IV B 4, 5*] Sarcoidosis does not present as a solitary lung nodule. Bronchogenic carcinoma, tuberculosis, metastatic colon cancer, and hamartoma can all result in a solitary pulmonary lesion. The most likely diagnosis among those listed is bronchogenic carcinoma.

11. The answer is A. [*Chapter 5 V B 1, 2, C 2, E 1 f, 2 c, d*] The presence of pulmonary osteoarthropathy without other specific poor prognostic signs is not unfavorable in and of itself and should not alter treatment plans. Chest wall invasion by definition describes a T3 primary tumor and, therefore, a stage III lesion. Adenocarcinoma cell type is associated with a less favorable cell type than squamous cell or bronchoalveolar carcinoma. Hoarseness indicates metastases to the aortopulmonary lymph nodes, and this denotes poor prognosis (N2 or N3 disease). Pleural effusion of any type associated with carcinoma of the lung is a poor prognostic sign.

12. The answer is A. [*Chapter 5 V F 1, G 2*] The best chance for a cure in carcinoma of the lung is provided by expeditious thoracotomy with resection of the tumor. In a patient with no evidence of metastatic disease and with a less malignant histologic cell type, the likelihood of survival for 5 years postoperatively may be as high as 60%–80%. Preoperative radiation therapy has only been useful for superior sulcus tumor.

13. The answer is D. [*Chapter 5 X A, B 1, 2, C 2 d*] The commonest lesions of the middle mediastinum are enterogenous cysts, which have their origin from the embryonic foregut. These include bronchogenic cysts and esophageal duplication cysts. Pericardial cysts also occur in the middle mediastinum, most often found at the right cardiophrenic angle. Lymphomas can occur at any location in the mediastinum. Ascending aortic aneurysms are included as middle mediastinal masses. Ganglioneuromas, however, occur only in the posterior mediastinum.

14. The answer is C. [*Chapter 6 I A 6 b, c*] Immediate resuscitation, establishment of an airway, ventilatory support, closed-chest cardiac massage, and defibrillation are all appropriate protocols for the management of cardiac arrest. In addition, drug therapy may also be appropriate. Agents that may be useful include epinephrine and calcium for their cardiotonic effects, sodium bicarbonate to treat the associated acidosis, and vasopressors to support blood pressure. While open-cardiac massage is occasionally required for traumatic cardiac arrest or for arrest occurring after open-heart surgery, most instances are managed by closed-chest massage.

15. The answer is A. [*Chapter 6 I E 6*] Myocardial infarction and many of its complications are treated medically, including a variety of arrhythmias that can occur. However, some complications require surgery. The scarred myocardium of a ventricular aneurysm may produce akinesia or dyskinesia of the ventricular wall, which will decrease the ejection fraction. In addition, thrombosis can form in this area, and distal thromboembolization may result. Aneurysms should be corrected if either of these two complications are present. Rupture of the ventricle and rupture of the intraventricular septum carry extremely high mortality rates and require surgical correction as early as possible. Severe papillary muscle dysfunction or papillary muscle rupture results in mitral valvular incompetence. This should be corrected promptly with surgical replacement of the mitral valve.

16. The answer is B. [*Chapter 6 I H 1*] A pericardial effusion volume as small as 100 ml may produce symptomatic tamponade if the fluid accumulates rapidly. Large amounts may be tolerated if the accumulation is gradual. Chronically occurring effusions, such as those that occur with malignant involvement of the pericardium, may require creation of a pericardial window to allow drainage of fluid into the chest. Chronic constrictive pericarditis is most likely a sequela of prior viral infection, although a definite history is rarely obtained. It is also associated with tuberculous pericarditis.

17. The answer is A. [*Chapter 6 II B 3*] Hypoxia and certain prostaglandins may act to keep the ductus arteriosus patent in a newborn infant; it normally closes within the first few days of life. The history of patent ductus arteriosus is variable. Common presenting symptoms include dyspnea, fatigue, and palpitations, signifying congestive heart failure; however, many patients remain asymptomatic. On physical examination, a "machinery-like" murmur is usually heard; other signs include a widened pulse pressure and pounding peripheral pulses. Patent ductus may be seen in combination with other defects, such as ventricular septal defect and coarctation of the aorta, but it does not cause these defects. Since the direction of shunt is left-to-right, neither clubbing of the fingers nor cyanosis occurs.

18. The answer is E. [*Chapter 6 II C 1–4*] Coarctation is found twice as often in male as in female children. Associated intracardiac defects are commonly seen with this condition. Physical findings include upper extremity hypertension with absent or diminished pulses in the lower extremity. Surgical correction is the treatment of choice, ideally when the child is between 5 and 6 years old, although symptoms may mandate earlier repair. Residual hypertension may be a problem postoperatively. Spinal cord injury due to ischemia and postoperative mesenteric ischemia may also be seen in a small number of cases.

19–23. The answers are: 19-A, 20-B, 21-A, 22-D, 23-C. [*Chapter 6 I A 8*] Mechanical valves cause a higher incidence of thromboembolic events than do tissue valves. Therefore, life-long anticoagulation therapy is indicated for these valves. Mechanical valves can fail catastrophically (strut failure, disc dislodgement or embolization), while tissue valves tend to fail over weeks to months unless a paravalvular leak is present. Since both valves are foreign bodies, infection generally requires replacement regardless of valve type. However, there are a few reports of antibiotic sterilization of tissue valves without the need for reoperation.

24–27. The answers are: 24-D, 25-C, 26-A, 27-E. [*Chapter 5 X A 1, 2, B 1, 2, C 2; Chapter 16 IV B 1 c*] Neuroblastomas are highly malignant tumors, arising from the sympathetic chain located in the posterior mediastinum. Bronchogenic cysts and pericardial cysts are of mesothelial origin and are located in the middle mediastinum, usually at the cardiophrenic angle. Thymomas occur in the anterior mediastinum and are associated with the clinical syndrome of myasthenia gravis. Teratomas contain elements of all three germ cell layers and frequently calcify.

28–31. The answers are: 28-C, 29-A, 30-D, 31-B. [*Chapter 6 I B 1 b (2), 2 b (2), C 1 b (4) (a), 2 b (2)*] As a general rule, valvular obstruction causes hypertrophy in the proximal associated cardiac chamber, whereas valvular insufficiency causes dilatation in both proximal and distal associated cardiac chambers. Therefore, aortic stenosis would cause isolated left ventricular hypertrophy, and mitral stenosis would cause isolated left atrial hypertrophy (since the atria can only hypertrophy to a small degree, they mainly dilate). On the other hand, aortic regurgitation would cause both left ventricular and aortic dilatation, whereas mitral regurgitation would cause both left atrial and left ventricular dilatation.

Part III
Vascular Disorders

7

Peripheral Arterial Disease

R. Anthony Carabasi, III
Bruce E. Jarrell

I. GENERAL PRINCIPLES OF PERIPHERAL ARTERIAL DISEASE

A. Atherosclerosis is a disease process that involves both large and small arteries. Arterial lesions tend to occur at certain locations, such as the proximal internal carotid artery, the infrarenal aorta, and the superficial femoral artery. The supraceliac aorta and the distal deep femoral artery are rarely involved. The reason for this pattern is not known, but it is probably related to different flow patterns at various locations in the arterial system.

1. Types of lesions. Pathologically, arterial lesions can be divided into three general types.
   a. Fatty streaks are discrete, subintimal lesions, which are composed of cholesterol-laden macrophages and smooth muscle cells. These may occur early in life and are not hemodynamically significant.
   b. Fibrous plaques are more advanced lesions, which also contain an extracellular matrix. These may progress to cause an obstruction to flow.
   c. Complex plaques are characterized by intimal ulceration or intraplaque hemorrhage. These plaques may cause local occlusion of the vessel or may result in embolization of the clot or pieces of cholesterol, causing distal arterial occlusion.

2. Risk factors. There are certain risk factors, which predispose patients to develop atherosclerotic vascular lesions, including:
   a. Cigarette smoking
   b. Diabetes mellitus
   c. Hypertension
   d. Lipid abnormalities, most commonly familial hypercholesterolemia
   e. A strong family history of vascular disease

B. Clinical presentation. A thorough history and physical examination can confirm the diagnosis of peripheral vascular disease and can suggest the anatomic location of specific occlusive lesions.

1. Claudication is one of the most characteristic symptoms of peripheral vascular disease. It is described by the patient as profound fatigue, aching, or crampy pain in the extremity. It is always caused by exertion and never caused by standing or sitting for prolonged periods. It is promptly (within minutes) relieved by rest.
   a. Symptoms appear distally to the site of vascular occlusion.
      (1) In iliac occlusion, the discomfort is in the thigh or buttock.
      (2) In superficial femoral artery occlusion, the symptoms are found in the calf.
      (3) Pulses are usually absent or diminished distally to the lesion. Pulses that are palpable at rest may disappear after exercise.
      (4) At rest, the patient has no discomfort, indicating that limb-threatening ischemia is not present.
   b. Treatment
      (1) Initial therapy is usually nonoperative and includes cessation of smoking, control of hypertension and lipid abnormalities, weight loss, and exercise.
      (2) There is only one drug approved in the United States for the treatment of claudication, pentoxifylline, which acts by decreasing blood viscosity and increasing red cell flexibility, thereby increasing flow in the microcirculation.
   c. Prognosis. Claudication is an indication that systemic vascular disease is present.

(1) The prognosis of the affected limb is relatively good with only 10% of patients progressing to severe ischemia or limb loss in 10 years.

(2) The long-term survival of these patients is more guarded, being 73% at 5 years and 38% at 10 years.

(3) The commonest cause of death is atherosclerotic heart disease.

2. Ischemic rest pain results from severe compromise of arterial flow. Here the blood supply is inadequate even at rest.

  a. Symptoms. Patients describe intense pain, burning, or tingling, usually across the distal foot and arch, which is exacerbated by elevating the foot (i.e., while trying to sleep in bed). It may be relieved by keeping the foot in a dependent position or by walking slowly.

  b. Treatment. Serious consideration should be given to revascularization in these patients since the disability and discomfort are severe and the degree of ischemia is critical.

3. Gangrene (tissue necrosis) occurs when blood flow is inadequate to maintain tissue viability.

  a. Etiology

    (1) Gangrene may result from chronic progressive arterial disease or may result from embolization of cholesterol or an organized thrombus from a proximal source.

    (2) Occasionally, gangrene of the toes may occur without significant proximal arterial disease. This represents occlusion of small blood vessels from intrinsic obliterative disease and is seen most commonly in diabetics.

  b. Treatment is local debridement or amputation of nonviable tissue and revascularization or removal of the source of emboli to protect the remaining tissue at risk.

C. Diagnosis

1. Noninvasive tests. If the history and physical examination suggest the presence of vascular disease, there are various noninvasive tests that can confirm the diagnosis.

  a. Pulse volume recording is a technique that measures the volume changes in the extremity during the cardiac cycle. This is printed as a waveform for review. By pattern recognition, the presence and the location of occlusive lesions can be ascertained.

  b. Segmental arterial blood pressures can be obtained at various locations in the arm and leg.

    (1) A pressure drop distally in an extremity indicates arterial stenosis or occlusion.

    (2) The **ankle brachial index (ABI)** is the ratio of the systemic blood pressure at the ankle to that of the brachial artery in the arm.

      (a) Normally, the ratio should be 1.0 or slightly greater.

      (b) Patients complaining of claudication typically have an ABI of less than 0.8.

      (c) Patients with rest pain usually have an ABI of less than 0.5.

      (d) The ABI is *not* accurate in patients whose arteries are calcified (usually diabetics). These arteries cannot be compressed; thus, the ABI is falsely elevated.

  c. Doppler waveform analysis combined with **B-mode imaging** of the arteries is called a **duplex examination**.

    (1) This test is used most commonly to evaluate the carotid arteries and the large veins of the legs.

    (2) It has been used recently to follow patients after the placement of bypass grafts in the legs.

2. Invasive tests for assessment of peripheral vascular disease include digital subtraction angiography and percutaneous arterial angiography.

  a. Digital intravenous subtraction angiography (DIVA) is performed by injecting contrast into a large vein. The arterial system can be visualized by proper timing of the x-ray exposures.

    (1) Advantages. This technique is attractive because no arterial puncture is required; thus, it is safe for use on outpatients.

    (2) Disadvantages. This technique has not lived up to expectations since the resolution is only fair, the contrast volume is large, and if the patient moves or the timing of exposure is not correct, the images will not be satisfactory.

  b. Arterial digital subtraction angiography uses the same subtraction technique as the DIVA procedure, but the dye is placed into the affected artery. This produces excellent images with very small amounts of contrast.

    (1) Advantages. The patient experiences minimal discomfort, and the small amount of contrast required allows the injection to be repeated if necessary.

    (2) Disadvantages. This technique requires an arterial puncture, and the area that can be studied at one time is relatively small.

  c. Conventional arteriography is the current standard method for evaluating vascular diseases. Contrast material is injected into the artery of interest, usually by way of a femoral artery puncture, and sequential x-ray exposures are made. As the contrast moves distally, the filling of the arteries is recorded during the filming sequence.

    (1) Advantage. Arteriography provides large films that clearly reveal the area under investigation.

    (2) Disadvantages. This procedure is associated with several serious complications.

      (a) Acute renal failure can result from the nephrotoxicity of the dye, and **acute dehydration** can result from the brisk diuresis induced by the hyperosmotic contrast dye. Both complications can be minimized by adequate pre- and post-angiographic hydration and by limiting the total amount of dye injected. In addition, **allergic reactions** to the dye can occur.

      (b) Acute arterial occlusion occasionally follows an angiography.

        (i) Ischemia is most apt to be related to technical problems, including simple thrombosis of the artery at the site of needle insertion, distal embolization into the lower leg from a thrombus forming on the angiogram catheter or from a dislodged plaque, or subintimal dissection of an atherosclerotic plaque during catheter manipulation.

        (ii) Clinical symptoms of acute arterial occlusion following angiography include absent pulses, especially those present prior to the examination; severe, constant pain, numbness, or paresthesia in the extremity examined; and pallor of the skin and coolness to touch in the involved extremity.

        (iii) Treatment of acute arterial occlusion during angiography depends upon the underlying cause and should be initiated promptly. If flow is re-established within 2–6 hours, the results are excellent. For example, acute thrombosis can be treated with lytic therapy, using urokinase or streptokinase. Since this is a very fresh thrombosis, rapid lysis should occur. Intimal dissection that causes thrombosis requires thrombectomy and direct arterial repair or bypass, and embolization of an atherosclerotic plaque requires operative embolectomy.

        (iv) Although **arterial vasospasm** can explain this acute ischemic episode, it occurs in less than 3% of cases.

      (c) Pseudoaneurysms may develop following removal of the angiographic catheter. This is usually caused by an inability to apply adequate pressure at the arterial puncture site and is more likely to occur in patients with high blood pressure.

        (i) Pseudoaneurysms present as swelling following removal of the catheter.

        (ii) An ultrasound of the area should be obtained to distinguish a pseudoaneurysm from a simple hematoma. If pulsatile flow is seen outside the lumen of the artery, a pseudoaneurysm is present.

        (iii) Pseudoaneurysm should be repaired promptly in the operating room.

d. Brachial artery catheterization

  (1) This study is performed frequently for cardiac catheterization or for angiography when the lower extremity vessels are unsuitable.

  (2) Thrombosis of the brachial artery does not usually result in acute hand ischemia, but it can cause hand claudication. Thus, surgical repair is indicated.

e. Axillary artery catheterization

  (1) This study is performed occasionally when the femoral vessels are not adequate for angiography.

  (2) A periarterial hematoma may follow this study and compress the brachial plexus, causing arm disability if it is not surgically decompressed.

f. Translumbar aortography is performed by catheterizing the aorta with a long needle, which is inserted posteriorly in the lumbar area.

  (1) This study is useful when neither femoral nor upper extremity arteries are suitable for catheterization or when ulcerated plaques are present in the aorta because catheter manipulation could dislodge the plaques, resulting in distal embolization.

  (2) This study may be complicated, however, by retroperitoneal hematomas.

D. Nonoperative procedures to eliminate atherosclerotic plaques

1. **Arterial dilation** in areas of stenosis by means of an inflatable balloon catheter is a nonoperative technique that fractures atherosclerotic plaques. It may be used in most extremity vessels.
   a. The dilation is performed by a radiologist immediately following angiography. An inflatable balloon attached to an angiographic catheter is fluoroscopically guided to the stenotic area. The balloon is then inflated to 4–8 atm to fracture the plaque.
   b. Clinically significant distal emboli may follow this procedure in 3%–5% of the cases.
   c. The patency of balloon dilation varies according to the location. The results are very good in the common iliac arteries, but long-term patency decreases in small distal vessels.

2. **Atherectomy catheters** are capable of removing plaques from diseased arteries and restoring distal blood flow.

3. **Lasers** can be used to open small channels in diseased vessels. This opening can then be enlarged with a balloon or atherectomy catheter.

II. DIABETIC FOOT

A. Clinical presentation

1. **Infection in the toes and feet** of patients with diabetes mellitus can arise after minor trauma.

2. **Peripheral neuropathy,** which produces loss of sensation and proprioception, leading to the development of trophic ulcers on the plantar surface of the foot, is very common among diabetic patients. If the ulcers become infected, it is usually caused by mixed flora, including anaerobic bacteria, and may manifest itself by causing:
   a. A deep plantar space abscess
   b. Cellulitis of the dorsum of the foot
   c. Osteomyelitis of the metatarsal or phalangeal bones

3. **Atherosclerosis** occurs with increased frequency among diabetic individuals. It also occurs at a younger age and progresses more rapidly in diabetic than in nondiabetic individuals.

4. **Gangrene** develops among diabetic individuals with a much higher frequency than among nondiabetics as a result of:
   a. Large vessel occlusive disease in which pulses are absent
   b. Small vessel disease (microangiopathy) characterized by thickening of the capillary basement membrane. This process is very common in diabetics.

B. Prevention of injury and meticulous foot care is very important in the diabetic patient.

1. Any sign of infection demands immediate evaluation.

2. Properly fitted shoes are very important.

3. The diabetic patient should *never* walk barefoot as minor skin breaks can result in catastrophic infection.

C. Treatment of infection

1. Debridement of necrotic tissue

2. Bed rest, total avoidance of weight-bearing, and avoidance of pressure on the affected area

3. Systemic antibiotics

4. Close monitoring of blood sugar as control of the diabetes may be difficult during the acute stage of infection

III. AORTOILIAC OCCLUSIVE DISEASE

A. Clinical presentation

1. **Causes.** Aortoiliac occlusive disease is usually caused by atherosclerosis (Figure 7-1). Other less common entities that can occlude the aorta include Takayasu's arteritis and aortic coarctation.

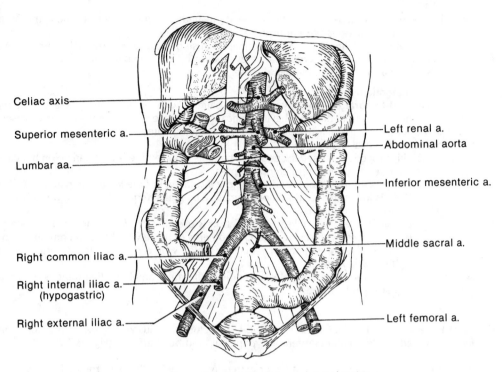

Figure 7-1. Arteries of the abdominal region.

2. Symptoms

a. Patients may be asymptomatic but more commonly have buttock and thigh claudication. Severe ischemia, leading to gangrene or limb loss, is rare with isolated aortoiliac disease.

b. Men with this condition may be impotent if blood flow to the pelvis is severely diminished.

B. Indications for surgery

1. Severe claudication or rest pain

2. Tissue loss

3. Peripheral arterial emboli

a. Causes. This is caused by occlusion of distal vessels in the skin or digits of the lower extremity by pieces of the plaque or platelet-fibrin clots.

b. Symptoms. The patient presents with a painful cyanotic digit ("blue toe" syndrome) or multiple small skin infarctions.

c. Treatment is exclusion of the diseased arterial segment in the proximal vessel.

4. Impotence in men if other organic or psychogenic causes have been ruled out and if a hemodynamically significant vascular lesion is present

C. Operative procedures

1. Endarterectomy consists of opening the artery and removing the portion of the intima and media containing the plaque. Currently, this technique is used only for short lesions of the distal aorta or common iliac arteries.

2. Aortofemoral bypass is the most commonly used procedure. It bypasses all intra-abdominal occlusions.

a. The distal anastomosis is usually performed on the common femoral artery with the toe of the graft extended over the proximal deep femoral artery. This technique results in the best long-term patency, which approaches 85%–90% at 5 years.

    b. The proximal anastomosis should be done near the renal arteries where the least amount of disease is present in the aorta.

    c. Operative mortality is 1%–5%. The major cause of death is myocardial infarction. All patients should have a preoperative evaluation by a cardiologist, even if they have no symptoms or history of cardiac disease.

  3. Extra-anatomic bypass

    a. Femoral-femoral bypass may be used in patients with unilateral iliac disease if the remaining iliac artery does not have significant obstructive disease. In well-selected cases, the results are good with 70%–75% 5-year patency rates.

    b. Axillobifemoral bypass

      (1) This procedure is used for poor-risk patients who require revascularization but cannot tolerate direct aortofemoral bypass.

      (2) This procedure is associated with a low mortality, but the long-term patency (60%–70%) is lower than aortofemoral bypass. The grafts frequently require thrombectomy to achieve long-term patency.

      (3) Despite these drawbacks, this operation is useful in the following circumstances:

        (a) In patients with severe medical problems or those who have had multiple prior abdominal operations or radiation, which would make standard aortofemoral bypass hazardous.

        (b) After removal of an infected aortic graft where an alternative route is required for revascularization.

IV. LOWER EXTREMITY OCCLUSIVE DISEASE includes occlusive disease of the common femoral, superficial femoral, deep femoral, popliteal, and tibial arteries (Figure 7-2).

  A. Cause. The commonest cause of lower extremity disease is **atherosclerosis** although other less common conditions can also cause obstruction.

    1. The superficial femoral artery is the artery most frequently involved. Occlusion usually occurs distally where the artery passes through the adductor hiatus. The commonest symptom is claudication, which may not be severe if good collateral vessels are present.

    2. The profunda femoris artery supplies blood to the thigh and collateral flow to the popliteal artery. The origin of this vessel frequently is stenotic, but the distal vessel is usually spared by atherosclerosis.

    3. The popliteal artery may be occluded by atherosclerosis, entrapment by the gastrocnemius or popliteus muscle, or by cysts in the adventitia of the artery. The latter two conditions should be considered if a young patient presents with claudication.

    4. The tibial arteries may be occluded by atherosclerosis or embolization. Patients with diabetes frequently have occlusion of these vessels.

  B. Clinical presentation

    1. Patients with lower extremity arterial occlusion present with claudication (commonest), rest pain, and tissue necrosis. If the arterial insufficiency is severe, tissue necrosis may produce nonhealing ulcers.

    2. Other physical findings include loss of hair, nail changes, pallor on elevation, and dependent rubor.

  C. Surgical treatment

    1. Indications for surgery. There are one relative and two absolute indications for surgery in patients with femoropopliteal occlusive disease.

      a. Tissue necrosis of the leg or foot is an urgent reason to proceed with surgery.

      b. Rest pain is a syndrome characterized by pain or aching across the distal foot, which occurs when the leg is elevated or when the patient is in bed. This is relieved by placing the leg in a dependent position. It indicates severe arterial insufficiency and is an indication for intervention.

      c. Claudication. This is a relative indication for intervention. If the symptoms interfere with a patient's ability to work or if they interfere severely with the patient's life-style,

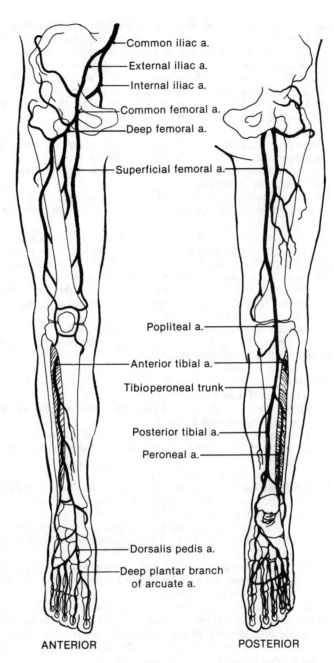

Figure 7-2. Arteries of the lower extremity.

surgery may be offered. This should only be done after a period of exercise, weight reduction, and abstinence from smoking.

2. Operative procedures

a. Femoropopliteal bypass, using autogenous saphenous vein, is the basic operation. If a vein is not available or is not suitable for bypass, an artificial prosthetic graft may be used.

(1) Although early results with prosthetic grafts are acceptable, they are not as durable as veins, and every reasonable attempt should be made to use autologous material.

(2) The 5-year patency of vein bypasses are 65%–80%, and the limb salvage rate is 90%.

(3) Mortality from the operation is primarily from myocardial infarction, and these patients should be evaluated for occult coronary artery disease.

  b. **Femorotibial artery bypass** is required in patients with occlusive disease in the popliteal and tibial vessels. Two technique are used, and the results are excellent with both.

(1) One technique uses a reversed saphenous vein.

(2) The other technique leaves the saphenous vein in its bed but renders its valves incompetent (in situ technique).

  c. **Profundaplasty** (repair of the origin of the profunda femoris artery) as an isolated procedure may result in relief of rest pain and healing of ulcers if applied properly. This procedure is used in poor-risk patients with occlusion of the superficial femoral arteries and severe stenosis of the origin of the profunda femoris artery. It can often be carried out under local anesthesia.

  d. **Lumbar sympathectomy** is useful in patients who have unreconstructable lower extremity arterial disease. It is an uncommon operation since the introduction of the femorotibial bypass.

(1) Good results may be obtained in patients with mild rest pain or small areas of superficial skin ulceration or in patients who have an ankle brachial index over 0.3.

(2) This procedure is rarely indicated in diabetics since many of these patients have an "autosympathectomy" as a result of their underlying disease.

(3) The L_2, L_3, and L_4 ganglion are removed via a retroperitoneal approach. In some centers, sympathectomy is accomplished by injecting irritating material percutaneously to destroy the ganglion.

  e. **Amputation.** If reconstruction cannot be accomplished or if a patient is debilitated and cannot ambulate, amputation may not only be lifesaving but may be expeditious in promoting the total rehabilitation of the patient. Occasionally, the result is better than that of an extensive vascular procedure. Approximately 50% of all amputations are performed on diabetics.

(1) **Indications for amputation**

  (a) The presence of extensive gangrene in the weight-bearing portion of the foot, especially beneath the heel

  (b) Systemic sepsis, particularly when caused by gas-forming organisms

  (c) A patient who has no potential for ambulation even after successful revascularization

  (d) Unreconstructable vascular disease

(2) **Rehabilitation.** The level of amputation should be below the knee if possible. This allows the greatest chance of rehabilitation. An absolute method for predicting amputation healing is not available.

  (a) A pulsatile pulse volume recording in the calf or a transcutaneous PO_2 greater than 40 mm Hg at the site of amputation usually indicate that the area will heal primarily.

  (b) The rehabilitation rate depends on the level of amputation and ranges from 60%–70% for unilateral below-the-knee amputations to 10% for bilateral above-the-knee amputations.

  (c) The healing failure rate is up to 20% for below-the-knee amputations.

(3) **Operative mortality rate** is about 13% with 50% of deaths occurring secondarily to cardiac problems and 25% secondarily to respiratory problems. The long-term mortality rate following amputation is 50% at 3 years and 70% at 5 years when the amputation is performed for vascular disease.

V. ACUTE ARTERIAL OCCLUSION OF THE LOWER EXTREMITY results in sudden cessation of arterial blood flow to the extremity (see Figure 7-2). Acute ischemia may be followed by necrosis if rapid intervention does not take place. The commonest site of occlusion is the femoral artery, followed by the iliac and popliteal arteries and aortic bifurcation.

  A. **Causes.** The recent onset of arrhythmia, especially atrial fibrillation, may give a clue to the source of the embolus. The commonest cause of acute occlusion is an embolus or, frequently, multiple emboli, which originate from several sources.

  1. **Atherosclerotic heart disease** is thought to be the source of emboli in 60% of cases. Atrial fibrillation is present in 50%–80% of patients who produce emboli.

2. Rheumatic valvular heart disease is the source of emboli in 21% of cases.

3. Abdominal aortic ulcerated plaques are the source of emboli in 1%–2% of cases. This small but significant group of patients may present with digital emboli, resulting in cyanotic toes ("blue toe" syndrome).

B. The clinical presentation of a lower extremity embolus results from ischemia of the tissues supplied by the occluded artery. Physical findings include:

1. Acute onset of severe pain and a sensation of coolness

2. Acute loss of motor and sensory function

3. A pale, pulseless extremity without edema

4. Ankle blood pressure that is very low or undetectable

C. Treatment. Management of acute arterial occlusion includes rapid diagnosis and expeditious surgical correction of the occlusion.

1. Heparin therapy. Patients should be heparinized immediately when the clinical diagnosis is made.

2. Hydration therapy. Patients should be given adequate hydration to maintain a high urine output (preferably 100 ml/hr). Alkalinization of the urine and osmotic diuresis (mannitol) are used to protect the kidney from damage due to myoglobinuria in cases of prolonged severe ischemia.

3. Preoperative arteriogram. If onset is acute, a cardiac source is present, and the patient has no prior history of claudication, an arteriogram preoperatively is not necessary.

4. Surgical treatment. Patients should undergo surgery within 6–8 hours of onset. The surgeon should perform an embolectomy, using a Fogarty balloon catheter. The catheter is passed down the occluded artery past the embolus. It is then inflated and pulled back through the artery, extracting the embolus as it is withdrawn.
  a. Limb salvage is accomplished in 75% of cases.
  b. Mortality is 12%–20% and can be prevented only by meticulous perioperative care and a rapid surgical procedure.

5. Medical treatment. The role of thrombolytic therapy for acute embolic disease is unclear. It is not applicable in patients with severe ischemia since it may require 12–24 hours for maximum benefit. Patients with intracardiac thrombus are also probably not candidates since lytic treatment may lead to further embolization.

6. Postoperative treatment. Patients should be given anticoagulant therapy to minimize the risk of recurrent embolization.

VI. MESENTERIC VASCULAR DISEASE may present as an acute life-threatening emergency or as a chronic debilitating problem.

A. Chronic mesenteric ischemia results from slowly progressive stenosis or occlusion of the visceral vessels (i.e., celiac, superior mesenteric artery, and inferior mesenteric artery) [see Figure 7-1].

1. Clinical presentation
  a. Usually two of the three vessels must be involved for symptoms to be present. The celiac and superior mesenteric arteries are the most commonly involved.
  b. The signs and symptoms of chronic mesenteric ischemia include:
   (1) Abdominal pain following a meal
   (2) Weight loss secondary to avoiding food due to pain
   (3) An epigastric bruit

2. Diagnosis
  a. Recently, duplex scanning of the visceral vessels has been used to screen patients with suspected chronic mesenteric ischemia.
  b. Arteriography is the most useful diagnostic study. Both anterior–posterior and lateral views of the aorta must be done to visualize the origins of the visceral vessels.

3. Treatment. If appropriate lesions are found, operation is recommended.
  a. Bypass from a healthy aorta to the visceral vessels or endarterectomy of the involved visceral vessels are the preferred treatments.
  b. In well-selected patients, the results of operation are excellent with 90% of patients cured of their symptoms.

B. Acute mesenteric ischemia is a surgical emergency, which has several causes.

  1. Etiology
    a. Embolization usually to the superior mesenteric artery is the commonest cause of acute mesenteric ischemia.
      (1) The heart is the commonest source.
      (2) These patients present with a triad of symptoms.
        (a) Severe pain out of proportion to the physical findings
        (b) A history of gut emptying, usually a massive bowel movement with or without vomiting
        (c) Atrial fibrillation or other cardiac conditions, which predisposes to embolus formation
    b. Thrombosis of visceral arteries
      (1) Sudden occlusion of preexisting atherosclerotic lesions of the visceral vessels may cause acute mesenteric ischemia.
      (2) Patients with suspected acute mesenteric ischemia should be questioned about preexisting symptoms of weight loss and pain with eating.
    c. Nonocclusive mesenteric insufficiency. This condition is the result of low flow to the visceral circulation due to low cardiac output.

  2. Treatment
    a. Salvage of these patients depends on a high index of suspicion and prompt diagnosis and treatment.
      (1) All patients suspected of having acute mesenteric ischemia should be hydrated and given broad-spectrum antibiotics.
      (2) An angiogram is performed to confirm the diagnosis. Treatment is then instituted based on the arteriographic findings.
        (a) If an embolus is found, the treatment is prompt surgical embolectomy.
        (b) If mesenteric thrombosis is found, the treatment is vascular reconstruction, which usually is a bypass to the superior mesenteric artery.
    b. Following embolectomy or reconstruction, the bowel is assessed for viability. Overtly necrotic bowel is resected. If marginal viability is present in the remaining bowel, it should be left in place. A "second look" operation should be done in 24 hours to ensure viability of the residual bowel.
    c. If the original angiogram reveals nonocculsive mesenteric ischemia, treatment is directed toward improving cardiac function.
      (1) Hydration and, if necessary, inotropic therapy is begun.
      (2) The angiographic catheter is left in place and vasodilating drugs can be infused into the mesenteric circulation after hydration has been accomplished.
      (3) A repeat angiogram is done in 24 hours to assess the success of treatment. Vasospasm should be reversed and normal arterial perfusion restored if treatment has been effective.
      (4) These patients may require celiotomy if peritoneal signs are present or develop during treatment. Operative management is as outlined in VI B 1.

C. Mesenteric venous thrombosis presents more insidiously than acute mesenteric ischemia. Typically it causes slowly progressive abdominal pain and distention and may be confused with intestinal obstruction.

  1. Etiology. It is usually caused by a hypercoagulable state, such as a neoplasm or a hematologic abnormality.

  2. Diagnosis. It can be diagnosed by computed tomography (CT scan), which reveals hyperconcentration of contrast in the wall of the mesenteric vein without flow in the lumen.

  3. Treatment
    a. Nonoperative treatment is anticoagulation (intravenous heparin) and treatment of the underlying disorder.

      b. Celiotomy may be necessary if peritonitis develops, but 75% of patients can be treated nonoperatively if the diagnosis is made promptly and appropriate treatment is given.

VII. RENAL ARTERY STENOSIS. Stenosis of the renal artery results in decreased perfusion pressure to the kidney. This stimulates the juxtaglomerular apparatus to release renin, which initiates the formation of angiotensin. This substance is a potent vasoconstrictor and also stimulates the release of aldosterone from the adrenal gland. The end result is systemic hypertension.

    A. Causes. The two commonest causes of renal artery stenosis are atherosclerosis and fibromuscular dysplasia. The latter is a disease that produces single or multiple stenoses of the renal arteries, particularly in women.

    B. Clinical presentation. This is a relatively rare entity and is found in only 1%–5% of hypertensive patients. The diagnosis should be suspected in patients with the following characteristics:

        1. Sudden onset of severe hypertension in patients less than 35 or more than 55 years of age

        2. Sudden worsening of hypertension in a patient who had been well controlled

        3. Inability to control blood pressure despite multiple drug therapy

        4. The presence of flank bruits associated with any of the above reinforces the likelihood of the diagnosis

    C. Diagnosis. Laboratory tests may be helpful in confirming the presence of hypertension caused by renal artery stenosis although no test is completely reliable.

        1. Renal vein renin ratio compares the renin output from the individual renal veins. Ideally this test is done under exacting conditions, including discontinuing antihypertensive medications. A renin ratio of 1.5 or greater is significant and has been predictive of a successful surgical cure of hypertension in about 85% of cases. Renin ratios may be unreliable if both renal arteries are stenotic.

        2. The renal/systemic renin index documents the contribution of each individual kidney to plasma renin and also documents suppression of the contralateral kidney in unilateral disease.

          a. The formula is:

$$\frac{\text{renal vein renin} - \text{systemic renin}}{\text{systemic renin}}$$

          b. An index over 0.48 indicates hypersecretion by that kidney.
          c. An index approaching 0 indicates suppression in that kidney.

        3. Duplex scanning has been used recently to evaluate patients for renal artery stenosis. The technique is demanding but holds promise as a useful screening test.

        4. Selective renal arteriography is the definitive examination to demonstrate stenotic lesions of the renal arteries and is essential in planning therapy.

    D. Treatment of renal artery stenosis depends on the etiology and location of the lesion, the status of the involved kidney, and the clinical status of the patient. Options include bypass, endarterectomy, percutaneous dilation, and nephrectomy.

        1. Percutaneous dilation is a very effective treatment for patients with lesions in the midportion of the renal artery. The lesions frequently occur in this location in patients with fibromuscular dysplasia. Early and late results in well-selected patients are excellent. The technique is not well suited for atherosclerotic lesions at the origin of the renal artery or for lesions that occur in distal branches of the renal artery.

        2. Renal artery endarterectomy can be used for unilateral or bilateral localized atherosclerotic osteal lesions of the renal arteries.

        3. Bypass to the renal artery distal to the lesion is the most commonly performed procedure.
          a. The saphenous vein in adults and the hypogastric artery in children are the preferred conduits.

    b. The aorta above or below the renal artery is usually used as the origin of the graft. Other sources of inflow are the hepatic, splenic, and iliac arteries.

    c. A small percentage of patients have multiple lesions, involving both the main renal artery and the hilar branches. In these patients, the kidney can be removed, cooled, and repaired ex vivo. The kidney is then replaced in its anatomic location or transplanted to the pelvis.

4. Nephrectomy is an alternative in patients with a unilateral vascular lesion and a normal contralateral kidney. The indication would be refractory hypertension with elevated renin from the involved kidney and suppression of the normal kidney. Nephrectomy is usually chosen for small, nonfunctioning kidneys.

5. Medical treatment. Antihypertensive drugs can be used to control mild to moderate hypertension from renal artery stenosis (when the diastolic blood pressure is in the 90–100 range).

    a. The risks of medical management are higher when blood pressure is erratic or difficult to control.

    b. Medical management is a more reasonable approach than surgery in patients with generalized atherosclerosis.

    c. Medical management is less desirable than surgery in children and in patients with fibromuscular dysplasia.

6. Results of treatment depend on the disease process, the accuracy of preoperative testing, and the ability to completely repair the arterial lesions.

    a. Fibromuscular dysplasia with localized arterial lesions do very well with improvement or cure of hypertension in 90% of patients.

    b. Repair of isolated atherosclerotic lesions also yield good results if the distal renal artery is normal.

    c. Nonlocalized lesions in patients with widespread atherosclerosis yield the poorest results.

VIII. EXTRACRANIAL CEREBROVASCULAR DISEASE

A. Overview. Cerebrovascular accident (stroke) is an injury to the central nervous system, resulting in death of brain tissue. It can be a silent event or can result in temporary or permanent loss of function.

1. Epidemiology

    a. There are approximately 600,000 new strokes per year in the United States, resulting in approximately 150,000 deaths (25% mortality).

    b. Cerebrovascular accidents are the third leading cause of death in the United States.

    c. Recurrent stroke is the leading cause of death in stroke patients and occurs at the rate of 9% per year.

2. Causes

    a. Cerebral infarction in 85% of cases due to:

        (1) Embolization (commonest)

        (2) Primary vessel occlusion

    b. Hemorrhage in 15% of cases, including:

        (1) Intracerebral hemorrhage (commonest)

        (2) Subarachnoid hemorrhage (usually due to rupture of an intercranial aneurysm)

3. Symptoms. Most surgically treatable lesions occur at the carotid bifurcation, and these lesions cause symptoms by producing emboli or by restricting flow to the brain. Embolization of atherosclerotic debris, fibrin, or platelets from a carotid plaque is the commonest cause of ischemic insult to the brain. These emboli can produce a range of symptoms.

    a. Transient ischemic attacks (TIAs) are episodes of focal neurologic symptoms. The classic TIA syndrome is characterized by abrupt onset, usually the maximal symptoms occur in less than 5 minutes. Rapid resolution occurs usually within 2–15 minutes and always within 24 hours. Neurologic symptoms correspond to a specific hemispheric arterial distribution. There are no residual neurologic deficits following resolution.

        (1) TIAs usually occur secondarily to an embolus originating from a carotid plaque, frequently associated with a bruit located high in the neck.

(2) TIAs are associated with hemispheric neurologic symptoms, including:
  (a) A motor deficit contralateral to the involved carotid artery
  (b) A sensory deficit contralateral to the involved carotid artery
  (c) Minor or global aphasia
  b. Amaurosis fugax is transient monocular blindness caused by an embolus to a retinal vessel. Examination of the fundus may show a grey fibrin plaque or a bright yellow (Hollenhorst) cholesterol plaque in a retinal artery.
  c. Cerebrovascular accident or completed stroke

B. Vertebrobasilar artery disease. A cause-and-effect relationship between the vertebrobasilar system (Figure 7-3) and neurologic symptoms can be very difficult to establish because the symptoms are not specific. The following symptoms are generally, but not exclusively, related to the posterior circulation of the central nervous system:

1. A motor deficit, involving any combination of extremities, and including drop attacks, which are loss of lower extremity motor function with no loss of consciousness

2. A sensory deficit involving any combination of extremities

3. Loss of vision

4. Ataxia or gait disturbance

C. Carotid bruits are caused by flow disturbances in the carotid artery. They may be confused with transmitted heart murmurs. Heart murmurs are usually heard bilaterally and in all positions in the neck. Bruits originating in the carotid artery are usually heard high in the neck and may be unilateral. Carotid bruits are *not* reliable indicators that severe carotid disease is present but should alert the examiner that vascular disease (particularly coronary artery disease) is present.

D. Workup of the patient with cerebrovascular disease. Patients who present with neurologic symptoms should be carefully evaluated.

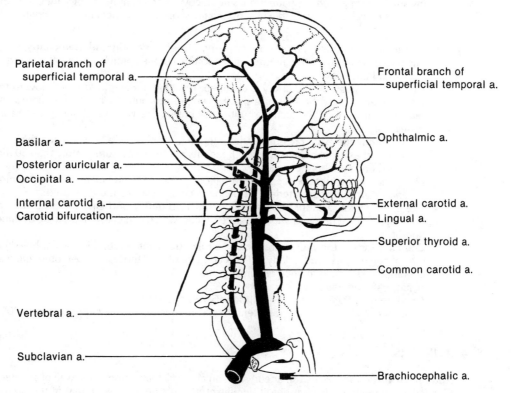

Figure 7-3. Arterial supply to the brain.

1. A noninvasive duplex examination of the carotid arteries detects significant lesions in the neck.

2. CT scan should be obtained to look for areas of cerebral infarction or intracranial pathology.

3. Cardiac evaluation should include an electrocardiogram (EKG), echocardiogram if a cardiac source is suspected, and a Holter monitor if a rhythm disturbance is suspected.

E. Medical treatment

1. **Warfarin.** Anticoagulation with warfarin is useful primarily in patients who have suffered a cerebral embolus originating from the heart. This occurs most commonly following a myocardial infarction (mural thrombus), in patients with rheumatic heart disease, or in patients with chronic atrial fibrillation.

2. **Aspirin** is beneficial in patients with cerebrovascular disease when the end points of stroke, TIA, and death are combined.

3. **Dipyridamole** has not been shown to be beneficial in patients with cerebrovascular disease.

F. Surgical treatment of cerebrovascular disease is currently under intense scrutiny.

1. **Indications for surgery**
   a. **TIAs or amaurosis fugax** are the most widely accepted indications for surgical treatment. Patients who are acceptable operative risks should undergo carotid arteriography. If a lesion is present in the appropriate carotid artery, surgery is recommended.
   b. **Asymptomatic carotid stenosis** (high grade, > 75%) is a controversial indication for surgery. Operation should only be recommended if the morbidity and mortality of the operation is less than 3%.
   c. **Stroke** followed by complete or near complete recovery is an acceptable indication for operation if the patient has an appropriate carotid lesion and is an acceptable candidate for surgery.
   d. **Acute dense neurologic deficit,** a totally **occluded internal carotid artery,** a **devastating stroke** from which the patient does not recover significant neurologic function, and **severe medical illness,** which will substantially shorten life expectancy, are contraindications for surgery.

2. **Procedures.** The operation most commonly employed is **carotid endarterectomy.**
   a. The operation removes the diseased inner portions of the common, internal, and external carotid arteries.
   b. During the operation, the artery is clamped, resulting in decreased blood flow to the brain. Cerebral protection, using a shunt, is employed routinely by some surgeons and selectively by others. If selective shunting is chosen, the need for shunting can be assessed by:
      (1) Measuring the back pressure in the internal carotid artery after clamping the common and external carotid arteries. If the mean arterial pressure is more than 50 mm Hg, shunting is not necessary.
      (2) Observing the electroencephalogram (EEG) for changes after clamping the common and external carotid arteries. If slowing occurs, a shunt should be used.
   c. The blood pressure should be carefully monitored during and after the procedure as these patients are prone to wide pressure swings, which can cause neurologic dysfunction or injury.
   d. Complications of the procedure include stroke, transient cerebral ischemia, bleeding, cranial nerve injury, particularly to CN X and CN XII, and those related to other medical conditions, especially myocardial infarction.
   e. A successful operation is very effective.
      (1) More than 90% of patients will be relieved of symptoms.
      (2) Future stroke risk in the ipsilateral hemisphere is reduced by approximately 70%.

IX. ANEURYSMS

A. **Abdominal aortic aneurysms.** An aneurysm is an abnormal dilatation of the wall of an artery. Generally, an aneurysm is considered significant if its diameter is twice that of the normal artery. An aneurysm of the aorta may rupture and cause death and should be repaired when detected. Most abdominal aortic aneurysms are caused by atherosclerosis.

1. **Diagnosis.** Abdominal aortic aneurysms most often occur below the level of the renal arteries and are usually discovered on physical examination or during evaluation of an unrelated abdominal condition in which the patient has a CT scan, ultrasound examination, or abdominal x-rays.
   a. **X-ray.** Calcification of part of the abdominal aorta seen on posteroanterior or lateral abdominal x-ray is present in 60% of patients.
   b. **Ultrasonography and CT scan** of the abdomen demonstrate the dilated aorta and are the most accurate tests for aneurysm size. CT is especially useful since it gives details about the relationship of the aneurysm to the renal and visceral vessels and demonstrates venous anomalies, which may be present.
   c. **Angiography** is useful for patients with hypertension due to associated renal artery stenosis, distal arterial occlusive symptoms, or suspected mesenteric ischemia.

2. **Surgical treatment.** Repair of aneurysms is done by replacing the diseased segments of the aorta with prosthetic grafts.
   a. All patients undergoing elective repair should have careful preoperative medical screening, including a cardiac evaluation. Patients with severe or unstable coronary artery disease should undergo coronary catheterization and, if necessary, aortocoronary bypass preoperatively.
   b. Intraoperatively, patients should be very carefully controlled.
      (1) A Swan-Ganz catheter is used to monitor cardiac filling pressure and cardiac output before, during, and after aortic clamping.
      (2) Mannitol is given to stimulate brisk diuresis.
      (3) Aortic clamp time is kept to a minimum. Clamps are removed slowly, and fluid status is adjusted to avoid blood pressure changes.
      (4) Acidosis and hyperkalemia may occur after clamps are removed and must be treated promptly.

B. Atypical aneurysms of the abdominal aorta

1. **Inflammatory aneurysms** are characterized by a dense fibrotic reaction, involving primarily the anterior and lateral walls of the aneurysm and the surrounding tissues.
   a. The duodenum is frequently densely adherent to the aneurysm wall and can be severely injured if attempts are made to mobilize the aneurysm. The aneurysm is repaired by incising it away from adherent bowel and visualizing the neck of the aneurysm from within the lumen of the aorta.
   b. The inflammatory reaction frequently recedes after repair of the aneurysm.

2. **Mycotic abdominal aortic aneurysms** are caused by bacterial inflammation of the arterial wall. In the infrarenal aorta, the commonest organism found is *Salmonella*.
   a. Mycotic aneurysms usually are saccular, occur in atypical locations, and lack calcification of the wall.
   b. Patients present with fever, elevated white blood cell counts, and positive blood cultures. Evidence of septic embolization may also be present.
   c. Treatment begins with culture and sensitivity directed antibiotics. The patients are then surgically explored.
      (1) If there is no periaortic purulence and Gram stain of the proximal and distal artery is negative, the aneurysm is repaired with an interposition graft.
      (2) If gross purulence is present, the aneurysm and surrounding tissue is resected, the aorta is closed, and an extra-anatomic bypass (i.e., axillobifemoral bypass) is constructed.
   d. Long-term antibiotic therapy is indicated in these patients.

C. Ruptured abdominal aortic aneurysms

1. **The risk of rupture** is related to the size of the aneurysm.
   a. Approximate rates of rupture in 5 years are:
      (1) If less than 4.5 cm in diameter, 9%
      (2) If 4.5–7 cm in diameter, 35%
      (3) If more than 7 cm in diameter, 75%

b. The expansion rate of an aneurysm is 0.4 cm in diameter per year. More rapid expansion indicates an unstable aneurysm and is an indication for repair.

2. **Clinical and laboratory findings**
   a. Severe central abdominal or back pain, occasionally localized to the lower abdomen, groin, or testes
   b. A pulsatile abdominal mass in over 80% of cases
   c. Shock in many cases. Some patients with small contained ruptures may have a stable blood pressure. They are at risk of catastrophic decompensation and should be treated urgently.
   d. Positive CT scan (possible only if the patient is stable and there is doubt about the diagnosis)

3. **Surgical repair** of a ruptured aortic aneurysm must be performed as soon as the diagnosis is made. The operative mortality rates range between 50% and 60%. Death is usually secondary to massive intraoperative hemorrhage and cardiac complications.

4. **Surgical complications** are not infrequent in either elective or emergency aortic surgery. Many of these complications can be minimized by careful management, and if recognized early, some can be successfully treated, preventing major morbidity and mortality.
   a. **Postoperative renal failure** occurs in 21% of cases of ruptured aneurysms and in 2.5% of aneurysms treated by elective surgery with mortality rates of up to 90%.
   b. **Ischemic colitis** results from ligation of the inferior mesenteric artery in both elective surgery for aneurysms and in surgery for ruptured aneurysms. It occurs to some degree in 6% of elective cases, but it results in full-thickness injury with necrosis in only 1%–2% of cases. Ischemic colitis should be suspected in any patient with postoperative diarrhea, especially when the stools are heme-positive. It can usually be diagnosed with sigmoidoscopy. The mortality rate can reach 50% if diagnosis and treatment are delayed. Treatment consists of resection of the dead colon, proximal colostomy, and closure of the distal colon (Hartmann's procedure).
   c. **Acute leg ischemia** occurs postoperatively in up to 7% of cases. It should be suspected if pulses that were present previously are absent. It is caused by clamp injury or embolization. Treatment is repair of the injury or embolectomy.
   d. **Spinal cord ischemia** is a **rare complication** (0.25% of cases) of aortic aneurysm surgery and is commonest in cases of ruptured aneurysm. It results from **injury to the artery of Adamkiewicz,** which supplies the spinal cord and arises from the left side of the abdominal aorta, usually at T_8 to L_1 but occasionally as low as L_4. Spinal cord ischemia produces a **classic anterior spinal artery syndrome,** which is characterized by:
      (1) Paraplegia
      (2) Rectal and urinary incontinence
      (3) Loss of pain and temperature sensation but preservation of vibratory and proprioceptive sensation (due to the independent anterior and posterior circulations of the middle and lower spinal cord)
   e. **Aortic graft infection** can occur in the body of the graft or at the anastomoses. It may **result from bacterial seeding** either at the time of graft implantation or at a later date as a result of bacteremia. The commonest infecting organism is *Staphylococcus aureus,* but *S. epidermidis* is not infrequently found. The lumina of all currently used grafts are covered with a pseudointima rather than endothelium and have a decreased resistance to infection compared to the native vessel.
      (1) The **incidence of infection** is between 1% and 4% of all grafts used. It may be decreased significantly by the perioperative use of antibiotics. First generation cephalosporins (i.e., cefazolin) are the drugs of choice.
      (2) Prosthetic grafts may become infected at anytime after implantation, even many years after the operation.
      (3) Infected grafts can present in several ways.
         (a) If the graft goes to the femoral arteries, the commonest presenting sign is an inflammatory mass or draining sinus in the groin.
         (b) Grafts that are totally in the abdomen may present only with fever and occasionally abdominal discomfort.
         (c) Multiple skin petechia may be seen in the lower extremities distal to an infected graft.

      (d) The graft anastomosis may erode into the gastrointestinal tract, a condition called an **aortoenteric fistula**. This condition must be suspected in any patient with gastrointestinal bleeding and a prosthetic vascular graft in the abdomen.

5. Diagnosis
    a. Endoscopy of the esophagus, stomach, and duodenum should be done if gastrointestinal bleeding is present to search for bleeding sites, such as an ulcer. The distal duodenum should be visualized as the aortoenteric fistula may be visible in this location.
    b. CT scan may demonstrate air or fluid around an infected graft or may show a false aneurysm.
    c. An indium tagged white blood cell scan may localize the area where the graft is infected.
    d. An aortogram may demonstrate a false aneurysm and also will guide the surgeon in vessels available for reconstruction at surgery.
    e. A **sinogram**, which outlines the graft, is diagnostic if a draining sinus is present.

6. Treatment depends upon the location of the infection.
    a. Local groin infection of an aortofemoral bypass can be treated by unilateral graft limb excision and, if necessary, extra-anatomic reconstruction of the involved leg.
    b. Infection of an intra-abdominal graft mandates bilateral extra-anatomic reconstruction followed by removal of the graft. Graft infection is a serious problem, which carries a 35%–50% mortality and a 20%–40% chance of major amputation.

7. Sexual dysfunction
    a. The sympathetic nerves controlling ejaculation cross the left common iliac artery near the aortic bifurcation. If injured, retrograde ejaculation will occur.
    b. Disturbance of pelvic blood flow during aortic reconstruction may result in impotence. Perfusion of at least one hypogastric artery should be maintained in planning the method of graft placement.

D. Other arterial aneurysms

1. Iliac artery aneurysms usually are extensions of aortic aneurysms. They may be diagnosed as pulsatile masses that are palpable on rectal examination; occasionally, they rupture into the sigmoid colon or another part of the gastrointestinal tract and present as gastrointestinal bleeding. They rarely occur as isolated aneurysms.

2. Splenic artery aneurysms are the commonest intra-abdominal aneurysm if abdominal aortic aneurysms are excluded. Causes include fibrous dysplasia, portal hypertension, multiparity, and inflammation (secondary to pancreatitis).
    a. Diagnosis is frequently incidental and is made when a plain film of the abdomen shows a left upper quadrant ring-shaped calcification.
    b. Rate of rupture of bland splenic aneurysms in nonpregnant females is 2%. The mortality of rupture is 25%. The rate of rupture in a pregnant female is 90%.
    c. Indications for repair include rupture, symptoms (pain in left upper quadrant), and the presence of an aneurysm in a woman of childbearing age.

3. Peripheral arterial aneurysms. The popliteal artery is the commonest location for peripheral aneurysms. The usual cause is atherosclerosis.
    a. Clinical presentation
      (1) Approximately 50% are bilateral. Of these, 25% have associated abdominal aortic aneurysms.
      (2) Rupture is rare, but embolization and thrombosis are common. These aneurysms should be repaired when discovered.
      (3) Physical examination detects hyperactive popliteal pulses, and the aneurysm can be seen on ultrasound. An arteriogram guides reconstruction.
    b. Treatment. Most popliteal aneurysms are treated by ligation and bypass. Attempts to completely remove the aneurysm are dangerous because injury to adjacent nerves and veins can occur.

X. VASOSPASTIC DISEASES chiefly affect the upper extremities and involve episodic vasoconstriction, usually of the small palmar and digital arteries and arterioles. Common symptoms include pain, numbness, coldness, and, occasionally, skin ulcers. Vasospasm may be associated with collagen vascular disease, atherosclerosis, trauma, and embolism from peripheral arterial lesions or without an identifiable associated disease.

A. Disorders

1. **Raynaud's phenomenon** is episodic vasoconstriction, most commonly of the fingers but occasionally of the feet. It is usually initiated by cold exposure or emotional stimuli and occurs mainly in women.
   a. The affected digits may go through a classic sequence of color changes, including:
      (1) **Pallor** due to severe vasospasm in the dermal vessels
      (2) **Cyanosis** due to sluggish blood flow and resultant marked blood desaturation
      (3) **Rubor** due to the reactive hyperemia
   b. **Symptoms** range from **numb discomfort,** which is usually localized in the fingers, to **ulceration** or **gangrene.**
   c. **Associated local or systemic disease.** Scleroderma is the disease most commonly associated with Raynaud's phenomenon.
   d. **Management** of Raynaud's phenomenon includes a number of different modalities.
      (1) Cold should be avoided. Hands should be protected by gloves or hand warmers in extreme, cold weather.
      (2) Tobacco should be avoided because it stimulates vasoconstriction.
      (3) Use of phenoxybenzamine for α-blockade may be therapeutic. Calcium channel blockers, such as nifedipine, are the drugs of choice. Intra-arterial reserpine may also be useful.
      (4) Emotional problems should be controlled.
      (5) Sympathectomy is rarely recommended in these patients since they have vascular occlusion of the digital vessels.

2. **Raynaud's disease** is similar to Raynaud's phenomenon; however, the condition shows no association with a systemic disease. The process rarely progresses to necrosis. Seventy percent of patients are young women, in whom the occurrence is usually bilateral and symmetrical. **Treatment** is similar to that of Raynaud's phenomenon, and nonoperative management controls 80% of patients. Sympathectomy is reserved for patients with disabling symptoms who are refractory to medical therapy. It may be effective because the digital vessels are spastic and not occluded.

3. **Cold hypersensitivity** may occur following frostbite. The affected area is bluish with a burning pain. Medical management and occasionally sympathectomy control the symptoms.

B. Associated disorders

1. Cryoglobulinemia or cold hemagglutinins

2. Myxedema

3. Ergotism

4. Thrombocytosis

5. Macroglobulinemia

6. Occupations where the hands suffer repeated trauma, such as jackhammer operators

7. Nerve compression syndromes, such as the carpal tunnel syndrome

8. Arterial compression syndromes, such as the thoracic outlet syndrome

C. Diagnosis. Tests may be performed to document vasospasm.

1. **Doppler** examination to measure arm and wrist blood pressure

2. **Digital plethysmography** to study the digital arteries. If they are diminished and unresponsive to temperature change, the arteries are occluded. If warming reverses the changes, vasospasm is likely.

3. The presence of a cervical or an axillary bruit suggests arterial occlusive disease. Arteriography may be necessary to eliminate this possibility totally. During arteriography, a vasodilator may be injected intra-arterially and the dye injection repeated. Demonstration of increased blood flow and vasodilation is strong support for the presence of vasospastic disease.

XI. VASCULAR GRAFTS. When arteries and veins develop occlusive lesions, the tissues they supply may need revascularization if an adequate collateral circulation fails to develop and supply enough nutrients to prevent ischemia. Revascularization is frequently performed by bypassing the occlusive lesion with either a biologic or a synthetic vascular prosthesis.

A. Biologic prostheses

1. **Autogenous vein grafts** are veins that are transplanted from one part of the body to another for use in bypassing an occlusion in either an artery or a vein. These grafts have a patency rate superior to that of synthetic grafts and are, therefore, the graft of choice.
   a. **Saphenous vein grafts** are as long as the lower extremity. Graft diameter is in the range of 2–8 mm; therefore, the vein can be used only for vessels of that size.
      (1) **Arterialization** of the saphenous vein results in thickening of the vein wall. Although the majority of these grafts do well, intimal and medial injury and proliferative fibroplasia do occur, resulting in long-term dysplasia with the development of stenotic lesions.
      (2) **Atherosclerotic lesions** appear in 2%–15% of the arterialized vein with time.
   b. **Treatment** with platelet-inhibiting drugs, such as aspirin, may increase long-term patency.

2. **Autogenous arterial grafts** are arteries that are removed from one area of a patient's vascular tree and inserted into another area (e.g., use of a hypogastric artery to bypass renal artery stenosis in a child).

3. **Vascular allografts** are vessels that are removed from one individual and implanted into another individual.
   a. **Arterial allografts** have a high rate of degeneration and are generally not used.
   b. **Venous allografts** may be used if they are modified to decrease the antigenicity by proteolytic digestion or freezing. If they are unmodified, immune rejection of the graft occurs across both the histocompatibility barrier and the blood group ABO barrier.
   c. **Human umbilical vein allografts** are currently used for bypass grafts. The grafts are rendered nonantigenic by a tanning procedure, using glutaraldehyde, and are supported externally by a polyester mesh. Results have shown excellent long-term patency for both lower extremity revascularization and hemodialysis vascular access.

4. **Vascular heterografts** are vessels that are removed from animals and rendered nonantigenic by the tanning process. The most commonly used graft is the dialdehyde starch-tanned bovine carotid artery. This graft has been used successfully for both vascular reconstruction and hemodialysis vascular access, but it has a tendency to develop aneurysms (in 3%–6% of cases) in certain applications.

B. Synthetic vascular prostheses

1. **Types**
   a. **Dacron grafts** are very successful when used for large-vessel replacements, such as in the aorta or iliac vessels. The long-term patency for grafts in the extremities is much less acceptable, however. Dacron may be knitted or woven into tubular grafts.
      (1) **Woven grafts** have tight structures of low porosity, which allow less ingrowth of tissue into the interstices.
      (2) **Knitted grafts** have looser structures with resultant higher porosity. The tissue ingrowth into the grafts is greater than in woven grafts, allowing a more stable pseudointima to form. The grafts require preclotting with nonheparinized blood to lessen blood loss at the time of implantation.
      (3) **Velour grafts** are Dacron grafts that, in addition to having the characteristics of knitted Dacron grafts, have loops of yarn occluding some of the pores and projecting onto the surfaces. This presumably allows the pseudointima to anchor more securely, preventing sloughing of these tissues into the graft lumen.

    b. Expanded polytetrafluoroethylene (PTFE) grafts are tubular grafts extruded from PTFE resin.

      (1) The porosity is low due to a strongly electronegative charge on the polymer surface caused by the fluoride atoms. Protein aggregates from blood adhere to the surface, and a thin, poorly adherent pseudointima forms on the luminal surface.

      (2) An outer reinforcing layer is present on some grafts. In addition to increasing the bursting strength of the graft, this layer also prevents the ingrowth of tissue into the graft structure.

      (3) The PTFE grafts give results superior to those of the Dacron grafts when they are used in the lower extremity. The PTFE grafts are the second choice to the autogenous saphenous vein grafts when use of the veins is not practicable.

2. Potential problems

    a. All of the currently used synthetic grafts fail to develop a true endothelialized blood lumen.

      (1) Instead, a **pseudointima** develops, consisting of leukocyte, platelet, and red blood cell debris combined with fibrin and other proteins. This surface is both intrinsically thrombogenic and susceptible to infection from blood-borne organisms.

      (2) Endothelium covers only 1–2 cm of graft adjacent to each anastomotic site. This region is called the **pannus**.

    b. Whenever a **bacteremia** is anticipated, the patient should be given **prophylactic antibiotics** to prevent seeding of the graft with organisms.

8

Venous Disease, Pulmonary Embolism, and Lymphatic System

Bruce E. Jarrell
R. Anthony Carabasi, III

I. VENOUS DISEASE OF THE LOWER EXTREMITIES

A. Overview

1. **Anatomy.** The venous system is divided into four general areas.
   a. **The deep venous system** includes the popliteal, femoral, and iliac veins.
   b. **The superficial venous system** is made up of subcutaneous veins and the greater and lesser saphenous veins.
   c. **The communicating venous system** is a network of veins (**perforating veins**) connecting the superficial and deep systems with valves that allow flow only from the superficial to the deep system.
   d. **Venous valves** are delicate web-like structures in all lower extremity veins that prevent reverse blood flow in the veins. The valves prevent venous hypertension from occurring when the patient is in an erect position. In addition, they assure that blood is pumped from the superficial to the deep system and back towards the heart when the patient is walking.

2. **Etiology.** Venous disease may be caused by either congenital or acquired disorders.
   a. **Valvular incompetence** is the congenital or acquired inability of the valves to prevent reflux and gravitational hypertension of the venous system.
   b. **Venous thrombosis** is the formation of thrombi in the venous system. The thrombi usually originate at the calf vein level and progress cephalad. They occur as a result of elements of **Virchow's triad**:
      (1) **Trauma** to the vein wall (e.g., caused by surgery or physical injury)
      (2) **Decreased velocity** of venous blood flow (e.g., due to postoperative immobility or drugs, such as estrogen, which decrease venous tone)
      (3) **Increased coagulability** or a change in the cellular components of blood (e.g., due to surgery or polycythemia vera)

B. Disorders

1. **Superficial thrombophlebitis** is inflammation or thrombosis of the superficial veins. A pulmonary embolus rarely is present with superficial thrombophlebitis.
   a. **Clinical presentation**
      (1) A tender palpable cord along the course of a vein
      (2) A red, indurated vein
      (3) Varicose (dilated) veins
   b. **Treatment**
      (1) Bed rest and elevation of the extremity
      (2) Local application of heat for relief of pain
      (3) Support hose worn both during the period of inflammation and for prophylaxis
      (4) Heparin administration (not necessary if only superficial phlebitis is present)
   c. **Complications. Chronic recurrent superficial thrombophlebitis** is treated with antibiotics in addition to the treatment described above because the syndrome often includes a streptococcal lymphangitis, which, if untreated, results in additional occlusion of the lymphatics, resulting in continued edema, dilatation, and inflammation, creating a vicious circle.

2. **Varicose veins** are dilated networks in the subcutaneous venous system that result from valvular incompetence. Deep venous thrombosis is not often a factor in the development of varicose veins.

a. Clinical presentation
  (1) Local pain and edema
  (2) Local inflammation
  (3) Local hemorrhage into the surrounding tissue
  (4) Dilated superficial veins
  (5) A positive **Trendelenburg test**, which is a method of proving incompetent valves by occluding the superficial vein and demonstrating filling from the deep system
b. Treatment
  (1) Nonoperative management principally involves the use of support hose, which keeps the superficial system collapsed and minimizes the effect of venous hypertension on venous dilatation.
  (2) Operative management
    (a) Indications for surgery
      (i) Previous or impending hemorrhage from an ulcerated varicosity. Painless exsanguination from these lesions may occur, especially during sleep, if there is bleeding.
      (ii) Cosmetic considerations
      (iii) Primary incompetence of the greater saphenous vein at the saphenofemoral junction with the development of varicosities along the course of the vein
      (iv) Severe recurrent pain over the varicosity
    (b) Surgical procedures
      (i) Preoperative evaluation of the patency of the deep venous system. Ligation of the saphenous vein in the presence of a thrombosed deep system could result in massive venous obstruction and venous gangrene.
      (ii) Ligation and removal of the greater saphenous vein when involved
      (iii) Ligation of incompetent perforating veins between the superficial and deep systems
3. Deep venous thrombosis is thrombosis of part or all of the deep venous system of an extremity. It occurs in 250,000 individuals a year.
  a. Etiology
    (1) Deep venous thrombosis usually originates in the lower extremity venous system, starting at the calf vein level and progressing proximally to involve the popliteal, femoral, or iliac system. Some 80%–90% of **pulmonary emboli** originate here.
    (2) Other veins in which thrombi occasionally develop include:
      (a) Pelvic veins, especially during pregnancy, pelvic surgery, and gynecologic cancer
      (b) Renal veins, especially when intrinsic renal disease is present
      (c) Inferior vena cava
      (d) Ovarian veins
      (e) Upper extremity and neck veins, especially with athletic activity and the use of intravenous cannulas
      (f) The right atrium in the presence of intrinsic cardiac disorders
  b. Clinical presentation
    (1) The classic clinical syndrome includes calf or thigh pain, edema, tenderness, and a positive **Homan's sign** (calf pain on dorsiflexion of the foot). In patients with venographically proven deep venous thrombosis:
      (a) Fifty percent have the classic clinical findings.
      (b) Fifty percent have no associated physical findings in the extremities.
    (2) Pulmonary embolism is the presenting symptom in many patients.
    (3) Evaluation must ascertain the presence or absence of arterial vascular insufficiency.
  c. Diagnosis of deep venous thrombosis is made by means of **laboratory tests.**
    (1) Venogram of the ascending venous system is the **most accurate diagnostic method for deep venous thrombosis**. Radiopaque dye is injected into the pedal veins, and a tourniquet is loosely applied at the ankle to direct the flow of dye into the deep venous system. Inflammation or thrombosis of the veins occurs in 3% of patients who undergo venography unless the vein is flushed with a heparin solution after infusion.
    (2) Doppler ultrasound examination has an accuracy rate of 80%–90% for the diagnosis of deep venous thrombosis above the knee. The test determines:
      (a) Variation of flow in the femoral vein with respiration, which indicates the patency of the venous system between the femoral vein and the heart
      (b) Increased femoral venous flow when the blood is rapidly squeezed from the calf veins, indicating patency between the calf veins and the femoral vein

     (c) The presence of normal venous velocity in the femoral, popliteal, and posterior tibial veins

     (d) The presence of a difference in ultrasound findings between the diseased and the normal extremity

  (3) **Impedance plethysmography** measures the variations in the volume of calf blood upon releasing a blood pressure cuff placed so as to cause temporary thigh venous occlusion. This test is accurate for about 90% of cases of deep venous thrombosis above the knee.

  (4) **Iodine-125 (^{125}I) labeled fibrinogen scanning** is serial scanning of both lower extremities to detect the uptake of radioactive fibrinogen into a clot. This method is best used for diagnosis of thrombosis of the calf veins, but due to a small risk of hepatitis transmission, the popularity of this procedure is decreasing.

d. Treatment

  (1) Continuous **heparin** infusion is given for 7–10 days followed by administration of **warfarin** or subcutaneous administration of heparin for 3–6 months.

  (2) Thrombolytic therapy with **streptokinase** or **urokinase** is used if extensive deep venous thrombosis results in impaired perfusion of the extremity. There is insufficient data to support the use of thrombolytic therapy to prevent or decrease the incidence or severity of postphlebitic therapy, although it seems logical.

  (3) **Inferior vena caval interruption** is used only if heparin is contraindicated or if a pulmonary embolus occurs in spite of adequate anticoagulation therapy. However, this treatment prevents only pulmonary embolism and does not treat the deep venous thrombosis.

e. Prevention

  (1) **Simple preventive measures** include early mobilization after surgery, the use of support hose, which compresses superficial veins in the legs and increases flow in the deep veins, and the correction of preoperative risk factors, such as polycythemia vera.

  (2) **Intermittent calf compression** by means of a pneumatic cuff increases leg blood flow velocity and helps to prevent stasis.

  (3) Venoconstrictive substances, such as **dihydroergotamine**, may also increase deep venous blood velocity.

  (4) Pre- and postoperative administration of prophylactic **heparin** may be effective in preventing deep thrombosis. An intermittent subcutaneous dose of 3000–6000 units is given every 8–12 hours. At this dose heparin activates antithrombin III, inhibits platelet aggregation, and decreases thrombin availability. In several large series, heparin decreased:

     (a) Postoperative phlebitis. There was a 25% incidence in controls versus a 7% incidence in patients treated with heparin.

     (b) Fatal pulmonary embolism. There was a 7% mortality rate in controls versus a 1% mortality rate in those treated with heparin.

f. Complications

  (1) **Postphlebitic syndrome** occurs in 10% of patients with deep venous thrombosis and is due to permanent obstruction of the deep venous system. (Recanalization of veins occurs late if at all and usually results in incomplete recanalization and valvular incompetence.)

     (a) **Clinical presentation**

       (i) Chronic venous insufficiency occurs due to the development of dilated and, therefore, incompetent venous collaterals around the venous obstruction.

       (ii) **Leg edema**, **pain**, and **nocturnal cramping** can be minimal or severe.

       (iii) Venous **claudication** (pain, cramps, and a sensation of heaviness during exercise) may also occur.

       (iv) Abnormal **skin pigmentation** and **dermatitis** usually occur.

       (v) **Stasis ulceration** of the pretibial calf skin due to local superficial venous hypertension (especially during ambulation) causes edema, local thrombosis, and blood extravasation into the subcutaneous tissue followed by necrosis and ulceration. This may occur years after the episode of deep venous thrombosis, but it can result in severe progressive disability.

     (b) **Treatment**

       (i) Support hose is worn chronically to prevent superficial venous hypertension.

      (ii) Ligation of local perforating veins is used to lower the venous pressure at the ulcer if it will not heal.

      (iii) An Unna boot, a medicated pressure bandage, is applied weekly or biweekly until the ulcer heals.

      (iv) A change of life-style to avoid leg dependency may improve the ulceration.

  (2) Phlegmasia alba dolens is caused by acute occlusion of the iliac and femoral veins due to deep venous thrombosis.

    (a) Clinical presentation. It results in a **pale cool leg** with a diminished arterial pulse due to spasm.

    (b) Treatment is **thrombolytic therapy** followed by **heparin administration** to prevent progression to phlegmasia cerulea dolens.

  (3) Phlegmasia cerulea dolens is secondary to acute and nearly total venous occlusion of the entire extremity outflow, including the iliac and femoral veins. It is commoner in the left leg. Association with another disease is common: For example, 30% of cases occur in postoperative and postpartum patients, and pelvic malignancy is not infrequent.

    (a) Clinical presentation

      (i) Physical findings include cyanosis of the extremity with massive edema, severe pain, and absent pulses, followed by venous gangrene.

      (ii) Shock may occur as a result of sequestration of a significant amount of blood in the leg.

    (b) Treatment

      (i) Thrombolytic therapy followed by heparin administration

      (ii) Thrombectomy occasionally if nonoperative therapy is unsuccessful

      (iii) Bed rest with leg elevation

II. PULMONARY EMBOLISM is a mechanical obstruction of the flow of blood in the pulmonary arterial system due to lodgment of a thromboembolus. The resultant effects include decreased cardiac output, pulmonary vasospasm, hypertension, impaired blood oxygenation, and bronchospasm.

  A. Overview. Pulmonary embolism is one of the commonest causes of **sudden death in hospitalized patients**.

    1. Normal individuals can tolerate a 60%–70% occlusion of the pulmonary vasculature, but patients with preexisting cardiac or pulmonary disease tolerate much smaller occlusions poorly.

    2. Pulmonary embolism is frequently sudden and seemingly unheralded, although it is often preceded by the development of small and clinically unrecognized emboli. Only 10% of all autopsy-proven cases of pulmonary embolism are diagnosed premortem.

    3. Ninety percent of deaths occur within 2 hours after the onset of the initial symptoms. Therefore, if the patient lives longer than 2 hours, the chance of survival is very high.

    4. Pulmonary embolism develops in 10%–40% of patients with **deep venous thrombosis** (see I B 3). However, approximately 33% of patients with pulmonary embolism have no antecedent symptoms of deep venous thrombosis.

      a. Thrombosis in the venous system is caused by situations described in **Virchow's triad** (see I A 2 b).

      b. Pulmonary embolus formation can be prevented through the early diagnosis and prevention of deep venous thrombosis.

  B. Risk factors

    1. Pregnant women and women in the postpartum period have an incidence of pulmonary embolism five times greater than the incidence in age-matched controls. Pulmonary embolus formation is a common cause of death after pregnancy.

    2. Estrogen therapy is associated with an increased risk of pulmonary embolism four to seven times that of controls. The risk is dose-dependent and is eliminated within several weeks after cessation of therapy.

    3. Heart disease is associated with a three to four times higher risk of pulmonary embolus formation. This risk is directly related to the severity of the heart disease.

4. Obesity is associated with one and one-half to two times greater risk of pulmonary embolism.

5. Carcinoma is associated with a two to three times greater risk of pulmonary embolism.

6. Major trauma, especially spinal cord injury and pelvic or femoral shaft fractures, carries an increased risk of pulmonary embolus formation.

7. A history of pulmonary embolism increases the risk of later pulmonary embolus formation, especially after surgery.

8. Varicose veins are associated with a two times greater risk of pulmonary embolism.

9. Older age-groups are associated with an increased risk of developing pulmonary emboli.

C. **Symptoms** of pulmonary embolism range from none to severe cardiopulmonary dysfunction. In general, the more complicated the symptoms, the more unreliable the clinical diagnosis.

  1. Classic signs—hemoptysis, pleural friction rub, cardiac gallop, cyanosis, and **chest splinting**—are present in only 24% of patients.

  2. Nonspecific findings, including **tachycardia** (in 60% of cases), **tachypnea** (in 85% of cases), and **dyspnea** (in 85% of cases), are common. **Bronchospasm** and **pleuritic chest pain** also occur frequently.

  3. Electrocardiographic changes, including **arrhythmias** and evidence of **right ventricular strain**, may appear.

  4. Chest x-ray may be abnormal or totally normal.
    a. Occasionally, there is a **marked diminution of the pulmonary vasculature**, producing increased radiolucency in the area of the embolus (**Westermark's sign**).
    b. **Pleural effusion**, which is usually hemorrhagic, or **pulmonary infiltration** may be present, especially in cases of pulmonary infarction, which occurs in 10%–25% of cases of pulmonary embolism.

  5. Arterial blood gases frequently show hypoxemia with a low carbon dioxide partial pressure (Pco_2) associated with hyperventilation.
    a. Although serial measurements may document a sudden drop in oxygen partial pressure (Po_2), a single measurement is unlikely to confirm the diagnosis of pulmonary embolism.
    b. A normal Po_2 does not eliminate the possibility of pulmonary embolism.

D. **Diagnosis** of pulmonary embolism is based upon the results of several tests.

  1. Pulmonary arteriogram is the best technique for diagnosing pulmonary embolism. This test is virtually 100% accurate, but it is invasive, as a radiopaque dye is injected directly into the pulmonary artery. The attendant risk of cardiac arrest is small in stable patients, but it can be unacceptably high in hypotensive, unstable patients.

  2. Pulmonary radioisotope scanning is less invasive than arteriography.
    a. **Perfusion lung scan.** A radioactive particle, small enough to block a small number of pulmonary capillaries temporarily, is injected. A camera records different views of the uptake in the vasculature.
      (1) A major difficulty with this test is that many acute and chronic pulmonary diseases can result in similar perfusion defects. It is critical to compare the chest x-ray with the scan to determine the presence of other abnormalities.
      (2) A normal scan is very reliable in determining the absence of a pulmonary embolus.
        (a) The presence of segmental or large defects predicts pulmonary embolism in 71% of cases.
        (b) A subsegmental or small perfusion defect is associated with pulmonary embolism in only 27% of cases.
    b. **Ventilation scan** performed simultaneously with the perfusion lung scan improves the accuracy of the latter. An inert radioactive gas, such as xenon, is inhaled, and the patency and ventilation of the bronchial tree are assessed.
      (1) **Ventilation-perfusion mismatch** occurs when a perfusion defect is present but the ventilation scan is normal. **Matched ventilation-perfusion defect** occurs when a defect in the same location is revealed by both tests.

      (a) A segmental or large perfusion defect mismatched with a normal ventilation scan is associated with pulmonary embolism in 91% of cases.

      (b) A subsegmental or small perfusion defect mismatched with a normal ventilation scan is associated with pulmonary embolism in only 27% of cases.

      (c) A perfusion defect matched with a ventilation defect is associated with pulmonary embolism in 23% of cases.

    (2) When pulmonary embolus is clinically suspected but the lung scan is equivocal, an additional test should be performed to increase the reliability of those results. A **pulmonary arteriogram** is most reliable. A **leg venogram** is also useful in this situation in documenting the presence of deep venous thrombosis and, therefore, the likelihood of pulmonary embolism.

E. Treatment of pulmonary embolism includes supportive measures to maintain circulatory function and administration of heparin for systemic anticoagulation.

  1. Cardiovascular support is frequently necessary in patients with significant pulmonary embolism and should be instituted immediately. The supportive measures include oxygen administration, assisted ventilation, correction of cardiac arrhythmias, and treatment of shock by means of adequate hydration and vasopressors. Introduction of a Swan-Ganz catheter is usually necessary for adequate cardiopulmonary monitoring.

  2. Heparin as an anticoagulant should be administered in an initial bolus of 10,000–20,000 units to halt the thrombotic process and to stabilize platelets in the embolus to prevent the release of vasoactive and bronchoactive substances. Administration begins with a continuous intravenous drip of heparin at approximately 1000 units an hour; the dosage is then adjusted to maintain the partial thromboplastin time at one and one-half to two times the control time. Heparin is continued for a minimum of 7 days and is followed by long-term anticoagulation therapy for 3–6 months.

  3. Thrombolytic therapy with streptokinase, urokinase, or tissue plasminogen activator may be used in cases of acute life-threatening pulmonary embolism when cardiopulmonary function is severely compromised as evidenced by shock, profound hypoxemia, or elevated pulmonary arterial pressure. Because thrombolytic therapy results in the lysis of pre-existing thrombi, this therapy may be even more dangerous than heparin therapy, and it is **absolutely contraindicated** in patients with recent intracranial hemorrhage, recent surgery, or conditions associated with bleeding, such as peptic ulcer disease, large tumors, or urinary tract diseases associated with bleeding.

  4. Pulmonary embolectomy is reserved for very ill patients. If patients remain significantly unstable despite rapid resuscitation and, in the opinion of the attending physician, are too unstable to endure the several hour treatment with thrombolytic therapy, then embolectomy should be considered. A closed embolectomy, using a suction catheter, as well as an open embolectomy on cardiopulmonary bypass are the two most acceptable methods.

  5. Long-term anticoagulation may be maintained by either oral administration of warfarin or subcutaneous intermittent administration of heparin. The warfarin dosage should be carefully regulated to maintain the prothrombin time at 18–21 seconds. However, warfarin interacts with many other drugs, and its effectiveness can be severely altered by these drugs and by hepatic disease.

F. Complications of anticoagulation therapy

  1. Major hemorrhage requiring transfusions occurs in 1%–2% of patients on anticoagulants; **minor bleeding episodes** are common in over 16%; and fatal hemorrhage occurs in 0.1%–1%. The risk of hemorrhage is greater if heparin is administered intermittently or is given to elderly or severely hypertensive patients.

  2. Pulmonary embolism recurs despite anticoagulation therapy in 1%–8% of patients.

  3. Heparin-induced thrombocytopenia occurs in up to 5% of patients on heparin and may be related to the development of heparin-induced antibodies directed towards platelets. All heparin infusions must be discontinued if thrombocytopenia occurs, because of the risk of either hemorrhage or heparin-induced necrosis, a form of tissue necrosis that is related to localized intravascular thrombosis.

III. LYMPHATIC SYSTEM

A. Lymphedema is a condition characterized by swelling of one or more extremities caused by lymphatic insufficiency.

1. Types. Lymphedema may be idiopathic (**primary lymphedema**) or may be caused by acquired insufficiency due to infections, obstructions, or surgical destruction of the lymphatics (**secondary lymphedema**).

a. Primary lymphedema. Three types of primary lymphedema are distinguished by age of onset.

(1) Congenital lymphedema is present at birth or occurs early in infancy.

(a) It accounts for fewer than 10% of primary lymphedema cases.

(b) Lymphedema that is both congenital and hereditary is known as **Milroy's disease**.

(c) If there are virtually no lymphatics present at birth, the symptoms occur at that time. If some functioning lymphatics are present at birth, symptoms may be minimal or absent. As growth takes place and with repeated normal damage from minor infection or trauma, the remaining normal lymphatics are no longer adequate and edema occurs.

(2) Lymphedema praecox occurs at any time from puberty until the end of the third decade.

(a) Most cases of primary lymphedema are of this type.

(b) It is three times commoner in women than in men.

(3) Lymphedema tarda occurs after age 30.

b. Secondary lymphedema is due to obstruction from a variety of causes, including infection (see III C), parasites, mechanical injury (including surgery), postphlebitic syndrome, and neoplasms.

(1) In developed countries, the commonest causes are obstruction by malignancies, postsurgical lymphedema (e.g., lymphedema following mastectomy), and lymphatic destruction from therapeutic radiation.

(2) In less well-developed countries, parasitic obstruction (elephantiasis) is a common cause. *Wuchereria bancrofti* is the commonest offending parasite.

2. Diagnosis of lymphedema is usually made clinically.

a. The history characteristically includes edema, which begins at the ankle and progresses proximally. Progression is slow, usually over the course of several months.

b. Physical examination. Unlike the edema secondary to venous disease, the swollen extremity in lymphedema has no dark brawny edema or ulceration of the skin.

c. Laboratory tests. The diagnosis can be proven by lymphangiography, but this is not done routinely because it is difficult and hazardous.

3. Treatment

a. Medical treatment. Simple measures are the first line of treatment.

(1) Elevation of the affected limb, weight reduction, and salt restriction may be helpful.

(2) Compressive stockings may be of benefit if applied properly.

(3) It is extremely important to avoid trauma and infection, as these will greatly exacerbate the condition.

(4) Pulsatile compression devices may help to "squeeze" the edema from the swollen extremity in severe cases.

b. Surgical treatment to palliate uncontrolled lymphedema includes the following:

(1) The **Thompson procedure** is based on the assumption that dermal lymphatics may be functional even though the deep lymphatics are incompetent. A dermal flap is buried deep in the swollen extremity to provide competent lymphatics for drainage.

(2) The omentum, which contains an extensive lymphatic network, can also be transposed from the abdomen to the extremity. Although some benefit has been observed clinically by this procedure, no lymphatic communications between the omentum and the extremity have been demonstrated to develop in laboratory experiments.

(3) The most durable operation for chronic lymphedema is a staged resection of subcutaneous tissue and redundant skin, including muscle fascia, which was described originally by Sistruck and refined by Homans.

(a) This procedure leaves a large amount of redundant skin. This skin is excised, and the remaining skin is closed over subcutaneous drains.

(b) The procedure is done in stages, first on the medial side and then on the outer aspect of the leg.

       (c) Approximately 80% of patients treated with this operation have a substantial reduction in extremity size.

       (d) Periodic elevation for 30 minutes twice a day and leg compression are necessary to complement the operative procedure.

    (4) Microsurgical anastomoses between a lymphatic and a small vein have been tried.

       (a) This procedure works well when proximal lymphatics in the groin or pelvis are obstructed.

       (b) Dilated lymphatics distal to the point of obstruction can be anastomosed to nearby veins, theoretically providing a decompression mechanism for lymphatic fluid.

B. Lymphatic tumors

1. Benign tumors are most commonly **cystic hygromas**.

    a. These are derived from embryonic lymph sacs and are seen during the first year of life.

    b. They are most commonly found in the neck but also occur in the groin, axilla, and mediastinum.

    c. Cystic hygromas in the neck may cause respiratory distress and, in this case, should be excised. Cranial nerves should not be sacrificed, since these are benign tumors.

2. Lymphangiosarcoma is an extremely rare **malignant lymphatic tumor**. It can occur in any extremity affected by chronic lymphedema, but it is seen most commonly after a mastectomy that is complicated by lymphedema of the arm [see Chapter 23 III G 1 c (3)].

3. Lymphatic metastases are seen with many kinds of primary tumor.

C. Lymphangitis and lymphadenitis

1. Causes. Inflammation in the lymphatic channels (**lymphangitis**) and in the lymph nodes (**lymphadenitis**) is caused by bacterial invasion, usually by β-hemolytic streptococci or by staphylococci.

2. Clinical presentation. Usually, an extremity is affected.

    a. There is hyperemia around the affected lymphatic, manifested by a red streak, which advances toward the draining lymph nodes.

    b. Movement of the affected extremity is painful and also propels the bacteria along the lymphatic channel, exacerbating the condition.

    c. If the process is not arrested by the lymph nodes, septicemia can occur.

3. Treatment consists of immobilizing the limb and giving antibiotics. If a source of bacterial seeding is present (e.g., a paronychia), it should be drained. Uncomplicated cases resolve promptly and usually without sequelae. Repeated insults can result in a chronic secondary lymphedema.

Part III Vascular Disorders

STUDY QUESTIONS

Directions: Each question below contains five suggested answers. Choose the **one best** response to each question.

1. Regions where atherosclerotic lesions are likely to occur include all of the following EXCEPT the

(A) infrarenal aorta
(B) superficial femoral artery
(C) proximal internal carotid artery
(D) supraceliac aorta
(E) proximal coronary arteries

2. Characteristics of arterial claudication include all of the following EXCEPT

(A) it causes profound fatigue in the leg, hip, and thigh
(B) it is regularly produced by exercise
(C) it is relieved by rest in several minutes
(D) it occurs after sitting for long periods of time
(E) extremity pulses are diminished

3. All of the following complications may commonly follow lower extremity angiography EXCEPT

(A) renal failure
(B) dehydration
(C) arterial occlusion
(D) pseudoaneurysm formation
(E) intracerebral hemorrhage

4. Foot ulcers secondary to arterial insufficiency are successfully treated by all of the following techniques EXCEPT

(A) debridement of devitalized tissue
(B) elevation of the affected extremity
(C) antibiotic administration
(D) bed rest
(E) avoidance of pressure on the heel

5. Aortoiliac vascular reconstruction is indicated by all of the following clinical presentations EXCEPT

(A) impotence related to bilateral internal iliac artery occlusion
(B) rest pain in the foot
(C) complete occlusion of the external iliac artery
(D) gangrene of the toes
(E) emboli in the leg originating from the distal aorta

6. The commonest cause of death following arterial reconstruction of the lower extremity is

(A) graft infection
(B) cerebrovascular accident
(C) myocardial infarction
(D) systemic sepsis secondary to skin necrosis
(E) none of the above

7. True statements concerning acute arterial occlusion include all of the following EXCEPT

(A) it is usually caused by emboli that originate from a cardiac source
(B) it results in severe pain
(C) it requires immediate heparinization
(D) a fasciotomy is always required following restoration of blood flow
(E) balloon catheter embolectomy is the most commonly used surgical procedure

8. A 65-year-old woman with a long history of atrial fibrillation presents to the emergency room with a history of sudden onset of severe abdominal pain. Following the onset of pain, she vomited once and had a large bowel movement. No flatus has been passed since that time. Physical examination reveals a mildly distended abdomen, which is diffusely tender, although peritoneal signs are absent. Ten years ago, she underwent an abdominal hysterectomy. The most likely diagnosis in this patient would be

(A) acute cholecystitis
(B) perforated duodenal ulcer
(C) acute diverticulitis
(D) acute embolic mesenteric ischemia
(E) small bowel obstruction secondary to adhesions

9. Characteristics of a patient with renovascular hypertension include all of the following EXCEPT

(A) sudden onset of severe hypertension in a patient younger than 35
(B) inability to control blood pressure despite multiple drug therapy
(C) sudden worsening of hypertension in a patient who had been well controlled
(D) presence of flank bruits
(E) elevated white blood cell count in the urine

10. All of the following statements concerning abdominal aortic aneurysm are true EXCEPT

(A) most abdominal aortic aneurysms are caused by atherosclerosis

(B) most abdominal aortic aneurysms begin just above the level of the renal arteries

(C) abdominal aortic aneurysms are most frequently discovered on physical examination

(D) a CT scan gives details about the relationship of the aneurysm to renal and visceral vessels and demonstrates accompanying venous anomalies

(E) angiography should be carried out in patients with suspected renovascular hypertension or mesenteric ischemia

11. All of the following statements concerning popliteal artery aneurysms are true EXCEPT

(A) the usual cause is atherosclerosis

(B) they are bilateral in 50% of cases

(C) many of these patients have an associated abdominal aortic aneurysm

(D) rupture is quite common so these aneurysms should be repaired when discovered

(E) most popliteal aneurysms are treated by ligation and bypass

12. Factors that increase the risk of pulmonary embolism in patients undergoing surgery include

(A) superficial phlebitis 1 year ago

(B) estrogen therapy

(C) obesity

(D) pregnancy

(E) deep venous thrombosis 1 year ago

13. Clinical findings associated with varicose veins include all of the following EXCEPT

(A) deep venous thrombosis

(B) a positive Trendelenburg test

(C) valvular incompetence

(D) local hemorrhage

(E) pain relief with support hose

14. Correct statements concerning deep venous thrombosis include all of the following EXCEPT

(A) it is most accurately diagnosed by venography

(B) about 50% of patients have no physical findings in the extremities

(C) iodine-125 fibrinogen scanning is highly accurate for iliac vein thrombosis

(D) it most often originates in the lower extremity venous system

(E) heparin infusion is the treatment of choice

15. Postphlebitic syndrome is associated with all of the following conditions EXCEPT

(A) chronic stasis ulceration

(B) venous valvular incompetence

(C) venous claudication

(D) recurrent pulmonary embolism

(E) dermatitis

16. True statements concerning diagnostic procedures for pulmonary embolism include all of the following EXCEPT

(A) a ventilation-perfusion scan is more accurate than a perfusion scan alone for detecting pulmonary embolism

(B) pulmonary arteriography is highly accurate in detecting clinically significant pulmonary emboli

(C) a normal lung scan essentially rules out a pulmonary embolus

(D) a perfusion lung scan is helpful in differentiating pulmonary embolism from chronic pulmonary disease

(E) a leg venogram documents the presence of deep venous thrombosis and, therefore, the possibility of pulmonary embolism

17. Which of the following statements concerning the treatment of pulmonary embolism with anticoagulation therapy is true?

(A) Thrombolytic therapy with streptokinase may be used with patients who have life-threatening pulmonary embolism complicated by intracranial hemorrhage

(B) Heparin is most effective when administered intermittently, especially to elderly patients

(C) Pulmonary embolism recurs despite anticoagulation therapy in 30% of cases

(D) Warfarin is most useful for long-term anticoagulation therapy, as associated drug interactions are mininal

(E) None of the above statements is true

18. All of the following statements about primary lymphedema are true EXCEPT

(A) Milroy's disease occurs in women over 30 years of age and tends to run in families

(B) the three types of primary lymphedema differ only in the age of the patient at onset

(C) lymphedema may be exacerbated by repeated damage from minor infections

(D) lymphangiography will confirm the diagnosis

(E) in mild cases, primary lymphedema will respond to compression stockings and elevation

Directions: Each question below contains four suggested answers of which **one or more** is correct. Choose the answer

A   if **1, 2, and 3** are correct
B   if **1 and 3** are correct
C   if **2 and 4** are correct
D   if **4** is correct
E   if **1, 2, 3, and 4** are correct

19. True statements concerning vascular grafts include which of the following?

(1) Atherosclerotic lesions may appear in arterialized saphenous vein bypass grafts
(2) Synthetic vascular grafts spontaneously develop a lining of endothelial cells in the midgraft region in humans
(3) Vascular heterografts have a tendency to form aneurysms
(4) Arterial allografts from human cadaver donors have a high rate of success when used for aortic bypass

20. A 65-year-old man presents with a history of melanotic stools for the past 3 days. Eight years prior to this office visit he underwent resection of an abdominal aortic aneurysm, which was corrected by placement of an aortobilateral iliac graft. He has no gastrointestinal complaints and has been in good health since his operation. Rectal examination reveals no masses in the ampulla, and the stool is grossly heme-positive. Which of the following studies would be useful in the evaluation of this patient?

(1) Upper gastrointestinal endoscopy
(2) CT scan
(3) Colonoscopy
(4) Arteriography

21. A child who was involved in a playground scuffle decided not to report it. Some time later, the teacher noticed the child protecting her elbow. Examination showed a laceration with a red streak extending toward the armpit. The school nurse diagnosed lymphangitis. Correct statements regarding this patient include which of the following?

(1) Septicemia may occur if the process is not arrested by the lymph nodes
(2) *Escherichia coli* is the most commonly isolated organism
(3) Any source of infection, such as a paronychia or other collections, should be drained
(4) Exercising the affected limb to promote lymphatic drainage is mandatory

22. True statements concerning cystic hygromas include which of the following?

(1) They are derived from embryonic lymph sacs
(2) They occur in the neck, groin, axilla, and mediastinum
(3) They may enlarge enough to cause respiratory distress
(4) Removal should include cranial nerve resection, since recurrence rates are high

Directions: The group of questions below consists of lettered choices followed by several numbered items. For each numbered item select the **one** lettered choice with which it is **most closely** associated. Each lettered choice may be used once, more than once, or not at all.

Questions 23 and 24

Match each description of a lymphatic neoplasm to the appropriate tumor or tumors.

(A) Lymphangiosarcoma
(B) Cystic hygroma
(C) Both
(D) Neither

23. This is a rare form of malignant lymphatic tumor

24. This tumor occurs most frequently in the mastectomy patient with lymphedema

ANSWERS AND EXPLANATIONS

1. The answer is D. [*Chapter 7 I A*] Atherosclerotic lesions occur at characteristic locations. Among the commonest are the coronary arteries, the infrarenal aorta, the superficial femoral artery, and the internal carotid artery. Areas that are frequently spared include the supraceliac aorta and the distal deep femoral artery. The exact reason that lesions form in these locations is unknown. The current theory is that lesions form in areas of low shear stress and low flow, which are characteristics of the locations mentioned above.

2. The answer is D. [*Chapter 7 I B 1 a (1)–(4), 2 a*] One of the most characteristic symptoms of peripheral vascular disease is claudication—that is, pain that commonly occurs in the calf muscles and less commonly in the buttocks and thigh muscles. Extremity pulses often are diminished or absent. The pain occurs after a predictable amount of exercise and is promptly relieved by rest. Pain that occurs after sitting or standing for prolonged periods is not due to arterial insufficiency but more likely is due to a musculoskeletal disorder.

3. The answer is E. [*Chapter 7 I C 2 c (2) (a)–(c)*] Angiography is a relatively safe procedure; however, an awareness of the complications that can occur is the first step toward prevention. The chances of renal failure or dehydration can be minimized by adequate pre- and post-procedure hydration. The appropriate choice of puncture site can minimize the chances for acute arterial occlusion. Usually, a large artery, such as the femoral artery, is chosen to avoid acute thrombosis around the indwelling catheter. Following removal of the catheter, pressure must be applied for 20–30 minutes to assure an adequate seal in the puncture site. Failure to do this allows blood to extravasate from the arterial puncture into the surrounding tissue, which may result in a hematoma or a pseudoaneurysm. Intracerebral hemorrhage is not a complication usually associated with angiography.

4. The answer is B. [*Chapter 7 II C 1–4*] Foot ulcers can develop secondary to arterial insufficiency; however, with early care, ulcers can be controlled and healed before they become extensive. Ulcers can be successfully treated by debridement of devitalized tissue, immobilization of the affected limb, systemic or local administration of antibiotics, amputation of necrotic tissue, avoidance of weight bearing on an affected limb, and bed rest without elevation of the affected limb; elevation of an ischemic limb will decrease arterial perfusion, thereby impeding the healing process. It is important to avoid decubitus ulcers in patients at bed rest. Prolonged pressure on the heel must be avoided by frequent changes in position and appropriate padding.

5. The answer is C. [*Chapter 7 III A, B 1–4*] Indications for surgery in aortoiliac occlusive disease include severe claudication or rest pain, tissue necrosis of the lower extremities or toes, formation of distal arterial emboli, and impotence secondary to bilateral internal iliac occlusion. Aortoiliac vascular reconstruction is an inadequate procedure for complete occlusion of the external iliac artery because it will not restore sufficient blood flow to the affected limb. Also, there is a high risk of thrombosis of the graft limb that feeds the affected side because of inadequate outflow.

6. The answer is C. [*Chapter 7 IV C 2 a (3)*] Myocardial infarction remains the leading cause of death in patients undergoing virtually any type of vascular reconstruction. For this reason, in elective circumstances, cardiac evaluation is recommended preoperatively. Should occult, severe coronary artery disease be present, consideration should be given to repair of the coronary artery disease prior to elective vascular surgery. Graft infection, systemic sepsis from gangrene, and cerebrovascular accidents are only occasional causes of morbidity and mortality in these patients.

7. The answer is D. [*Chapter 7 V A 1–3, B 1–4, C 1, 4*] Acute arterial occlusion is the sudden cessation of arterial blood flow to an extremity, which results in ischemia that may be followed by necrosis if rapid intervention does not occur. The most frequent cause of the occlusion is the lodgment of emboli that originate from atherosclerotic heart disease (60%), rheumatic heart disease (21%), or abdominal aortic ulcerated plaques (1%–2%). Clinical findings include sudden severe pain; a pale, cool, pulseless extremity; acute loss of motor and sensory function; and low or undetectable ankle blood pressure. Patients should be heparinized immediately (i.e., when the clinical diagnosis is made) and operated on within 6 hours of the onset of symptoms. The surgeon usually will perform an embolectomy, using a Fogarty balloon catheter. Fasciotomy is not always required, especially if the revascularization is done promptly and is uncomplicated. If the patient develops swelling, pain in the leg out of proportion to physical findings, and elevated compartment pressure in the leg that has been ischemic for a prolonged period, fasciotomy is performed.

8. The answer is D. [*Chapter 7 VI B 1 a–c*] The triad of a cardiac arrhythmia, the sudden onset of severe abdominal pain, and gut emptying is classic for embolic mesenteric ischemia. This constitutes a surgical emergency, and the patient described in the question should be treated with vigorous rehydration followed by arteriography to confirm the diagnosis. Prompt embolectomy of the superior mesenteric artery could salvage this patient provided that there is no delay in her definitive surgical treatment.

9. The answer is E. [*Chapter 7 VII B 1–4*] Patients with renovascular hypertension generally have a diastolic blood pressure greater than 110 mm Hg. Sudden onset at the extremes of age should be a clue that this condition may be present. Patients who have been stable and suddenly develop severe uncontrolled high blood pressure also merit consideration of this diagnosis. The presence of flank bruits is a nonspecific finding but is highly suggestive in a patient who meets the above criteria.

10. The answer is B. [*Chapter 7 IX A 1 a–c*] Abdominal aortic aneurysms most commonly originate below the level of the renal arteries. They are usually found on physical examination or during evaluation for an unrelated abdominal condition for which the patient has a CT scan, ultrasound, or abdominal x-rays. A CT scan demonstrates the relationship of the aneurysm to renal and visceral vessels and shows associated venous anomalies. Angiography shows associated severe renal artery lesions or lesions of the visceral vessels and should be done in patients who manifest signs or symptoms of these conditions.

11. The answer is D. [*Chapter 7 IX D 3 a, b*] Rupture of popliteal artery aneurysms is quite rare, but embolization and thrombosis are common; thus, these aneurysms should be repaired when discovered. The commonest cause is atherosclerosis, and these are bilateral in 50% of cases and frequently associated with aneurysms in other locations, such as the abdominal aorta. Complete excision of these aneurysms is risky since they are usually adherent to the accompanying veins and nerves. For this reason, most popliteal artery aneurysms are treated by ligation and bypass.

12. The answer is A. [*Chapter 8 I B 1; II B 1–9*] Pulmonary embolism is one of the commonest causes of sudden death in hospitalized patients. Patients who are at increased risk for pulmonary embolism include the following: patients with deep venous thrombosis or varicose veins, pregnant women and women in the postpartum period, women undergoing estrogen therapy, obese patients, cancer patients, trauma patients, and patients who have had previous pulmonary embolism. Previous episodes of superficial phlebitis are not associated with pulmonary embolism.

13. The answer is A. [*Chapter 8 I B 2*] Varicose veins are dilatated networks in the subcutaneous venous system that result from valvular incompetence. Deep venous thrombosis is not often a factor in the development of varicose veins. Clinical findings associated with varicose veins include edema, pain, inflammation, dilated superficial veins, local hemorrhage into the surrounding tissue, and a positive Trendelenburg test, which indicates incompetent valves.

14. The answer is C. [*Chapter 8 I B 3 a (1), b (1), c (1), (4), d (1)*] The origin of deep venous thrombosis is most often in the lower extremity venous system. The classic clinical picture includes calf or thigh pain, edema, tenderness, and a positive Homan's sign; however, 50% of patients with proven venous thrombosis have no physical findings in the extremities. While venography is the most accurate diagnostic technique, Doppler ultrasonography and impedance plethysmography are also highly accurate, provided that the thrombosis occurs above the knee. Iodine-125 fibrinogen scanning is less accurate in upper leg thrombosis. The treatment of choice for uncomplicated deep venous thrombosis is continuous heparin infusion for 7–10 days, followed by administration of warfarin or subcutaneous administration of heparin for 3–6 months.

15. The answer is D. [*Chapter 8 I B 3 f (1)*] The postphlebitic syndrome generally presents as a lower leg complication due to a permanent obstruction of the deep venous system. It occurs in 10% of patients with deep venous thrombosis. Physical findings include chronic venous insufficiency, venous valvular incompetence, leg edema, pain, nocturnal cramping, venous claudication, abnormal skin pigmentation, and dermatitis. Stasis ulceration may occur years after the episode of deep venous thrombosis, but it can result in severe progressive disability. Pulmonary embolism is not likely to occur as part of this syndrome, although it can occur after any episode of deep venous thrombosis.

16. The answer is D. [*Chapter 8 II D*] Pulmonary ventilation is assessed with an inert radioactive gas, such as xenon, which is inhaled; the technique improves the accuracy of the perfusion scan. Pulmonary arteriography is diagnostic in almost all cases, but it is an invasive procedure with a risk of causing cardiac arrest. A perfusion lung scan can show similar results with pulmonary embolism or chronic pulmonary disease; however, a normal scan rules out an embolus. A leg venogram documents the presence of deep venous thrombosis, which is the most common origin of pulmonary embolism.

17. The answer is E. [*Chapter 8 II E 1–5, F 1, 2*] Thrombolytic therapy with streptokinase or urokinase may be used in patients with acute life-threatening pulmonary embolism; however, it is contraindicated in patients with recent intracranial hemorrhage, recent surgery, or other bleeding disorders. Heparin as an anticoagulant should be administered as an initial bolus of 10,000–20,000 units and continued as an intravenous drip at approximately 1000 units an hour for a minimum of 7 days. The risk of hemorrhage is greatest if heparin is administered intermittently or is given to elderly or severely hypertensive patients. Although warfarin can be used for long-term anticoagulation therapy, its effectiveness can be severely altered by its interactions with other drugs. Despite anticoagulation therapy, pulmonary embolism recurs in 1%–8% of patients.

18. The answer is A. [*Chapter 8 III A 1 a, 2 c, 3 a*] The three types of primary lymphedema are congenital lymphedema, lymphedema praecox, and lymphedema tarda; all three types appear to be similar except for the age of the patient at onset. Repeated lymphatic damage from minor infections and trauma reduces the number of normal lymphatics, thereby exacerbating the disorder. Most mild cases are controlled by elevating the affected limb and by using compression stockings; more advanced cases are controlled by pneumatic compression devices. Milroy's disease is a form of congenital lymphedema and, thus, is present at birth or early in life. It is also hereditary. Lymphedema in a 30-year-old woman would be classified as lymphedema tarda.

19. The answer is B (1, 3). [*Chapter 7 XI A 1, 3 a, 4, B 2 a*] Arterialization of the saphenous vein grafts results in thickening of the vein wall. Although most of these grafts do well, atherosclerotic lesions appear in 2%–15% of arterialized veins with time. Vascular heterografts, vessels removed from animals and rendered nonantigenic by the tanning process, have been used successfully for both vascular reconstruction and hemodialysis vascular access; however, they have a tendency to develop aneurysms (in 3%–6% of cases) in certain applications. Arterial allografts have a high rate of degeneration and are generally not used. All of the currently used synthetic grafts fail to develop a true endothelialized blood lumen; instead, a pseudointima develops that is thrombogenic and susceptible to infection.

20. The answer is E (all). [*Chapter 7 IX C 4 e (3) (d), 5*] A patient who presents with gastrointestinal bleeding and a history of an intra-abdominal aortic graft must be presumed to have an aortoenteric fistula until proven otherwise. This patient should undergo upper gastrointestinal endoscopy in an attempt to visualize the entire stomach and duodenum. This will rule out peptic ulcer and gastritis. If the distal duodenum can be seen, erosions in this area would be highly suggestive of an aortoenteric fistula. A CT scan may demonstrate the presence of a false aneurysm and fluid or gas surrounding the infected aortic prosthesis. If these studies are negative, the patient should undergo colonoscopy to evaluate for the presence of colonic neoplasms or diverticulosis and to visualize arteriovenous malformations. Arteriography is useful to plan reconstruction should graft excision be necessary and to demonstrate a pseudoaneurysm if the aortic or iliac anastomosis is disrupted secondary to infection. These symptoms should be evaluated emergently, however, because of the risk of spontaneous free rupture and exsanguination.

21. The answer is B (1, 3). [*Chapter 8 III C 2 a*] Lymphangitis is an acute inflammation of the lymphatic channels. Staphylococci and β-hemolytic streptococci are the usual causative pathogens. Septicemia can occur if the lymph nodes do not arrest the infection. Any source of infection must be adequately drained. The extremity should be at rest, and exercise is contraindicated since it will propel the bacteria through the lymph channels, which is likely to exacerbate the situation.

22. The answer is A (1, 2, 3). [*Chapter 8 III B 1*] Cystic hygromas are the commonest benign tumors of the lymphatics. Derived from embryonic lymph sacs, they are seen during the first year of life. They occur most often in the neck, where they can become large enough to cause respiratory distress. Other, less common, sites are the groin, axilla, and mediastinum. Cranial nerves should not be sacrificed since these tumors are benign.

23 and 24. The answers are: 23-A, 24-A. [*Chapter 8 III B 1, 2*] Lymphangiosarcoma is a very rare neoplasm of the lymphatic system. Most neoplasms in the lymphatics are metastatic tumors. Lymphangiosarcoma most often occurs after a mastectomy in an arm that has been complicated by lymphedema.

Cystic hygroma is the most commonly occurring benign tumor of the lymphatic system. It occurs during the first year of life, most often in the neck but also in the groin, axilla, and mediastinum. Cystic hygroma in the neck may cause respiratory distress and, thus, should be excised.

Part IV
Gastrointestinal Disorders

9

Common Life-Threatening Disorders

Vincent T. Armenti
Bruce E. Jarrell

I. ACUTE ABDOMEN

A. Definition. The acute abdomen is the term used for an episode of severe abdominal pain that lasts for several hours or longer and requires medical attention. Prompt diagnosis is important because an acute abdomen is caused by an intra-abdominal emergency in most patients.

B. Symptoms. The history obtained from the patient should elicit both specific symptoms typical of a disease process and nonspecific symptoms.

1. Nonspecific symptoms should be elicited first.
  a. Pain
    (1) Gradual periumbilical pain indicates visceral peritoneal irritation, such as appendicitis, diverticulitis, or other inflammatory conditions. The pain may become more specifically localized as the disease process progresses.
    (2) Severe, explosive pain indicates a process that immediately soils the parietal peritoneum, such as perforation of a hollow viscus. The pain may be either localized or generalized.
    (3) Progressive, severe pain suggests a worsening intra-abdominal condition, such as occurs with ischemic necrosis of the bowel or other organs.
    (4) Localized pain that recurs as a generalized pain suggests that the inflamed organ has perforated. Acute appendicitis, for example, causes right lower quadrant pain, which then becomes generalized if perforation occurs.
    (5) Crampy pain indicates an obstruction in the gastrointestinal tract. This type of pain has a crescendo component, building up to intense pain, followed by a decrescendo component; the patient may then have an interval with no pain.
      (a) Distinguishing between crampy pain versus constant or other types of pain is very important because crampy pain is associated with bowel obstruction.
      (b) If crampy pain develops into constant severe pain, it suggests that the involved bowel segment is now ischemic or gangrenous.
  b. Anorexia, nausea, and vomiting are common accompanying symptoms in acute inflammatory abdominal processes. Although they are reliably present when a problem is surgical, they also accompany nonsurgical diseases, in which case they often precede the pain (as in gastroenteritis).
  c. Changes in bowel habits are so common that they are seldom helpful unless very specific changes occur. For example:
    (1) Bloody diarrhea suggests colitis, *Salmonella* infestation, or colonic ischemia.
    (2) Patients with intestinal obstruction usually pass no flatus or bowel movement by rectum for 1–2 days prior to seeking medical attention.
  d. Symptoms of sepsis, such as **chills** and **fever,** may be nonspecific, although certain patterns are typical of certain diseases. For example:
    (1) The fever of uncomplicated appendicitis rarely exceeds 101° F, whereas that of perforation often exceeds 101° F.
    (2) Cholangitis with choledocholithiasis is often accompanied by a shaking chill.

2. Specific symptoms should be elicited as clues to specific diseases.
  a. Previous surgery. A history of previous surgery yields important information.
    (1) Adhesions may have formed within the peritoneal cavity, leading to intestinal obstruction.

      (2) If the surgery was for malignant disease, the malignancy may have recurred, causing pain, sepsis, intestinal obstruction, and other symptoms.

      (3) Previous removal of any organ (most likely the appendix, the gallbladder, or the uterus, ovaries, and fallopian tubes) eliminates that organ from consideration.

      (4) Previous surgery may point to a specific problem; for example, suppurative cholangitis in a patient with previous choledocholithiasis and retained common duct stone.

   b. Previous episodes of similar pain warrant questions about the subsequent disease course and the results of any diagnostic studies that were performed.

   c. Characteristic maneuvers in certain diseases that provide temporary relief of pain must be sought.

      (1) A patient with acute peritonitis will lie very still; any movement results in excruciating pain.

      (2) A patient with a common duct stone or a kidney stone will pace the floor, unable to find a comfortable position.

      (3) The pain of an acute peptic ulcer may be relieved by food or antacids, whereas pain from acute cholecystitis or pancreatitis may be exacerbated by food.

   d. Previous illnesses. A history of disease in other body systems may be very useful.

      (1) Urinary tract. Symptoms such as dysuria, hematuria, or changes in urinary habits should be sought.

      (2) Reproductive tract in the female. The patient should be asked about a past or present vaginal discharge, dysmenorrhea, a history of pelvic inflammatory disease, time of last menstrual period, and so forth.

      (3) Cardiovascular system. Atrial fibrillation of recent onset or digitalis therapy might suggest intestinal ischemia.

      (4) Diabetes mellitus is associated with sepsis.

C. Physical examination of the patient with acute abdominal pain should yield new information that reinforces impressions obtained from the history. As with the history, there are both specific and nonspecific findings.

  1. Complete physical examination must be performed so that an important related or unrelated extra-abdominal diagnosis will not be missed. Points requiring particular attention include the following:

   a. Changes in vital signs, particularly fever, tachypnea, hypotension, or cardiac rhythm irregularities

   b. Inspection for jaundice, dehydration, feculent breath, pneumonia, or mental disorientation or obtundation

   c. Examination of the extremities for loss of pulses

  2. Abdominal examination

   a. Overall inspection

      (1) A distended abdomen with visible peristalsis suggests small bowel obstruction.

      (2) Prominent muscle guarding or rigidity will be visible, particularly if it is localized to one area of the abdomen.

      (3) A scaphoid abdomen may suggest herniation of the abdominal contents through the diaphragm and into the thoracic cavity, particularly after blunt abdominal trauma.

      (4) Hernias are frequently visible, particularly when the patient is standing.

   b. Palpation of the abdomen should be done gently and should begin away from the area of maximum tenderness.

      (1) The inguinal area should be examined for hernias or inflammatory conditions.

      (2) The abdomen should be examined to determine the points of maximum tenderness or the presence of referred tenderness. **Rebound tenderness** is tenderness that occurs when the examining hand is quickly removed from the abdominal wall. It is indicative of acute peritoneal irritation.

      (3) Spasm is determined by gently depressing the abdominal wall muscles.

         (a) Comparing two areas simultaneously allows the examiner to distinguish an abnormal area from a normal one.

         (b) A spasm is **voluntary** if the patient is tensing the muscle in response to pain and **involuntary** if the muscle is taut secondary to the underlying inflammatory process.

    (4) Palpation for abdominal masses should be done systematically. A mass in a particular abdominal quadrant suggests a specific diagnosis.

        (a) Right upper quadrant: Acute cholecystitis or a complication of this diagnosis, such as subhepatic or intrahepatic abscess

        (b) Left lower quadrant: Acute diverticulitis or peridiverticular abscess

        (c) Right lower quadrant: Acute appendicitis or appendiceal abscess

        (d) Left upper quadrant (uncommon in the acute abdomen): Complication of gastric or colonic malignancy, subphrenic abscess, or some acute inflammatory process related to the spleen, such as infarction

        (e) Midabdominal area: Pancreatic malignancy or abscess, complication of a perforated ulcer, or leaking abdominal aortic aneurysm

  c. Percussion of the abdomen

    (1) Percussion is useful because it confirms areas of maximum tenderness and the presence of rebound tenderness.

    (2) On rare occasions, the hollow sound of **tympany** indicates free intraperitoneal air, but it usually is present because of air in the intestine.

    (3) A large area of tympany in the left upper quadrant suggests acute gastric dilation, a condition that can cause reflex hypotension through vagal pathways.

  d. Auscultation is useful in many acute abdominal problems.

    (1) A silent abdomen indicates the absence of peristalsis, suggesting diffuse peritonitis, which occurs with major abdominal sepsis, intestinal ischemia or gangrene, or prolonged (longer than 3 days) mechanical obstruction with marked distention of the bowel. Absent peristalsis may also indicate an ileus, resulting from some other process, such as pneumonia, a renal stone, or trauma.

    (2) Intermittent peristaltic rushes that have a crescendo followed by silence suggest an intestinal obstruction. This sign is particularly useful when the peristaltic rush coincides with the onset of episodic abdominal pain. Certain nonsurgical inflammatory conditions, such as gastroenteritis, produce **high-pitched intermittent peristaltic rushes**. The pain pattern is usually not synchronous with the rushes.

3. Rectal examination should be performed routinely in patients with acute abdominal pain.

  a. Rectal palpation may localize the tenderness. In acute appendicitis, if the patient's appendix is located in the pelvis, the only physical finding may be a right pelvic tenderness found on rectal examination.

  b. The presence of blood in the stool suggests either a malignancy, hemorrhoids, or an acute inflammatory gastrointestinal process, such as an ulcer or colitis.

  c. A mass palpable on rectal examination may be a pelvic abscess secondary to a perforated viscus, a sign of pelvic inflammatory disease, or a metastatic malignancy.

  d. Acute prostatitis in men is diagnosed rectally even though it may present with vague abdominal pain.

4. Gynecologic examination should be performed in all women and girls with abdominal pain. (The patient's bladder should be empty.)

  a. Cervical or parauterine tenderness suggests pelvic inflammatory disease.

  b. A uterine, ovarian, or pelvic mass suggests:

    (1) Intrauterine pregnancy

    (2) Ectopic pregnancy with rupture and hemorrhage

    (3) Pelvic, ovarian, or tubal inflammatory disease with or without abscess formation

    (4) Pelvic or gynecologic malignancy

  c. Cervical discharges should be examined microscopically for gonococci.

5. Examination of the genitalia should be performed in all men and boys. Torsion of the testicle, a urologic emergency, may present as sudden onset of lower quadrant or scrotal tenderness.

6. Special signs are useful in diagnosing acute abdominal pain.

  a. Tenderness to percussion over the liver or kidney suggests acute hepatitis or pyelonephritis.

  b. Iliopsoas sign is pain in the lower abdomen and psoas region that is elicited when the thigh is flexed against resistance. It suggests that an inflammatory process, such as appendicitis or perinephric abscess, is in contact with the psoas muscle. Patients may also limp while walking and may lie with the ipsilateral hip flexed to minimize psoas muscle use.

c. Obturator sign is pain elicited when the thigh is flexed and then rotated internally and externally. It suggests an inflammatory process in the region of the obturator muscle, such as an obturator hernia.

d. Murphy's sign is elicited by palpating the right upper quadrant during inspiration: As the gallbladder descends during inspiration, acute pain is elicited. It suggests acute cholecystitis.

e. Cough tenderness occurs in the area of maximum tenderness when the patient coughs. The tenderness may also be elicited by shaking the patient or by any other sudden jarring movement.

f. Ecchymosis in the flank, periumbilical region, or back suggests a retroperitoneal hemorrhage. Possible causes include trauma, acute hemorrhagic pancreatitis, a leaking abdominal aortic aneurysm, and intestinal gangrene.

g. Subcutaneous, subfascial, or pelvic crepitus suggests a rapidly spreading gas-forming infection. These infections must be rapidly diagnosed and explored surgically if they are to be cured.

D. Medical illnesses that can cause an acute abdomen

1. Life-threatening medical illness, such as lower lobe pneumonias, acute myocardial infarction, diabetic ketoacidosis, and acute hepatitis, should be sought.

2. Acute polyserositis (occurring with collagen vascular diseases), rheumatic fever, porphyria, and chronic lead intoxication are uncommon causes of acute abdominal pain that can be exceedingly difficult to diagnose preoperatively. A careful history and physical examination may, however, raise them as possibilities.

3. Musculoskeletal problems, particularly vertebral compression of abdominal wall nerves, can also mimic acute general surgical conditions.

4. A high index of suspicion is necessary for acute abdominal emergencies in immunosuppressed patients (i.e., transplant or steroid-dependent patients) whose symptoms and findings may be minimal.

E. Laboratory tests provide important information in many diseases.

1. Complete blood count
   a. A red cell count may reveal anemia or suggest hemoconcentration secondary to dehydration.
   b. A white cell differential count is usually shifted to the left.
   (1) Leukocytosis in the 20,000–40,000 range suggests a major septic process in need of rapid surgical intervention. However, the white cell count may be misleading. For example, a normal white cell count in an elderly or diabetic patient may in fact accompany a major septic episode because advanced age can bring on an inability to generate a leukocytosis.
   (2) Profound leukopenia, particularly with a lymphocytic predominance, suggests a viral illness.
   (3) Other conditions, such as leukemia or lead intoxication, may also be diagnosed from the complete blood count.

2. Urine examination generally rules out urinary tract infection or kidney stone disease. Pelvic inflammatory processes in contact with the ureter or bladder may produce a few white cells and red cells in the urine. If there is doubt, intravenous pyelography should be performed prior to surgery.

3. Serum amylase should be measured in all patients with acute abdominal pain. In general, if the level is high, it usually indicates acute pancreatitis, although other surgical illnesses, such as mesenteric thrombosis and perforated ulcer, should not be overlooked.

4. Arterial blood gases may be very helpful in identifying a profound metabolic acidosis. This suggests either septic shock or severely ischemic or necrotic tissue, which indicates the necessity for surgery if no other obvious cause, such as diabetic ketoacidosis, can be found.

5. Serum electrolytes, serum creatinine, coagulation profile, and liver function tests are other studies that are often obtained.

F. X-ray studies

1. **Upright chest x-ray and flat and upright x-ray of the abdomen** should be obtained in most cases of acute abdominal pain. A chest x-ray is essential to rule out other diseases, such as pneumonia, that can mimic conditions associated with an acute abdomen. Additionally, a chest x-ray is superior to an abdominal x-ray in demonstrating intraperitoneal free air below the diaphragm.

   a. **Bony structure abnormalities.** These frequently overlooked clues may be important in trauma or malignant disease.

   b. **Gastrointestinal gas pattern.** Air is commonly present in the stomach and colon. However, air in the small intestine is abnormal and suggests an intra-abdominal process.

      (1) **Paralytic ileus** (see II B)

         (a) Air that is **evenly distributed** throughout the small and large intestine usually signifies paralysis of the bowel secondary to a process that is not primarily surgical.

         (b) Ileus may be **localized** to a specific area, such as the **"sentinel" loop,** an area of localized duodenal ileus adjacent to the pancreas in acute pancreatitis.

      (2) **Acute gastric dilation** is indicated by a **markedly dilated gastric bubble.** (This condition can result in severe abdominal pain and vasovagal hypotension but is easily treated by nasogastric tube decompression.)

      (3) **Mechanical obstruction of the intestine** (see II A) is revealed by the presence of **distended air- and fluid-filled loops of bowel proximal** to the obstruction and **decompressed intestine distally.** This air may be absent in the distal tract, particularly the rectum, unless air has been introduced by an enema given in the past 24 hours.

         (a) Mechanical bowel obstruction is an important diagnosis because it may be associated with strangulation of the bowel with resultant ischemia and necrosis. When both ends of a loop of bowel are obstructed, such as occurs with a volvulus, this is termed a closed loop obstruction and represents a surgical emergency due to the high risk of rupture and generalized peritonitis.

         (b) Postoperative adhesions, carcinoma of the colon, and inguinal hernias are the three commonest **causes of bowel obstruction.** Specific causes may be diagnosed by the intestinal gas pattern.

            (i) **Hernias** may result in intestinal air located in a nonanatomic location. For example, an inguinal hernia may show gas-filled intestine extended below the inguinal ligament.

            (ii) **Volvulus** is a segment of bowel that has twisted upon itself, resulting in both mechanical obstruction and vascular compromise. It may appear on the plain film as an isolated distended loop of bowel with tapered ("bird-beak") margins. A sigmoid volvulus is treated by sigmoidoscopy and decompression. Other types of volvulus are treated operatively.

            (iii) An **ischemic** or **gangrenous bowel** may produce few radiologic findings. If the colon is affected, however, the mucosal edema may be seen as "thumbprinting" on the wall of a dilated colon.

            (iv) Isolated **distention of the colon by large amounts of air** may be seen on x-ray. It may be due to any of the acute processes, such as **distal colonic obstruction,** which may be secondary to malignancy, profound constipation, stricture, or volvulus; **"toxic megacolon,"** a massive colonic dilation, which is associated with acute colitis; and **colonic ileus,** a condition of obscure etiology, which results in marked distention of the cecum. If the cecum enlarges past 10–12 cm in diameter, there is a significant risk of perforation.

   c. **Abnormal air collections outside the intestinal lumen**

      (1) **Free air within the peritoneal cavity** signals a perforation of a hollow viscus and indicates a surgical emergency.

         (a) It is present in about 80% of gastroduodenal perforations but in fewer than 25% of colonic perforations.

         (b) Free peritoneal air is rarely secondary to other causes. However, it may be present in patients undergoing peritoneal dialysis and for up to 1 week following a laparotomy.

      (2) **Air collections within the wall of the colon,** a condition termed **pneumatosis cystoides intestinalis,** generally indicate an isolated, walled-off intestinal perforation.

      (3) **Air stippling within soft tissue structures** may indicate the dissection of air into the tissues from a thoracic source, such as a pneumothorax. It may, however, be due to

a rapidly progressive, catastrophic gas-forming infection (see Chapter 2 II), which is a true surgical emergency.

(4) Air–fluid level outside the intestinal tract is associated with a subphrenic or subhepatic abscess.

(5) Air within the biliary tree indicates an abnormal communication between the biliary tree and the intestinal tract. Causes include:

(a) A surgical connection created to provide biliary drainage (e.g., choledochoduodenostomy)

(b) A gas-forming infection within the biliary tree (**cholangitis**). Cholangitis is associated with biliary obstruction and should be treated with antibiotics followed closely by surgery to drain the biliary tract.

(c) Large gallstones, particularly in the elderly, which can erode into the adjacent intestine (usually the duodenum), allowing air to enter the biliary tract and the gallstone to enter the bowel. Usually, this produces transient symptoms initially, until several days later when the gallstone impacts upon and obstructs the distal ileum, producing small bowel obstruction.

(6) Air within the portal vein is seen when a gas-forming infection affects the portal system (**pylephlebitis**). The infection usually derives from necrotic tissue, particularly from the small intestine, appendix, or left colon.

d. Abnormal calcifications

(1) Renal stones are calcified in up to 85% of cases and appear along the path of the ureter.

(2) Fecaliths (calcified material within the appendix) are strong evidence for acute appendicitis in patients with abdominal pain.

(3) Pancreatic calcification suggests chronic pancreatitis.

(4) Gallstones are calcified in 15% of cases.

(5) Heavily calcified vessels may be present in mesenteric ischemia.

(6) Masses, such as teratomas or malignant neoplasms, may calcify.

e. Soft tissue shadows

(1) Peritoneal fat lines and **psoas muscle shadows** may be lost in rapidly spreading infections, hematomas, or abscesses.

(2) Margins of solid organs (liver, kidney, or spleen) may be displaced from their normal locations by an abnormal mass.

(3) A **distended bladder** may be visible and may be responsible for marked abdominal pain.

2. Contrast roentgenography can be highly useful in patients with an acute abdominal process that remains undiagnosed after other studies.

a. Intravenous pyelogram (IVP) should be obtained if a renal stone is suspected. It is also useful in identifying acute pyelonephritis, perinephric abscess, or renal infarction. When a patient suspected of having appendicitis has microscopic hematuria, the IVP is particularly useful to verify that the hematuria is due to the periappendiceal inflammation rather than to a renal stone.

b. Barium swallow is helpful if it is suspected that the patient's esophagus has ruptured during a violent episode of vomiting. Known as **Boerhaave's syndrome,** this unusual accident may result in a left pleural effusion, which communicates with the esophageal rent, as demonstrated by the barium swallow.

c. Upper gastrointestinal (GI) series, using diatrizoate meglumine (Gastrografin), a water-soluble radiopaque dye, should be performed if a perforation of the stomach or duodenum is suspected but cannot be proven because free air is not visible on the plain film.

d. Placing contrast materials into the colon and rectum should be done very cautiously when an inflammatory condition or a perforation is suspected, because even a small increase in pressure could easily convert friable tissue into a frank perforation.

(1) This procedure is best used when the diagnosis of colon perforation is suspected and especially in a patient taking anti-inflammatory or immunosuppressive drugs, particularly corticosteroids.

(2) In such cases, diatrizoate meglumine should be used because barium sulfate, when it mixes with stool and detritus from an infection, becomes firmly attached to the peritoneal cavity. Extensive abscess formation results, even after the surgeon attempts to irrigate the area thoroughly.

e. Small bowel follow-through contrast study tracks the barium through the small intestine after an upper GI series. It is useful in identifying a point of small bowel obstruction when either the history, the physical examination, or plain x-ray fails to verify the diagnosis of small bowel obstruction.

G. **Abdominal ultrasonography** is usually of little diagnostic value in the patient with abdominal distention and severe pain, but it can be helpful when acute cholecystitis, cholelithiasis, biliary obstruction, or an abscess is suspected. **Computed tomography** may also be helpful but is generally reserved for the patient whose condition remains undiagnosed after other studies have been exhausted.

H. **General principles** employed in the approach to the patient with acute abdominal pain are discussed below.

1. **A careful and systematic evaluation** of the patient should be routinely followed. Most patients will have a well-documented diagnosis if this principle is fulfilled.

2. **Statistically speaking, certain diagnoses are very common,** such as appendicitis and gastroenteritis, while **other diagnoses are quite rare,** such as pylephlebitis. The physician should not search for an occult diagnosis when a common diagnosis is more likely to be correct.

3. **When the diagnosis is not initially clear, continued observation and repeated blood studies** (complete blood count, arterial blood gases, amylase, and electrolytes) may lead to the correct diagnosis as the disease process evolves.
   a. Although this practice might be desirable in a patient with gastroenteritis, **delay can be catastrophic** in acute appendicitis, ischemic bowel, small bowel obstruction, volvulus, or incarcerated hernia.
   b. If the diagnosis is not certain, but the patient may have a potentially lethal condition that could be cured by an early operation, then an early operation should be performed—that is, a small percentage of negative laparotomies are justified in patients with acute abdomen. This premise is best illustrated by the case of a patient with acute appendicitis. Here, a policy of watchful waiting may convert a simple appendicitis into a perforated appendicitis with generalized peritonitis and septic shock. The risk of death from this complication is many times higher than the risk from a small right lower quadrant incision in a patient who proves to have a normal appendix and mesenteric adenitis.

4. **Analgesics, particularly narcotics, should be withheld** from the patient until the diagnosis is established or until the decision to proceed to surgery has been made. Serial physical examinations will be totally useless if the patient has been given narcotics.

5. **Antibiotics should also be withheld** until a diagnosis has been made and the antibiotic therapy is needed. The only exception to this is the patient who presents in septic shock from an unknown cause. In that situation, broad-spectrum antibiotics should be part of the patient's resuscitation.

6. **Fluid deficits and electrolyte imbalances should be corrected** before surgery. The few **exceptions** are:
   a. Conditions that threaten immediate exsanguination, such as a ruptured abdominal aortic aneurysm
   b. Conditions in which the fluid or electrolyte abnormality cannot be corrected in a reasonable amount of time—that is, conditions that cause profound acidosis, such as necrotic bowel, where the acidosis cannot be corrected until the bowel is surgically removed

7. **Nasogastric tubes** should be placed before the induction of anesthesia to empty the stomach, thus minimizing the risk of pulmonary aspiration.

II. **INTESTINAL OBSTRUCTION.** The normal flow of intestinal contents can be blocked by a mechanical obstruction or by a functional obstruction that occurs because of impaired intestinal motility. An acute abdomen often ensues.

A. **Mechanical obstructions** are common and have various benign and malignant causes. If not treated expeditiously (usually by surgical removal of the cause), mechanical obstructions can rapidly become lethal. **Acute obstruction** occurs over hours to days and has a rapidly evolving course, whereas **chronic obstruction** may have a slow course with malnutrition, constipation, and other signs of chronic illness.

1. **Types**
   a. **Simple obstruction.** There are no complicating factors, such as ischemia or perforation.
   b. **Strangulating obstruction.** The blood supply to the involved segment of bowel is significantly impaired. The ischemia may result from a twisting of the intestinal blood supply upon itself (**volvulus**) or from a constriction of the blood flow by a tight band or hernial opening.
   c. **Closed loop obstruction.** The colon is obstructed but the ileocecal valve remains intact, permitting intestinal contents to enter the obstructed region and greatly distend the cecum. This may result in cecal perforation if not treated expeditiously.
   d. **Intussusception.** The bowel invaginates itself, causing a narrowing of the lumen and subsequent obstruction. It may result from either viral infections or intraluminal polypoid tumors.
   e. **Perforating obstruction.** The bowel proximal to the obstruction overdistends and perforates. The commonest area of perforation when the colon is obstructed is the cecum.

2. **Causes**
   a. **Intestinal adhesions** are the commonest cause of obstruction.
      (1) They may result from a previous surgical exploration, particularly when talc was used to lubricate the surgeon's gloves, or their etiology may be obscure.
      (2) They may be diffuse, involving all peritoneal structures, or solitary, blocking only one area of the intestine.
   b. **Hernias** (see Chapter 2 V and Chapter 29 II) are a second very common cause of intestinal obstruction. A segment of intestine migrates through a defect in the abdominal wall (**external hernia**) or through a mesenteric or omental defect (**internal hernia**) and becomes blocked by the narrow ring that is present at the peritoneal communication of the hernia.
   c. **Intestinal tumors** are the third commonest cause of obstruction. The commonest obstructing tumor is an adenocarcinoma of the colon or rectum. Benign lesions of the small bowel and colon, such as lipomas, can become the leading point of an intussusception. Other malignant tumors, such as carcinoid or lymphoma, can obstruct the intestinal lumen.
   d. **Other intrinsic lesions** within the bowel wall or the lumen can cause acute obstruction.
      (1) **Congenital lesions:** Webs, malrotations, and atresias
      (2) **Inflammatory lesions:** Crohn's disease, diverticulitis, ulcerative colitis, and infections, such as tuberculosis
      (3) **Luminal foreign bodies:** bezoars, parasites, and gallstones
      (4) **Radiation injury,** other **trauma,** or **endometriosis**
   e. **Other extrinsic lesions** can compress the intestinal lumen, such as large intra-abdominal tumors or abscesses.

3. **Treatment**
   a. Intestinal adhesions are treated by surgical lysis of the obstructing bands.
   b. Hernias are treated by a reduction of the contents of the hernia and subsequent repair. The bowel must always be examined for necrosis.
   c. Intestinal tumors are treated by surgical removal.
   d. Treatment of intrinsic and extrinsic lesions depend on the lesion.

B. **Functional obstructions** are blockages in the intestinal flow that result from impaired motility (**paralytic** or **adynamic ileus**). These are usually **treated** by observation and by fluid and nutritional support until the causal agent resolves. Possible **causes** include:

1. **Direct irritation of the intestine,** such as generalized peritonitis. Irritation may also be a factor in the postoperative adynamic ileus that can last for 3–7 days following surgery.

2. **Extraperitoneal causes,** such as a retroperitoneal hematoma or nerve root compression. Retroperitoneal dissections, such as a nephrectomy or sympathectomy, can cause a prolonged ileus.

III. UPPER GASTROINTESTINAL HEMORRHAGE

A. **Causes** of massive upper gastrointestinal hemorrhage as shown by endoscopy are given in Table 9-1.

B. **Types of bleeding.** The diagnosis of hemorrhage is generally obvious, but **locating the site of bleeding** may be difficult. The **type of gastrointestinal bleeding** may give a clue to its source.

1. **Hematemesis** is the vomiting of blood, either bright red or resembling coffee grounds in appearance. Hematemesis usually indicates a bleeding source proximal to the ligament of Treitz. **Coffee-grounds hematemesis** indicates that the blood has been in contact with gastric acid long enough to become converted from hemoglobin to methemoglobin.

2. **Hematochezia** is the passage of bright red blood by rectum. Although it indicates gastrointestinal bleeding, it does not specify the level within the gastrointestinal tract.

3. **Melena** is the passage of black, usually tarry, stools. Although the melena signifies a longer time within the gastrointestinal tract than bright red blood, it does not guarantee that the bleeding is from the upper tract.

4. Blood mixed with stool and mucus can produce a characteristic jelly-like or "currant-jelly" stool. This may originate from a Meckel's diverticulum, particularly in children.

C. **History.** The history should include information about previous episodes of gastrointestinal bleeding, current medications (e.g., aspirin or Coumadin use), and related diseases (e.g., hematologic disorders, alcoholism, peptic ulcer disease, and recent episodes of vomiting).

D. **Physical examination** should specifically include a search for evidence of nasopharyngeal bleeding, portal hypertension, weight loss, malignancy, or systemic diseases, such as chronic hepatic or renal failure.

E. **Diagnosis.** The cause and the location of the bleeding must be confirmed unless imminent exsanguination calls for immediate measures (see Chapter 21 I C 3). In less urgent circumstances, once the patient has been stabilized, one may continue with diagnostic procedures.

1. **Fiberoptic endoscopy** of the upper gastrointestinal tract has become the optimal diagnostic procedure because it allows direct visualization of the lesion in over 80% of cases.
   a. Endoscopy allows:
      (1) Determination of the size and number of lesions in most cases (lesions are multiple in 15% of cases)
      (2) Assessment of which site is actively bleeding
      (3) Assessment of the rate of bleeding. If, for example, an arterial vessel is visibly bleeding in the base of a large duodenal ulcer, then there is a good chance that it will not stop bleeding.
      (4) Distinction between an ulcer, varices, gastritis, and a tear in the esophagus (Mallory-Weiss syndrome) that follows forceful vomiting
      (5) Determination of whether a lesion is benign or malignant
   b. Endoscopy is only safe if the patient's vital signs are relatively stable. Sedation is dangerous because it increases the risk of vomiting followed by aspiration of the gastric contents into the pulmonary bed.

Table 9-1. Causes of Upper Gastrointestinal Hemorrhage

Cause	Incidence
Duodenal ulcer	40%
Gastric ulcer	10%–20%
Diffuse erosive gastritis	15%–20%
Esophageal varices	10%
Mallory-Weiss tear of the gastro-esophageal junction	10%
Gastric carcinoma	Lower than 5%

2. Upper GI series helps to define anatomy or pathology more completely, but unfortunately it sheds little light on the relationship of a particular lesion to the hemorrhage.

3. Passage of a nasogastric tube aids considerably in determining that the source of bleeding is proximal to the ligament of Treitz.

4. Angiography and radionuclide scanning may occasionally help to locate the site of bleeding, but both procedures are more useful in lower gastrointestinal hemorrhage.

F. Treatment. If treated expeditiously in a systematic fashion, the patient with upper gastrointestinal hemorrhage has an excellent chance for recovery. Treatment is aimed at supporting the patient's vital signs as well as stopping the hemorrhage. **Resuscitation measures** should begin immediately when the patient is first seen.

1. Medical treatment of aggravating factors can then begin.
   a. A nasogastric tube is inserted, and the residual thrombus in the stomach is removed with an iced saline solution.
   b. Clotting factors. Any clotting abnormalities are corrected with appropriate factors (see Chapter 1 IV C 3).
      (1) Fresh frozen plasma if the prothrombin time is abnormal
      (2) Platelets if thrombocytopenia is present
      (3) Vitamin K if bleeding is from esophageal varices
   c. Antacids. An aggressive antacid regimen is begun.
      (1) Hourly antacid therapy with gastric pH monitoring is probably the most effective method of stopping hemorrhage.
      (2) Histamine$_2$-(H$_2$-) receptor antagonists, such as ranitidine, are less effective than antacids in stopping a hemorrhage. They are useful, however, for preventing the development of secondary erosive gastritis.
   d. Vasopressin, a powerful vasoconstrictor, may be useful.
      (1) It can be infused through a peripheral vein at a rate of up to 1 unit a minute, or it can be infused directly into the bleeding vessel by means of angiography.
      (2) Vasopressin temporarily controls bleeding in 75% of patients; by contrast, bleeding was stopped in 30% of patients treated conventionally without vasopressin. However, vasopressin is contraindicated in patients with significant coronary artery disease. It reduces cardiac output, an effect that can be partially corrected by isoproterenol (given with caution in patients with portal hypertension).
   e. Fiberoptic endoscopy, in addition to being a diagnostic procedure, may also be useful when esophageal varices are to be sclerosed (see Chapter 14 II E) or small bleeding sites are to be coagulated.
   f. Angiography similarly may be a therapeutic aid. It allows bleeding from small vessels to be controlled either by embolization of the bleeding vessel or by intra-arterial administration of vasopressin.
   g. Balloon tamponade (see Chapter 14 II E 3 c) can be important in controlling bleeding from varices.

2. Surgical treatment. The type of surgery performed is discussed in Chapter 11.
   a. The patient's cardiovascular status, as well as the amount and duration of bleeding, is particularly important. For example, a patient with heart disease may tolerate continued bleeding poorly and, thus, may need early surgery.
   b. Only about 10% of patients will require surgery.
   c. Indications for surgery are as follows:
      (1) Exsanguinating hemorrhage. A patient with uncontrollable hemorrhage who is losing blood faster than it can be replaced must be sent to the operating room immediately for control of the site of bleeding.
      (2) Profuse bleeding, especially in association with **hypotension.** Patients should be treated surgically:
         (a) If more than 4 units of blood are required for initial resuscitation
         (b) If bleeding continues at a rate greater than 1 unit every 8 hours
         (c) If a brief hypotensive episode could have catastrophic results, as in patients with coronary artery disease or cerebrovascular disease or in patients older than 60 years of age
      (3) Continued hemorrhage despite resuscitation and other treatment
         (a) The mortality rate of upper gastrointestinal bleeding is low among patients who need less than 6–7 units of blood.

         (b) The rate rises dramatically with requirements above 7 units. Thus, surgery should be undertaken before the blood loss reaches that point.

      (4) Recurrent bleeding after its initial cessation. About one-fourth of patients rebleed, and the mortality rate for these patients is as high as 30%, in contrast to a mortality rate of about 3% among patients who do not rebleed.

      (5) Pathologic features of the bleeding site that **increase the risk** of recurrent bleeding include:

         (a) A posterior duodenal ulcer with the gastroduodenal artery visible in its base

         (b) A giant gastric ulcer

   3. Special situations may call for a modification of the usual routines of management.

     a. A patient with a rare or hard-to-find blood type should be operated upon while blood is still available.

     b. A patient who refuses blood transfusion for any reason should be explored early.

     c. A patient with a coagulopathy should have the disorder corrected, if possible, prior to surgical exploration.

 G. Prognosis. The prognosis for patients who are bleeding from a source other than esophageal varices is as follows:

   1. Some 25%–50% will have a recurrence of bleeding during the next 5 years, and about 20% will require surgery.

   2. The mortality rate is low (about 3%) if the bleeding stops spontaneously, whereas it is as high as 33% in patients who soon rebleed.

IV. LOWER GASTROINTESTINAL HEMORRHAGE

 A. Overview. Acute lower gastrointestinal hemorrhage is managed initially in much the same way as upper gastrointestinal hemorrhage.

   1. Resuscitation with blood and intravenous fluids is begun immediately.

   2. The history is taken and a **physical examination** is performed.

   3. Diagnostic studies are begun to identify the site and cause of the bleeding.

   4. Vasopressin may be used as in upper gastrointestinal bleeding (see III F 1 d).

 B. Initial studies

   1. Anorectal examination is performed to determine if the source of bleeding is a hemorrhoid, anal fissure, anal carcinoma, or other anorectal lesion.

   2. A bleeding site in the upper gastrointestinal tract must be ruled out.

     a. A nasogastric tube is passed to ascertain that no bleeding is present in the gastroduodenal region. On occasion, however, duodenal bleeding will not reflux into the stomach because of a closed pyloric sphincter.

     b. Endoscopy (see III E 1) is, therefore, required to rule out upper gastrointestinal bleeding with absolute certainty. Most physicians will withhold endoscopy when a highly probable source of the bleeding is found in the lower gastrointestinal tract. However, if surgery is anticipated, particularly when one is not sure of the diagnosis, endoscopy of the upper gastrointestinal tract should be performed to exclude any bleeding site there.

   3. A bleeding site in the lower gastrointestinal tract must be located. Once the upper tract has been eliminated as a source of bleeding, the lower tract should be investigated, including the distal small bowel, colon, and anorectal area.

     a. Sigmoidoscopy should be performed.

       (1) The presence of a mass lesion, such as rectal carcinoma, is visualized in about 3% of patients with massive lower gastrointestinal bleeding.

       (2) Discrete bleeding sites from ulcers or hemorrhoids may be seen.

       (3) A diffusely hemorrhagic mucosa suggests colitis, a platelet deficiency, or a hematologic disorder.

       (4) Even if no lesion is visualized, it is important to make certain that the lower 15 cm of the rectum is normal, because this region is inaccessible intraperitoneally if laparotomy is necessary. Additionally, if it is normal, it gives presumptive evidence that the bleeding is coming from a more proximal site.

  b. Anoscopy is frequently overlooked, but should be routinely performed because bleeding lesions in the anal canal may be missed on sigmoidoscopy.

C. Subsequent diagnostic tests will depend upon whether the bleeding stops or continues. About 75% of the patients will spontaneously stop bleeding without further intervention.

  1. If bleeding stops, the following steps are taken.
   a. A **"barium enema,"** a **colonoscopy,** or both procedures should be performed
    (1) To identify or rule out diverticulosis or colon carcinoma
    (2) To provide indirect evidence for colonic mucosal ischemia
   b. The patient should be monitored thereafter.

  2. If bleeding continues, further diagnostic studies should be done to identify the source more precisely in preparation for surgery if it becomes necessary.
   a. If bleeding continues slowly, a barium enema may be useful to determine the presence, number, and location of diverticuli. However, if bleeding is more rapid, the residual barium in the colon may make subsequent angiography difficult or impossible.
   b. If bleeding is profuse, angiography and **radionuclide scanning** are useful.
    (1) Selective mesenteric angiogram will identify the bleeding site (or sites) in up to 80% of patients when the rate of bleeding exceeds 0.5 ml/min. Angiography is also highly useful for identifying angiodysplastic lesions of the colon.
    (2) Radionuclide scan, which uses red blood cells labeled with technetium 99m (^{99m}Tc), is sensitive enough to detect a bleeding site when the rate is as low as 0.10 ml/min.
   c. Colonoscopy is unsatisfactory and may be dangerous when lower gastrointestinal bleeding is rapid: Visualization is poor, and there is a risk of colon perforation.

D. Indication for surgery is persistent bleeding.

  1. The patient's cardiovascular status and amount and duration of bleeding are taken into consideration, as for upper gastrointestinal hemorrhage (see III F 1, 2).

  2. The surgical procedure is aimed at removing the underlying cause of the bleeding.

  3. On occasion, the precise point of bleeding cannot be established.
   a. In these instances, the stomach, duodenum, and small intestine should be carefully examined. Meckel's diverticulum, Crohn's disease, and other inflammatory or malignant lesions should not be overlooked.
   b. A "blind" total colectomy may be necessary if no other source of the bleeding is found.

  4. The **mortality rate** for lower gastrointestinal bleeding is currently about 10%.

V. SHOCK is a clinical condition that occurs as a result of inadequate tissue perfusion. Four types are recognized: hypovolemic, septic, cardiogenic, and neurogenic. Use of invasive monitoring, including pulmonary arterial pressure monitoring (i.e., Swan-Ganz catheter), helps to distinguish the different types of shock. Some of these measurements include cardiac output, peripheral vascular resistance, and central venous pressure.

A. Hypovolemic shock is characterized by a loss of circulating volume. The type of fluid lost includes blood, plasma, extracellular, extravascular, or water.

  1. Etiology. Common causes include hemorrhage, as in trauma, dehydration, and burns.

  2. Clinical manifestations. Patients have pale, cool skin and slow capillary refill. They are frequently apprehensive and restless.

  3. Hemodynamics. There is low or normal cardiac output, high peripheral vascular resistance, and usually low central venous pressure.

  4. Treatment is directed at restoring the blood or fluid loss. Regardless of the type of loss, initial treatment involves crystalloid replacement. The source of fluid or blood loss must be identified. Surgical intervention is often necessary.

B. Septic shock occurs in the setting of invasive infection. Chemical mediators have peripheral vascular effects and probably direct myocardial effects, resulting in decreased systemic vascular resistance, organ dysfunction, and myocardial depression.

     1. Etiology. Common causes include genitourinary tract infections, pulmonary infections, wound and soft tissue infections, abscesses, and invasive catheters.

     2. Clinical manifestations. Early (hyperdynamic state), the patient is flushed, warm, and confused. Later, the patient may have a depressed sensorium.

     3. Hemodynamics. Early in the course, there is high cardiac output, low peripheral vascular resistance, and usually low central venous pressure.

     4. Treatment is aimed at controlling the septic focus, including antibiotic therapy. Surgical intervention is often necessary. Additional support includes fluid resuscitation, sometimes vasoactive drugs, and diuretics.

C. Cardiogenic shock is due to an inadequacy of the heart as a pump.

     1. Etiology. Common causes may be intrinsic, as in myocardial contusion and infarction, or extrinsic, as in cardiac tamponade and tension pneumothorax.

     2. Clinical manifestations. Patients have pale, cool skin and slow capillary refill. They may be quiet or apprehensive.

     3. Hemodynamics. There is usually low cardiac output, high peripheral vascular resistance, and high central venous pressure in tamponade.

     4. Treatment consists of ensuring adequate volume while treating the underlying cause (i.e., pericardiocentesis in tamponade).

D. Neurogenic shock can occur in severe cerebral, brain stem or spinal cord injury. An interference in the balance of vasodilator and vasoconstrictor influences to vessels results in hypotension. Contrasted to hypovolemic shock where there is volume loss, the patient tends to be in a normovolemic state.

     1. Etiology. Common causes include spinal anesthesia, spinal cord injury, anaphylactic shock, and fainting (vasovagal reaction).

     2. Clinical manifestations. There is little change in skin color and temperature and normal capillary refill. There are varied effects on mental status, which is often normal.

     3. Hemodynamics. Cardiac output may be high with low peripheral vascular resistance and low central venous pressure with normal circulating volume.

     4. Treatment is directed at excluding other causes of shock and giving volume and vasoconstrictor drugs if needed. Surgical intervention is not usually necessary.

10
Esophagus

Frederick R. Armenti
Richard N. Edie

I. INTRODUCTION

A. Anatomy

1. Location. The esophagus is approximately 24 cm in length. It extends from the C_6 vertebral level to the T_{11} level.

  a. It originates at the **upper esophageal sphincter**, which is made up of the cricopharyngeal muscle, then courses behind the arch of the aorta, and descends into the thorax on the right.

  b. It deviates anteriorly and enters the abdomen via the **esophageal hiatus**, which is formed by the right crus of the diaphragm.

  c. The tubular esophagus meets the saccular stomach at the **gastroesophageal junction**, where the esophagus is anchored by the phrenoesophageal ligament. The gastroesophageal junction is approximally 40 cm from the incisors.

2. Histology

  a. The esophageal mucosa consists of squamous cell epithelium except for the distal 1–2 cm, which is junctional columnar epithelium.

  b. There are two layers of muscle throughout the esophagus, an inner circular and outer longitudinal layer. The upper one-third is striated muscle whereas smooth muscle predominates in the lower two-thirds.

  c. The esophagus, unlike the rest of the gastrointestinal tract, lacks a serosal covering.

B. Vasculature

1. Arterial supply to the esophagus is from branches of the inferior thyroid, the bronchial, intercostal inferior phrenic, and left gastric arteries.

2. Venous return is more complicated.

  a. An extensive subepithelial venous plexus empties superiorly into the hypopharyngeal veins and inferiorly into the gastric veins. The left gastric vein is also known as the coronary vein.

  b. The left gastric vein is an important portosystemic connection, especially in patients with portal hypertension.

3. Lymphatic drainage is to the nearest lymph nodes. Lymphatics of the upper esophagus drain into the cervical or mediastinal nodes, whereas drainage of the distal lymphatics is more often to the celiac nodes.

C. Innervation.
The esophagus is supplied by the sympathetic and parasympathetic system via the pharyngeal plexus, the vagus, upper and lower cervical sympathetic, and splanchnic nerves. Meissner's and Auerbach's plexuses are present in the normal esophagus.

D. Physiology

1. The upper esophageal sphincter is a high-pressure zone at the upper border of the esophagus. It is 3–5 cm in length, and it relaxes during swallowing.

2. Peristalsis in the central portion of the esophagus consists of wave-like movements that pass down the body of the esophagus and become stronger toward the lower portion. Esophageal peristaltic pressures range from 25–80 mm Hg.

3. **The lower esophageal sphincter** is a high-pressure zone at the lower portion of the esophagus. It is 3–5 cm in length and functions to prevent gastroesophageal reflux. The lower esophageal sphincter pressure is influenced by a number of factors and substances.
    a. Lower esophageal sphincter **pressure is increased** by a protein meal, alkalinization of the stomach, gastrin, vasopressin, and cholinergic drugs.
    b. Lower esophageal sphincter **pressure is decreased** by secretin, nitroglycerin, glucagon, chocolate, fatty meals, and gastric acidification.

II. DISORDERS OF ESOPHAGEAL MOTILITY

A. Cricopharyngeal dysfunction

1. **Pathophysiology**
    a. Cricopharyngeal dysfunction is caused by a failure of the upper esophageal sphincter to relax properly.
    b. The problem may be an incoordination between relaxation in the upper esophageal sphincter and simultaneous contraction of the pharynx, which may result in a pharyngoesophageal (Zenker's) diverticulum. This is a false diverticulum composed only of mucosa that herniates posteriorly between the fibers of the cricopharyngeal muscle.
    c. Cricopharyngeal dysfunction is frequently associated with **hiatal hernia** and **gastroesophageal reflux**.

2. **Symptoms** include dysphagia; reflux of undigested food; and, if a Zenker's diverticulum has developed, a mass in the neck, usually on the left side, which occasionally causes tracheal compression.

3. **Diagnosis**
    a. **The history and physical examination** are usually adequate to diagnose cricopharyngeal dysfunction.
    b. **X-rays**, which include a barium swallow, are helpful in delineating a diverticulum.
    c. **Endoscopy** is indicated to rule out other esophageal disorders, including gastroesophageal reflux or neoplasm.

4. **Treatment**
    a. **Cricopharyngeal myotomy** is the treatment of choice for cricopharyngeal dysfunction.
    b. Excision or resuspension of the diverticulum may be combined with the myotomy.

B. Achalasia

1. **Pathophysiology**
    a. Achalasia is an esophageal disease of unknown etiology, although it may be secondary to ganglionic dysfunction. It consists of abnormal peristalsis in the body of the esophagus, which causes:
        (1) High resting lower esophageal sphincter pressure
        (2) Failure of the lower esophageal sphincter to relax during swallowing
    b. The body of the esophagus becomes dilated, and the muscle hypertrophies in an attempt to force material through the dysfunctional lower esophageal sphincter. A similar symptom complex can be caused by **Chagas' disease**, which is due to the organism *Trypanosoma cruzi*.
    c. Carcinoma of the esophagus is 10 times commoner in patients with achalasia than in the general population.

2. **Symptoms** of achalasia include dysphagia, followed by regurgitation and weight loss. Frequently, respiratory symptoms are present due to aspiration.

3. **Diagnosis**
    a. **X-ray studies** reveal a dilated esophagus with a beak-like extension into the lower narrowed segment at the lower esophageal sphincter.
    b. **Esophageal manometry** reveals the high resting lower esophageal sphincter pressure, failure of relaxation during swallowing, and lower than normal pressure in the body of the esophagus.
    c. **Esophagoscopy** is required to rule out neoplasia and to document the extent of esophagitis.

4. Treatment for achalasia is palliative since lower esophageal function can never be restored to normal.
   a. Nonsurgical treatment consists of forceful pneumatic dilatation of the contracted lower esophageal stricture, which is just above the gastroesophageal junction.
   b. Surgical treatment is **esophagomyotomy** by the **modified Heller procedure**, usually via a left thoracotomy. Care is taken not to disturb the vagus nerve attachments to the esophagus to prevent reflux. The myotomy is confined to the lower portion of the esophagus, usually 7–10 cm in length.
      (1) Surgical results with the Heller procedure are generally better than with pneumatic dilatation for relief of dysphagia.
      (2) Esophagomyotomy can be combined with an antireflux procedure.

C. Diffuse esophageal spasm

   1. Pathophysiology
      a. Diffuse esophageal spasm is a disorder of esophageal motility that consists of **strong nonperistaltic contractions**.
      b. Unlike achalasia, this condition has normal sphincteric relaxation and may be associated with gastroesophageal reflux.

   2. Symptoms consist of chest pain, which can radiate to the back, neck, ears, jaw, or arms, and may be confused with typical angina pectoris. The pain usually occurs spontaneously, and many patients are considered to have a psychoneurosis.

   3. Diagnosis
      a. Manometry reveals high-amplitude repetitive contractions with a normal sphincteric response to swallowing.
      b. X-rays are normal in half of cases but may reveal diverticula, segmental spasm, and a corkscrew-appearance of the esophagus.

   4. Treatment
      a. Surgery is moderately effective with good results obtained in over two-thirds of the patients. The best results are obtained in emotionally stable patients with severe disease and without associated lower gastrointestinal problems.
         (1) Surgery consists of a long esophagomyotomy that extends from the arch of the aorta to just above the lower esophageal sphincter.
         (2) Care is taken to preserve lower esophageal sphincter function, which is usually normal in these patients.
         (3) If significant gastroesophageal reflux is present, an antireflux procedure is performed.
      b. Medical treatment. Calcium channel blockers and smooth muscle relaxants, such as nitrates, may ameliorate symptoms.

D. Esophageal reflux

   1. Etiology. Esophageal reflux is secondary to **dysfunction of the lower esophageal sphincter,** which results in recurrent reflux of the gastric contents into the lower esophagus. Lower esophageal sphincter dysfunction may be related to:
      a. Decreased endogenous gastrin production
      b. Operations on or near the esophageal hiatus (e.g., vagotomy and gastrectomy)
      c. A sliding-type esophageal hiatal hernia. However, many patients with this type of hiatal hernia have no evidence of reflux, and many patients with normal lower esophageal anatomy suffer from esophageal reflux.
      d. Scleroderma, a systemic cause of lower esophageal sphincter dysfunction through weakening of the esophageal smooth muscle
      e. Exogenous causative agents, including tobacco and alcohol

   2. Symptoms of esophageal reflux are substernal pain, heartburn, and regurgitation, all of which may worsen with bending and lying down.

   3. Diagnosis is made by:
      a. Manometry, which reveals decreased lower esophageal sphincter pressure
      b. Esophagoscopy, which reveals varying degrees of esophagitis
      c. Twenty-four–hour pH measurements in the lower esophageal area, which demonstrate increased acidity
      d. Cineradiography, which correlates the amount of reflux via motion pictures

4. Treatment
  a. Medical treatment
    (1) Antacids
    (2) Metoclopramide, which increases both lower esophageal sphincter pressure and gastric motility, thus increasing the rate of gastric emptying
    (3) Histamine$_2$-receptor antagonists to reduce acidity
    (4) Weight reduction
    (5) Abstinence from smoking and alcohol
    (6) Elevation of the head of the bed at night
  b. Surgical treatment
    (1) Indications for surgery include:
      (a) Symptoms refractory to medical treatment
      (b) Additional problems, such as esophageal webs (see VII B) or severe esophagitis, stricture formation, or **Barrett's esophagus** (i.e., replacement of the normal epithelial lining with columnar epithelium in the lower esophagus secondary to esophagitis)
    (2) Antireflux operations are designed to increase lower esophageal sphincter tone. All of the operations involve wrapping the lower esophagus with gastric fundus and restoring the distal esophagus to its original intra-abdominal position with the gastroesophageal junction below the diaphragm. The three most commonly used operations are:
      (a) The **Belsey Mark IV operation**, which is a 270° wrap performed through a left thoracotomy
      (b) The **Nissen fundoplication**, which is a 360° wrap of the stomach around the esophagus performed through the abdomen
      (c) The **Hill repair**, or posterior gastropexy, which uses the arcuate ligament to reestablish the intra-abdominal position of the distal esophagus.

III. ESOPHAGEAL STRICTURES

A. Caustic stricture

1. Etiology. Caustic stricture is caused by the ingestion of caustic agents, such as lye, drain openers, and oven cleaners.

2. Diagnosis
  a. A history of caustic ingestion and the **presenting symptoms**, which may be mild or very severe, including shock from severe burning of the esophagus, are sufficient to make the diagnosis. It is important to identify the etiologic agent.
  b. Endoscopy is indicated as soon as possible to determine the extent of damage.

3. Treatment
  a. A neutralizing agent (usually milk) is given as soon as possible to counteract the effects of the caustic agent.
  b. Corticosteroids and broad-spectrum antibiotics are administered for 3–6 weeks.
  c. X-rays of the esophagus are performed at 10–14 days to determine if **strictures** are developing.
    (1) Strictures occur in 5%–10% of patients who have ingested lye.
    (2) If strictures have formed, a program of dilatation, using esophageal dilators, is begun 3–4 weeks after ingestion.
  d. Esophageal replacement with stomach or colon may be necessary.

B. Strictures secondary to esophagitis and reflux

1. Pathophysiology. These strictures are caused by a recurrent alternating pattern of mucosal destruction secondary to gastric acid reflux and subsequent healing.
  a. The strictures most often occur at the gastroesophageal junction.
  b. In severe cases, a long stricture may result.

2. Diagnosis
  a. A **history** of reflux symptoms and dysphagia is suggestive of strictures.
  b. X-ray of the esophagus confirms the diagnosis.
  c. Esophagoscopy is important to determine the extent of the disease and to rule out malignancy.

   3. Treatment
   a. Dilatation of the esophagus is attempted first, and then an antireflux operation is performed.
   b. If dilatation and an antireflux operation do not relieve the esophageal obstruction, a reconstructive procedure, using either the stomach or colon for esophageal replacement, may be necessary to restore adequate swallowing function.

IV. TUMORS OF THE ESOPHAGUS

A. Benign tumors

   1. Leiomyomas account for two-thirds of all benign tumors of the esophagus.
   a. Symptoms. Dysphagia occurs when leiomyomas exceed a diameter of 5 cm as they grow within the muscular wall, leaving the overlying mucosa intact.
   b. Diagnosis
      (1) A **history** of dysphagia is typical.
      (2) A **barium swallow** reveals a localized smooth filling defect in the esophageal wall.
      (3) **Esophagoscopy** is performed to confirm the diagnosis.
      (4) **Biopsy** of the lesion is contraindicated because it violates the mucosa, making subsequent surgical therapy difficult.
   c. Surgical treatment
      (1) In symptomatic patients, the **tumor is enucleated** from the esophageal wall without violating the mucosa.
      (2) A limited esophageal resection is indicated if the tumor lies in the lower esophagus and cannot be enucleated.

   2. Benign intraluminal tumors are usually **mucosal polyps, lipomas, fibrolipomas,** or **myxofibromas.**
   a. Symptoms are dysphagia, occasionally regurgitation, and weight loss.
   b. Diagnosis
      (1) **X-rays** of the esophagus suggest the diagnosis.
      (2) **Esophagoscopy** is performed to confirm the diagnosis and to rule out malignancy.
   c. Surgical treatment
      (1) Esophagotomy, removal of the tumor, and repair of the esophagotomy comprise the surgical treatment.
      (2) Endoscopy should not be used to remove these tumors because of the possibility of esophageal perforation.

B. Malignant tumors

   1. Incidence. In the United States, the incidence of esophageal carcinoma ranges from 3.5/1,000,000 for whites to 13.5/100,000 for blacks. The highest incidence of esophageal carcinoma is noted in the Hunan Chinese population with as many as 130/100,000 individuals affected.

   2. Etiology. The exact cause is unknown. Associated factors are tobacco use, excessive alcohol ingestion, nitrosamines, poor dental hygiene, and hot beverages. Certain preexisting conditions also increase the likelihood of developing esophageal cancer, including achalasia, esophagitis, and Barrett's esophagus.

   3. Pathology
   a. Type
      (1) **Squamous cell carcinoma** is the commonest form.
      (2) **Adenocarcinoma,** the next commonest, is the type that occurs in patients with Barrett's esophagus.
      (3) **Rare tumors** of the esophagus include **mucoepidermoid carcinoma** and **adenoid cystic carcinoma.**
   b. Tumor spread. Esophageal malignancies metastasize both through the lymphatic system and the bloodstream with metastases occurring in liver, bone, and brain.

   4. Diagnosis
   a. A **history** of dysphagia and weight loss is almost always present.
   b. Contrast study of the esophagus demonstrates the location and extent of tumor.

    c. Esophagoscopy is essential for tissue diagnosis and determination of the extent of the tumor.

    d. Bronchoscopy is performed to assess the possibility of invasion of the tracheobronchial tree.

    e. Computed tomography (CT scan) of the chest and abdomen is done to evaluate local lymphatic spread, and a thorough search is made for distant metastases.

5. Treatment

    a. Surgical treatment provides the only cure.

      (1) The operation consists of total thoracic esophagectomy with reconstruction of gastrointestinal continuity with either the stomach or colon.

      (2) Operation is the best treatment for the patient as it allows normal or near normal swallowing.

      (3) Overall, surgical therapy is associated with a 5%–15% 5-year survival rate. As high as a 30% 5-year survival rate has been reported for patients who are in the early stages of disease with no demonstrable lymph node metastases.

    b. Radiotherapy and chemotherapy are currently being investigated as adjuncts to surgery. Neoadjuvant chemotherapy given prior to surgical resection appears to shrink the tumor mass and may have an impact on long-term survival. Studies are now underway.

      (1) In some poor-risk patients, radiotherapy alone has been used for carcinoma of the esophagus with some palliative effects.

      (2) In patients who have advanced disease with either invasion of the tracheobronchial tree or advanced metastases, palliative effects may be obtained by placing a permanent, large-diameter tube through the area of esophageal obstruction, to allow swallowing of saliva and soft foods.

V. PERFORATION OF THE ESOPHAGUS

A. Etiology

    1. Perforations of the esophagus have two basic **causes:**
    a. Instrumentation (e.g., esophagoscopy or dilatation)
    b. Boerhaave's syndrome (postemetic rupture of the esophagus)

    2. Rupture of the esophagus results in mediastinitis, which, if not corrected, is almost always fatal.

B. Diagnosis

    1. History. Patients give a recent history of instrumentation of the esophagus or severe vomiting. All patients complain of severe chest pain, which usually is most prominent in the area of the rupture.

    2. Physical examination
    a. Crepitation in the neck results from mediastinal air.
    b. Occasionally, a crunching sound can be heard over the heart (Hamman's sign) due to air in the mediastinum behind the heart.
    c. Septic shock also can occur.

    3. Chest x-ray reveals air in the mediastinum and, possibly, a widened mediastinum.
    a. If the perforation is in the lower esophagus, air may be present under the diaphragm within the abdomen.
    b. If the pleura has been violated, a pneumothorax may be present.

    4. A barium swallow should be performed if perforation is suspected. This study is better than esophagoscopy for identifying a perforation.

C. Treatment is primarily an attempt to provide wide drainage of the mediastinum and is best approached by a thoracotomy.

    1. If diagnosed early (6 hours), perforation can be treated with simple drainage, esophageal repair, and appropriate antibiotic coverage.

    2. If the diagnosis is delayed, the esophagus is impossible to repair because of the massive inflammation and tissue edema in the area. In this case, drainage and esophageal diversion are performed with the hope that esophageal reconstruction can be performed later.

VI. MALLORY-WEISS SYNDROME

A. Pathophysiology. This condition presents as acute massive upper gastrointestinal hemorrhage. The bleeding occurs in the lower esophagus, usually near the gastroesophageal junction, and is secondary to a partial thickness tear in the lower esophagus, which follows a prolonged period of severe vomiting and retching. The tear usually extends into the stomach and may involve the greater curvature of the cardia.

B. Diagnosis is made by endoscopy, which is performed to locate the tear and rule out other causes of bleeding.

C. Treatment is by supportive measures as blood volume replacement, antacids, and gastric lavage.

    1. In most cases the bleeding subsides spontaneously.

    2. Exploratory laparotomy is performed with gastrotomy and suture of the tear of the esophagus from within the stomach if the bleeding persists. The lacerations are closed using continuous nonabsorbable sutures. Recurrence is extremely rare.

VII. ESOPHAGEAL WEBS

A. Upper esophageal webs are part of the **Plummer-Vinson syndrome**, which presents in middle-aged, edentulous women with atrophic oral mucosa, anemia, and dysphagia. The web occurs just below the esophageal introitus. **Treatment** is usually by esophageal dilatation.

B. Lower esophageal webs, or **Schatzki's rings**, commonly occur in patients with reflux. Patients complain of dysphagia. **Treatment** consists of esophageal dilatation and an antireflux procedure.

11
Stomach and Duodenum

R. Anthony Carabasi, III
Diane R. Gillum

I. INTRODUCTION

A. Stomach

1. Anatomy. The stomach is a muscular organ that functions in food storage and digestion. It has four parts and two sphincteric mechanisms.

a. Parts (Figure 11-1)
   (1) The **cardia** is the area near the gastroesophageal junction.
   (2) The **fundus** is the extension of the stomach above the gastroesophageal junction.
   (3) The **body** is the area between the fundus and the antrum.
   (4) The **antrum** is the distal quarter of the stomach. It begins at the incisura angularis and ends at the pylorus.

b. Sphincteric mechanisms
   (1) The **gastroesophageal sphincter** is a high-pressure zone of muscular activity in the distal esophagus. It relaxes with swallowing to allow food to enter the stomach. When contracted, it prevents the reflux of food from the stomach into the esophagus.
   (2) The **pylorus** is a well-defined muscular sphincter that controls the movement of food out of the stomach. It also prevents the reflux of duodenal contents into the stomach.

2. Innervation. The nervous supply of the stomach is via parasympathetic and sympathetic fibers.

a. The parasympathetic supply is through the **vagus nerves**. The anterior or left vagus supplies the anterior portion of the stomach. The posterior or right vagus supplies the posterior stomach. The vagi contribute to gastric acid secretion both by direct action on parietal cell secretion and by stimulating the antrum to release gastrin. They also contribute to gastric motility.

b. The sympathetic innervation is via the **greater splanchnic nerves**. These terminate in the **celiac ganglion,** and postganglionic fibers travel with the gastric arteries to the stomach. The sympathetic afferent fibers are the pathway for perception of visceral pain.

3. Vasculature
a. Arterial supply to the stomach is via the right and left gastric arteries, the right and left gastroepiploic arteries, and the vasa brevia.
   (1) The **right gastric artery** is a branch of the common hepatic artery and supplies the lesser curvature.
   (2) The **left gastric artery** is a branch of the celiac axis and supplies the lesser curvature.
   (3) The **right gastroepiploic artery** is a branch of the gastroduodenal artery and supplies the greater curvature.
   (4) The **left gastroepiploic artery** is a branch of the splenic artery and supplies the greater curvature.
   (5) The **vasa brevia** arise from either the splenic artery or the left gastroepiploic artery and supply the fundus.
b. Venous drainage of the stomach is both portal and systemic.
   (1) The right and left **gastric** and **gastroepiploic veins** accompany their corresponding arteries. They drain into the portal system.
   (2) The **left gastric vein** also has multiple **anastomoses** with the **lower esophageal venous plexus**. These drain systemically into the azygous vein.

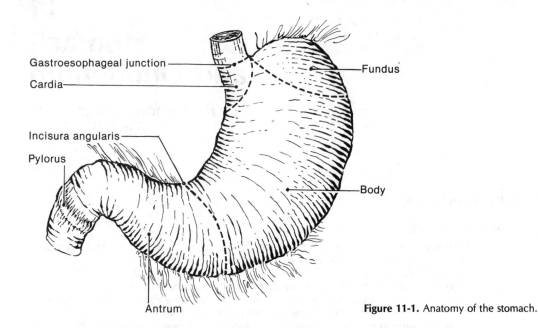

Gastroesophageal junction

Cardia

Incisura angularis

Pylorus

Fundus

Body

Antrum

Figure 11-1. Anatomy of the stomach.

   c. Lymphatic drainage of the stomach is extensive. Lymph nodes that drain the stomach are found at the cardia, along the greater and lesser curvatures, and near the pylorus.

  4. Microscopic anatomy. The stomach has four layers and three distinct mucosal areas.
    a. The layers of the stomach wall are **serosa, muscularis, muscularis mucosae,** and **mucosa.** The **layers of muscle fibers** are **longitudinal, oblique,** and **circular.**
    b. The divisions of the mucosa correspond to the gross divisions of cardia, body, and antrum.
      (1) The cardiac gland area is a ½- to 4-cm zone beginning at the cardia. These shallow glands secrete mucus.
      (2) The parietal cell area comprises the proximal three-quarters of the stomach. Four **types of cells** are found **in its glands:**
        (a) Mucous cells secrete an alkaline mucous coating for the epithelium. This 1mm–thick coating primarily facilitates food passage. It also provides some mucosal protection.
        (b) Zygomatic or **chief cells** secrete pepsinogen. They are found deep in the fundic glands. **Pepsinogen** is the precursor to **pepsin,** which is active in protein digestion. Chief cells are stimulated by cholinergic impulses, by gastrin, and by secretin.
        (c) Oxyntic or **parietal cells** produce **hydrochloric acid** and **intrinsic factor.** They are found exclusively in the fundus and body of the stomach. They are stimulated to produce hydrochloric acid by gastrin.
        (d) Argentaffin cells are scattered throughout the stomach. Their function is unclear.
      (3) The pyloroantral mucosa is found in the antrum of the stomach.
        (a) Parietal and chief cells are absent here.
        (b) G cells, which secrete gastrin, are found in this area. They are part of the **amine precursor uptake and decarboxylase (APUD) system** of endocrine cells. **Gastrin** is a hormone that causes the secretion of hydrochloric acid and pepsinogen in the stomach. It also influences gastric motility.

B. Duodenum

  1. Anatomy. The duodenum is the first portion of the small intestine. It is divided into four **portions** (Figure 11-2).
    a. The first portion of the duodenum, the **duodenal cap,** is the horizontal portion distal to the pylorus. It is approximately 5 cm in length and is partially retroperitoneal at its distal margin.

b. The second or **descending portion** of the duodenum is approximately 7 cm in length. The **common bile duct** and **pancreatic duct** empty into the duodenum here.

c. The third or transverse portion of the duodenum is 12 cm long. It runs horizontally to the left and ends to the left of the third lumbar vertebra.

d. The fourth portion of the duodenum runs superiorly and to the left for 2½ cm. At its terminal portion, the **duodenojejunal flexure,** it changes direction sharply and becomes the **jejunum.** This area of the duodenum is fixed in position by the **ligament of Treitz.**

2. Vasculature

a. Arterial supply of the duodenum is via the **superior pancreaticoduodenal artery,** a branch of the hepatic artery, and the **inferior pancreaticoduodenal artery,** a branch of the superior mesenteric artery.

b. Venous drainage is via anterior and posterior **pancreaticoduodenal venous arcades.** These drain into the portal and superior mesenteric veins.

3. Microscopic anatomy of the duodenum is similar to that of the rest of the small intestine.

a. Walls of the duodenum

(1) The **anterior wall** of the duodenum has four **coats**—the **serosa,** the **muscular layer,** the **muscularis mucosae,** and the **mucosa.**

(2) The **posterior wall** is retroperitoneal and lacks serosa.

(3) The **muscular layer** consists of inner **longitudinal** and outer **circular muscle fibers.**

b. Specialized glands of the duodenum, **Brunner's glands,** are found in the proximal duodenum and secrete an alkaline mucus. This mucus is thought to protect the mucosa.

C. Gastric acid secretion is mediated by a complex interplay of neuronal and hormonal influences. The **secretory response during eating** is divided into three **phases.**

1. The cephalic phase is mediated by vagal stimulation. It is provoked by the sight, smell, and thought of food.

a. Vagal stimulation has a direct effect on parietal cells, causing acid secretion.

b. Vagal stimulation also causes release of gastrin from the antrum. **Gastrin** is the most potent stimulator of gastric acid secretion.

2. The gastric phase of secretion is provoked by mechanical distention of the antrum by food. This stimulates additional gastrin release.

3. The intestinal phase of secretion is not well understood. Intestinal factors, such as cholecystokinin are mild stimulators of acid production.

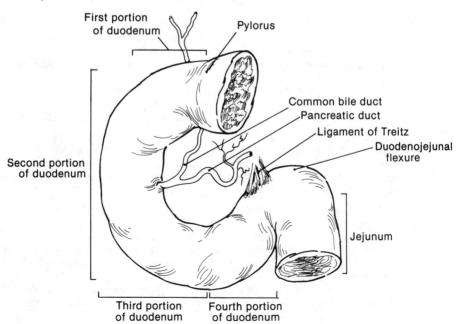

Figure 11-2. Anatomy of the duodenum.

4. **Feedback mechanisms** that inhibit gastric acid secretion include a decline in vagal stimulation. At an antral pH of 2, gastrin release is inhibited. Finally, as acid chyme enters the duodenum, it triggers the release of secretin. This further inhibits gastrin secretion.

II. **ULCER DISEASE.** Ulcers may be found in the stomach or duodenum. The etiology of the ulcer and its treatment depend on its location.

A. **Gastric ulcers**

1. **Classification**
   a. **Type I.** Most gastric ulcers occur within the body of the stomach in an area termed the locus minoris resistentiae. This refers to the histologic transitional zone between the parietal cells of the body and the gastrin-secreting cells of the antrum.
   b. **Type II.** These gastric ulcers are associated with duodenal ulcers.
   c. **Type III.** These are pyloric channel ulcers or gastric ulcers located near the pylorus. They tend to behave more like duodenal ulcers than gastric ulcers and are discussed in II B 1 c.
   d. **Type IV.** These ulcers are located near the gastroesophageal junction high on the lesser curve. Though they act like type I gastric ulcers, they are classified separately since the surgical approach is different.

2. **Incidence.** Gastric ulcers are commoner in men, in the elderly, and in lower socioeconomic groups. Duodenal ulcers are commoner than gastric ulcers, although the ratio has been decreasing (2:1).

3. **Etiology.** The etiology of gastric ulcers is multifactorial and not completely delineated. Damage to the gastric mucosal barrier appears to be the key.
   a. **Reflux of bile** into the stomach is thought to change the mucosal barrier, allowing gastric acid to enter the mucosa and injure it. This appears to be a major factor in gastric ulcer formation.
   b. **Drugs** can alter the mucosal barrier to hydrogen ion.
      (1) Ethanol, indomethacin, and salicylates are examples, though none has been proven to cause gastric ulcers.
      (2) The combination of smoking and salicylate ingestion is strongly implicated in the development of gastric ulcers.
   c. **Acid secretion.** Persons with gastric ulcers tend to have lower than normal rates of acid secretion, both basal and stimulated. Their serum gastrin levels are approximately twice the normal levels.

4. **Diagnosis**
   a. **History of burning epigastric pain** that is relieved by food but recurs ½ to 1½ hours later is the usual presentation of gastric ulcers.
   b. **Upper gastrointestinal (GI) series** is the initial diagnostic test. It can detect about 70% of gastric ulcers.
   c. Endoscopy follows if the radiologic examination is positive.
      (1) **Multiple biopsies** must be done to rule out malignancy.
      (2) **Gastric washings** and **cytology** are useful adjuncts in ruling out malignancy.

5. **Gastric ulcers and cancer**
   a. Evidence suggests that gastric ulcer does not degenerate into carcinoma.
   b. However, gastric cancer will ulcerate in 25% of cases, and it is, therefore, mandatory to prove histologically that suspicious or nonhealing gastric ulcers are not carcinoma. Approximately 10% of gastric ulcers are malignant.

6. **Medical treatment** of gastric ulcers is indicated initially. Most gastric ulcers will heal within 12–15 weeks.
   a. **Antacid therapy** has not been demonstrated to be superior to placebo.
   b. **Histamine$_2$-(H$_2$-) receptor antagonists,** such as **cimetidine** and **ranitidine,** may be effective in speeding the healing of ulcers, particularly in those patients who have a high or normal rate of acid secretion.
   c. **Cytoprotective agents,** such as **sucralfate,** have been shown to be effective. Sucralfate, when exposed to acid, forms a viscous substance that binds to damaged mucosa. It also can neutralize small amounts of acid.
   d. **Avoidance of** ethanol, tobacco, and **drugs that irritate** the gastric mucosa is important.

7. **A recurrence rate** of 25%–60% in 5 years is associated with gastric ulcers treated with short-term medical therapy. Most recurrences are within 6 months of the first event.

8. **Surgical treatment**
   a. **Indications for surgery**
      (1) Malignancy cannot be ruled out.
      (2) The ulcer fails to heal after 12–15 weeks of medical therapy.
      (3) A recurrent ulcer develops despite adequate medical therapy.
      (4) Complications develop (e.g., perforation or severe hemorrhage).
   b. **Operative procedures** (Figure 11-3)
      (1) **Hemigastrectomy** (excision of the distal 50%–60% of the stomach with excision of the ulcer) is historically the procedure of choice.
         (a) Reconstruction is accomplished with a gastroduodenal anastomosis known as a Billroth I gastrectomy (Figure 11-3*A*) whenever technically possible.
         (b) A gastrojejunal anastomosis, a Billroth II gastrectomy (Figure 11-3*B*) is done whenever the duodenum cannot be mobilized well enough to create a tension-free gastroduodenal anastomosis.
      (2) **Vagotomy with antrectomy,** a lesser resection, is also an alternative, but it tends to be associated with a high recurrence rate. Vagotomy is important in types II and III gastric ulcers.
      (3) **Mortality** from surgery is approximately 1%, and the recurrence rate is less than 1%.

B. **Duodenal ulcers**

1. **Location**
   a. Most duodenal ulcers are found in the first portion of the duodenum, as often on the posterior as the anterior wall.
   b. About 5% of duodenal ulcers are postbulbar, located in the more distal duodenum.
   c. **Pyloric channel ulcers** occur in duodenal mucosa and are treated like duodenal ulcers although they are anatomically located in the stomach. They frequently do not respond to medical therapy and often require surgery, largely because of the development of gastric outlet obstruction.

2. **Etiology.** The major cause of duodenal ulcer is increased acid production. Duodenal ulcer patients are capable of secreting larger amounts of acid than normal controls.
   a. **Gastrin secretion** has also been shown to be a factor. The parietal cells in duodenal ulcer patients are more sensitive to gastrin and require significantly less gastrin to stimulate the maximal secretion of acid. The feedback inhibition, by acid, of gastrin release may be impaired in some patients.
   b. **Tobacco, caffeine, alcohol, and aspirin** use are all associated with an increased incidence of duodenal ulcer but have not been proven to be causative.
   c. **Persons with blood group O,** particularly those who do not secrete blood group substances in their saliva, are more likely to have duodenal ulcer.
   d. **The Zollinger-Ellison syndrome** (see Chapter 17 II C), caused by a gastrin-secreting tumor of the pancreas, is associated with a virulent form of duodenal ulcer disease.

3. **Diagnosis**
   a. **History of epigastric pain** that may radiate to the back is the usual presentation. The pain is relieved by food; however, the period of relief becomes shorter as symptoms progress. The pain typically wakes the patient at night.
   b. **Upper GI series** is the mainstay of diagnosis.
   c. **Endoscopy** is not necessary routinely, as the incidence of carcinoma is very small. Endoscopy is indicated in patients with typical symptoms but a negative barium study.
   d. **Gastric analysis** provides useful baseline data in patients requiring surgery.
   e. **Serum gastrin levels** are obtained in patients with recurrent ulceration after surgery, in those who fail to respond to medical management, and in those with suspected endocrine disorders, such as the Zollinger-Ellison syndrome. Normal serum gastrin levels are less than 200 pg/ml.

4. **Medical treatment** of uncomplicated duodenal ulcer disease is usually successful.
   a. **Avoidance of aspirin, caffeine, alcohol, and tobacco** is recommended. Stress should also be avoided.

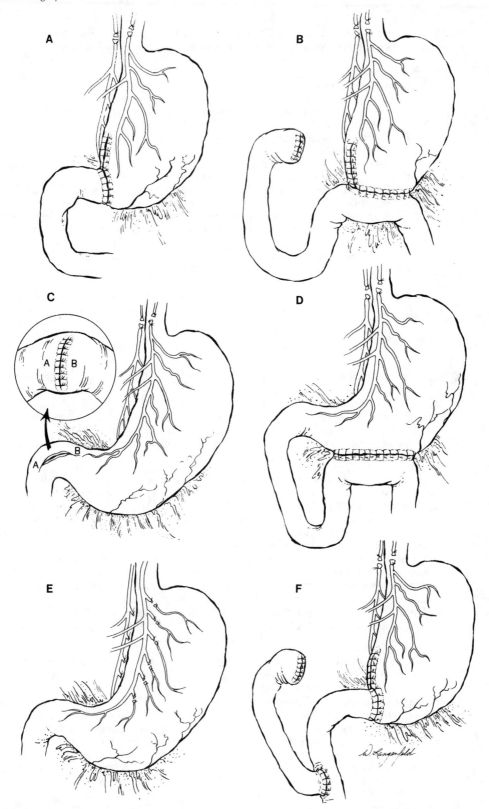

Figure 11-3. Common gastric surgical procedures: *A*, vagotomy and antrectomy (Billroth I); *B*, vagotomy and antrectomy (Billroth II); *C*, vagotomy and pyloroplasty; *D*, vagotomy and gastrojejunostomy; *E*, parietal cell vagotomy; and *F*, Roux-en-Y gastrojejunostomy.

    b. H₂-receptor antagonists (i.e., cimetidine, ranitidine) have become the **mainstays** of duodenal ulcer therapy. Most duodenal ulcers will heal in 4–6 weeks with such therapy. Because there is a high recurrence rate after discontinuation of medical therapy, maintenance therapy is often advised following ulcer healing.

    c. Antacids can also be used as an adjunct to help control gastric pH and to promote healing.

  5. Surgical treatment of duodenal ulcer is reserved for patients who fail to respond to medical therapy or who have complications. There are a number of surgical options. The goal of each is to reduce acid secretion; therefore, most approaches concentrate on abolishing vagal stimulation, antral gastrin secretion, or both.

    a. Vagotomy with antrectomy (see Figures 11-3*A* and 11-3*B*) is the procedure associated with the lowest recurrence rate.

    b. Vagotomy with drainage is associated with a recurrence rate of 6%–7%. After vagotomy the motility of the stomach and pylorus is impaired, creating a functional obstruction. For this reason, a drainage procedure, such as a **pyloroplasty** (see Figure 11-3C) or **gastrojejunostomy** (see Figure 11-3*D*), is required.

    c. Parietal cell vagotomy (see Figure 11-3*E*), also known as highly selective vagotomy, is gaining in popularity, especially when the indication for surgical intervention is intractable pain. Only the gastric branches of the vagus nerve are divided. Because innervation of the pylorus is maintained, a drainage procedure is not necessary. Recurrence rates with this procedure are somewhat higher (approximately 10%), but the morbidity is less as compared to truncal vagotomy with antrectomy.

C. Complications of ulcers include perforation, hemorrhage, and obstruction.

  1. Perforations occur most commonly with ulcers on the anterior surface of the duodenum. Gastric perforations are less common. Occasionally, ulcers can perforate posteriorly into the lesser sac.

    a. Signs and symptoms

      (1) Typical symptoms of perforation include sudden onset of severe abdominal pain, radiation of pain to the shoulder, nausea, and vomiting.

      (2) Signs include a rigid abdomen and shock. An upright chest x-ray frequently demonstrates air under the diaphragm.

    b. Treatment. Simple operative closure of the perforated ulcer, often with a patch of omentum, is the usual treatment. Definitive treatment of the ulcer (e.g., by vagotomy with antrectomy) may be indicated in low-risk patients with minimal soilage of the peritoneal cavity, especially if they give a long history (more than 3 months) of ulcer symptoms.

  2. Hemorrhage occurs in approximately 15%–20% of patients with ulcers. Medical management controls the hemorrhage in most cases.

    a. Endoscopy is necessary to evaluate the site of the hemorrhage.

    b. Electrocautery through the endoscope can sometimes be used to control bleeding ulcers. Vessels, visible in the ulcer crater, however, should be approached cautiously with the endoscope. They more often require surgical intervention.

    c. Surgery. Surgical intervention is usually needed to control **massive hemorrhage,** defined as blood loss that requires transfusion of more than 1500 ml of blood products without stabilization of vital signs, or continued blood loss, requiring more than 6 units of transfused blood in a 24-hour period. If the site of bleeding is a **duodenal ulcer:**

      (1) Oversewing of the bleeding point is done via a longitudinal opening through the pylorus.

        (a) If this fails to control the vessel, it is necessary to isolate and ligate the gastroduodenal artery.

        (b) The incision through the pylorus is then closed transversely, which is known as a **pyloroplasty,** or **widening of the pylorus**.

        (c) A **truncal vagotomy** (division of the two main vagal trunks) is also done (see Figure 11-3C)

      (2) Vagotomy with antrectomy is another option in low-risk patients.

  3. Gastric outlet obstruction can be caused by **prepyloric ulcers** and by chronic **scarring of the pyloric channel**. Patients respond poorly to medical therapy.

    a. Symptoms. Obstruction causes symptoms of crampy abdominal pain, nausea, and vomiting. The stomach is usually markedly dilated. Prolonged vomiting due to obstruction can lead to electrolyte disorders, particularly hypokalemic metabolic alkalosis from the large hydrochloric acid losses.

b. Initial treatment consists of several days of nasogastric suction to allow the stomach to return to normal size.

c. Surgery. Vagotomy with antrectomy or **vagotomy with drainage** is done.

III. GASTRITIS is a mucosal lesion. It is classified as acute or chronic.

A. Acute gastritis

1. **Acute diffuse gastritis** can be due to a number of irritating agents, particularly aspirin and ethanol. Hemorrhage can occur and can be massive. Removal of the inciting agent and antacid therapy usually result in prompt healing.

2. **Stress ulceration (acute hemorrhage gastritis)** is another form of acute gastritis. Ischemia of the gastric mucosa is the inciting event. The injury is compounded by the effect of the intraluminal acid.

   a. Location. Stress ulcers are characteristically shallow mucosal lesions that start in the fundus. They then spread distally and can involve the entire stomach.

   b. Clinical presentation. Affected patients frequently have sepsis, multiple organ system failure, severe trauma, or a complicated postoperative course. Stress ulceration that occurs in burn patients is known as **Curling's ulcer.** Though stress ulceration is common in critically ill patients, only 5% develop significant gastric bleeding.

   c. Prophylaxis against stress ulceration can be achieved with antacids given as needed to keep the gastric pH above 5. H_2-receptor antagonists are equally effective at maintaining an adequate gastric pH.

   d. Treatment

   (1) **Medical treatment** involves correcting the underlying problems (e.g., sepsis) and vigorous use of antacids. Cimetidine is not helpful once bleeding has occurred.

   (2) **Surgical treatment** is rarely necessary and is associated with a high mortality. In the case of uncontrollable bleeding, near total gastrectomy is usually the best option.

B. Chronic gastritis (atrophic gastritis). Atrophy of the gastric tubules and inflammatory infiltration of the lamina propria are the lesions found in atrophic gastritis. Intestinal metaplasia may occur. There are two **types** of chronic gastritis. Both are associated with an increased risk of gastric carcinoma. Their etiology is unknown.

1. **Type A gastritis** involves the proximal stomach diffusely but spares the antrum. This gastritis is associated with parietal cell antibodies in the serum. Acid secretion is markedly reduced, and vitamin B_{12} absorption is impaired.

2. **Type B gastritis** is the commoner type. It is found in association with duodenal and gastric ulcers, and its incidence increases with age. No parietal cell antibodies are found, and acid production is only slightly reduced.

IV. GASTRIC AND DUODENAL TUMORS

A. Gastric tumors

1. **Malignant tumors.** Approximately 90%–95% of gastric tumors are malignant and of the malignancies, 95% are carcinomas.

   a. Gastric cancer

   (1) The **incidence** of carcinoma of the stomach has been decreasing.

   (2) **Symptoms** include pain, anorexia, and weight loss. Symptoms tend to occur late in the course of the disease.

   (3) **Diagnosis** can be made with an upper GI series and confirmed with endoscopic biopsy.

   (4) **Classification.** Gastric carcinoma is classified according to its gross characteristics.

   (a) **Fungating.** These are the least common lesions and have a better prognosis.

   (b) **Ulcerating.** These are the commonest.

   (c) **Diffusely infiltrating (linitis plastica).** The tumor causes extensive submucosal infiltration.

(5) Surgical treatment depends on nodal disease and distant metastases.

  (a) Potentially curable lesions are treated with subtotal or total gastrectomy, depending on tumor location. Wide margins on the stomach are necessary since extensive submucosal tumor spread can occur. Lesions of the fundus and cardia may require resection of the spleen.

  (b) The role of lymphadenectomy is controversial, but for favorable lesions, there is some advantage to removing the draining nodes. Removal of the omentum and its nodes is included.

  (c) Palliative resections are indicated in the presence of obstructing or bleeding gastric cancers.

(6) Adjuvant therapy after potentially curative resection is controversial, but some benefit may be obtained from a regimen of 5-fluorouracil, doxorubicin, and mitomycin. Unresectable tumors may show some response to combined chemotherapy and radiation therapy.

(7) Prognosis depends largely on the depth of invasion of the gastric wall, involvement of regional nodes, and the presence of distant metastases but still remains poor. Tumors not penetrating the serosa and not involving regional nodes are associated with approximately 70% 5-year survival. This number drops dramatically if the tumor is through the serosa or into regional nodes. Only 40% of patients have potentially curable disease at the time of diagnosis.

b. Gastric lymphoma can be primary or can occur as part of disseminated disease. The stomach is the commonest site of **primary intestinal lymphoma**. The tumors may be bulky with central ulceration.

  (1) Diagnosis preoperatively is crucial since the surgical approach differs markedly from that used with gastric cancer.

  (2) Surgical treatment involves local resection (partial gastrectomy). Most lesions also require treatment with radiation therapy, chemotherapy, or both.

  (3) Prognosis is good with 5-year survival up to 90%.

c. Leiomyosarcomas are bulky, well-localized tumors. They are slow to metastasize and can be treated with partial gastrectomy.

2. Benign tumors are uncommon.

  a. Leiomyomas are the commonest benign gastric tumors. They are usually asymptomatic but may undergo hemorrhage or cause a mass effect. They are submucosal and well encapsulated.

  b. Gastric polyps are of two types. They often can be excised via the endoscope.

   (1) Hyperplastic polyps are the commonest and are not premalignant.

   (2) Adenomatous polyps are associated with a high risk of malignancy, especially those greater than 1.5 cm.

  c. Other benign tumors are fibromas, neurofibromas, aberrant pancreas, and angiomas.

B. Duodenal tumors, both benign and malignant, are rare.

1. Malignant tumors are usually adenocarcinomas. Treatment of resectable lesions is pancreaticoduodenectomy (**Whipple's procedure**).

2. Benign tumors include lipomas, leiomyomas, and adenomas. They can be locally excised if necessary.

V. ACQUIRED OBSTRUCTIVE DISORDERS OF THE STOMACH AND DUODENUM

A. Gastric outlet obstruction (see II C 3)

B. Gastric volvulus is an uncommon entity. The volvulus may be intermittent. It is caused by laxity of the ligaments supporting the stomach and is frequently associated with diaphragmatic hernias.

1. Types

  a. Organoaxial volvulus is a rotation around the cardiopyloric line, a line drawn along the length of the stomach between the cardia and pylorus.

  b. Mesentericoaxial volvulus occurs around a line perpendicular to the cardiopyloric line.

  c. Volvulus may also occur as a combination of these two types.

2. Surgical treatment includes reducing the torsion and fixation of the stomach.

C. **Superior mesenteric artery syndrome.** Especially in young, thin women, the third portion of the duodenum can be obstructed by the superior mesenteric artery, which takes a sharp angle from the aorta and courses over the duodenum. This anatomic configuration is combined with **predisposing factors,** such as a lack of the retroperitoneal fat cushion, prolonged immobilization, and pressure (e.g., from a body cast). The syndrome is also known as **cast syndrome** because of its association with patients in body casts.

1. **Symptoms** include vomiting and postprandial pain.

2. **Treatment**
   a. **Medical treatment** consists of eliminating all contributing factors, such as casts, girdles, and lying in the supine position. Weight gain may alleviate symptoms.
   b. **Surgical treatment** includes either releasing the ligament of Treitz, which moves the duodenum out from beneath the superior mesenteric artery, or bypassing the obstruction.

VI. MISCELLANEOUS DISORDERS OF THE STOMACH AND DUODENUM

A. **Mallory-Weiss tears** are linear mucosal lesions found at the gastroesophageal junction. They are caused by repeated forceful vomiting and can result in profuse hemorrhage. Diagnosis is made by endoscopy. Only 10% of patients require surgery to stop the bleeding, which consists of oversewing the mucosal tear (see Chapter 10 VI).

B. **Bezoars** are agglutinated masses of hair **(trichobezoars),** vegetable matter **(phytobezoars),** or a combination of the two that form within the stomach.

1. **Trichobezoars** occur most commonly in young, neurotic women. **Phytobezoars** are seen after a partial gastric resection and tend to be commoner in older men.

2. **Symptoms** of a bezoar include nausea, vomiting, weight loss, and abdominal pain. **Complications** include obstruction and ulceration.

3. **Treatment** generally requires surgical removal, although enzymatic dissolution of some bezoars has been successful.

C. **Menetrier's disease** is an abnormality of the gastric mucosa with an unknown etiology.

1. Characteristics include the following:
   a. A hypertrophic gastric mucosa is seen on x-ray.
      (1) Giant rugae are characteristic; these spare the antrum.
      (2) Mucous cells are increased in number, and parietal and chief cells are decreased.
   b. There is gastric hypersecretion of mucus with a high protein and low acid concentration; systemic hypoproteinemia is the result.

2. **Treatment.** Total gastrectomy is required in patients with severe hypoproteinemia.

D. **Duodenal diverticula** are frequently asymptomatic. The commonest location is opposite the ampulla of Vater. These are **pulsion diverticula,** caused by "pulling" of muscles. Severe hemorrhage or perforation can occur, but in the absence of such complications, no treatment is indicated.

VII. COMPLICATIONS SPECIFIC TO GASTRIC SURGERY. These symptom complexes, known as **postgastrectomy syndromes,** can be disabling.

A. **Alkaline reflux gastritis** is the commonest problem after a gastrectomy, occurring in about 25% of all patients.

1. **Symptoms** are postprandial epigastric pain, nausea, vomiting, and weight loss.

2. **Diagnosis. Endoscopy** demonstrates the gastritis and a free reflux of bile.

3. **Treatment** is conversion of the Billroth I or II gastrectomy (see Figures 11-3A and 11-3B) to a Roux-en-Y anastomosis (see Figure 11-3F).

B. **Afferent loop syndrome** is caused by intermittent mechanical obstruction of the afferent loop of a gastrojejunostomy.

1. **Symptoms** include early postprandial distention, pain, and nausea, which are relieved by vomiting of bilious material not mixed with food.

2. **Treatment** consists of providing good drainage of the afferent loop, usually by conversion to a Roux-en-Y anastomosis.

C. **Dumping syndrome** affects most postgastrectomy patients but is a significant problem in only a few.

1. **Etiology.** It is caused by the release of hypertonic chyme into the small bowel. This in turn causes rapid accumulation of fluid and consequent jejunal distention.

2. **Signs and symptoms**
   a. **Symptoms** may include epigastric fullness or pain, nausea, palpitations, dizziness, and diarrhea.
   b. **Signs** include tachycardia and elevated blood pressure.

3. **Treatment**
   a. **Conservative measures** control most patients' symptoms. They are advised to avoid a high-carbohydrate diet and not to drink fluids with meals.
   b. **Surgical treatment** is used to delay gastric emptying, including interposition of an anti-peristaltic jejunal loop between the stomach and small bowel.

D. **Postvagotomy diarrhea** is common in its mild form but seldom is a disabling problem. Symptoms usually improve during the first year after surgery.

12
Small Intestine

Michael J. Moritz
R. Anthony Carabasi, III

I. INTRODUCTION

A. Anatomy

1. **External structure.** The small intestine is the length of bowel that extends from the pylorus to the cecum.
   a. **The duodenum**, which is retroperitoneal, extends from the pylorus to the ligament of Treitz.
   b. **The jejunum** (proximal 40%) **and ileum** (distal 60%), which are intraperitoneal, make up the remainder of the small intestine.

2. **Internal structure**
   a. The **total length** of small bowel is approximately 3 m (duodenum 30 cm, jejunum 110 cm, and ileum 160 cm). Length is proportionate to body size (total jejunoileal length is approximately 160% of body height).
   b. The **jejunum** is larger in diameter, thicker walled, has more prominent plicae circulares (mucosal folds), and has less mesenteric fat than the ileum.
   c. The lymphoid tissue (Peyer's patches) found in the submucosa becomes more prominent distally in the ileum.

3. **Vasculature.** The **arterial supply** to the small intestine is primarily from the jejunal and ileal branches of the superior mesenteric artery.
   a. **Jejunal mesenteric arteries** have only one or two arcades and a long vasa recta (the small arteries directly adjacent to the bowel wall).
   b. Ileal arteries have multiple arcades that extend closer to the bowel and have short vasa recta.

4. **Layers of the wall of the small intestine**
   a. **The mucosa** is composed primarily of columnar epithelium with goblet cells. The absorption of nutrients takes place through the mucosa. The mucosa covers the intestinal villi and has an absorption area of approximately 500 m². Mucosal cells proliferate rapidly and have a life span of 5 days.
   b. **The submucosa** is the strongest layer and provides strength to an intestinal anastomosis. It contains nerves, Meissner's plexus, blood vessels, and fibrous and elastic tissue.
   c. **The muscularis**—the muscle layer—is composed of an outer longitudinal layer and an inner circular layer with Auerbach's myenteric plexus of ganglion cells in between.
   d. **The serosa** is the outermost layer and derives embryologically from the peritoneum.

B. Physiology.
The **primary functions** of the small intestine are **digestion** and **absorption**. All ingested food and fluid, and also secretions from the stomach, liver, and pancreas, reach the small intestine. The total volume may reach 9 L a day, and all but 1–2 L will be absorbed.

1. **Motility**
   a. **Two types of contractions** occur following a meal.
      (1) **To-and-fro motion** mixes chyme with digestive juices and provides prolonged exposure to the absorptive mucosa.
      (2) **Peristaltic contractions** move food distally.
   b. In the fasting state, a strong contraction beginning in the duodenum occurs every 2 hours. This completes the emptying of residual food from previous meals.
   c. Parasympathetic stimulation promotes contractions while sympathetic stimulation inhibits them.

2. **Absorption.** Vitamins, fat, protein, carbohydrates, water, and electrolytes are all absorbed in the small intestine.
   a. **Water** is absorbed throughout the small intestine, although most water is absorbed in the jejunum. Passive absorption is the mechanism.
   b. **Electrolytes**
      (1) **Potassium** is absorbed by passive diffusion.
      (2) **Sodium** is actively transported, and once a gradient is established, **chloride** follows passively.
      (3) **Calcium** is actively transported in the jejunum (regulated by vitamin D).
   c. **Fat** absorption occurs chiefly in the duodenum and jejunum. Fat is digested by pancreatic lipase and becomes emulsified in bile acid micelles. The micelles release fatty acids and monoglycerides to the mucosal cells. After absorption, the mucosa **resynthesizes** triglycerides, which are assembled into **chylomicrons** and transported into the lymphatics. (All other absorbed nutrients are transported directly into the portal venous system.)
   d. **Carbohydrates** are digested by salivary and pancreatic amylase. Enzymes of the mucosal cell surface further reduce sugars to the monosaccharides fructose, galactose, and glucose, which are absorbed by active transport.
   e. **Protein** digestion begins in the stomach (by pepsin) and continues in the small bowel by pancreatic enzymes. The process is completed at the brush border, yielding tripeptides, dipeptides, and amino acids. All are absorbed by active transport.
   f. **Vitamins A, D, E, and K** are fat-soluble and are absorbed in micelles from the intestine. Most water-soluble vitamins are absorbed by passive diffusion. **Vitamin B$_{12}$** is complexed with intrinsic factor and absorbed by pinocytosis at the distal ileum. Vitamin C, thiamine, and folic acid are actively transported.
   g. **Iron** is absorbed as the ferrous (reduced) ion Fe^{2+}. Conversion of the ferric to the ferrous ion is enhanced by the presence of reducing substances in the diet, such as vitamin C (ascorbic acid). Absorption is via active transport and occurs primarily in the jejunum.

II. SMALL BOWEL DISEASES

A. **Tumors of the small intestine**

1. **Benign neoplasms** are usually asymptomatic. They are 10 times commoner than malignant tumors (autopsy data).
   a. **Polyps**
      (1) **Adenomatous polyps** are rare in the small intestine. They may be seen in the **familial polyposis** syndromes and have malignant potential in this setting.
      (2) **Hamartomatous polyps** are found in patients with **Peutz-Jeghers syndrome** (mucocutaneous pigmentation accompanied by widespread intestinal polyposis). There is virtually no malignant potential in this syndrome.
      (3) **Juvenile (retention) polyps** are benign hamartomas and not true neoplasms. They are commoner in the rectum and usually autoamputate. They may cause bleeding or obstruction and are resected if symptoms occur.
   b. **Other benign tumors** include leiomyomas, lipomas, adenomas, hemangiomas, fibromas, and neurofibromas (in descending order of frequency), any of which require resection if symptomatic.

2. **Malignant neoplasms**
   a. **Overview**
      (1) **Incidence.** The commonest tumors are adenocarcinoma (40%), carcinoid (30%), lymphoma (20%), sarcoma, and metastases from distant malignancies.
      (2) **Symptoms. Malignant tumors constitute 75% of symptomatic small bowel tumors** and usually present with bleeding, diarrhea, perforation, or obstruction (which may be due to intussusception).
      (3) **Diagnosis** is frequently made late in the course of disease as symptoms are often subtle and insidious in onset.
      (4) **Treatment** is segmental resection, including adequate margins proximally and distally and as much mesentery as possible without compromising the blood supply to the remaining small intestine.
   b. **Adenocarcinoma** is commonest in the duodenum and proximal jejunum. Metastases are present in a large percentage of patients at operation. Patients with resectable tumors have a 25% 5-year survival rate.

    c. **Carcinoid tumors** are derived from enterochromaffin cells. These cells are part of the **a**mine **p**recursor **u**ptake and **d**ecarboxylation system (APUD cells), and hence, carcinoid tumors are classified as **apudomas**. Carcinoid tumors are commonest in the appendix, then the small bowel (usually the ileum), then the rectum. Other sites are uncommon.

      (1) **Prognosis** is related to size (i.e., diameter). Both carcinoid tumors and metastases are slow growing, and prolonged survival is common.

        (a) Tumors less than 1 cm (75% of total) have a 2% incidence of metastases.

        (b) Tumors 1–2 cm (20% of total) have over a 50% rate of metastases.

        (c) Tumors over 2 cm (5% of total) have an 80%–90% rate of metastases.

      (2) Only small bowel carcinoids have a tendency to multicentricity (30%).

      (3) **Carcinoid syndrome**—flushing, diarrhea, bronchoconstriction, and tricuspid and pulmonary valvular disease—is caused by serotonin and other vasoactive substances secreted by the tumor.

        (a) These substances are cleared by the liver, so only liver metastases, which drain into the systemic veins, or primary extraintestinal carcinoids (e.g., bronchial carcinoids) cause the syndrome. About 10% of patients with small bowel carcinoids develop the syndrome.

        (b) **Diagnosis** is made by finding elevated levels of 5-hydroxyindoleacetic acid (5-HIAA), the breakdown product of serotonin, in the urine.

        (c) **Treatment** includes resection of the primary tumor and resection or "debulking" of metastases. Liver metastases can be resected (when solitary) but usually require palliative therapy with (intra-arterial) chemotherapy or hepatic arterial ligation or embolization to decrease the blood flow to the metastases.

        (d) **Prognosis.** The overall 5-year survival rate for small bowel carcinoid patients is 70%. If liver metastases are present, the 5-year survival rate is 20%.

    d. **Primary small bowel lymphomas** usually arise in the ileum.

      (1) Perforation is a frequent presentation; however, lymphomas can also present with fever of unknown origin or with malabsorption.

      (2) Biopsies of lymph nodes and the liver are necessary for staging.

    e. **Leiomyosarcoma** is the commonest of the small bowel sarcomas.

    f. **Metastases** to the small bowel are present in 50% of malignant melanoma patients at autopsy. Many other carcinomas can also metastasize to the small bowel.

B. Crohn's disease (regional enteritis; granulomatous ileitis) is a chronic, transmural granulomatous inflammatory disease that can involve any area of the gastrointestinal tract. Its cause is unknown. It is the **commonest surgical disease of the small intestine.**

  1. **Distribution.** The small bowel alone is involved in 25% of patients, both the small and the large bowel in 50%, and the colon alone in almost 25%. The distal ileum, the commonest site, is involved in 70% of all cases, which accounts for the older name, **terminal ileitis.**

  2. **Diagnosis**

    a. **Peak age of onset** is between the second and fourth decades.

    b. **Symptoms** include diarrhea (usually not bloody), abdominal pain, lethargy, fever, weight loss, and anorectal disease. Anal fissures, fistulas, or ulcers, or perirectal abscesses, are seen in 50% of patients with colonic involvement and 20% of patients with small bowel disease.

    c. **Signs** include an abdominal mass, anemia, and malnutrition. Extraintestinal manifestations include inflammatory ocular, joint, skin, and biliary disease.

    d. **X-ray findings** on contrast study characteristically include segmental areas of stricture separated by "skip areas" of uninvolved bowel, cobblestone appearance of the mucosa, and fistulas.

  3. **Differential diagnosis** includes ulcerative colitis, lymphoma, and infectious enteritides (tuberculosis, amebiasis, and *Yersinia*, *Campylobacter*, and *Salmonella* infections).

  4. **Medical treatment** is preferred and can include rest, a low-residue diet, prednisone and oral antibiotics (sulfasalazine or metronidazole), sedatives, antispasmodics, and, when necessary, total parenteral nutrition. Although antibiotics and steroids are helpful in acute active disease, their effectiveness in preventing relapse of symptoms has not been established.

  5. **Surgical treatment**, which is reserved for **complications** of the disease, ultimately becomes necessary in most cases. Surgical therapy is conservative—resecting as little bowel

as necessary. If resection is hazardous, bypass or exclusion of the involved segment may be necessary.

    a. Intestinal obstruction, usually due to stricture and inflammation, is the commonest complication.

    b. Abscesses and fistulas are also common. Abscesses may be intra- or retroperitoneal. Fistulas (see Chapter 2 IV) form from bowel to skin, to bladder, to vagina, to urethra, or to other loops of bowel.

    c. Perianal disease is best treated with oral metronidazole.

        (1) Perirectal abscesses require drainage. Anal fistulas or fissures may need surgery if they are multiple or severe.

        (2) In general, surgery for perianal disease should be as limited as is practical, because wound healing in these patients is poor and recurrence is common.

    d. Perforation, hemorrhage, intractable symptoms, cancer, and growth retardation (in children) are less common indications for surgery.

6. Prognosis is only fair. Roughly 50% of patients who require surgery will require it again within 5 years. The likelihood of recurrence after each reoperation is again approximately 50%.

C. Diverticulosis

1. Duodenal diverticula are common (seen on 10%–20% of upper gastrointestinal x-rays), but over 90% are asymptomatic.

    a. Approximately 70% of duodenal diverticula are in the periampullary region, and they frequently cause symptoms.

    b. Periampullary diverticula can cause cholangitis, pancreatitis, and recurrent common bile duct stones.

2. Jejunoileal diverticula are rare.

    a. They may cause obstruction, bleeding, or perforation.

    b. They may also cause malabsorption due to bacterial overgrowth within the diverticulum.

3. Meckel's diverticulum is the commonest diverticulum of the gastrointestinal tract (incidence 3%). It is located within 2–3 feet of the ileocecal valve.

    a. Most symptomatic Meckel's diverticula are seen in childhood, usually causing bleeding. The bleeding is from heterotopic gastric mucosa in the diverticulum, causing "peptic" ulceration in adjacent ileal mucosa.

    b. Problems in adults include bowel obstruction, bleeding, and acute diverticulitis, which may be indistinguishable from appendicitis.

    c. Asymptomatic Meckel's diverticulum should *not* be resected.

D. Small bowel fistulas (see Chapter 2)

E. Short bowel syndrome is a complication of small bowel resection.

1. Symptoms. It is characterized by malabsorption with diarrhea and excessive loss of fat and protein in the stool. Inadequate absorption of water, electrolytes, minerals, and vitamins also invariably occurs. The length of bowel necessary to avoid the syndrome is variable, but patients with less than 100 cm (3.5 feet) of small bowel are most susceptible.

2. Total parenteral nutrition (TPN; see Chapter 1 II F 3) is essential postoperatively. The small bowel will hypertrophy with time, and most patients can be weaned from parenteral nutrition gradually. For refractory cases, long-term total parenteral nutrition **(home TPN)** is available.

3. Oral nutrition. Ensuring that oral nutrition is adequate requires attention to several points.

    a. The total calories ingested must increase, to compensate for that portion not absorbed.

    b. A low-residue or elemental diet is needed. An **elemental diet** contains only components that are directly absorbed by the intestinal mucosa without any enzymatic digestion (medium- and short-chain triglycerides, mono- and disaccharides, and mono- and dipeptides), plus vitamins and minerals. It contains *no* residue (undigestible material).

    c. Antiperistaltic agents should be given.

    d. Reflex gastric hypersecretion should be controlled with histamine$_2$-(H$_2$-) receptor antagonists.

    e. Fat- and water-soluble vitamin supplementation is needed.

    f. Parenteral vitamin B_{12} is needed if the distal ileum has been resected.

    g. Calcium and magnesium supplementation should be given.

    h. Medium-chain triglycerides should replace dietary fats because they do not require micelles for absorption.

  4. Surgical therapy is available, consisting of reversal of a short segment of distal small bowel to slow the intestinal transit time if adequate oral nutrition cannot be attained.

F. Radiation injury to the small bowel occurs in two phases.

  1. Acute phase injury is due to mucosal injury. Symptoms, which include nausea, vomiting, and diarrhea, are transient. Rarely, bleeding or perforation occurs and requires surgery.

  2. Chronic effects appear months to years later and are due to an obliterative vasculitis. The symptoms and signs are similar to those associated with recurrent malignancy, and, indeed, this possibility must always be fully evaluated.

    a. Minor symptoms—abdominal pain, malabsorption, and diarrhea—require symptomatic therapy only.

    b. Major complications that require surgery include bowel obstruction (unrelieved by decompression with a nasogastric or long tube), perforation, abscess, fistula, and hemorrhage. Hemorrhage may be from mucosal erosion or an enteroarterial fistula.

    c. Surgery is technically difficult due to fibrosis and scarring. With resection or bypass, unirradiated bowel must be used for any anastomosis. Even so, the anastomosis or surgical wound is likely to break down with subsequent fistula formation or other complications.

  3. Prognosis. The perioperative mortality rate is less than 15%, but the long-term mortality rate is high. The 5-year survival rate is less than 50%.

13
Colon, Rectum, and Anus

Maryalice Cheney
Anthony V. Coletta

I. INTRODUCTION

A. Gross anatomy

1. **Large intestine.** The large intestine is divided into five parts: the **ascending colon, transverse colon, descending colon, sigmoid colon,** and **rectum.** The colon begins at the **cecum,** where it is joined by the **terminal ileum** at the **ileocecal valve,** which is a bilobed structure. The **appendix** projects from the convergence of the teniae coli (the three muscular bands comprising the outer longitudinal muscle of the colon) at the lowest part of the cecum. Although the commonest site of the appendix is retrocecal (65%), it may also be located in the pelvis, in front of (prececal), behind (postcecal), or below (subcecal) the cecum.

   a. The colon continues cephalad in a retroperitoneal course as the **ascending colon** to the **hepatic flexure.** It is suspended from above at the hepatic flexure by the hepatocolic ligament.

   b. It becomes intraperitoneal and courses from right to left as the **transverse colon** to the **splenic flexure,** where it is again suspended from above by the linocolic, splenocolic, and gastrocolic ligaments.

   c. The colon turns to course downward as the **descending colon** in a retroperitoneal position to the sigmoidocolic junction, where the **sigmoid colon** begins (as an intraperitoneal structure).

   d. At approximately the level of the sacral promontory (S3), the **rectum** begins. It is the rectosigmoid junction where the teniae coli diverge to form the single longitudinal outer muscle layer of the rectum.

      (1) The rectum measures 12–15 cm in length and, for descriptive purposes, is divided into upper, middle, and lower thirds.

      (2) It descends along the curvature of the sacrum and coccyx, passing through the pelvic diaphragm and ending in the anal canal.

      (3) The rectum describes three lateral curves, the inner aspect of which forms the **valves of Houston.**

         (a) These valves are excellent sites for rectal biopsy because their protrusion makes an easy target, and perforation is less likely after biopsy because they do not contain all layers of the bowel wall.

         (b) The middle valve of Houston marks the anterior peritoneal reflection.

      (4) The rectal ampulla is the most distal portion of the rectum, which functions as a reservoir because of its characteristic distensibility.

      (5) The rectum lacks a mesentery, sacculations, and appendices epiploicae.

2. **Peritoneal relations**

   a. Although the peritoneal reflection shows considerable personal and sexual variation, in general, it is 7–9 cm from the anal verge in men and 5–7 cm above the anal verge in women.

   b. The posterior peritoneal reflection is usually 12–15 cm from the anal verge.

   c. The rectum ends at the **anorectal junction**.

   d. The **anal canal** is the terminal portion of the intestinal tract. It begins at the anorectal junction, is 4 cm in length, and ends at the anal verge. It is surrounded by two muscular tubes, which are involved in the mechanism of continence.

      (1) The innermost muscular tube is the **internal sphincter muscle,** which is a continuation of the inner circular muscle of the rectum. It is smooth muscle with involuntary control and autonomic innervation.

(2) The outer muscular tube is comprised of the **external sphincter muscle** (subcutaneous, superficial, and deep portions), which is a striated muscle under voluntary control and somatic innervation.

B. Histologic anatomy. The colonic wall is composed of four **layers: mucosa, submucosa, muscularis propria,** and **serosa.**

1. **The mucosa** is the innermost layer of the colon and rectum and is lined by columnar epithelium. Malignant cells confined to the mucosa are referred to as carcinoma-in-situ.
   a. At the level of the anal canal, extending approximately 1–2 cm above the dentate line, is a zone of transitional epithelium, having both columnar and squamous components.
   b. Below the dentate line, the anal canal is lined by modified skin (**anoderm**), which is squamous epithelium. If differs from the perianal skin in that it contains no hair follicles or sebaceous glands.

2. **The submucosa,** a layer of connective tissue containing blood vessels and lymphatics, is the strongest layer of the bowel wall. Neoplasms must penetrate the submucosal layer to gain access to the lymphatic system, enabling metastatic spread.

3. **The muscularis propria** is made up of the inner circular and outer longitudinal muscles. The rectum lacks a serosal layer. The clinical significance of the layers of the bowel wall lie in the staging of colorectal cancer where the depth of invasion is the basis of the Duke's staging system and the most significant prognostic indicator.

C. Vasculature

1. **Arterial supply**
   a. The three branches of the **superior mesenteric arteries** listed below have many anastomotic connections.
      (1) **Ileocolic artery** is a terminal branch of the superior mesenteric artery, and supplies blood to the appendix, via the **appendicular artery,** and to the cecum and the proximal ascending colon.
      (2) The **right colic artery,** which may originate from the superior mesenteric artery or the ileocolic artery, supplies the remainder of the ascending colon and the hepatic flexure.
      (3) The **middle colic artery** originates from the proximal superior mesenteric artery and supplies the transverse colon.
   b. The left colic branch of the **inferior mesenteric artery** supplies the splenic flexure and the descending colon. It communicates with the middle colic artery (and thus the superior mesenteric artery) via the **marginal artery of Drummond**. This anastomosis may be variable.
      (1) **Sigmoid** and **rectosigmoid arteries,** branches of the inferior mesenteric artery, supply the sigmoid colon. They communicate with the **left colic artery** via the marginal artery.
      (2) The rectum is supplied by branches of the **superior rectal** (hemorrhoidal) **artery,** which is a branch of the inferior mesenteric artery (portal blood supply), by the **middle rectal** (hemorrhoidal) **artery,** a branch of the internal iliac artery (systemic blood supply), and by the **inferior rectal** (hemorrhoidal) **artery,** a branch of the internal pudendal artery. There is a rich submucosal anastomotic network among these vessels.

2. **Venous return.** The veins that drain the colon and rectum in general parallel the arteries similarly named.
   a. The colon drains into the portal venous system.
   b. The rectum is drained by both the portal and systemic venous systems. The middle and lower thirds of the rectum communicate directly with the systemic venous system via the internal iliac veins and the portal venous system via the inferior mesenteric vein.

3. **Lymphatic drainage**
   a. In general, the lymphatic vessels follow the arterial blood supply.
   b. Below the dentate line, lymph from the anal canal usually drains to the inguinal lymph nodes.

D. Innervation. The two main neural pathways are the autonomic and visceral afferent systems.

1. **Autonomic system**
   a. **Parasympathetic division**
      (1) The vagus nerve provides parasympathetic innervation into the lower gastrointestinal tract to the level of the splenic flexure.

       (2) From the splenic flexure to the dentate line, parasympathetic innervation arises from nervi erigentes (i.e., the pelvic splanchnic nerves), which originate from levels S2, S3, and S4.

       (3) The parasympathetic nerves provide motor innervation to the wall of the bowel.

    b. **The sympathetic division,** via the greater and lesser splanchnic nerves, innervates the blood vessels to the lower gastrointestinal tract.

  2. **Visceral afferent system**

    a. **Parasympathetic nerves** carry afferent reflex arcs along the vagal and splanchnic pathways.

    b. **Sympathetic nerves** for the most part carry pain and pressure afferents along sympathetic pathways and are responsible for referred pain.

E. Physiology. The major function of the large bowel is storage, transport, and concentration of intestinal waste products. Sodium, chloride, and water are actively absorbed. The absorptive capacity of the colon is approximately 2 L/day. The colonic mucosa secretes potassium and bicarbonate. Excessive diarrhea may result in potassium and bicarbonate losses and metabolic acidosis. **Colonic gas** originates from both swallowed air and the by-products of bacterial reactions with colonic contents.

II. EVALUATION OF THE COLON, RECTUM, AND ANUS

A. The history should always include a description of the following:

  1. Recent and past bowel habits (noting any change)

  2. Patterns of rectal bleeding

  3. Consistency of the stools

  4. Personal or family history of inflammatory bowel disease, colonic polyps, or cancer of the colon, breast, uterus, or ovaries

  5. Characterization of pain if present

B. Physical examination

  1. The standard techniques for examination of the abdomen are followed.

  2. An **anorectal examination,** most comfortably performed in the lateral decubitus position, should include:

    a. Inspection of the perianal region

    b. Digital rectal examination

    c. Anoscopy

    d. Rigid sigmoidoscopy

    e. Flexible fiberoptic sigmoidoscopy

    f. Examination of stools for occult blood

C. X-ray studies

  1. **Plain abdominal x-rays** can assess patterns of air and fluid, such as free intra-abdominal air as well as small bowel and colonic gaseous extension.

  2. **Contrast enema.** A routine contrast study of the colon is performed using barium. When perforation is suspected, Gastrografin is substituted. Intraperitoneal barium results in acute peritonitis and, combined with fecal contamination, is a life-threatening condition associated with a high mortality.

    a. **Three phases of barium contrast studies**

       (1) **Barium filled phase.** Films are taken with the patient in both the prone and supine positions.

       (2) **Postevacuation phase.** Films are taken with the patient in the prone position. These films are especially useful in diagnosing inflammatory disorders.

       (3) **Air contrast phase,** performed by the insufflation of air after barium evacuation, provides mucosal detail that is most useful in detecting small polypoid lesions.

    b. **Bowel preparation.** Incomplete cleansing of the colon is a major source of diagnostic error. Colon preparation for a routine barium contrast study includes:

       (1) **Clear liquid diet** for 24 hours

(2) **Oral cathartics** on the afternoon and evening before the examination (except in patients with evidence of colonic obstruction)

(3) **Suppository** or **enema** on the morning of the examination

c. **Complications of barium contrast studies**

(1) **Perforation of the bowel**

(a) Most commonly, perforation is related to the insertion of the enema tip or inflation of a retention balloon. Perforation secondary to instrumentation is most often seen in the rectum below the peritoneal reflection.

(b) Less commonly, perforation is related to excessive colonic pressure generated during the study. In the absence of associated colonic disease, perforation resulting from excessive pressure usually occurs in the cecum.

(2) **Barium impaction** results from incomplete evacuation of barium following the examination.

(3) **Barium granulomas,** nonspecific ulcerative or polypoid lesions, which are often subclinical, are caused by tearing of the rectal mucosa during administration of the contrast.

D. Endoscopic studies

1. **Anoscopy** enables the evaluation of the anal canal.

2. **Rigid proctosigmoidoscopy.** The rigid sigmoidoscope is 25 cm in length. It enables evaluation of the rectum and sigmoid colon to this level.

   a. The examination is most commonly performed in the lateral decubitus or prone jackknife position. Preparation for the examination requires two Fleet enemas only.

   b. For over 100 years, rigid sigmoidoscopy remained the time-honored method for examining the rectum and sigmoid colon. However, it was uncomfortable for the patient and resulted in poor patient and physician compliance.

3. **Flexible fiberoptic sigmoidoscopy.** In 1968, the first successful examination of the colon beyond 25 cm was performed. The flexible fiberoptic sigmoidoscope is 65 cm in length, allowing the evaluation of a significantly greater length of colon than the rigid sigmoidoscope.

   a. The position of the patient as well as the preparation for this examination is the same as that for rigid sigmoidoscopy.

   b. With a trend towards a more proximal distribution of colonic neoplasms came the need to examine a greater length of colon.

   (1) In the 1930s, 1940s, and 1950s, 50% of all colorectal cancers were detectable by digital rectal examination, and about 65% by the 25-cm rigid sigmoidoscope.

   (2) By the mid-1970s, only 35% of all cancers arose in the distal 20 cm.

   c. The flexible fiberoptic sigmoidoscope is superior to the rigid sigmoidoscope with respect to patient comfort and diagnostic yield.

4. **Colonoscopy.** The flexible fiberoptic colonoscope is approximately 160 cm in length and enables visualization of the entire colonic mucosal surface in more than 90% of examinations. Concurrent biopsy and polypectomy are possible.

   a. **Indications.** Colonoscopy is indicated for:

   (1) The initial treatment of patients with adenomas detected by flexible fiberoptic sigmoidoscopy. All polyps are removed to eliminate neoplastic tissue and identify foci of malignancy.

   (2) The preoperative evaluation of patients with known colorectal cancer. Synchronous cancers have been found in 7% of these patients and synchronous polyps in 29%.

   (3) Evaluation of a positive fecal occult blood test

   (4) Follow-up in patients with inflammatory bowel disease to determine disease activity and rule out malignancy

   b. **Bowel preparation.** A complete bowel preparation is required. Patients are permitted nothing to eat or drink for 8 hours prior to the procedure. Although the specific bowel preparation may vary from physician to physician, all preparations include oral cathartics and a clear liquid diet as well as enemas prior to the procedure.

   (1) One liter of 10% mannitol may be given orally over 1 hour on the morning of the examination preceded by a clear liquid diet the evening before. Mannitol provides an osmotic purging of the colon.

   (2) Alternatively, 1 gal of polyethylene glycol (Golytely) is ingested (i.e., 8 oz every 10 minutes until complete) the night before the procedure.

    c. Complications. Bleeding and perforation are the commonest complications but occur in less than 2% of cases.

E. Fecal occult blood is obtained by placing stool on guaiac paper, which contains a compound that is oxidized when a peroxide-containing developer solution is added to it, resulting in a blue color change. The reaction is catalyzed by peroxidase and pseudoperoxidase (including hemoglobin).

    1. Antioxidants, such as vitamin C, can block pseudoperoxidase activity. Red meat and peroxidase-containing vegetables (i.e., turnips, radishes, and tomatoes), as well as iron, may result in a false-positive test.

    2. Normal gastrointestinal blood loss varies from 0.5–2 ml a day. Approximately 20 ml of bleeding daily is required for a consistently positive fecal occult blood test, using standard technique.

    3. If a properly performed fecal occult blood test is positive, a diagnostic evaluation of the entire colon is indicated.

F. Bowel preparation for elective colon and rectal surgery will vary from physician to physician; however, all physicians should combine a low-residue diet with mechanical and antibiotic bowel preparation.

    1. The low-residue diet is begun 2 days prior to surgery and is followed by mechanical preparation.

    2. Oral antibiotic therapy, using a neomycin and erythromycin base, is begun 1 day prior to surgery.

    3. A single dose of intravenous broad-spectrum antibiotic is given on call to surgery.

    4. The greatest disagreement concerns the use of postoperative antibiotics. At least one dose of postoperative antibiotics is required.

III. CONSTIPATION. The magnitude of this problem, particularly in women and the elderly, is great.

A. Definition. The meaning of the term constipation varies from patient to patient. It is used to describe hard stools, stools that are difficult to evacuate, or incomplete evacuation. The term should be applied to define stool frequency only. Constipation is considered less than three bowel movements a week.

B. Etiology. Frequent causes of constipation include:

    1. A poor diet that is low in fiber in combination with decreased fluid intake and physical inactivity and a failure to acknowledge the urge to defecate (the most frequent cause)

    2. Abnormal motility, such as irritable bowel syndrome or slow transit

    3. Anatomic disorders, such as anal fissure, rectal prolaspe, rectocele, or stricture

    4. Drugs, such as antidepressants, narcotics, or iron

    5. Neurologic disorders, such as Hirschsprung's disease, spinal cord injury, multiple sclerosis, diabetes mellitus, or scleroderma

    6. Endocrine and metabolic disorders, such as hypothyroidism, pregnancy, or premenstrual syndrome

C. Diagnosis is based on the following:

    1. History

    2. Physical examination

    3. Barium enema

    4. Anorectal manometry

    5. Transit studies, such as ingestion of radiopaque pellets followed by serial abdominal films

    6. Laboratory studies

D. Treatment

1. Most patients can be managed with dietary modification, counseling regarding activity, and laxatives, enemas, or suppositories.

2. Persistent symptoms despite conservative treatment require further evaluation.

3. With the exception of Hirschsprung's disease (see Chapter 29 VIII), the surgical indications for treatment of constipation are not clearly defined. Subtotal colectomy with ileorectal anastomosis has been used to treat chronic and intractable constipation with good results.

IV. DIARRHEA. Excessive loose stools may be due to a number of causes, including infection, inflammation, or metabolic, neural, gastric, pharmacologic, and motility disorders.

A. Diagnosis is based on the following:

1. History, including recent travel as well as antibiotic therapy

2. Physical examination

3. Laboratory studies, including stool for routine culture, ova, parasites, *Campylobacter, Yersinia, Clostridium difficile,* viral culture, and white and red blood cells

4. Endoscopy (and biopsy when indicated)

B. Types

1. **Noninfectious diarrhea** may result from neutropenic enterocolitis (e.g., ileocecal syndrome and typhilitis), bowel wall necrosis associated with the treatment of hematologic disorders, and severe neutropenia. Symptoms include diarrhea, abdominal pain, and sepsis.

2. **Infectious diarrhea.** Colonic involvement results in diarrhea, pain, and tenesmus. Episodic diarrhea is most commonly caused by the ingestion of fecally contaminated foods. *Escherichia coli* is the commonest cause.

3. **Antibiotic-associated diarrhea** (pseudomembranous colitis) is a potentially lethal illness. Although clindamycin, tetracycline, and ampicillin are the most frequent antibiotics implicated, almost all antibiotics have been associated with this condition.
   a. **Clinical presentation.** Bloody diarrhea and abdominal pain may begin up to 6 weeks after antibiotic therapy.
   b. **Diagnosis.** A stool culture reveals *C. difficile* toxin. Proctosigmoidoscopy and biopsy reveal whitish raised plaques and pseudomembranes.
   c. **Treatment.** Offending antibiotics are discontinued. Oral vancomycin, or alternatively oral metronidazole, is the treatment of choice.

V. INCONTINENCE is the inability to control the passage of stool or flatus.

A. Etiology

1. Aging

2. Obstetric injury

3. Iatrogenic causes, such as previous anorectal surgery

4. Trauma

5. Neurologic disorders

6. Rectal prolapse

7. Overflow secondary to fecal impaction

B. Diagnosis is based on the following:

1. History

2. Anorectal examination

3. Anorectal manometry

4. Electromyography (EMG)

C. Treatment is directed toward the specific etiology.

　1. Nonoperative treatment includes biofeedback as well as measures that will improve the consistency of the stool.

　2. Operative treatment includes:
　　a. Overlap sphincteroplasty and Park's postanal repair
　　b. Gracilis muscle transposition, which is reserved for the unusual situation in which the bulk of the patient's sphincter mechanism has been destroyed
　　c. Colostomy, which is used as a last option

VI. ANORECTAL DISEASE. Ninety percent of all anorectal surgical procedures can be performed under local anesthesia combined with intravenous sedation.

　A. Anal fissures are linear tears (ulcers) commencing at or just below the dentate (pectinate) line and extending distally to the anal verge. In 90% of cases, they are located in the posterior midline.

　　1. Nonoperative treatment includes sitz baths, suppositories, and fiber supplements.

　　2. Operative treatment is lateral partial internal sphincterotomy. Indications for operative management include persistent pain, lack of healing, and recurrence.

　B. Hemorrhoids. Tissue commonly referred to as hemorrhoids is formed by three radially oriented arteriovenous tufts. There is an internal component covered by mucosa and an external component covered by skin.

　　1. Internal hemorrhoids. Although the normal location is within the anal canal, these can present with bleeding and prolapse.
　　　a. Classification. Internal hemorrhoids are classified into four categories.
　　　　(1) First-degree hemorrhoids. Prominent internal hemorrhoidal tissue
　　　　(2) Second-degree hemorrhoids. Internal hemorrhoidal prolapse, which reduces spontaneously
　　　　(3) Third-degree hemorrhoids. Internal hemorrhoidal prolapse, which requires manual reduction
　　　　(4) Fourth-degree hemorrhoids. Incarcerated internal hemorrhoidal prolapse
　　　b. Treatment
　　　　(1) Sclerotherapy is used in the treatment of first-degree and second-degree internal hemorrhoids with symptoms of bleeding or prolapse.
　　　　(2) Rubber band ligation is used in the treatment of first-degree, second-degree, and third-degree internal hemorrhoids presenting with bleeding or prolapse.
　　　　(3) Operative excision is used in the treatment of third-degree and fourth-degree hemorrhoids presenting with prolapse.

　　2. External hemorrhoids are covered by perianal skin. These often present with painful thrombosis.
　　　a. Nonoperative treatment of external hemorrhoidal thrombosis. It can be anticipated that in 1–3 weeks there will be resolution of the clot and associated symptoms.
　　　b. Operative treatment. Pain, bleeding, and the desire to avoid perianal skin tags are indications for operative excision.

　C. Anorectal fistulous abscess

　　1. Etiology. Most anorectal fistulous abscesses are cryptoglandular in origin. Almost all originate posteriorly in the region of maximum density of the anorectal gland.

　　2. Treatment
　　　a. All anorectal abscesses require prompt drainage at the time of diagnosis. Delay in treatment (to allow time for "pointing") results in further destruction of normal tissue and possibly incontinence.
　　　b. Even chronic asymptomatic fistulas require operative treatment. Two-thirds of all anorectal abscesses treated by simple incision and drainage will recur as fistula in ano. One-third will be cured.

VII. POLYPS

A. Types

1. **Pedunculated** polyps are suspended from the bowel wall via a stalk.

2. **Sessile** polyps have a broad base with no definitive stalk.

B. Classification

1. **Inflammatory polyps.** These polyps are outgrowths of mucosa in response to active inflammation; thus, they are referred to as pseudopolyps. They are non-neoplastic.

2. **Hyperplastic polyps.** These polyps are small tumors of no clinical significance, which are most commonly seen in the rectum of as many as 50% of adult colons, making them the commonest polyp among adults. They are non-neoplastic.

3. **Hamartomatous polyps.** These polyps are comprised of normal tissue in an abnormal configuration. Juvenile polyps are the commonest type of hamartomatous colonic polyps. They are non-neoplastic.

4. **Adenomatous polyps.** Only adenomatous polyps have **certain malignant potential,** which is related to size (Table 13-1) and type of polyp.
   a. **Tubular adenomas.** These are characterized by a smooth firm surface and pink color.
   b. **Villous adenomas.** These are characterized by multiple frond-like projections from their surface. They are soft and sessile. Although usually asymptomatic, they may present with watery diarrhea and hypokalemia. Because of their markedly increased cellularity, they have a higher incidence of malignant change than tubular adenomas.
   c. **Tubulovillous adenomas.** Both tubular and villous components prevail.

C. Malignant transformation.
Approximately 95% of all colorectal cancers arise from polyps. The polyp to cancer sequence takes 5–15 years.

D. Treatment

1. Polyps can be removed nonoperatively, using an endoscopic polypectomy.

2. Polyps not amenable to endoscopic removal because of size, configuration, or malignancy are removed operatively.

3. Certain malignant polyps can be definitively treated with endoscopic polypectomy; however, these polyps must have the following characteristics:
   a. They must be pedunculated.
   b. The carcinoma must be limited to the head of the polyp.
   c. There must be no venous or lymphatic invasion.
   d. They must not be poorly differentiated.

E. Polyposis syndromes

1. **Familial polyposis** is an autosomal dominant disorder characterized by greater than 100 adenomatous polyps of the colon and rectum. Approximately 50% of the children of affected parents have this disorder, and only individuals with polyps transmit the disease. Left untreated, the disease is uniformly fatal with carcinoma developing in 100% of affected patients by the fifth decade.
   a. **Clinical presentation**
      (1) Polyps usually present by early adult life.
      (2) Approximately 20% of cases are sporadic.

Table 13-1. Malignant Potential of Adenomatous Polyps

Polyp Size	Incidence of Malignancy
<1 cm	1%
1–2 cm	10%
>2 cm	30%–40%

(3) Although it has been theorized that polyps exist for at least a decade before causing symptoms, the commonest complaints are bleeding, diarrhea, and abdominal pain.

b. **Diagnosis** is confirmed by proctosigmoidoscopy and biopsy. Once the disorder has been diagnosed in one family member, examination of the entire family is indicated.

c. **Treatment** is operative and directed towards eradicating the polyps. Surgical options include:
   (1) Proctocolectomy with distal rectal mucosectomy and ileal pouch–anal anastomosis
   (2) Subtotal colectomy and ileorectal anastomosis with eradication (fulguration) of rectal polyps and continued rectal surveillance
   (3) Panproctocolectomy and ileostomy

2. **Gardner's syndrome** is a variant of familial polyposis. It is transmitted by an autosomal dominant gene with varying penetrance.

   a. **Clinical presentation**
      (1) Gardner's syndrome is characterized by colorectal polyposis. Polyps are frequently present in the small bowel (gastric polyps, 70%; duodenal polyps, nearly 100%).
      (2) Additional features include:
         (a) Osteomata (usually mandible and skull)
         (b) Cysts
         (c) Soft tissue tumors
         (d) Desmoid tumors of the abdominal wall and mesentery
         (e) Dental abnormalities
         (f) Periampullary carcinoma
         (g) Thyroid cancer

   b. **Treatment** is operative as described for the familial polyposis syndrome (see VII E 1 c) with additional surveillance of the upper gastrointestinal tract and management of extraintestinal manifestations if they occur independently.

3. **Peutz-Jeghers syndrome** is an autosomal dominant disorder.

   a. **Clinical presentation**
      (1) Hamartomatous polyps appear throughout the gastrointestinal tract.
      (2) Cutaneous pigmentation appears on the buccal mucosa, lips, and digits.
      (3) Presenting symptoms may be those of intussusception, including colicky abdominal pain.

   b. **Treatment** is designed to remove symptomatic polyps, minimizing intestinal resection.

4. **Turcot syndrome** is familial polyposis in association with malignant tumors of the central nervous system.

VIII. BENIGN AND MALIGNANT NEOPLASMS OF THE COLON AND RECTUM

A. Carcinoma of the colon and rectum

1. **Incidence and distribution**
   a. Carcinoma of the colon and rectum is the commonest visceral cancer in the United States. The peak incidence is in the seventh decade of life.
   b. Over 60% of colorectal cancers are located in the distal colon. There has been a recent trend towards a more proximal distribution.

2. **Etiology.** The cause is unknown.

3. **Risk factors**
   a. Genetic: Family cancer syndrome
   b. Environmental: Low-fiber, high-fat diet
   c. Inflammatory bowel disease
   d. Polyposis syndromes
   e. Personal history of colon polyps or colon cancer

4. **Classification**
   a. Adenocarcinoma is the predominant type of cancer.
   b. Squamous cell carcinoma is rare.
   c. Adenosquamous carcinoma is rare.

5. **Clinical presentation** depends upon the location of the tumor, size of the tumor, and metastatic disease.
    a. **Right-sided lesions** often present with anemia from slow chronic blood loss. Although pain and mass may be present, the large diameter of the right colon and the liquid nature of the stool make obstruction a late occurrence.
    b. **Left-sided lesions** are more likely to present with obstruction, which is described by the patient as a change in bowel habits. A small bowel lumen, a solid stool, and frequent occurrence of annular lesions contribute to this presentation.

6. **Workup of the patient** comprises the following:
    a. Barium enema
    b. Endoscopy with biopsy
        (1) Proctosigmoidoscopy
        (2) Colonoscopy
    c. Computed tomography (CT scan), intravenous pyelogram (IVP), SMA-12 (for enzymes), endorectal ultrasound (for rectal cancer), and flat plate and upright abdominal x-rays (when obstruction is suspected)

7. **Staging.** The most widely accepted pathologic staging system is the Astler-Coller modification of Duke's classification.
    a. **Stage A:** Confined to the mucosa
    b. **Stage B₁:** Extension into but not through the muscularis propria but no nodal involvement
    c. **Stage B₂:** Extension through the muscularis propria but no nodal involvement
    d. **Stage C₁:** Extension into but not through the muscularis propria with positive nodal involvement
    e. **Stage C₂:** Extension through the muscularis propria with positive nodal involvement
    f. **Stage D:** Metastatic disease

8. **Treatment.** Operative therapy is the preferred treatment for colorectal cancer. Resection involves the removal of the diseased bowel, encompassing the lymphovascular pedicle to the corresponding segment of bowel. Historically, a 5-cm margin of distal rectum beyond the cancer was thought to be essential for an adequate resection, but it has been determined that a 2-cm distal margin is adequate. This fact along with newer surgical techniques (e.g., the availability of surgical stapling devices) has allowed low rectal lesions to be treated by resection and anastomosis, avoiding a permanent colostomy without compromising survival.
    a. **Operative procedures—rectal cancer**
        (1) **Upper-third lesions.** Low anterior resection
        (2) **Middle-third lesions.** With the presently available techniques and instrumentation, almost all middle-third rectal lesions can be treated definitively by low anterior resection.
        (3) **Lower-third lesions.** Several surgical options exist.
            (a) Miles' resection is the traditional treatment of choice.
            (b) Sphincter-saving operations, including:
                (i) Low anterior resection
                (ii) Pull-through procedures
                (iii) Local treatment (for select favorable low rectal cancers), including fulguration, local excision, and contact radiotherapy
    b. **Adjuvant therapy**
        (1) The role of radiotherapy for colorectal cancer is evolving. Presently, both pre- and postoperative radiotherapy are being evaluated in the treatment of both colon and rectal cancer (particularly rectal cancer) to determine the effect on survival as well as local recurrence.
        (2) The role of chemotherapy has not been clearly defined.

9. **Prognosis** is related to the Astler-Coller stage, specifically the depth of bowel wall invasion and lymph node involvement.

10. **Recurrent disease**
    a. Determination of **carcinoembryonic antigen (CEA) levels** has become an accepted means of screening for the recurrence of colorectal cancer. CEA levels are followed serially every 3 months for the first 2 years postoperatively. A persistent rise in the CEA level warrants a metastatic workup.
    b. Recurrence of colorectal cancer is often painful, debilitating, and difficult to treat.
        (1) Surgery can provide palliation and relieve obstruction.

(2) Chemotherapy is of indeterminate value.

(3) Radiation therapy is palliative.

(4) Hepatic resection for isolated liver metastasis has been associated with a 25% 5-year survival.

(5) Pulmonary resection for isolated pulmonary metastasis has been associated with a 20% 5-year survival.

B. Carcinoid tumors

1. Overview. Carcinoid tumors of the colon are rare (2% of all gastrointestinal carcinoids). They are most commonly found in the appendix, followed by the small bowel and rectum.

a. The malignant potential of carcinoid tumors is related to their size.

(1) Tumors less than 1 cm in size have a 1% chance of malignancy.

(2) Tumors between 1 and 2 cm in size have a 10% chance of malignancy.

(3) Tumors greater than 2 cm in size have an 80% chance of malignancy.

b. Midgut carcinoid tumors (mid-duodenum to midtransverse colon) are:

(1) Argyrophil- and argentaffin-positive

(2) Frequently multicentric

(3) Associated with the carcinoid syndrome

c. Hindgut carcinoid tumors are:

(1) Rarely argyrophil- or argentaffin-positive

(2) Unicentric

(3) Not associated with the carcinoid syndrome

d. Patients with carcinoid tumors have an increased incidence of gastrointestinal adenocarcinoma.

2. Treatment. Local excision is the treatment of choice except in demonstrably invasive or large (greater than 2 cm) carcinoids where a traditional cancer operation is indicated.

C. Tumors of the appendix

1. Carcinoid (see VIII B)

2. Adenocarcinoma

3. Mucocele. Perforation or contamination during resection can result in the unusual disease, **pseudomyxoma peritonei**. This disease is characterized by accumulation of large amounts of mucus within the abdomen. It is also associated with neoplasms of the ovary.

D. Other neoplasms (benign and malignant) are rare and are named for their tissue of origin.

1. Lymphoid (lymphoma and lymphosarcoma)

2. Adipose (lipoma and liposarcoma)

3. Muscle (leiomyoma and leiomyosarcoma)

IX. NEOPLASMS OF THE ANAL CANAL AND ANAL MARGIN

A. Anal margin (below the dentate line) [Table 13-2]

1. Squamous cell carcinoma

2. Basal cell carcinoma

3. Perianal Paget's disease

4. Bowen's disease

B. Anal canal (above the dentate line)

1. Histology

a. Squamous cell carcinoma (epidermoid carcinoma)

b. Mucoepidermoid carcinoma

c. Cloacogenic (transitional cell) carcinoma

d. Adenocarcinoma

Table 13-2. Anal Margin Neoplasms

Location	Presentation	Treatment
Squamous cell carcinoma	Central ulcerating lesion, bleeding, itching, or mass	Local excision or radiotherapy; abdominal perineal resection (for extensive lesions)
Basal cell carcinoma	Central ulceration, mild discomfort, or bleeding	Local excision or radiotherapy
Paget's disease	Erythematous, scaly plaques and incessant itching; 85% of cases develop a visceral cancer	Wide local excision; may consider abdominal perineal resection or multimodality therapy for more advanced lesions
Bowen's disease	Chronic dermatosis; erythematous, crusty plaques; itching; burning; or bleeding. Squamous cell cancer will develop in 10% of lesions; 70%–80% of patients will develop other malignancies in life	Wide local excision

      (1) Rectal origin
      (2) Anal gland origin
    e. Malignant melanoma
2. **Clinical presentation.** Bleeding, pain, mucus discharge, mass, or itching. Malignant melanoma may be completely asymptomatic, appearing as a dark pigmented hemorrhoid-type lesion, or it may present as a large fungating, ulcerating mass.

3. **Diagnosis** is based on the following:
    a. History
    b. Anorectal examination, including biopsy

4. **Treatment.** With the exception of small, superficial, squamous cell carcinoma of the anal canal treated with wide local excision, the traditional treatment of all malignant neoplasms of the anal canal was abdominal perineal resection (Miles' resection). Recently, several alternatives to the classic treatment have been used with encouraging results. These include:
    a. External beam radiotherapy
    b. Interstitial radiotherapy
    c. Combined multimodality therapy (radiotherapy and chemotherapy) [**Nigro protocol**]. At this time, first line treatment for carcinoma of the anal canal (e.g., squamous cell carcinoma, cloacogenic carcinoma, and mucoepidermoid carcinoma) is combined multimodality therapy. With regard to malignant melanoma—although early diagnosis and Miles' resection represent the only chance for cure, the survival rates after Miles' resection and local excision have been similar, making local excision a consideration in many cases.

X. INFLAMMATORY BOWEL DISEASE

  A. Crohn's colitis (see Chapter 12 II B)

    1. **Clinical presentation.** The major diagnostic consideration is the differentiation of Crohn's colitis (granulomatous colitis) from ulcerative colitis. Among the characteristics of Crohn's colitis that distinguish it from ulcerative colitis are:
      a. Transmural involvement
      b. Skip areas of normal mucosa
      c. Higher incidence of fistulas
      d. Perianal disease
      e. A greater likelihood of proximal colonic involvement
      f. Less frequent bleeding

2. Treatment
  a. Medical treatment
   (1) Sulfasalazine, systemic or local (enema)
   (2) Steroids, systemic or local (enema)
   (3) Metronidazole for the treatment of perianal disease
  b. Operative treatment. Surgical options include:
   (1) Panproctocolectomy and ileostomy
   (2) Subtotal colectomy and ileoproctostomy
   (3) Segmental resection (reserved for isolated ileocolic disease)

B. Ulcerative colitis is an uncommon inflammatory disorder involving the mucosa of the large bowel.

1. Incidence
  a. In the United States, the incidence is higher among Jews than non-Jews.
  b. Women are affected slightly more frequently than men.
  c. There is a bimodal incidence between 15 and 30 years of age and then again between 50 and 80 years of age.

2. Etiology is unknown. Infectious, immunologic, genetic, and environmental causes have been implicated.

3. Histology
  a. The disease begins at the dentate line and extends proximally. When the rectum alone is involved, the disorder is called ulcerative proctitis. Extension is continuous with no skip areas of normal bowel.
  b. Unlike Crohn's disease, only the mucosa and submucosa are involved.
  c. Pseudopolyps (inflammatory polyps) are seen.

4. Clinical presentation
  a. The onset may be acute or insidious.
  b. The patient commonly presents with watery diarrhea mixed with blood, pus, and mucus and accompanied by tenesmus and urgency.
  c. Pain, fever, weight loss, and dehydration occur to varying degrees.
  d. Extraintestinal manifestations include: arthritis, spondylitis, ocular lesions (episcleritis and uveitis), oral lesions, hepatobiliary disease (cholangitis, cirrhosis, and cholelithiasis), cutaneous lesions (pyoderma gangrenosum, erythema nodosum, and polyarteritis nodosum).

5. Diagnosis
  a. Physical examination. Depending on the acuteness and severity of the presentation, findings range from a normal abdominal examination to peritoneal signs.
  b. Endoscopy with biopsy is contraindicated if toxic megacolon is present.
   (1) Mild colitis presents as mucosal granularity.
   (2) Moderate colitis presents as mucosal contact friability, ulcers, and mucus exudate.
   (3) Severe colitis presents as spontaneous mucosal bleeding, extensive ulceration, and pseudopolyps.
  c. Barium enema
   (1) Barium enema may reveal mucosal irregularity, colonic shortening, and loss of haustration (long-standing disease).
   (2) Barium enema is contraindicated in the presence of toxic megacolon.
  d. Laboratory findings. Anemia and leukocytosis are present to varying degrees.
  e. Differential diagnosis
   (1) Ulcerative colitis must be differentiated from other inflammatory or infectious disorders of the colon, particularly Crohn's disease.
   (2) Malignancy and diverticular disease may also mimic ulcerative colitis.

6. Complications
  a. Toxic megacolon is present in 3%–5% of cases. The transverse colon exceeds 6 cm in diameter. This condition, which is associated with severe prostration, can be fatal.
  b. Colonic perforation is seen in 3% of cases and is often fatal.
  c. Hemorrhage
  d. Colon cancer. There is an increased risk of colon cancer in patients with pancolitis (disease extending to the hepatic flexure) for more than 10 years. The risk increases by 2%–3% a year after 10 years of continuous pancolitis.

> **(1)** Colon cancer associated with ulcerative colitis is more frequently multicentric and poorly differentiated than colon cancer not associated with this disease.
> **(2)** Routine colonoscopic surveillance with disparate mucosal biopsies, looking for dysplasia, is mandatory in patients with long-standing pancolitis.
> **(3)** Colonic carcinoma may be difficult to diagnose in patients with ulcerative colitis because of chronic bleeding, mucus diarrhea, and mucosal abnormalities.

7. Treatment
   a. Medical treatment is the mainstay for uncomplicated disease, using the following:
   (1) Sulfasalazine, systemic or local (enemas)
   (2) Steroids, systemic or local (enemas)
   b. Operative treatment is indicated for failures of medical management; complications, such as hemorrhage, perforation, obstruction, or colon cancer; and in long-standing pancolitis where mucosal biopsies confirm dysplasia. Surgical options include:
   (1) Panproctocolectomy with permanent ileostomy
   (2) Subtotal colectomy with ileoproctostomy and lifelong surveillance of the rectum
   (3) Proctocolectomy with distal rectal mucosectomy and ileal pouch–anal anastomosis. This procedure is never performed in an emergency setting.

XI. ISCHEMIC COLITIS

A. Clinical presentation

1. Individuals with ischemic colitis are usually elderly and have complicating medical problems.

2. The onset is usually characterized by acute abdominal pain followed by bloody bowel movements. The clinical presentation depends on the extent, duration, and location of the vascular occlusion.

3. Proctosigmoidoscopic examination almost always reveals rectal sparing.

B. Classification

1. **Transient ischemia**
   a. The affected area of bowel receives vascular compensation from the collateral circulation, and associated symptoms are mild.
   b. Barium enema may reveal "thumbprinting."
   c. Ischemia results in mucosal sloughing, followed by regeneration.

2. **Ischemic stricture** is due to a more prolonged impairment of blood flow.
   a. Symptoms regress slowly.
   b. "Thumbprinting" as well as stricture may be seen on barium enema.
   c. Secondary invasion by intestinal bacteria induce an inflammatory cycle that ends in healing fibrosis.

3. **Gangrene**
   a. Symptoms progress rapidly to peritonitis and septic shock.
   b. Barium enema is contraindicated.
   c. Perforation and gangrene are grave complications, warranting immediate operative intervention.

C. Treatment

1. Antibiotics, bowel rest, and intravenous hydration should be administered initially.

2. Strictures, if symptomatic, can be resected electively.

3. Gangrene and perforation are treated by resection of the involved segment.

XII. DIVERTICULAR DISEASE

A. Incidence. Approximately 50% of adults in this country have diverticular disease by 60 years of age.

B. Pathogenesis. Presumably, the generation of high intercolonic pressure precipitates mucosal protrusion through the circular muscle coat of the bowel wall at points of weakness. The points of weakness occur on the antimesenteric wall between tenia where blood vessels perforate the bowel wall. By the law of LaPlace, the pressure generated within the bowel lumen is greatest in the sigmoid colon where the lumen is narrowest. For this reason, diverticula are most commonly seen in the sigmoid colon. Their proximity to blood vessels explains their propensity for bleeding. Diverticular disease is not seen in the rectum.

C. Etiology. A diet low in fiber appears to be a cause.

D. Histology. The diverticula are comprised of mucosa and serosa (these are pulsion diverticula, not true diverticula).

E. Clinical presentation. Most patients with diverticular disease are asymptomatic. Diverticulitis manifests as fever and abdominal pain. Urinary symptoms often occur.

F. Diagnosis

1. Contrast enema. Traditionally, the barium enema has been the most valuable diagnostic study for evaluating patients with diverticular disease in both the acute and chronic setting. In the acute setting, a water-soluble contrast enema (Gastrografin) is used (see II C 2).

2. CT scan is used in the acute setting to evaluate the colonic wall and pericolonic tissue planes and for guided drainage of intra-abdominal abscesses. CT scan is presently being evaluated for its superiority over barium enema in the acute setting.

3. Endoscopy is an invaluable tool for confirming the diagnosis of diverticular disease and for evaluating strictures and bleeding in nonacute cases.

4. Cystoscopy/cystogram is used for evaluating colovesicle fistulas.

5. IVP is obtained preoperatively to determine the position and possible involvement of the ureters.

6. Leukocyte count is obtained serially during an acute attack.

7. Differential diagnosis
   a. Irritable bowel syndrome
   b. Carcinoma
   c. Crohn's disease

G. Complications

1. Hemorrhage (see Chapter 9 IV). Diverticular disease is second only to arteriovenous malformation as a cause of massive gastrointestinal bleeding of colonic origin.

2. Diverticulitis and its complications, including:
   a. Perforation
   b. Obstruction
   c. Stricture
   d. Fistulas of the bladder, bowel, uterus, or vagina

H. Treatment of diverticulitis

1. Nonoperative treatment
   a. Bowel rest with or without nasogastric suction, parenteral hydration, and broad-spectrum antibiotics are the mainstays of medical treatment. Substantial clinical improvement should occur within 24–48 hours.
   b. Abscesses can be localized and drained, using CT guidance.

2. Operative treatment. The need for urgent or emergency operative intervention is a matter of clinical judgment and is based on the severity of the patient's disease and the direction of the clinical course.
   a. Indications
      (1) In general, a rising temperature, worsening physical examination, or worsening or persistent leukocytosis, despite adequate medical management is an indication for operative intervention.

(2) Patients with recurrent attacks or patients whose first attack occurs before age 50 as well as those patients with complications of diverticulitis are best managed by operative therapy.

b. Operative procedures

(1) Elective resection with primary anastomosis is the preferred operative procedure. After an acute attack of diverticulitis, a 6–12 week waiting period is recommended before elective colon resection.

(2) Operative management of perforated diverticulitis should be individualized and includes:

(a) Sigmoid colon resection with primary anastomosis. This is the most effective treatment for localized diverticular abscess. A localized abscess does not preclude primary anastomosis if the ends of the bowel are free of disease and the patient is not immunosuppressed.

(b) Sigmoid colon resection with primary anastomosis and proximal diverting stoma

(c) Sigmoid colon resection with end colostomy and Hartmann's pouch. This is the operation of choice if there is any doubt that an anastomosis will not heal.

(i) The diseased bowel is removed, a proximal end-diverting colostomy is created, and the distal rectum is oversewn (Hartmann's pouch) or brought out to the skin as a mucous fistula.

(ii) Once the acute process has subsided, which usually takes several months, the patient returns for reconstitution of the bowel.

(d) Transverse colostomy and drainage alone. This staged procedure has been associated with a consistently high morbidity and mortality.

(3) Technical considerations include ureteral stent placement and preoperative marking of the stoma site.

XIII. RECTAL PROLAPSE is a rare condition in which the entire rectal wall prolapses to varying degrees through the anus.

A. Etiology. Rectal prolapse involves an intussusception of the rectosigmoid colon. Contributing anatomic defects include an elongated and redundant rectosigmoid colon, loss of support of the pelvic floor musculature, and loss of the normal curvature of the rectum along the anterior sacrum.

B. Diagnosis is by physical examination and cinedefecography.

C. Treatment

1. Although many different operative procedures have been described, the treatment of choice in the healthy, low-risk patient is high anterior resection (removing redundant sigmoid colon), posterior mobilization of the rectum to the levator ani muscles, and rectopexy.

2. In the high-risk patient who would not tolerate an abdominal procedure, perineal proctosigmoidectomy is the treatment of choice.

3. Other options include placement of a foreign body to narrow the anal orifice (i.e., Tiersch wire or Silastic sling).

XIV. VOLVULUS

A. Overview

1. Volvulus occurs when mobile segments of large bowel rotate on the mesenteric axis, causing luminal obstruction and varying degrees of vascular compromise.

2. This condition is seen most commonly in the sigmoid colon (90%), followed by the cecum (10%). It rarely occurs in the transverse colon.

B. Sigmoid volvulus

1. Pathogenesis. An elongated mobile sigmoid colon on a narrow mesenteric root is the classic setting. This anatomic state is often associated with chronic constipation, which can cause dilatation and lengthening of the sigmoid colon. Patients with neurologic disorders and elderly patients with prolonged periods of inactivity are at risk.

2. Clinical presentation. Symptoms are those of colonic obstruction, including abdominal pain and distention.

3. Diagnosis
  a. Plain x-rays of the abdomen may be diagnostic, revealing a markedly distended sigmoid loop.
  b. Contrast enemas show the typical "bird's beak" deformity.

4. Treatment
  a. Operative treatment
    (1) The treatment of choice is immediate decompression, followed by elective sigmoid resection.
      (a) Decompression is performed, using a rigid sigmoidoscope and placement of a rectal tube.
      (b) Elective resection is performed during the same hospitalization after a complete bowel preparation.
    (2) Emergency resection and end colostomy are performed if peritoneal signs suggest vascular compromise. Reconstitution can be carried out electively.
  b. Nonoperative treatment is associated with a high recurrence rate.

C. Cecal volvulus

  1. Pathogenesis. An abnormally mobile cecum and ascending colon, which are usually attached retroperitoneally, are prerequisites for cecal volvulus. Twisting is usually around the pedicle of the ileocolic artery, and thus, closed loop obstruction and ischemia occur early.

  2. Clinical presentation. Acute small bowel obstruction with peritoneal signs indicate vascular compromise.

  3. Diagnosis is based on the following:
    a. Plain abdominal films
    b. Barium enema

  4. Operative treatment is indicated. Delay in diagnosis and treatment of cecal volvulus contributes significantly to the mortality rate (approximately 10%).
    a. In the presence of vascular compromise, resection of the right colon with or without anastomosis (depending on the condition of the patient) is indicated.
    b. In the absence of vascular compromise, right hemicolectomy with ileotransverse colostomy or detorsion and fixation of the cecum to the lateral abdominal wall (cecopexy) are the most commonly performed procedures.

XV. MISCELLANEOUS COLONIC DISORDERS

A. Colonic ileus (intestinal pseudo-obstruction, Ogilvie's syndrome)

  1. Etiology. Although many factors are thought to be involved, the etiology is not completely understood. Although colonic ileus is often seen in association with underlying disease, this syndrome may be seen in the postoperative period following abdominal or orthopedic surgery.

  2. Diagnosis
    a. Plain abdominal x-rays reveal colonic distention (most marked proximally) out of proportion to small bowel distention.
    b. Differential diagnosis
      (1) Volvulus
      (2) Mechanical obstruction
      (3) Hirschsprung's disease
      (4) Toxic megacolon
      (5) Fecal impaction

  3. Treatment
    a. Nonoperative treatment entails the restoration of fluids and electrolytes, nasogastric suction, and colonoscopic decompression.
    b. Operative treatment is indicated for vascular compromise and failure of colonoscopic decompression. Cecostomy provides operative decompression.

B. Acute appendicitis is the commonest condition requiring acute abdominal surgery.

1. **Incidence.** The peak incidence of this disease is in the second and third decades of life. It is rare in very young children.

2. **Etiology**
   a. Obstruction of the lumen of the appendix is the principal cause.
      (1) Fecaliths (inspissated stool) are the commonest cause of the obstruction.
      (2) Less common causes include:
         (a) Lymphoid hypertrophy
         (b) Barium
         (c) Intestinal worms
         (d) Cecal cancer
   b. Persistent appendiceal mucosal secretions, gradual distention with inflammation of the appendix, bacterial overgrowth, and if the condition is allowed to progress, ischemia, gangrene, and perforation follow obstruction of the lumen.

3. **Diagnosis** is based on the history, physical examination, laboratory findings, and x-rays (when necessary).
   a. **History**
      (1) The classic history includes pain as the prime symptom.
         (a) The pain begins in the epigastrium, gradually moves to the periumbilical region, and finally over a period of 1–12 hours, localizes in the right lower quadrant.
         (b) This pain sequence may differ considerably from the above description, especially in light of the varied anatomic locations of the appendix (see I A 1).
      (2) Anorexia is a second prominent symptom and is nearly always present to some degree. Vomiting occurs in about three-fourths of the patients.
      (3) The sequence of symptoms is important in contributing to the diagnosis. Anorexia followed by pain and then by vomiting (when it occurs) is the classic course. Vomiting preceding pain should call the diagnosis into question.
   b. **Physical examination.** Physical findings depend primarily on the stage of the disease and the location of the appendix.
      (1) Temperature and pulse are only slightly elevated early in the disease. Higher elevations may indicate a complication, such as perforation or abscess.
      (2) Pain on palpation over McBurney's point (two-thirds of the distance from the umbilicus to the anterior iliac spine) is usually present when the appendix is located anteriorly. When it is located in the pelvis, abdominal findings may be minimal, and only rectal examination may yield significant findings.
      (3) Abdominal muscle guarding and rebound tenderness reflect the stage of the disease since progression is associated with peritoneal irritation.
      (4) Several signs, if present, assist in the diagnosis.
         (a) **Rovsing's sign** is pain in the right lower quadrant on palpation of the left lower quadrant.
         (b) **Psoas sign** is pain on extension of the right thigh with the patient lying on the left side.
         (c) **Obturator sign** is pain on internal rotation of the flexed right thigh with the patient supine.
   c. **Laboratory studies**
      (1) A moderate leukocytosis (10,000–16,000 white blood cells) with a predominance of neutrophils is usual. A normal white blood cell count does not rule out appendicitis, however.
      (2) Urinalysis may show a few red blood cells.
   d. **X-ray studies** are usually used only when the diagnosis is in question.
      (1) Plain abdominal films may show a localized right lower quadrant ileus or a radiopaque fecalith.
      (2) Barium enema may be helpful in difficult cases when an accurate diagnosis remains elusive. A filling defect in the cecum is the most reliable indicator of appendicitis with this study.
   e. **The differential diagnosis** for right lower quadrant pain includes:
      (1) Mesenteric lymphadenitis
      (2) Regional ileitis
      (3) Pelvic inflammatory disease

      (4) Gastroenteritis
      (5) Ruptured ovarian cyst (or other ovarian disorders)
      (6) Urinary tract disorders (infection, calculus)
      (7) Cecal or sigmoid diverticulitis

4. Treatment
  a. Appendectomy is the treatment of choice.
  b. Antibiotics are used in appendicitis
      (1) Preoperatively, broad-spectrum intravenous antibiotics are indicated to lessen the incidence of postoperative wound infection.
      (2) Postoperatively, antibiotics are continued for 24 hours for patients with uncomplicated appendicitis.
          (a) Antibiotics are usually continued for 5–7 days postoperatively for cases of appendiceal rupture with abscess formation.
          (b) Antibiotics are usually continued for 7–10 days for cases of appendiceal rupture with diffuse peritonitis.

5. Complications
  a. Clinical course
      (1) Left untreated, some cases of appendicitis proceed to perforation.
      (2) Following perforation, the contents of the abdominal cavity will attempt to contain the process, forming a phlegmon, an inflamed mass of matted intestine and omentum. A phlegmon may progress to a fibrous walling off of a collection of pus secondary to the rupture, and appendiceal abscess.
      (3) If the body's attempts to contain the perforation are unsuccessful, the entire abdominal cavity may become contaminated, causing a diffuse peritonitis.
      (4) Significant temperature and pulse elevation, marked leukocytosis, and findings typical of peritoneal inflammation, with or without a mass (phlegmon or abscess) in the right lower quadrant, indicate perforation. The mass may sometimes be appreciated only on rectal examination.
      (5) Appendiceal perforation significantly increases postoperative morbidity and mortality rates. The approach to acute appendicitis should be timely intervention to prevent progression to this complication.
  b. Abdominal ultrasonography may assist in the differential diagnosis of a right lower quadrant mass.
  c. Treatment of perforated appendicitis includes intravenous antibiotics and hydration, and surgical intervention including appendectomy and abscess drainage. The timing of such intervention is individualized to each patient.

14
Liver, Portal Hypertension, and Biliary Tract

Michael J. Moritz
Bruce E. Jarrell

I. LIVER

A. Anatomy. The liver is the largest, heaviest intra-abdominal organ, weighing about 2% of total body weight.

1. **Segmentation.** The liver is composed of two lobes (left and right), and each lobe has two segments (Figure 14-1).
   a. These lobes are divided by the **interlobar fissure,** an invisible line between the gall-bladder fossa anteriorly and the inferior vena cava posteriorly.
   b. The **falciform ligament,** the only externally visible boundary, marks the **segmental fissure** between the median and lateral segments of the left lobe.
   c. The right lobe segmental fissure has no external landmarks.

2. **Vascular supply (hepatic arterial and portal venous).** The segmental anatomy of the liver is determined by the vascular supply and biliary tree.
   a. **Arterial supply** is from the common **hepatic artery,** a branch of the celiac axis.
      (1) The hepatic artery carries fully oxygenated blood and comprises 25% of the liver blood flow.
      (2) The common hepatic artery enters the porta hepatis medially to the common bile duct, gives off the gastroduodenal artery to become the proper hepatic artery, and bifurcates into right and left hepatic arteries.
      (3) The **cystic artery** usually arises from the right hepatic artery.
      (4) In 25% of the population, the left hepatic artery arises from the left gastric artery. In approximately 20%, the right hepatic artery arises as a branch of the superior mesenteric artery.
   b. **Venous supply and return**
      (1) The **portal vein** carries partially oxygenated blood as it drains the entire splanchnic circulation (all structures that receive blood from the celiac, superior mesenteric, and inferior mesenteric arteries) and comprises 75% of the liver blood flow.
         (a) It is formed by the confluence of the superior mesenteric, splenic, inferior mesenteric, and coronary veins (Figure 14-2).
         (b) It enters the liver hilum, where it divides to form **right** and **left branches,** which supply the right and left hepatic lobes.
         (c) It lies posteriorly in the porta hepatis.
      (2) Blood leaves the liver via the hepatic veins.
         (a) The hepatic veins course **between segments** (rather than into segments like the segmental vascular supply). For example, the middle hepatic vein lies between the right and left hepatic lobes and is exposed when opening the interlobar fissure (Figure 14-3).
         (b) The hepatic veins drain directly into the inferior vena cava just inferior to the diaphragm.
   c. **The biliary tree** follows the segmental divisions of the hepatic artery and portal vein intrahepatically. The bile ducts lie anterolaterally in the porta hepatis.

3. **Hepatic resections** are based upon the segmental anatomy. The surgeon divides the vascular–biliary supply to the portion to be removed and preserves the vascular–biliary structures to the portion to be retained.
   a. **Right hepatic lobectomy** transects the liver through the interlobar fissure between the gallbladder fossa and the inferior vena cava (see Figure 14-3).

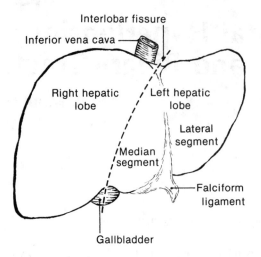

Figure 14-1. Surgical anatomy of the liver: left and right lobes.

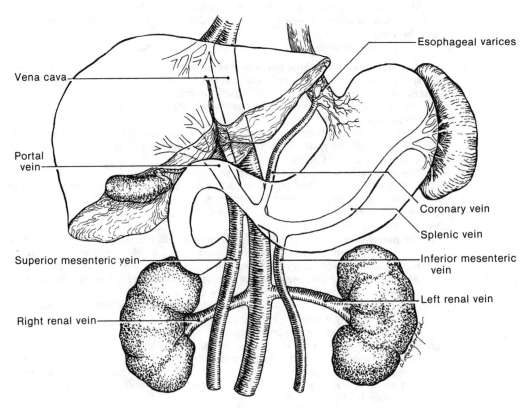

Figure 14-2. Portal circulation.

b. **Left hepatic lobectomy** uses the same guidelines.

c. **Trisegmentectomy** removes the entire right lobe and the median segment of the left lobe across the anatomic division of the falciform ligament (leaving only the left lateral segment).

d. **Left lateral segmentectomy** removes the segment of liver to the left of the falciform ligament.

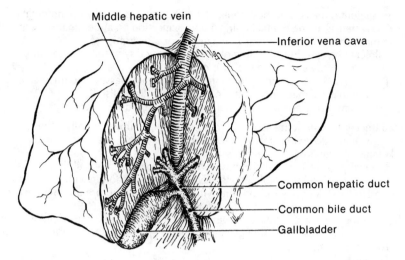

Figure 14-3. Plane of resection for right and left hepatic lobectomy.

  e. Wedge resections are performed for small lesions near the liver surface that do not require a full lobectomy. These resections do not adhere to anatomic boundaries but are safe because a limited amount of tissue is transected.

B. Studies of the liver

  1. Liver function tests are blood tests of a few of the myriad of functions that the liver performs.
    a. Synthetic function of hepatocytes is reflected by:
      (1) Serum proteins, such as albumin or fibrinogen
      (2) Clotting factors, as measured by coagulation tests (see Chapter 1 IV)
      (3) Cholesterol
      (4) Blood glucose
    b. Clearance function of hepatocytes is estimated by:
      (1) Ammonia
      (2) Indirect bilirubin, which is taken up from the blood by hepatocytes
    c. Excretory function of hepatocytes and patency of the biliary tree is reflected by:
      (1) Direct bilirubin
      (2) Enzyme levels, such as alkaline phosphatase and gamma glutamyl transferase
    d. Extent of injury to the hepatocytes is reflected by the serum levels of the enzymes, aspartate transaminase (AST), also called glutamic oxalacetic transaminase (GOT), and alanine transaminase (ALT), also called glutamic pyruvic transaminase (GPT).

  2. Imaging of the liver is used to define parenchymal lesions and plan liver resections when appropriate.
    a. The sulfur-colloid **liver–spleen scan,** which visualizes the reticuloendothelial system, is rarely used as more accurate studies are now available.
    b. Ultrasound is excellent for detecting the texture of the parenchyma and any lesions within the parenchyma.
    c. Computed tomography (CT) and **magnetic resonance imaging (MRI)** visualize the parenchyma and adjacent tissues with great clarity.
    d. Arteriography is used to determine the arterial supply and can detect large parenchymal lesions.
    e. Hepatobiliary scanning is a nuclear medicine scan used to visualize the liver and biliary tree (see III B 6).

  3. Needle biopsy (either percutaneous or at surgery) provides liver tissue for histologic study.

C. Benign tumors of the liver. In women, oral contraceptive use has increased the incidence of benign primary liver tumors.

1. **Hemangioma,** the commonest benign hepatic tumor, is usually asymptomatic. Usually, it is discovered as an incidental finding (i.e., calcification on abdominal x-ray or a characteristic mass on ultrasound) and is managed by observation.
   a. **Clinical presentation.** Hemangiomas can produce symptoms by compressing adjacent structures or by stretching the liver capsule.
   b. **Pathology.** Grossly, there may be single or multiple masses, and microscopically, there are vascular lacunae lined with normal endothelial cells.
   c. **Treatment.** Only symptomatic hemangiomas should be resected.

2. **Hepatocellular adenoma** is an uncommon benign tumor usually seen in women and strongly associated with oral contraceptive use. It is also found in men and women who take anabolic (androgenic) steroids.
   a. **Clinical presentation.** There may be no symptoms or physical findings.
      (1) Approximately 25% of patients have a palpable abdominal mass or abdominal pain.
      (2) Up to 30% of patients present with spontaneous rupture and hemorrhage into the peritoneal cavity. The mortality rate for rupture is about 9%.
   b. **Pathology.** Hepatocellular adenomas are soft tumors with sharply circumscribed edges but no true capsule. Histologically, normal hepatocytes are present, and there is no evidence of malignancy.
   c. **Diagnosis**
      (1) The tumor is usually suspected when a mass is seen on ultrasound or other scan of the liver.
      (2) Angiography is useful because hypervascularity or arterial splaying is frequently present.
      (3) Liver function studies are generally normal.
      (4) Biopsy is needed to exclude malignancy.
   d. **Treatment**
      (1) Oral contraceptives, anabolic steroids, and pregnancy should be avoided, and in the absence of these, the tumor frequently regresses. If the diagnosis is confirmed and the lesion is small, intrahepatic, and associated with oral contraceptive use, it may be safely observed.
      (2) Occasionally, the tumor is exophytic on a narrow pedicle and can be easily excised.
      (3) If the tumor is large and superficial or if a woman anticipates pregnancy in the near future, it should be resected because of the risk of spontaneous rupture and hemorrhage.
      (4) In cases of **spontaneous rupture with hemorrhage** into the peritoneal cavity, the patient should initially be resuscitated. Surgical intervention is indicated when cardiovascular stability is attained.
         (a) The recommended procedure is hepatic artery ligation. This frequently controls the bleeding and is associated with only minor aberrations in liver function when the liver is not cirrhotic.
         (b) Hepatic resection in the presence of acute rupture has a high mortality rate. Elective resection should, however, be performed at a later date.
         (c) If the patient is very unstable after rupture in spite of major resuscitative efforts, open packing or angiographic embolization of the hepatic artery may control the hemorrhage.

3. **Focal nodular hyperplasia** is the third commonest benign liver tumor. It occurs most often in women and has a weak association with oral contraceptive use.
   a. **Clinical presentation.** Symptoms and physical findings, when they occur, are similar to those seen with hepatocellular adenoma; however, focal nodular hyperplasia is usually asymptomatic and discovered as an incidental finding. Spontaneous rupture is rare.
   b. **Pathology.** Single or multiple lesions with a nodular appearance externally and a central scar with radiating septa on cut section are seen.
   c. **Histology.** The tumors are composed of hyperplastic hepatocytes with inflammatory cells. Bile duct epithelium is a prominent finding in contrast to hepatocellular adenoma. Overall, the lesions resemble regenerating nodules of cirrhosis.
   d. **Diagnosis and treatment** are similar to those for hepatocellular adenoma.

4. **Infantile hemangioendothelioma** is a benign liver tumor of children, which has malignant potential.
   a. **Clinical presentation.** It may present as hepatomegaly and high-output cardiac failure in an infant with a large arteriovenous fistula.

b. Pathology. Grossly, it is a nodular lesion, and microscopically, it shows dilated vascular spaces lined by endothelium.

c. Treatment is by excision or hepatic artery ligation.

D. Primary malignant tumors of the liver account for 0.7% of all cancers. In men, 90% of primary liver tumors are malignant; in women, only about 40% are malignant.

1. Hepatocellular carcinoma (hepatoma) is the commonest primary malignant liver tumor.

a. Incidence of hepatocellular carcinoma varies geographically, being highest in Africa and Asia and lowest in the Western world.

(1) Men are affected twice as often as women.

(2) The average age of affected individuals is 50 years, but hepatocellular carcinoma can occur at any age.

b. Associations. The tumor shows an association with a number of preexisting diseases and environmental substances, such as:

(1) Chronic hepatitis B virus (HBV) infection (present in as many as 80% of cases worldwide). The risk of developing hepatocellular carcinoma is increased 200-fold for chronic HBV carriers. The risk in male carriers is as high as 50%.

(2) Cirrhosis of the liver (present in approximately 60%–90% of patients), especially macronodular cirrhosis

(3) Hemochromatosis with iron overload and cirrhosis

(4) Schistosomiasis and other parasitic infestations

(5) Environmental carcinogens

(a) Industrial substances, including polychlorinated biphenyls (PCBs); chlorinated hydrocarbon solvents, such as carbon tetrachloride; nitrosamines; vinyl chloride and polyvinyl chloride (PVC); and organochloride pesticides

(b) Organic materials, including aflatoxins (produced by *Aspergillus flavus* or *A. fumigatus* and found on foods, such as peanuts)

(c) Thorotrast, an intravenous contrast agent that is no longer used

c. Clinical presentation

(1) Hepatocellular carcinoma often presents as a dull aching pain in the right upper quadrant; malaise, fever, and jaundice may also be present.

(2) Physical examination reveals hepatomegaly (present in 88% of cases), weight loss (in 85%), a tender abdominal mass (in 50%), or findings associated with cirrhosis (60%).

(3) About 10%–15% of patients present with acute hemorrhage into the peritoneal cavity with resultant shock.

(4) Paraneoplastic syndromes also may occur in which tumor cells secrete hormone-like substances that cause unusual syndromes, such as Cushing's syndrome.

d. Diagnosis. Liver function tests are usually abnormal, but there is no particular diagnostic pattern.

(1) Alpha-fetoprotein, a protein made by embryonal hepatocytes, is elevated in 70%–90% of cases.

(2) Hepatic ultrasound, CT scan, or MRI are the most reliable studies to determine the presence and operability of the lesions. These studies are positive in up to 90% of cases and can detect lesions as small as 1 cm in diameter.

e. Pathology. Hepatocellular carcinoma occurs as a solitary mass or as multiple masses. Local invasion, especially into the diaphragm, is common, as are distant metastases with the lung being most commonly involved (in up to 45% of cases).

f. Surgical treatment includes biopsy and exploration to determine resectability. To increase the potential for resectability, high-risk individuals (e.g., those with chronic HBV) should be periodically screened by measuring alpha-fetoprotein.

(1) If lesions are resectable, the average survival is approximately 3 years; the 5-year survival rate is about 20%.

(2) The operative mortality rate is as high as 20% but can be nearly 60% in patients with coexistent cirrhosis.

(3) If lesions are unresectable, patients have a mean survival time of 4 months.

(4) Attempts to induce tumor necrosis by hepatic artery ligation have shown poor results.

g. Chemotherapy has been ineffective when given systemically, but administration of drugs into the hepatic artery has given some promising preliminary results.

2. Hepatoblastoma

    a. Clinical presentation. Hepatoblastoma is the commonest primary malignant liver tumor in children and presents with abdominal distention, failure to thrive, and other symptoms of liver failure. Alpha-fetoprotein is frequently positive.

    b. Pathology. Approximately 80% are solitary liver masses that microscopically show nests and cords of primitive cells, resembling embryonic hepatocytes.

    c. Treatment is surgical excision. Inoperable tumors are treated with irradiation or chemotherapy but with poor results.

3. Cholangiocarcinoma is a tumor that arises from the bile duct epithelium; it represents 5%–30% of all primary hepatic malignancies.

    a. Clinical presentation. Signs and symptoms include right upper quadrant pain, jaundice, hepatomegaly, and occasionally a palpable mass. Patients are usually 60–70 years of age.

    b. Pathology. A hard greyish mass is found that microscopically shows adenocarcinoma of the biliary epithelium. Metastasis occurs initially to the regional lymph nodes or to the liver.

    c. Etiology. Associated conditions include parasitic infections (e.g., Clonorchis sinensis), primary sclerosing cholangitis, or Thorotrast exposure.

    d. Treatment of intrahepatic tumors is resection when feasible. Overall survival is poor.

4. Angiosarcoma, or **malignant hemangioendothelioma** is a highly malignant liver tumor composed of irregular spindle cells lining the lumina of hepatic vascular spaces.

    a. Etiology. Most cases (85%) occur in men, and there is a high association with chemical agents, especially vinyl chloride, Thorotrast, arsenicals, and organochloride pesticides.

    b. Clinical presentation. The tumor commonly spreads locally to the spleen (80% of cases) and distantly to the lungs (60% of cases).

    c. Treatment is resection when feasible, but patients rarely survive 1 year.

5. Sarcomas other than angiosarcoma are rare but are highly malignant and frequently not curable.

E. Metastatic tumors of the liver are much commoner than primary tumors (ratio 20:1).

1. Overview. The liver is the second commonest site of metastasis (exceeded only by regional lymph nodes) for all primary cancers of the abdominal viscera. Over two-thirds of all colorectal cancers ultimately involve the liver, and up to 50% of cancers outside the abdomen metastasize to the liver. Fully one-third of all cancers ultimately spread to the liver, which is the commonest site of hematogenous spread.

2. Diagnosis may be difficult because liver metastases are often asymptomatic.

    a. Laboratory studies. In a recent National Cancer Institute study, no single laboratory blood test could predict liver metastases in more than 65% of patients with subclinical disease. This percentage can only be raised by using imaging techniques.

        (1) Liver function studies (e.g., AST or alkaline phosphatase) detect only 50%–65% of subclinical metastases.

        (2) Testing for carcinoembryonic antigen (CEA) has been valuable for predicting the presence of liver metastasis in colorectal cancer as it is positive in over 85% of patients with proven disease. Unfortunately, this test lacks specificity.

    b. Imaging techniques are expensive as screening tests but are currently the most reliable nonsurgical method of finding liver metastases.

        (1) CT scan is the most accurate imaging technique, but it is expensive as a screening test.

        (2) Ultrasonography is almost as reliable as a CT scan, and it provides a reasonable screening test.

3. Treatment for metastatic disease to the liver depends on the type of primary tumor. Because colorectal cancer has generated the most reliable statistics, those figures are cited here.

    a. Chemotherapy for liver metastasis from colorectal cancer has been disappointing.

        (1) Systemic 5-fluorouracil (5-FU) therapy has resulted in a response rate of 9%–33% and a median survival of 30–60 weeks. (A response is defined as a 50% decrease in the size of an existing tumor and the development of no new lesion for a period of 1–2 months.)

(2) Hepatic arterial infusion of floxuridine (FUDR) has shown an increase in response rate but little or no improvement in patient survival.
b. Radiation therapy is poorly tolerated by the liver but may be palliative for painful liver metastases.
c. Hepatic artery ligation may cause a dramatic shrinkage in tumor size, but this is only transient. (Although most splanchnic primary cancers metastasize via the portal vein, they quickly become vascularized by the hepatic artery.)
d. Surgical resection is the most effective mode of therapy but is limited to the few patients who have unilobar liver lesions and no evidence of extrahepatic disease.
　(1) The incidence of liver metastasis at the time of surgery for primary colorectal cancer is 8%–25%, and approximately one-fourth of these lesions are solitary and resectable, so that about 5% of patients are potential resection candidates.
　(2) The 5-year survival rate approaches 20%–30% in patients with these criteria. The operative mortality rate is less than 6%, an acceptable risk.

F. Hepatic abscesses and cysts

1. Nonviral liver infections (i.e., bacterial, protozoal, or parasitic) generally localize as abscesses or cysts. Mortality without prompt, appropriate treatment is high.
　a. Etiology is dependent upon environmental factors, particularly geographic location and the presence of endemic parasites.
　b. Clinical presentation. Abscesses and cysts produce few localizing symptoms (i.e., chiefly pain and a mass in the right upper quadrant), while causing major systemic effects (i.e., fever, malnutrition, sepsis, or anemia).
　c. Diagnosis. Diagnostic tests used are similar to those used for tumors of the liver (see I B 2).

2. Bacterial abscesses are the commonest hepatic abscesses in the Western world.
　a. Etiology
　　(1) These are most commonly secondary to infectious processes in the abdomen, particularly cholangitis, appendicitis, or diverticulitis.
　　(2) They may also result from seeding from a distant infectious source, such as endocarditis.
　　(3) In 10%–50% of cases, no source can be identified.
　　(4) The **infecting organism** is related to the primary source.
　　　(a) When the source is abdominal, the commonest organisms are gram-negative rods (especially *Escherchia coli*), anaerobes (typically a *Bacteroides* species), and anaerobic streptococci (*Enterococci*).
　　　(b) When the source is extra-abdominal, gram-positive organisms predominate.
　b. Clinical presentation includes sepsis, fever and chills, leukocytosis, and anemia.
　　(1) Liver function studies show elevated enzyme levels, particularly alkaline phosphatase.
　　(2) The patient may have right upper quadrant pain, and the liver may be tender or enlarged.
　　(3) On occasion, sepsis may be overwhelming.
　　(4) Hemobilia may also occur due to erosion of the abscess into the biliary tree.
　c. Treatment
　　(1) The standard treatment for hepatic abscess is operative surgical drainage and antibiotic therapy, which have good results.
　　(2) Recently, hepatic abscesses have been managed by percutaneous drainage, using catheter aspiration guided by ultrasonic or CT imaging. This closed procedure may be curative, particularly for abscesses with minimal accompanying necrotic debris. Periodic sinograms of the abscess cavity are used to monitor healing and the adequacy of drainage.
　　(3) Multiple abscesses are difficult to manage and rely heavily on appropriate antibiotic coverage. It is important to determine the antibiotic sensitivity of the infecting organisms and to administer a full course of antibiotics to reduce the risk of recurrent or persistent infection.
　d. Mortality rate for hepatic abscess may be as high as 40% in difficult cases. This high rate is related principally to three factors.
　　(1) Delay in diagnosis. The possibility of an abscess is often overlooked in the critically ill patient. The use of CT scans and ultrasonography should improve this situation.

(2) Multiple abscesses. These are more difficult to drain properly, and, therefore, the patient may continue to be septic.

(3) Malnutrition. Patients with sepsis are very catabolic. Caloric supplementation, either orally or parenterally, is critical for the patient's well-being, wound healing, and immunocompetence.

3. Amebic abscess is the second commonest hepatic abscess in the Western world and is commoner than bacterial abscesses in third world countries.

   a. Etiology. Amebic abscess is due to infection with the protozoan *Entamoeba histolytica*, which typically reaches the portal vein from intestinal amebiasis.

   b. Clinical presentation includes fever, leukocytosis, hepatomegaly, and right upper quadrant pain. Occasionally, liver enzyme levels are elevated.

     (1) The abscess is usually solitary and affects the right lobe of the liver in 90% of patients.

     (2) Indirect hemagglutination titers for *Entamoeba* are elevated in up to 85% of patients with intestinal infestation and in 98% of patients with hepatic abscess.

     (3) The pus within the abscess is usually sterile and has the appearance of anchovy paste. Trophozoites are occasionally present in the periphery of the abscess.

   c. Treatment of choice is parenteral antibiotics, particularly metronidazole. The abscess is aspirated if it is large or adjacent to important structures, but surgical drainage is not usually necessary. Complications include secondary bacterial infection of the cavity and rupture into adjacent structures, such as the pleural, pericardial, or peritoneal spaces.

4. Hydatid cysts of the liver

   a. Etiology. Hydatid cysts result from infection with the parasite *Echinococcus granulosus*. Dogs are the definitive host, shedding ova in the feces, which infect intermediate hosts, such as man, sheep, and cattle. This infection is endemic in Southern Europe, the Middle East, Australia, and South America—all areas where sheep are raised.

   b. Clinical presentation

     (1) Hydatid cysts can develop anywhere in the body, but two-thirds occur in the liver.

       (a) The cyst and cyst lining contain parasites fully capable of spreading the infection.

       (b) The adjacent compressed liver tissue and scar form the ectocyst, which is not infective and should be retained when evacuating the cyst.

     (2) Hydatid cysts undergo progressive enlargement and may rupture.

       (a) Close to 50% rupture within the hepatic parenchyma to form daughter cysts.

       (b) Cysts may rupture into bile ducts, where the debris can cause biliary obstruction.

       (c) Cysts may rupture into the free peritoneal cavity, resulting in urticaria, eosinophilia, or anaphylactic shock, and with implantation into other viscera.

       (d) About 30% of patients develop cysts in the lungs or other extrahepatic organs.

     (3) Symptoms include liver enlargement and right upper quadrant pain in a patient with a history of exposure to an endemic area. Eosinophilia is present in 40% of patients, and serum tests for the parasite antigen are diagnostic.

       (a) All symptomatic cysts require surgery.

       (b) Small cysts deep within the parenchyma should be followed (for months to years) until they are sufficiently superficial to be removed.

       (c) When pericystic calcification is visible on an abdominal x-ray, it signifies the death of the parasite, a condition that requires no further treatment.

   c. Treatment

     (1) Because the cyst is quite fragile and easily ruptured, a hydatid cyst can rarely be removed intact. If the scoleces spill into the peritoneal cavity, the parasite will multiply and form new cysts.

     (2) The current method of treatment is controlled rupture of the cyst, followed by its removal.

       (a) This is accomplished by careful isolation of the operative field to prevent spillage, followed by aspiration of the cyst.

       (b) Once decompressed, the cyst and its contents are peeled off the ectocyst lining and removed, thus removing all living cyst elements.

       (c) The residual space is then sterilized with fresh 0.5% silver nitrate solution, which is a potent scolicide and relatively nontoxic. (There is no systemic scolicidal agent currently in use.)

(d) The residual cavity is carefully inspected for bile leakage from cyst–biliary communications, and these are sutured closed.

(e) If the cyst ruptured into a major bile duct, common bile duct exploration is done to remove all debris.

(f) The cyst is closed. No drains are used.

G. Trauma. Due to its large size, the liver is frequently injured by both blunt and penetrating trauma.

1. Mortality. Due to its high blood flow, proximity to the inferior vena cava, nearby vital structures, and propensity to develop infections, the overall mortality of liver trauma remains about 10%–20%. Injury to the hepatic veins and retrohepatic inferior vena cava has a mortality of over 50%, regardless of the method used to obtain control of the bleeding.

2. Diagnosis is usually related to intraperitoneal bleeding. Ongoing bleeding mandates surgery.

3. Surgical management. At surgery, initial hemostasis is obtained via **packing** or the **Pringle maneuver** (control and compression of the porta hepatis). Definitive control of bleeding requires exposure and ligation of individual parenchymal bleeders. This may require:

a. Tractotomy or opening of a missle tract or fracture to expose bleeding parenchyma

b. Resectional debridement, the removal of nonviable parenchyma without an anatomic (i.e., segmental or lobar) resection

c. Less common methods to control bleeding

(1) Anatomic resection has a high mortality (about 50%) when done as an emergency.

(2) Hepatic artery ligation may control arterial bleeding but is associated with infectious complications in the compromised parenchyma.

(3) Definitive packing can be useful when other methods are unavailable or fail. Ideally, it provides time (24–48 hours) to restore normothermia and clotting factors.

4. Late complications are common.

a. Subcapsular and intrahepatic hematomas can be carefully observed, but many ultimately require drainage.

b. Perihepatic collections, whether of blood or bile, usually become infected and must be drained.

c. Biliary fistulas may track to the skin or into the chest (biliary–pleural, bronchobiliary fistula). Treatment is similar to the treatment for gastrointestinal fistulas (see Chapter 2 IV).

d. Traumatic arteriovenous fistulas may result from penetrating trauma. Large fistulas are best treated by arterial embolization.

e. Hemobilia is due to arteriobiliary fistula formation.

(1) Patients present late (more than 1 month after injury) with gastrointestinal bleeding (hematemesis or melena), jaundice, biliary colic, or fever.

(2) Diagnosis and treatment are via arteriography and embolization.

II. PORTAL HYPERTENSION

A. Anatomy (see I A 2 b and Figure 14-2)

B. Pathophysiology. Portal hypertension is an abnormal elevation in portal venous pressure (normal is 5–6 mm Hg).

1. The increase in pressure stimulates the development of venous collaterals, which attempt to bypass the portal system.

2. The collateral veins are very fragile. They form portosystemic connections between the portal system and the inferior vena cava or the superior vena cava via the azygos system.

3. When portal pressure exceeds 20 mm Hg, **dilated veins** or **varices** are likely to develop. When the varices form in a submucosal location, such as at the gastroesophageal junction, they are subject to rupture and hemorrhage.

C. Etiology

1. Intrahepatic causes are commonest.

    a. Cirrhosis of the liver causes 85% of portal hypertension in the United States. The commonest etiology of cirrhosis is alcohol abuse, followed by postnecrotic cirrhosis and biliary cirrhosis.

      (1) Pathologically, cirrhosis produces:

        (a) Progressive narrowing of sinusoidal and postsinusoidal vessels due to centrilobular collagen deposition

        (b) Distortion of the sinusoidal anatomy by cirrhotic regenerative nodules

      (2) The resultant sinusoidal block increases resistance to portal blood flow through the liver and increases portal pressure.

    b. Schistosomiasis is a common cause worldwide. Portal hypertension develops when parasitic ova in small portal venules cause a presinusoidal block.

    c. Wilson's disease, hepatic fibrosis, and hemochromatosis are occasional causes of portal hypertension.

2. Prehepatic causes of portal hypertension are rare but are commoner in children. They are caused by portal vein obstruction due to either thrombosis, congenital atresia or stenosis, or extrinsic compression, such as occurs with tumors.

3. Posthepatic causes of portal hypertension are also rare.

    a. Budd-Chiari syndrome is characterized by hepatic vein thrombosis, which causes a postsinusoidal block with resultant hepatomegaly and ascites. This syndrome may be idiopathic or due to a hypercoagulable state as occurs with tumors, hematologic disorders, oral contraceptive use, and trauma. In the Orient, inferior vena caval webs are the commonest cause of hepatic vein obstruction. Oddly, this syndrome is not uncommon after bone marrow transplantation.

    b. Constrictive pericarditis produces a markedly elevated inferior vena cava pressure, resulting in resistance to hepatic venous outflow. It should be suspected when calcification of the pericardium is present.

4. Increased portal venous flow may result in portal hypertension. This is due to primary splenic disease and splenic arteriovenous fistulae or shunts.

5. Splenic vein thrombosis may cause hypertension of the veins at the splenic hilum, resulting in varices confined to the gastric fundus. This is usually due to pancreatitis or a pancreatic tumor (see II J 2 c).

D. Clinical presentation. The following are common findings in portal hypertension:

1. Encephalopathy

    a. This is secondary to portosystemic collaterals (with shunting of portal blood around the liver) and hepatic insufficiency.

    b. It may be related to elevated serum levels of ammonia in some patients, but the correlation is unreliable.

2. Gastrointestinal hemorrhage, frequently from gastroesophageal varices and complicated by impaired coagulation

3. Malnutrition, particularly in alcoholic cirrhosis

4. Ascites (see II K) secondary to hepatic sinusoidal hypertension, hypoalbuminemia, and hyperaldosteronism

5. Other manifestations of **collateral venous development,** such as a periumbilical caput medusae or hemorrhoids

6. Splenomegaly, which may be associated with hypersplenism (see II J)

7. Severe abdominal pain, acidosis, and leukocytosis if mesenteric venous gangrene develops secondarily to acute portal vein thrombosis. This is usually lethal.

E. Medical management of acute variceal hemorrhage. Variceal hemorrhage is life-threatening and is the principal complication of portal hypertension that requires emergency intervention.

1. The management of acute upper gastrointestinal hemorrhage is described in Chapter 9 III F.

2. Gastroesophagoscopy should be performed as soon as possible to find the site of bleeding and determine the presence of varices.

a. The cause of an upper gastrointestinal hemorrhage in cirrhotic patients is varices in 20%–50%, erosive gastritis in 20%–60%, peptic ulcer disease in 6%–19%, and esophageal tears (Mallory-Weiss syndrome) in 5%–18%.

b. Up to 8% of the patients have two bleeding sites.

3. Measures for controlling proven variceal bleeding include the following:

a. Injection sclerotherapy

(1) Injection of a sclerosing agent into a varix results in thrombosis of the vein.

(2) The procedure is done endoscopically and controls bleeding temporarily in 80% of patients; it is associated with a mortality rate of 10%–20%.

(3) This is currently the preferred method of acutely managing variceal bleeding in most centers.

b. Vasopressin (see Chapter 9 III F 1 d)

(1) This potent vasoconstrictor lowers portal pressure by mesenteric arterial vasoconstriction with resultant diminished mesenteric blood flow.

(2) It is equally effective intravenously or intra-arterially.

(3) Vasopressin is useful only for short-term hemorrhage control; it does not improve patient survival rates.

c. Balloon tamponade. The Sengstaken-Blakemore tube is a nasogastric tube with esophageal and gastric balloons for tamponade of varices.

(1) These tubes control bleeding in up to 35% of patients, but bleeding may resume when the balloon is deflated.

(2) Pneumonia, due to the inability to clear salivary secretions, is common unless a proximal suction tube is placed above the esophageal balloon.

(3) Esophageal rupture may result from mechanical disruption or ischemia of the esophagus.

(4) To minimize these complications, this tube should be used for a limited period of time, such as 48 hours.

F. Surgical management of acute massive bleeding. Acute massive bleeding that fails to respond to nonsurgical maneuvers requires emergency surgery, especially if hypotension is present.

1. The decision to proceed with surgery is made if bleeding continues despite transfusion of 5 units or more of blood, especially within 24 hours. The risk of death rises dramatically after 10 units of blood have been transfused, due both to sepsis and to the worsening of cirrhotic coagulopathy from the use of banked blood.

2. Surgery is not advisable in the presence of pneumonia, moderate or severe encephalopathy, severe coagulopathy, alcoholic hepatitis (II G 1 b), or severe liver failure.

3. Type of surgery performed may either be to decompress the portal venous system or directly ligate the bleeding varices.

a. Emergency portacaval shunting, although very effective in controlling hemorrhage (over 95% of patients stop bleeding), has a high operative mortality related to the Child classification of the patient (see Table 14-1).

(1) The usual procedure performed is an end-to-side portacaval shunt or a mesocaval shunt (see II H).

(2) The acute reduction of portal blood flow to the liver following shunting may lead to hepatic failure, accounting for two-thirds of the perioperative deaths. Pneumonia, renal failure, and delirium tremens are contributing lethal factors.

b. Ligation of varices [see II G 2 b (1)], either directly or by esophageal transection using a stapling device, usually stops the bleeding.

(1) Ligation is associated with an operative mortality rate of up to 30%.

(2) Bleeding recurs within several months in up to 80% of survivors.

4. The possibility of bleeding from sources other than varices should be clearly eliminated **before beginning** any surgical procedure.

G. Elective surgical management of esophageal varices is used when patients are not actively bleeding. The goal of this type of surgery is to prevent rebleeding with its concomitant risk of death.

1. Preoperative evaluation includes the following:

a. Endoscopy is used to prove that the esophageal varices bled.

b. Acute alcoholic hepatitis must be excluded.
   (1) This syndrome presents as liver failure with a diffusely tender liver.
   (2) Histologically, hepatocyte necrosis is seen with discrete hyaline bodies (Mallory's bodies) in hepatic cells.
   (3) Liver enzyme levels and liver function improve if the patient survives the acute episode.
   (4) A liver biopsy should be performed if the diagnosis is in question, since the operative mortality rate exceeds 50% when surgery is performed in the presence of alcoholic hepatitis.
c. The **Child classification** (Table 14-1) is used to evaluate the operative risk.
d. The patient's portal venous anatomy is determined, verifying the presence of a patent portal vein by:
   (1) Splenic and superior mesenteric arteriography followed by delayed venous-phase imaging is the most accurate method.
   (2) Doppler ultrasound examination to identify the portal vein and its tributaries and ascertain patency and direction of flow is simple and noninvasive.
   (3) Splenoportography, the injection of radiopaque dye into the spleen followed by imaging of the portal system, is reserved for specific visualization of the splenic vein.
e. The portal venous pressure can be measured indirectly by measuring the wedged hepatic venous pressure.

2. Type of elective surgery depends on the surgeon's preference and on the patient's pathologic and physiologic status. The choices are as follows:
a. Shunting procedures (see II H)
b. Direct occlusion of varices
   (1) Endoscopic variceal sclerosis (sclerotherapy) is initially effective in up to 80% of patients and has become the principal initial method of management for esophageal varices.
      (a) Many patients require resclerosis procedures because nothing has been done to lower the portal pressure.
      (b) Major risks include esophageal ulceration in the area of sclerosis, endoscopic perforation of the esophagus, pleural effusion, and esophageal stricture.
   (2) Simple ligation of varices may be performed by gastrotomy and suture ligation, transthoracic variceal ligation, or esophageal transection and reanastomosis with a stapler.
      (a) Although ligation usually controls bleeding, the incidence of rebleeding is very high.
      (b) It can be used for the initial control of bleeding to be followed by some form of portal decompressive surgery.
   (3) Paraesophageal devascularization combined with **esophageal transection** and **reanastomosis (Sugiura** procedure) has, in some series, been highly effective in preventing bleeding and has shown a low operative mortality rate.
      (a) The procedure may be performed in two stages: transthoracic esophageal devascularization, followed in 4–6 weeks by transabdominal proximal gastric devascularization, splenectomy, selective vagotomy, and pyloroplasty.
      (b) The operative mortality rate has been as low as 5%, and the rebleeding rate as low as 4% in the Japanese series. These excellent results have not been duplicated for European or American individuals with cirrhosis.

Table 14-1. The Child Classification for Determining the Operative Risk of a Shunting Procedure in a Patient with Portal Hypertension

	Child Group		
	A	**B**	**C**
Serum bilirubin (mg/dl)	< 2	2–3	> 3
Serum albumin (g/dl)	> 3.5	3–3.5	< 3
Presence of ascites	Absent	Easily controlled	Refractory
Presence of encephalopathy	Absent	Minimal	Severe
Presence of malnutrition	Absent	Mild	Severe
Operative mortality rate	2%	10%	50%

H. Shunting procedures are designed to lower the portal venous pressure, thereby decompressing esophageal varices and diminishing their propensity to bleed. **Portosystemic shunts** may be prophylactic or therapeutic and may be nonselective or selective.

1. **Prophylactic shunts** are performed on patients with proven varices, but prior to any episodes of esophageal variceal bleeding.
   a. Only 30%–40% of these patients ultimately bleed from their varices, making 60% of the procedures unnecessary.
   b. Nonselective shunts decrease hepatic portal venous flow, increasing the risk of hepatic decompensation.
   c. In randomized trials, prophylactic shunts have not improved survival rates. They are currently not recommended.

2. **Therapeutic shunts** are performed on patients who have had a variceal hemorrhage. Patient survival is principally a function of the Child classification (see Table 14-1) prior to surgery. Long-term survival in the alcoholic patient is principally determined by whether or not the patient continues to abuse alcohol.

3. **Nonselective portosystemic shunts** decompress the entire portal venous system into the inferior vena cava, lowering portal pressure.
   a. **The end-to-side portacaval shunt** (Figure 14-4) is the shunt most commonly performed.
      (1) The hepatic end of the portal vein is ligated, and the inferior end of the portal vein is sutured to the inferior vena cava, which results in dramatic lowering of portal pressure and decompression of varices.
      (2) The rebleeding rate is less than 5%, but the major problem is that portal flow into the liver is reduced to zero, which increases the risk of encephalopathy and hepatic failure.
   b. **The mesocaval shunt** is constructed with a large diameter (16–18 mm) prosthetic vascular graft to connect the superior mesenteric vein to the inferior vena cava (Figure 14-5).
      (1) With this shunt and the side-to-side portacaval shunt, the effect on portal blood flow into the liver is unpredictable; as portal pressure falls, portal flow into the liver falls. In fact, blood may flow out of the liver via the portal vein, thereby stealing hepatic arterial flow. Thus, the risk of hepatic failure may be higher than for end-to-side portacaval shunts.
      (2) The advantage of this shunt is the relative ease of exposing the mesenteric vein.
      (3) The disadvantages are two:
         (a) This shunt uses prosthetic material, which has the potential for infection.
         (b) There is a somewhat lower long-term patency rate as compared to shunts without prosthetic material.
      (4) As with all shunts, **thrombosis of the shunt returns the patient to a high risk of variceal hemorrhage.**

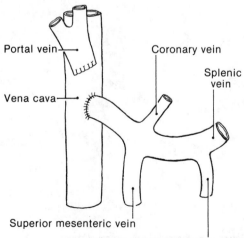

Figure 14-4. End-to-side portacaval shunt.

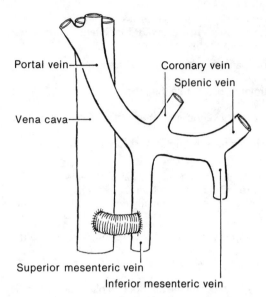

Portal vein

Coronary vein

Splenic vein

Vena cava

Superior mesenteric vein

Inferior mesenteric vein

Figure 14-5. Inferior vena cava–superior mesenteric vein (mesocaval) shunt.

    c. The side-to-side portacaval shunt is technically more difficult as a longer length of both veins must be prepared (Figure 14-6). Its use is reserved for situations where it is necessary to decompress the liver (see II K 1).

        (1) In the Budd-Chiari syndrome, this shunt or a mesocaval shunt converts the portal vein into an outflow vessel, replacing the thrombosed hepatic veins.

        (2) With refractory ascites and variceal hemorrhage, this shunt decompresses the liver and decreases ascites.

  4. Selective portosystemic shunts decrease the pressure in the gastroesophageal bed only and reduce the risk of gastroesophageal varices by shunting only gastroesophageal venous blood into the systemic circulation. Prospective trials have shown a significant decrease in the incidence of postoperative encephalopathy with the selective shunt as compared to the nonselective shunts. The **distal splenorenal (Warren) shunt** is most commonly performed (Figure 14-7).

    a. In this procedure, the distal end of the splenic vein (i.e., the portion coming directly from the splenic hilum) is anastomosed to the left renal vein, a low-pressure vein. The proximal splenic vein is ligated.

    b. The coronary vein, the right gastroepiploic vein, and other collaterals between the portal system and the gastric, pancreatic, and splenic region are ligated.

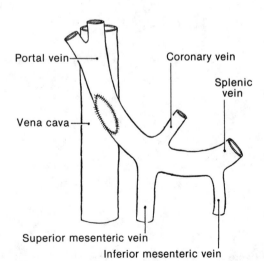

Portal vein

Coronary vein

Splenic vein

Vena cava

Superior mesenteric vein

Inferior mesenteric vein

Figure 14-6. Side-to-side portacaval shunt.

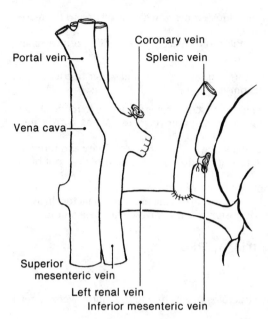

Portal vein

Coronary vein

Splenic vein

Vena cava

Superior
mesenteric vein

Left renal vein

Inferior mesenteric vein

Figure 14-7. Distal splenorenal (Warren) shunt.

c. As can be seen from Figure 14-7, portal venous flow into the liver is maintained, thus minimizing the problem of hepatic insufficiency and consequent encephalopathy.

d. Because portal sinusoidal pressure remains high, ascites is common after this procedure.

e. Chylous ascites may also occur as a result of surgical dissection in the retroperitoneum adjacent to major lymphatic channels.

I. Prognosis. Ultimately, in alcoholic patients with cirrhosis, regardless of the treatment, the potential for hepatic failure and death depend on whether or not the patient continues to consume alcohol. The prognosis for other causes of cirrhosis is not quite as poor, though the trends are the same. The overall statistics for alcoholic cirrhotic patients are as follows:

1. Approximately 15% of alcoholics develop cirrhosis, and 30% of these individuals die within a year of the diagnosis.

2. Approximately 40% (i.e., 13%–70%) of cirrhotic individuals develop bleeding varices, and without definitive treatment, 66% of these individuals die within a year.

a. Approximately 50%–80% of patients die from their first variceal hemorrhage without definitive treatment.

b. Of those patients who survive the initial hemorrhage to bleed a second time, the same proportion will die from their second hemorrhage.

J. Hypersplenism is common in patients with portal hypertension.

1. It should be treated conservatively (i.e., nonoperatively). Approximately half of patients who undergo shunting show improvement of the hypersplenism.

2. Splenectomy should be performed rarely for portal hypertension.

a. It is associated with a variceal hemorrhage recurrence rate as high as 90%.

b. Sepsis and death may follow splenectomy, especially in children.

c. Indication for splenectomy in a patient with variceal bleeding is radiographic proof of **splenic vein thrombosis**.

(1) This occurs as a result of an obstruction in the vein due to a pancreatic disorder, such as pancreatitis or a neoplasm.

(2) The varices are generally limited to the stomach (gastric varices) and, therefore, are **curable** by splenectomy.

K. Ascites is a complication of hepatic disease.

1. Etiology. It results from sinusoidal hypertension, hypoalbuminemia, abnormal hepatic and abdominal lymph production, and abnormal salt and water retention by the kidneys.

    a. Salt and water retention are due to **hyperaldosteronism,** which is related to decreased breakdown of aldosterone by the liver.

    b. Ascites may be worsened by portosystemic shunts [except side-to-side portacaval and mesocaval shunts (see II H 3 b, c)].

2. Medical management of ascites is efficacious and involves salt and water restriction and diuretics, especially the aldosterone antagonists.

3. Peritoneal–jugular shunting may be used to treat ascites that is refractory to medical management. Its efficacy in either controlling ascites or improving survival has not yet been definitely demonstrated.

    a. A plastic tube is implanted surgically, originating in the peritoneal cavity and terminating in the jugular vein. A valve in the tubing controls the direction of flow out of the peritoneal cavity.

    b. Diuretics should be continued for optimal shunt results.

    c. Peritoneal–jugular shunts may result in bleeding due to the presence of factors in ascitic fluid that stimulate the development of disseminated intravascular coagulation.

III. GALLBLADDER AND EXTRAHEPATIC BILIARY TREE

A. Overview

  1. Embryology

    a. Development of the liver and biliary structures begins during the fourth week of fetal life.

    b. The hepatic diverticulum forms as an outpouching of the foregut.

      (1) The **cranial portion** forms the liver, the larger branches of the intrahepatic ducts, and the proximal extrahepatic biliary tree.

      (2) The **caudal portion** forms the gallbladder, cystic duct, and common bile duct.

  2. Anatomy (Figure 14-8)

    a. Extrahepatic biliary tree

      (1) Structure

        (a) The **left** and **right hepatic ducts** join together after leaving the liver. This confluence forms the **common hepatic duct** (3–4 cm in length).

        (b) The common hepatic duct is joined at an acute angle by the cystic duct to form the common bile duct (10 cm in length; 3–10 mm in diameter).

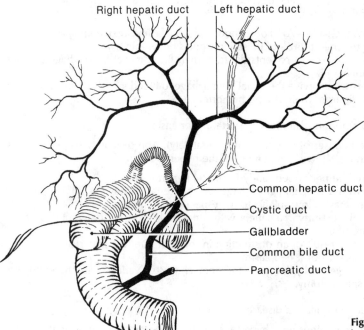

Right hepatic duct   Left hepatic duct

Common hepatic duct

Cystic duct

Gallbladder

Common bile duct

Pancreatic duct

Figure 14-8. Gallbladder and extrahepatic biliary tree.

(c) The **common bile duct** is lateral to the common hepatic artery and anterior to the portal vein. The distal one-third of the common bile duct passes behind the pancreas to the **ampulla of Vater,** also called the papilla.

(d) The common bile duct joins the **pancreatic duct** in one of three ways.

(i) Most commonly, the ducts unite outside the duodenum and traverse the duodenal wall and papilla as a single duct.

(ii) They may join within the duodenal wall and have a short common channel.

(iii) Least commonly, they enter the duodenum independently.

(2) The **sphincter of Oddi** surrounds the common bile duct as it traverses the ampulla of Vater and controls bile flow.

(3) **Blood supply to the ducts**

(a) The **hilar ducts** within the liver parenchyma are supplied primarily from the hepatic arteries.

(b) The blood supply to the **supraduodenal common bile duct** is variable, but generally blood flows superiorly. The most important vessels (the **"three o'clock"** and **"nine o'clock"** arteries) run along the sides of the duct, as their names imply.

b. **The gallbladder** is located on the inferior aspect of the liver and marks the division of the liver into its right and left lobes.

(1) **Anatomic portions**

(a) **Fundus** (most anterior)

(b) **Body,** which serves as the storage area

(c) **Infundibulum (Hartmann's pouch),** located between the neck and the body (most posterior)

(d) **Neck,** which connects with the cystic duct

(2) The **wall of the gallbladder** is composed of smooth muscle and fibrous tissue; the lumen is lined with high columnar epithelium.

(3) **Vasculature**

(a) **Arterial supply.** The gallbladder is supplied by the **cystic artery,** which is usually (95% of the time) a branch of the right hepatic artery that passes behind the cystic duct.

(b) **Venous return** is via cystic veins to the portal vein and small veins that drain directly into the liver.

(c) **Lymphatic drainage** from the gallbladder goes both to the liver and to hilar nodes.

(4) **Innervation** is from the **celiac plexus**.

(a) **Motor innervation** travels via vagal and postganglionic fibers from the celiac ganglia. The preganglionic sympathetic level is T_8–T_9.

(b) **Sensory innervation** travels from sympathetic fibers coursing to the celiac plexus through the right posterior root ganglion at levels T_8–T_9.

(5) The **valves of Heister** are mucosal folds in the cystic duct. Despite their name, they have no valvular function.

c. **Anomalies** of the arterial and biliary systems are common. Because "normal" anatomy occurs in fewer than 50% of individuals, the surgeon must have a thorough knowledge of both normal and anomalous anatomy.

3. **Physiology.** Bile is produced by the liver and transported via the extrahepatic ducts to the gallbladder where it is concentrated and released in response to humoral and neural control.

a. **Hepatic production of bile** is under neural and humoral control. Vagal and splanchnic stimulation, secretin, theophylline, phenobarbital, and steroids all increase bile flow. Approximately 600 ml of bile are produced daily (normal range: 250–1000 ml/day).

b. **Composition of bile.** Because the electrolyte concentration of bile approximates that of plasma, **lactated Ringer's solution** is a good replacement fluid for biliary losses. Bile is composed of

(1) Electrolytes and water

(2) Bile pigments

(3) Protein

(4) Lipids

(a) Phospholipids, primarily lecithin

(b) Cholesterol

(c) Bile acids (bile salts); chenodeoxycholic acid and cholic acid conjugated with taurine and glycine

    c. Functions of the gallbladder include:

      (1) Storage of bile

      (2) Concentration of bile

        (a) The absorption of water and electrolytes by the gallbladder mucosa results in a 10-fold increased concentration of lipids, bile salts, and bile pigments compared to hepatic bile.

        (b) The **secretion of mucus** protects the gallbladder mucosa from the irritant effects of bile and facilitates the passage of bile through the cystic duct. This mucus secretion represents the "**white bile**" seen with **hydrops of the gallbladder,** following cystic duct obstruction.

      (3) Release of bile

        (a) The coordinated release of bile requires simultaneous contraction of the gallbladder and relaxation of the sphincter of Oddi.

        (b) This process is under predominantly humoral control (via cholecystokinin), but vagal and splanchnic nerves also play a role.

B. Radiologic diagnosis of biliary tract disease

  1. Plain abdominal films demonstrate the 15% of gallstones that are radiopaque.

  2. Oral cholecystography (OCG) is the best method of demonstrating biliary calculi.

    a. This technique identifies abnormalities (visualization of stones or nonvisualization of the gallbladder) with a 95%–98% accuracy.

    b. This procedure requires the ingestion of iopanoic acid (Telepaque) tablets on the evening before the study. The chief disadvantages lie in its reliance on:

      (1) Absorption of the contrast medium from the gastrointestinal tract

      (2) Uptake and excretion of contrast medium from the hepatocytes

      (3) Concentration of contrast medium in the gallbladder

      (4) Patency of the hepatic and cystic ducts

  3. Cholecystokinin stimulation is used to diagnose gallbladder disease in symptomatic patients with a normal OCG. A **positive study** is represented by either of the following:

    a. Failure of the gallbladder to contract more than 40% at 20 minutes after cholecystokinin injection

    b. Reproduction of the patient's right upper quadrant pain when the cholecystokinin is injected

  4. Real-time ultrasonography has a 90%–93% accuracy in identifying calculi but is limited in detecting small stones. The technique is useful for the evaluation of acute cholecystitis.

  5. CT scans and MRI are expensive but delineate dilated ducts as well as retroperitoneal lymphadenopathy and lesions of the pancreatic head and the liver.

  6. Hepatobiliary iminodiacetic acid (HIDA) scan makes use of a gamma-emitting radioisotope (^{99m}Tc) attached to a substance excreted in the bile.

    a. It provides images of the liver, the biliary tree, and the intestinal transit of bile.

    b. The HIDA scan is the study of choice for the diagnosis of acute cholecystitis.

  7. Percutaneous transhepatic cholangiography (using the Chiba needle) is useful in the evaluation of the jaundiced patient. It localizes disease and allows the preoperative placement of biliary drainage catheters.

  8. Endoscopic retrograde cholangiopancreatography (ERCP) is also useful in evaluating the jaundiced patient.

    a. This procedure permits evaluation of the stomach, duodenum, ampulla of Vater, pancreatic duct, and common bile duct.

    b. If stones are present within the common bile duct, endoscopic papillotomy can be performed.

  9. Intravenous cholangiography is no longer performed.

C. Cholelithiasis (gallstones)

  1. Types and mode of formation. Gallstones form as a result of biliary solids precipitating out of the solution. Most stones (70%) are made up of cholesterol, bilirubin, and calcium with cholesterol as the major component.

    a. Cholesterol stones are large and smooth.

(1) The solubility of cholesterol in bile depends on the concentration of bile salts, lecithin, and cholesterol. Lecithin and cholesterol are insoluble in aqueous solution but dissolve in bile salt-lecithin micelles.

(2) Failure of the liver to maintain a micellar liquid can be caused by an increase in the concentration of cholesterol or a decrease in the concentration of bile salts or lecithin; either can result in cholesterol stone formation.

(3) Conversely, increasing the biliary concentration of lecithin and bile salts should hinder cholesterol stone formation.

   (a) This theory has been investigated by treating patients with cholesterol stones with oral bile salts.

   (b) In the National Cooperative Gallstone Study, patients with cholesterol gallstones were treated with chenodeoxycholic acid over a 2-year period. Complete resolution of stones was found in 13% of the patients, and partial dissolution in 41%.

b. Pure pigment (bilirubin) stones are smooth and are green or black in color; they are associated with hemolytic disorders, such as sickle cell anemia or spherocytosis.

c. Calcium bilirubinate stones are associated with infection or inflammation of the biliary tree.

   (1) Infection results in an increase in biliary calcium as well as an increase in β-glucuronidase (which converts conjugated bilirubin to the unconjugated form).

   (2) The calcium binds to the unconjugated bilirubin and precipitates to form calcium bilirubinate stones.

   (3) Normal bile contains glucaro-1,4-lactone, which inhibits the conversion of conjugated to unconjugated bilirubin and, thus, deters calcium bilirubinate stone formation.

2. **Clinical presentation** of cholelithiasis varies. It can present as (in increasing order of severity):

   a. Asymptomatic cholelithiasis

   b. Chronic cholecystitis

   c. Acute cholecystitis

   d. Complications of cholecystitis

   e. Choledocholithiasis (common bile duct stones)

3. **Asymptomatic cholelithiasis.** The treatment of asymptomatic cholelithiasis is controversial.

   a. Excluding diabetics and patients with sickle cell disease, truly asymptomatic cholelithiasis may be amenable to dietary management alone.

   (1) In several studies, however, up to 50% of patients ultimately developed symptoms, and 10%–20% developed biliary complications.

   (2) Criticism of the study is based on the assumption that these patients were not truly asymptomatic at the onset or that the symptoms that they developed were not truly biliary symptoms.

   b. Diabetic patients with cholelithiasis should definitely undergo cholecystectomy because of the higher risk of complications and a mortality rate as high as 15% from acute cholecystitis.

D. Cholecystitis is acute inflammation of the gallbladder associated with obstruction of the cystic duct. In 85%–95% of cases, cholecystitis is due to calculi. Bile stasis, bacteria, and pancreatic juice irritation may play a lesser role.

1. **Chronic cholecystitis**

   a. Clinical presentation. The patient complains of moderate intermittent pain in the right upper quadrant and epigastric region, nausea, and vomiting. The pain may radiate to the back or right scapular region. Symptoms are associated with eating fatty foods.

   b. Diagnosis. Laboratory studies are generally normal. On OCG, the gallbladder fails to visualize or shows a filling defect. Ultrasonography shows stones.

   c. Treatment is elective cholecystectomy. About 75% of patients operated on for cholecystitis secondary to cholelithiasis are completely relieved of their symptoms; approximately 25% retain mild symptoms that presumably are unrelated to the biliary tree.

   d. Nonoperative treatment (e.g., oral bile salts or lithotripsy) may be appropriate for select patients with small stones and functioning gallbladders (by OCG) and are being investigated.

2. Acute cholecystitis
  a. Pathophysiology
    (1) Most cases are due to an impacted stone in the gallbladder neck or the cystic duct with cyst duct obstruction. Direct pressure from the stone on the mucosa or duct obstruction causes ischemia, ulceration, edema, and impaired venous return, all of which leads to extensive inflammation in and around the gallbladder.
    (2) In 75% of cases, bacterial infection of the bile and gallbladder wall occurs.
    (3) Unchecked, these changes can lead to complications of acute cholecystitis
  b. Clinical presentation
    (1) The greatest incidence of acute cholecystitis is in adults aged 30–80; women are affected more often than men.
    (2) Most patients give a history consistent with prior chronic cholecystitis except this episode is worse or lasts longer.
    (3) Fever, nausea, and vomiting, and right upper quadrant tenderness with or without rebound tenderness are common. The gallbladder may be palpable.
  c. The differential diagnosis includes:
    (1) Perforated or penetrating peptic ulcer
    (2) Myocardial infarction
    (3) Pancreatitis
    (4) Hiatal hernia
    (5) Right lower lobe pneumonia
    (6) Appendicitis
    (7) Hepatitis
    (8) Herpes zoster
  d. Diagnosis
    (1) A radionuclide scan is the diagnostic study of choice.
    (2) Other mandatory studies include a complete blood count; measurement of serum amylase, serum bilirubin, and liver enzymes; an electrocardiogram; and chest x-ray.
    (3) Levels of the following may be elevated in patients with acute cholecystitis:
      (a) Serum alkaline phosphatase in 23%
      (b) Bilirubin in 45%
      (c) AST in 40%
      (d) Amylase in 13%
  e. Treatment
    (1) Cholecystitis should be treated with cholecystectomy. As the bile is usually infected, perioperative antibiotics are needed. There are two approaches to the timing of surgery.
      (a) Immediate surgery, that is, within 72 hours of the onset of symptoms
      (b) Delayed surgery, that is, after recovery from the acute attack with intravenous fluids and antibiotics. Surgery should be performed 6 weeks after the acute inflammation has resolved.
    (2) Most surgeons now advocate **early surgical intervention** in the treatment of acute cholecystitis. This is due to the improved safety of current techniques, the effectiveness of perioperative antibiotics, and the high risk (at least 50%) of recurrent acute cholecystitis if surgery is delayed. Our **approach** is as follows.
      (a) If symptoms began within 72 hours of the time of presentation, cholecystectomy is performed.
      (b) If symptoms began more than 72 hours before the time of presentation and the patient is responding to medical management (i.e., a nasogastric tube, intravenous fluids, nothing by mouth, and antibiotics), then surgery is delayed for 4–6 weeks.
      (c) Deterioration or failure to improve on medical management is an indication for surgery.

3. Acalculous cholecystitis is acute or chronic **cholecystitis in the absence of stones**. It occurs as a complication of burns, sepsis, trauma, or collagen vascular disease.
  a. Etiology. Possible causes include:
    (1) Kinking or fibrosis of the gallbladder
    (2) Thrombosis of the cystic artery
    (3) Sphincter spasm with obstruction of the biliary and pancreatic ducts
    (4) Prolonged fasting
    (5) Dehydration

(6) Systemic disease, such as the multiorgan failure associated with trauma
(7) Generalized sepsis
b. Treatment is cholecystectomy or cholecystostomy if the patient is too ill to tolerate cholecystectomy.

4. Complications of cholecystitis (and cholelithiasis) require urgent surgery.
  a. Emphysematous cholecystitis is an acute, usually gangrenous cholecystitis complicated by secondary invasion by gas-forming organisms.
    (1) Unlike acute cholecystitis, emphysematous cholecystitis is three times more prevalent in men than women and may occur without cholelithiasis.
    (2) Radiologically, the gallbladder is filled with gas in the absence of any communication between the gallbladder and the gastrointestinal tract.
    (3) Treatment is early cholecystectomy. Antibiotics effective against *Clostridia* and coliform organisms are given.
  b. Gangrenous cholecystitis results when extensive inflammation causes thrombosis of the cystic artery and resultant necrosis of the gallbladder. Bile cultures and appropriate antibiotics are essential.
  c. Perforated cholecystitis results from necrosis of the gallbladder wall and leakage of bile into the subhepatic space. Peritonitis, or more commonly subhepatic abscess, may result.
  d. Biliary-enteric fistula and gallstone ileus are complications of cholelithiasis, cystic duct obstruction, recurrent cholecystitis, adhesions to the surrounding viscera, perforation, fistula formation, and passage of the stone into the bowel.
    (1) The **site of fistula** with the gallbladder is most commonly the duodenum, but the colon or any other intra-abdominal viscera may be penetrated.
    (2) Site of bowel obstruction
      (a) As the stone travels in the gastrointestinal lumen, the terminal ileum is the commonest site of obstruction as this is the narrowest portion of the small bowel. Stones smaller than 2–3 cm are usually passed per rectum.
      (b) If a stone is passed free into the peritoneal cavity, extraluminal obstruction secondary to inflammation and adhesions can occur anywhere.
    (3) Clinical presentation
      (a) This is a disease of the elderly, and concomitant multisystem disease is common.
      (b) The patient presents with symptoms of small bowel obstruction (i.e., nausea, vomiting, obstipation, pain, and distention).
      (c) About 25% of patients have symptoms of acute cholecystitis immediately preceding the episode of obstruction. About 70% of the patients have a history of cholelithiasis.
    (4) Diagnosis
      (a) The correct diagnosis is made preoperatively in fewer than 25% of cases.
      (b) The diagnosis is suggested by the history and by plain films of the abdomen. These may show small bowel obstruction accompanied by air in the biliary tree, or a radiopaque stone in the right lower quadrant (seen in only 15% of cases).
    (5) Treatment
      (a) As these patients are often extremely ill, emergency laparotomy may permit only localization of the stone, proximal enterotomy, stone extraction, and closure of the enterotomy.
      (b) The whole small bowel, common bile duct, and gallbladder must be palpated for stones as recurrent gallstone ileus (due to other stones) develops in 5%–9% of patients.
      (c) Cholecystectomy and closure of the biliary fistula can be performed either concomitantly, or after an interval, depending on the patient's condition.

5. Treatment of cholecystitis. Cholecystectomy is designed to remove the gallbladder without damage to structures in the porta hepatis. Key features include:
  a. In the absence of severe inflammation, the cystic artery and duct can be identified early. Otherwise, they are not dissected until the gallbladder has been dissected off of the liver from the top downward.
  b. A common bile duct cholangiogram via the cystic duct (**operative cholangiogram**) is performed by filling the ducts with radiopaque dye and taking an x-ray. Operative cholangiography is done whenever there is suspicion that stones may have escaped the gallbladder into the common bile duct.
  c. Cholecystectomy can be performed via open or laparoscopic techniques.

   d. Cholecystostomy is an alternative procedure when extensive inflammation makes cholecystectomy too dangerous. In this procedure, the gallbladder fundus is opened, bile and stones are removed, and a tube is placed in the gallbladder for external drainage.

E. Postcholecystectomy syndrome is the term given to symptoms that develop after or persist despite cholecystectomy.

   1. In patients who have undergone cholecystectomy for chronic cholecystitis and cholelithiasis, postcholecystectomy symptoms are usually **extrabiliary** in origin and caused by:
   a. Hiatal hernia
   b. Peptic ulcer
   c. Pancreatitis
   d. Irritable bowel
   e. Food intolerance

   2. Symptoms may be **biliary** in origin and caused by:
   a. A stone in the common bile duct
   b. A stone in the stump of the cystic duct
   c. Stenosis of the sphincter of Oddi
   d. Biliary stricture

F. Bile duct disorders

   1. Choledocholithiasis (stones in the common bile duct) can be single or multiple and are found in 10%–20% of patients who undergo cholecystectomy. Most stones are formed in the gallbladder and pass into the duct. However, **primary common duct stones** can form in the absence of a gallbladder.
   a. Clinical presentation. Some patients are asymptomatic. Most patients present with right upper quadrant pain that radiates to the back and right shoulder, intermittent obstructive jaundice, acholic stools, or bilirubinuria.
   b. Diagnosis
      (1) In contrast to neoplastic obstruction of the common bile duct, the gallbladder is not palpable.
      (2) Diagnostic studies include ultrasonography, transhepatic cholangiography, or a radionuclide scan.
      (3) Liver function test results are consistent with obstructive jaundice and include elevations in bilirubin and alkaline phosphatase.
   c. Treatment involves cholecystectomy, choledochotomy (opening the common duct), common bile duct exploration, stone removal, T-tube placement, and T-tube operative cholangiography.
      (1) Operative cholangiography has decreased the need for common bile duct exploration but increased the proportion of positive explorations, that is, explorations in which stones are found.
      (2) The only absolute indication for common bile duct exploration is a palpable stone in the common bile duct.
      (3) When any of the following are present, operative cholangiography is performed, although these were at one time considered to be indications for duct exploration:
         (a) Increased size of the common bile duct
         (b) History of jaundice
         (c) Small stones in the gallbladder with a large cystic duct
         (d) A history of cholangitis or pancreatitis
      (4) Common bile duct exploration is not necessary if the operative cholangiogram is of good quality and demonstrates both:
         (a) No filling defects
         (b) Free flow of contrast medium into the duodenum
      (5) Common bile duct exploration is indicated if the operative cholangiogram shows either:
         (a) Filling defects within the intra- or extrahepatic biliary tree
         (b) Obstruction of the flow of bile into the duodenum
   d. Complications. Stones that remain after surgery complicate up to 10% of common bile duct explorations.
      (1) No treatment is necessary for small stones as they usually pass spontaneously.

(2) If stones are large, treatment options are:
(a) Chemical dissolution by intraduct administration of sodium cholate or mono-octanoin
(b) Mechanical extraction under radiographic guidance
(3) Primary or recurrent common bile duct stones can be treated surgically with a **biliary-enteric** connection to allow other stones easy passage out of the biliary tree. The two commonest are choledochoduodenostomy and transduodenal sphincteroplasty.

2. **Cholangitis,** or **infection of the bile ducts,** is a potentially life-threatening disease that results from concurrent biliary infection and obstruction. *E. coli* is the commonest offending organism.
   a. **Etiology.** Benign postoperative strictures and common bile duct stones account for 60% of the cases. Neoplasms, sclerosing cholangitis, plugged biliary drainage tubes, and biliary contrast studies are other causes.
   b. **Clinical presentation. Charcot's triad** of fever, jaundice, and right upper quadrant pain is present in 70% of cases. In severe cases, hypotension may be present.
   c. **Treatment** includes antibiotics, resuscitation with fluids and electrolytes, and relief of the obstruction (usually surgery).
   d. **Prognosis** depends on the cause of the obstruction; from best prognosis to worst, the order is stones, benign stricture, sclerosing cholangitis, and neoplasm.

3. **Primary sclerosing cholangitis** is a disease of unknown etiology that affects the biliary tract, resulting in stenosis or obstruction of the ductal system. Progressive obstruction, if not relieved, results in biliary cirrhosis and liver failure.
   a. **Clinical presentation**
      (1) Symptoms and signs include right upper quadrant pain or painless jaundice, usually without fever or chills, pruritus, fatigue, nausea, and symptoms of hepatic failure.
      (2) Other inflammatory conditions, particularly ulcerative colitis, may be present.
   b. **Histology.** The bile ducts show edema and areas of inflammation and fibrosis.
   c. **Diagnosis**
      (1) The diagnosis is made either by exploratory laparotomy and common bile duct exploration or preferably by endoscopic retrograde cholangiography or percutaneous transhepatic cholangiography.
      (2) Criteria needed to fulfill the diagnosis are:
         (a) Thickening and stenosis of a major portion of the biliary ductal system
         (b) Absence of prior surgery, choledocholithiasis, malignancy, or congenital biliary anomalies
         (c) No evidence of primary liver disease, particularly primary biliary cirrhosis
   d. **Treatment.** Operative management is dependent upon the level of bile duct involvement and the amount of fibrosis present. Restoration of adequate and permanent biliary drainage is the goal of operative management.
      (1) **Internal biliary drainage,** via either a hepaticoenteric or choledochoenteric anastomosis, is the preferred method of management. This is successful only when the major area of involvement is the extrahepatic bile ducts.
      (2) **External biliary drainage,** using a T tube or other percutaneous stent, establishes adequate drainage initially, but inevitably it becomes contaminated and results in bacterial cholangitis.
      (3) Cholecystectomy is performed only when gallbladder disease requires it.
   e. **Postoperative treatment** is strongly dependent upon the presence of preoperative sepsis and the adequacy of drainage. Steroids are not beneficial and could potentially complicate the postoperative course.
   f. **Prognosis** is poorly defined at present. If the liver parenchyma has been damaged or if the intrahepatic ducts are significantly involved, only hepatic transplantation offers a real chance of longevity, and this procedure is only possible when the patient is free of sepsis.

4. **Fibrosis of the sphincter of Oddi** is a disorder of uncertain etiology that causes colicky right upper quadrant pain, nausea, vomiting, and frequently recurrent pancreatitis. Treatment is by endoscopic papillotomy or transduodenal sphincteroplasty.

G. Neoplasms

1. **Benign tumors of the gallbladder** are rare. They include papilloma, adenomyoma, fibroma, lipoma, myoma, myxoma, and carcinoid.

2. Carcinoma of the gallbladder accounts for 4% of all carcinomas. It is the commonest cancer of the biliary tract and occurs in 1% of all patients undergoing biliary tract surgery.

  a. Etiology. Although the cause is not known, 90% of the patients have cholelithiasis. About 80% of the tumors are adenocarcinomas. Metastases occur by lymphatic spread to the pancreatic, duodenal, and choledochal nodes, and by direct extension to the liver.

  b. Clinical presentation. The commonest complaint is right upper quadrant pain. This is often associated with nausea and vomiting. The diagnosis is rarely made preoperatively.

  c. Treatment. The only truly curable cases are those where the tumor is found incidentally at cholecystectomy for other reasons. If there is microscopic invasion of the gallbladder, cholecystectomy with wedge resection of the liver and regional lymphadenectomy may improve the survival.

  d. Prognosis is poor: The 5-year survival rate ranges from 0–10%.

3. Common bile duct malignant tumors are rare and difficult to cure.

  a. Clinical presentation

  (1) The patient usually complains of pruritus, anorexia, weight loss, and an aching right upper quadrant pain. Jaundice is usually severe.

  (2) The following diseases may be associated with this malignancy:

  (a) Sclerosing cholangitis

  (b) Chronic parasitic infection of the bile ducts

  (c) Gallstones (present in 18%–65% of cases)

  (d) Prior exposure to Thorotrast

  b. Diagnosis may be made by percutaneous transhepatic cholangiography or ERCP. Both procedures are capable of biopsy for pathologic examination.

  c. Pathology. These tumors are called cholangiocarcinoma.

  (1) The gross pathologic finding is a mass involving a portion of the bile ducts. The microscopic appearance is that of adenocarcinoma, although the distinction from sclerosing cholangitis may be difficult.

  (2) The tumor may be located in the distal common bile duct (one-third of cases), the common hepatic duct or cystic duct (one-third of cases), or the right or left hepatic duct. When the confluence of the hepatic ducts is involved, the tumor is termed a **Klatskin tumor**.

  (3) The tumor initially metastasizes to the regional lymph nodes (16% of cases), spreads by direct extension into the liver (14%), or metastasizes to the liver (10%).

  d. Treatment. The management of common bile duct tumors is generally surgical, although fewer than 10% are resectable at the time of the initial diagnosis.

  (1) Tumors in the distal duct may be resected by pancreaticoduodenectomy (Whipple procedure) with biliary and gastrointestinal reconstruction. More proximal lesions can sometimes be locally resected with biliary reconstruction. The average length of survival after resection is 23 months. Postoperative radiation may improve the life expectancy.

  (2) Unresectable lesions should have rigid stents placed to provide palliation of the biliary obstructive symptoms.

  (a) Laparotomy with no bypass is associated with an average survival time of less than 6 months.

  (b) With stenting, the average survival time is 19 months.

  (i) In this procedure, either a transhepatic stent is placed percutaneously or a U tube is placed surgically.

  (ii) The U tube passes from the skin, through the liver, through the tumor, into the common bile duct, and then out through the abdominal wall.

  e. Prognosis

  (1) Metastatic spread of the tumor is usually slow and is not responsible for death.

  (2) The usual cause of death is related to the following:

  (a) Progressive biliary cirrhosis due to inadequate biliary drainage

  (b) Persistent intrahepatic infection and abscess formation

  (c) General debility

  (d) Sepsis

H. Choledochal cysts are congenital malformations of the pancreaticobiliary tree.

  1. Classification

  a. Type I: fusiform dilatation of the common bile duct

  b. Type II: diverticulum of the common bile duct
  c. Type III: choledochocele involving the intraduodenal portion of the common bile duct
  d. Type IV: cystic involvement of the intrahepatic bile ducts (**Caroli's disease**)

2. **The pathogenesis** is not known. Pathologically, patients show cystic dilatation of the common bile duct, a normal liver parenchyma, and (except in Caroli's disease) a normal intrahepatic biliary tree, and partial obstruction of the terminal common bile duct.

3. **Clinical presentation.** The commonest presenting symptom is intermittent jaundice. The classic triad of pain, jaundice, and an abdominal mass occurs in only 30% of the cases.

4. **Diagnosis.** Ultrasonography is the best initial investigative study followed by radionuclide scanning. Transhepatic cholangiography and ERCP can define the extent of the disease but are not necessary.

5. **Treatment.** Due to the risk of malignancy, cyst excision (rather than bypass) is the cornerstone of surgery.
   a. Type I patients are treated with cholecystectomy, cyst excision, and a Roux-en-Y choledochojejunostomy.
   b. Type II patients are treated by excision of the common bile duct diverticulum.
   d. Type III patients are treated by cyst excision and choledochoduodenostomy or by transduodenal sphincteroplasty.
   e. The type IV anomaly may be fatal. Patients require liver transplantation.

I. Congenital biliary atresia (see Chapter 29 IX B)

J. Trauma

1. **Gallbladder injuries** are uncommon but are seen after both penetrating and nonpenetrating trauma. Associated visceral injuries are common and most frequently (72%) involve the liver.
   a. Types of injuries to the gallbladder include contusions, avulsion, rupture, and traumatic cholecystitis.
   b. Clinical presentation. Right upper quadrant pain, right chest pain, biliary leakage through a penetrating wound, and shock are the commonest presenting symptoms.
   c. Diagnosis is most frequently made at laparotomy. A peritoneal tap may be negative.

2. **Extrahepatic bile duct injuries**
   a. Operative injury. Most extrahepatic bile duct injuries are iatrogenic, occurring during cholecystectomy.
      (1) Clinical presentation. Only 15% of intraoperative injuries are diagnosed at the time of surgery, and 85% present days to years later with progressive jaundice, cholangitis, or cirrhosis and its complications.
      (2) Diagnosis is by transhepatic cholangiography or ERCP.
      (3) Treatment. End-to-end (duct-to-duct) anastomosis may be done at the time of initial injury; otherwise a Roux-en-Y choledochojejunostomy is necessary.
      (4) The mortality rate after repair of a chronic biliary stricture is 8%–10%, and death is usually secondary to liver failure.
   b. Other extrahepatic bile duct injuries almost always accompany other visceral injuries and result from trauma, such as gunshot wounds. Isolated bile duct injuries are rare.
      (1) Clinical presentation is the same as those in gallbladder injuries.
      (2) Diagnosis is made at laparotomy.
      (3) Treatment, besides administration of antibiotics, involves meticulous exploration of the ducts. Either a primary end-to-end (duct-to-duct) anastomosis, or, more commonly, a Roux-en-Y choledochojejunostomy is appropriate.
   c. Intraperitoneal extravasation of bile
      (1) The extravasation of **sterile bile** results in chemical peritonitis.
         (a) This may be a mild peritonitis, producing ascites, or a localized collection.
         (b) Continuous outpouring of sterile bile may produce an extensive chemical peritonitis and shock.
      (2) Infected intraperitoneal bile induces a fulminant and frequently fatal peritonitis.

15
Pancreas

Jerome J. Vernick

I. ANATOMY. The pancreas (Figure 15-1) is a retroperitoneal, pistol-shaped organ. The handle of the pistol lies in the duodenal C-loop, and the barrel extends to the left upper quadrant. The average **weight** of the pancreas is 85 g, and the usual **length** is 12–15 cm. The normal anteroposterior thickness of the head is less than 2.5 cm; the neck, 1.5 cm; the body, 2 cm; and the tail, 2.5 cm.

A. Relations

    1. The head of the pancreas lies over the aorta and under the stomach and transverse colon, posteromedially to the inferior vena cava.
        a. The superior limit of the head is the **portal vein**. The anterior limit is the **gastroduodenal artery**.
        b. The **common bile duct** courses posteriorly to the head of the pancreas and partially within it.
        c. The head of the pancreas has a common blood supply with the medial wall of the **duodenal C-loop**. The serosal surface of the duodenum is intimately related to the capsule of the pancreas in that area.

    2. The uncinate process lies posteriorly to the superior mesenteric vein and anteriorly to the inferior vena cava.

    3. The tail of the pancreas is in close relation to the spleen and most accessory spleens and contains the splenic artery and vein (see Chapter 22 VII C).

    4. The neck of the pancreas lies at the confluence of the splenic and inferior mesenteric veins. The **posterior aspect of the pancreas** lies over this confluence at the origin of the portal vein.

    5. The anterior aspect of the pancreas lies against the posterior wall of the **stomach,** forming the posterior border of the lesser omental bursa, or lesser sac.

B. Vasculature

    1. The splenic artery and vein provide the **blood supply** to the pancreas. The pancreatic body and tail are related to these vessels, which run posteriorly and superiorly into the hilus of the spleen.

    2. The **superior mesenteric artery** and the **superior mesenteric vein** exit below the pancreas at the junction of the body and head and are surrounded by the uncinate process.

C. Functions. The **pancreatic ducts** drain pancreatic secretions into the duodenum. They comprise two separate systems:

    1. The duct of Wirsung, which empties into the ampulla of Vater in conjunction with the common bile duct, is the major system.

    2. The duct of Santorini, which empties into a minor papilla approximately 2 cm above and medial to the ampulla of Vater, is the minor system.

II. PANCREATITIS is an inflammatory process in the pancreas.

A. Overview

    1. Classification
        a. Pancreatitis was classified into four different categories in 1963 to clarify the different

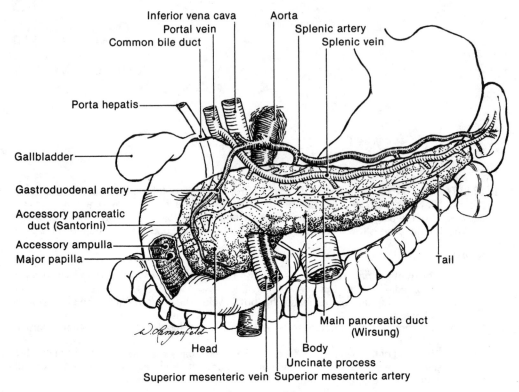

Inferior vena cava — Aorta
Portal vein — Splenic artery
Common bile duct — Splenic vein

Porta hepatis

Gallbladder

Gastroduodenal artery

Accessory pancreatic duct (Santorini)

Accessory ampulla

Major papilla — Tail

Main pancreatic duct (Wirsung)

Head — Body

Uncinate process

Superior mesenteric vein Superior mesenteric artery

Figure 15-1. Anatomy of the pancreas.

syndromes that are seen and to improve the standardization of treatment and prognosis. The four categories of pancreatitis are as follows:

(1) **Acute pancreatitis** arises in a previously asymptomatic patient and subsides to normalcy after treatment.

(2) **Acute relapsing pancreatitis** is a series of recurrent episodes of acute pancreatitis in an otherwise asymptomatic patient. A quiescent, asymptomatic phase always precedes and follows each attack.

(3) **Chronic relapsing pancreatitis** is a chronic inflammation of the pancreas with chemical evidence of pancreatitis, which fluctuates in its intensity and does not return to normal.

(4) **Chronic pancreatitis** shows unrelenting symptoms that are due to inflammation and fibrosis of the pancreas; the pancreatic duct and parenchyma usually show calcification. Chronic pancreatitis is often associated with malabsorption and even with pancreatic endocrine insufficiency.

b. Other classification systems based on etiology and pathology are also in use.

2. **Etiology.** Approximately 75% of pancreatitis cases can be explained on the basis of biliary tract disease or alcohol abuse, although the exact mechanism for the production of pancreatitis remains theoretical.

a. Biliary pancreatitis is thought to be induced by the inflammation that results from continued passage of stones through a common channel.

(1) The pancreatic duct and the bile duct empty into a common papilla, which is subject to trauma in a patient with biliary calculi.

(2) The entire common channel can be obstructed if a large calculus becomes impacted in the papilla. This can cause reflux of bile into the pancreatic duct, and experiments have shown that such reflux can induce pancreatitis. However, it is not clear whether this actually occurs in humans.

b. Alcohol is thought to cause pancreatitis by inducing an increase in gastric acidity.

(1) The combination of alcohol plus gastric acid causes:

(a) Increased pancreatic secretion

(b) Spasm of the sphincter of Oddi

(2) The increased intraductal pressure combined with the sphincteric spasm then presumably results in pancreatitis.

B. Acute pancreatitis

1. **Clinical presentation** of acute pancreatitis may vary from mild abdominal discomfort to profound shock with hypotension and hypoxemia. Usually the patient presents with epigastric pain that radiates to the back and is associated with nausea and vomiting. Findings vary with the severity of the inflammatory process.

   a. Most patients have mild to moderate abdominal tenderness.

   b. In severe cases, a rigid abdomen with epigastric guarding, rebound tenderness, and marked abdominal pain may be present.

   c. Severe pancreatic inflammation and necrosis may cause **retroperitoneal hemorrhage,** which can lead to large third-space fluid losses, hypovolemia, hypotension, tachycardia, and blood dissection along different tissue planes.

      (1) When blood dissection extends to the flank tissues, resulting in flank ecchymoses, it is known as **Grey-Turner's sign**.

      (2) When blood dissects up the falciform ligament and creates a periumbilical ecchymosis, it is known as **Cullen's sign**.

2. **History.** There is often a history of recent consumption of a heavy meal, many times with generous quantities of alcoholic beverages. The pain typically begins 1–4 hours after a meal and is often less severe when the patient sits slumped forward.

3. **Diagnosis** of acute pancreatitis is aided by the following studies:

   a. Serum amylase level. This is elevated in 95% of patients with acute pancreatitis.

      (1) Approximately 5% of all amylase determinations are falsely positive, and only 75% of patients with abdominal pain and an increased amylase level have pancreatitis.

      (2) The rise in amylase level is not proportional to the severity of the pancreatitis. Some inferences, however, can be made from the degree of elevation.

         (a) An amylase level over 1000 Somogyi units usually indicates biliary tract disease with pancreatitis.

         (b) An amylase level between 200 and 500 units often indicates alcoholic pancreatitis. Some 17% of patients with amylase levels in this range have no other evidence of pancreatitis.

      (3) The pancreas must be intact and functional to synthesize amylase and release it into the circulation. Thus, patients with acute pancreatitis superimposed on chronic pancreatitis may not demonstrate a rise in serum amylase.

      (4) A significant amount of circulating amylase is not of pancreatic origin. The major alternative source is salivary.

   b. Amylase:creatinine clearance ratio. Amylase determinations are more sensitive when the amylase clearance rate is compared to the creatinine clearance rate and a ratio is established.

      (1) An amylase:creatinine clearance ratio above 5 is strongly suggestive of pancreatitis.

      (2) Using this ratio avoids the problem of rapid renal clearance of amylase, which tends to reduce serum levels below the point where a simple serum amylase determination would be positive.

      (3) Impaired renal function affects the creatinine clearance rate sooner than the amylase clearance rate. Even in this situation, however, the amylase:creatinine clearance ratio appears to be more sensitive than the serum amylase level if urine specimens are collected for at least 1 hour.

   c. Radiographic imaging

      (1) Plain films of the upper abdomen are relatively insensitive with regard to diagnosing pancreatitis. Significant findings include the following:

         (a) Calcification in the area of the lesser sac and pancreas may indicate chronic pancreatitis, which is most often seen in association with alcoholism.

         (b) A gas collection in the lesser sac suggests abscess formation in or around the pancreas.

         (c) Blurred psoas shadows from retroperitoneal pancreatic necrosis may be seen on plain films.

         (d) Soft tissue shadows and gas-containing viscera may be visibly displaced by collections and edema in the lesser sac and structures adjacent to the pancreas.

         (e) An area of colonic spasm adjacent to an inflamed pancreas will cause the gas in the transverse colon to end abruptly (the "cutoff" sign).

         (f) Focal duodenal and jejunal ileus in the area of the pancreas can cause the "reversed 3" or "inverted 3" sign.

      (2) Barium studies may demonstrate upper gastrointestinal abnormalities.

         (a) The duodenal C-loop may be widened by pancreatic edema.

        (b) Hypotonic duodenography may demonstrate the **"pad" sign,** a smoothing out or obliteration of the duodenal mucosal folds by the edematous pancreas and the inflammatory response on the medial aspect of the C-loop.

    (3) **Angiography** is useful for delineating pancreatic and hepatic blood supply prior to radical surgery. Diagnostic aspects have been superceded by computed tomography (CT scan) and magnetic resonance imaging (MRI).

  d. **Ultrasound imaging** of the pancreas is especially useful in the diagnosis of pancreatitis.

    (1) Changes from the normal anatomy of the pancreas and its vascular landmarks can be delineated.

        (a) Acute pancreatitis is suggested by swelling beyond the normal anteroposterior thickness and loss of tissue planes between the pancreas and the splenic vein.

        (b) Other anomalies of the pancreas may also be seen. For example, a change in duct size or calcification may be shown.

        (c) Chronic pancreatitis is often manifested by the presence of calcification or pseudocysts containing fluid or showing a complex cystic structure.

        (d) Ascites, which is easily diagnosed by ultrasound, may or may not be present in chronic pancreatitis.

    (2) Various pancreatic disorders can change the ultrasound echogenicity.

        (a) Most diseases decrease the echogenicity in the pancreas; this is due to the presence of edema and inflammation. Tumors are also often hypoechogenic.

        (b) Increased echogenicity is generally due to gas or calcification.

    (3) Fluid densities lying within the pancreas indicate cysts, abscesses, or possibly lymphoma.

    (4) Ultrasound may also demonstrate the presence of gallbladder pathology, such as cholecystitis, cholelithiasis, or a dilated common bile duct.

    (5) Ultrasound has a major limitation in that it cannot be performed when excessive bowel gas is present as occurs with an ileus.

  e. **CT scan** of the pancreas may also be helpful. It provides higher resolution than ultrasonography, and it is not limited by blocking of intestinal gas.

    (1) The criteria for findings are similar to those described for ultrasound.

    (2) Dilute barium ingestion may help to outline the pancreas.

4. **Prognosis** in acute pancreatitis is aided by certain signs, which are associated with a higher mortality rate and are, therefore, useful prognostic indicators (Ranson's sign).

  a. **Signs at admission**

    (1) Patient's age over 55 years

    (2) White blood cell count over 16,000/mm³ of blood

    (3) Fasting blood sugar level over 200 mg/dl

    (4) Lactic dehydrogenase (LDH) over 350 units/ml

    (5) Glutamic oxaloacetic transaminase (GOT) over 250 units/ml

  b. **Signs 48 hours after admission**

    (1) A 10% drop in hematocrit

    (2) An increase of 5 mg/dl in blood urea nitrogen (BUN)

    (3) Serum calcium levels under 8 mg/dl

    (4) Arterial oxygen partial pressure (PaO_2) below 60 mm Hg

    (5) Anion base deficit greater than 4 mEq/L

    (6) Third-space fluid loss greater than 6 L

  c. **Determining prognosis.** If 0–2 of the above signs are present, the mortality rate is 0.9%; if 7–8 signs are present, it is 100%.

    (1) The poor prognostic signs at 48 hours are generally related to the severe local effects of pancreatitis, which result in massive third-space fluid loss and hemorrhage.

    (2) Systemic effects, such as shock and hypoxia, may also be a consequence of circulating toxins released by the pancreas.

5. **Medical treatment of acute pancreatitis.** Certain measures are considered standard. Not all of them are indicated in each case, however, and the patient's symptoms dictate much of the treatment required.

  a. **Nasogastric suction** is used to control nausea and vomiting, decrease pancreatic stimulation, and decrease gastrointestinal distention from an ileus. It also makes the patient more comfortable, although it does not appear to shorten the hospital stay.

  b. **Intravenous fluids** are used to replace the third-space fluid loss from edema and extravasation into the peripancreatic spaces. Crystalloid solutions are usually adequate.

    (1) Monitoring similar to that for burn patients should be initiated.

(2) This should include the use of a Foley catheter to measure urine output.

(3) In severe cases with unstable hemodynamics, the patient's fluid status should be monitored accurately with a Swan-Ganz catheter.

c. Antibiotics may reduce the risk of abscess formation and of lesser sac collections, which often progress to abscess formation.

(1) The early use of antibiotics is thought to promote the maturation of these collections into pseudocysts (see II E) rather than abscesses.

(2) Antibiotics also act as prophylaxis against cholangitis, which can develop if a swollen pancreatic head obstructs the biliary tract.

(3) If the pancreatitis is due to biliary calculi, the bile is almost certainly contaminated with bacteria, and antibiotics are indicated.

d. PaO$_2$ monitoring and chest x-ray. In severe pancreatitis, respiratory distress is common as are **pleural effusions**. These are more often on the left and contain high concentrations of amylase. The PaO$_2$ should, therefore, be monitored closely in patients with severe pancreatitis, and serial chest x-rays should be obtained to rule out the presence of effusions and parenchymal disease.

e. Withhold oral feedings until laboratory test results return to normal, and pain is gone for 48 hours. Exacerbations of the pancreatitis are common with premature feedings and removal of the nasogastric tube.

6. Surgery in acute pancreatitis

a. Indications for surgery

(1) To confirm the diagnosis in severe cases that do not respond to medical management

(a) The symptoms of severe acute pancreatitis can be mimicked by visceral perforation, mesenteric arterial occlusion, and other intra-abdominal catastrophes.

(b) Surgery may be needed to establish the diagnosis before the situation is irreversible.

(2) To relieve biliary or pancreatic duct obstruction

(a) Early biliary tract surgery may increase the mortality rate in severe pancreatitis. If possible, therefore, surgery should be delayed until the pancreatitis has subsided. The offending stone will have passed by the time of exploration in more than 90% of cases.

(b) If the patient's status continues to deteriorate, surgical exploration may become necessary.

(i) Cholecystostomy or common bile duct drainage should be considered with definitive dissection deferred, when there are acute severe inflammatory changes in the duodenum and region of the ampulla.

(ii) Definitive biliary tract surgery to correct the cause of the pancreatitis (e.g., removal of common bile duct stones or gallstones; repair of the sphincter of Oddi) should be done during the same admission as for the treatment of the acute pancreatitis to prevent recurrence.

(3) To drain the lesser sac

(a) Pancreatic or lesser sac drainage increases morbidity if it is done before septic complications have occurred. It is not effective as a prophylactic measure.

(b) Drainage has been shown to improve the prognosis when sepsis has occurred and lesser sac collections are present.

(c) For drainage of established lesser sac abscesses, drains can be inserted after wide opening of the lesser omentum. Irrigation catheters can be used as part of the therapeutic plan.

b. Operative procedures

(1) Resection for acute pancreatitis is a dangerous procedure and is not indicated. It has not been shown to decrease morbidity; in some studies, resection increased the mortality rate.

(2) Peritoneal lavage may be useful in excluding other severe intra-abdominal processes and may be therapeutic in severe pancreatitis. However, peritoneal lavage appears to improve early mortality rates but not ultimate survival rates in acute severe pancreatitis.

(a) Catheters may be placed percutaneously, and antibiotics may be included in the lavage solution.

(b) Peritoneal lavage can be undertaken as part of a laparotomy performed for diagnosis and lesser sac exploration.

      (c) Complications include a deterioration of pulmonary function, which may be compromised by abdominal distention from the dialysis solutions.

      (d) A high glucose load in the dialysis solution may induce severe hyperglycemia.

C. Relapsing pancreatitis frequently occurs in nonalcoholic patients and results from biliary tract disease—either calculi in the ducts or inflammation and spasm of the sphincter of Oddi.

  1. Diagnosis of relapsing pancreatitis may be made by demonstrating the presence of biliary stones or biliary sphincter dysfunction.

    a. Ultrasound (see II B 3 d) is useful for diagnosing biliary calculi.

    b. Microscopic examination of the bile is useful.

      (1) Bile is aspirated through a suction tube placed in the duodenum.

      (2) The bile is examined for white blood cells, cholesterol crystals, and microspheroliths.

      (3) These are signs of occult biliary disease and are an indication for cholecystectomy.

    c. Provocative testing (i.e., the **Nardi test**) can be done to determine if narcotic-induced stimulation or spasm will reproduce the abdominal pain and amylase elevation.

      (1) Morphine and neostigmine are given intramuscularly, and baseline levels are obtained for GOT and glutamic pyruvic transaminase (GPT), γ-glutamyl transpeptidase (GGT), amylase, and lipase.

      (2) Determinations are repeated at hourly intervals for 4 hours, and a final determination is made at 8 hours.

      (3) The test is positive if biliary pain is reproduced within 15–20 minutes after the injection and if the enzyme levels increase at least four times over the baseline levels.

      (4) In the presence of sphincteric disease:

        (a) Amylase levels will rise whether or not the gallbladder is present.

        (b) Liver-related enzymes will not rise if the gallbladder is present and can distend to relieve pressure on the hepatic ductal system.

        (c) The test can, therefore, be used to infer sphincteric disease in any pancreatic or biliary ductal system if the gallbladder is absent.

      (5) Although the test is controversial, it has been accurate in the diagnosis of perisphincteric disease.

      (6) At the time of surgery, the test results can be confirmed by measuring the pressure and flow in the common bile duct.

    d. Ultrasonic observation on duct dilatation after secretin administration has shown promise in the diagnosis of sphincteric disease.

  2. Treatment of relapsing pancreatitis is based on the etiology.

    a. In a patient with biliary calculi, the following procedures may be performed:

      (1) Cholecystectomy

      (2) Common bile duct exploration

      (3) Biliary manometry

      (4) Sphincteroplasty plus pancreaticobiliary septum resection, if indicated

    b. The **treatment of perisphincteric disease** is removal of the gallbladder, if it is present, and a wide sphincteroplasty that includes the pancreaticobiliary septum. The results have been very good in patients with a positive Nardi test.

    c. Many patients have had a cholecystectomy in the past, yet continue to have recurrent pancreatitis, biliary tract disease symptoms, or both.

      (1) These patients often have a positive provocative test and can be treated successfully by sphincteroplasty.

      (2) Patients with a negative provocative test require further workup, including endoscopic retrograde cholangiopancreatography (ERCP; see III A 3 b). Alcohol abuse should be ruled out.

    d. Patients with severe intrinsic pancreatic disease respond poorly to sphincteroplasty.

D. Chronic pancreatitis is often progressive.

  1. Pathologic findings include fibrosis and calcification throughout the gland.

    a. Early pancreatic changes may consist of plugging of the small pancreatic ducts with proteinaceous material containing eosinophils.

    b. With progression of the disease, the calcification becomes prominent and multiple areas of ductal dilatation may result.

    c. The ductal dilatation in its end stages produces a "chain-of-lakes" appearance.

    d. Common bile duct obstruction or duodenal obstruction can occur in advanced cases of chronic pancreatitis as a result of inflammation in surrounding areas.

2. **The etiology** is almost always alcohol-related. There are, however, congenital anomalies that can produce chronic ductal obstruction and chronic pancreatitis.

3. **Clinical presentation**
   a. A history of unrelenting pain is usual in advanced cases of chronic pancreatitis. The pain is usually the major indication for surgical intervention.
   b. Pancreatic damage may be severe enough to cause pancreatic endocrine insufficiency with impaired glucose tolerance or true diabetes.
   c. Exocrine pancreatic insufficiency results in malabsorption with consequent weight loss and steatorrhea.
   d. Plain films may show the calcifications in the ductal system or may aid in delineating neighboring areas that are caught in the inflammatory process.
   e. Severe disease in the head of the pancreas can mimic carcinoma and cause bile obstruction.

4. **Medical treatment** of chronic pancreatitis consists of:
   a. Analgesia
   b. Endocrine replacement as needed
   c. Exocrine replacement with pancreatic enzymes, such as pancrelipase (Viokase or Pancrease) or cholecystokinin (pancreozymin). High-dose pancreatic enzymes (i.e., 5 g four times daily) can suppress pancreatic secretion by feedback phenomenon.
   d. General measures, such as avoidance of alcoholic beverages and correction of malnutrition

5. **Surgical treatment** of chronic pancreatitis depends on the condition of the pancreatic ducts, as determined by ERCP. If ERCP is not possible and the patient must be operated upon, operative pancreatograms can be obtained.
   a. **Puestow operation.** A dilated, "chain-of-lakes" duct is treated by wide unroofing of the duct and dilated ductules with drainage of the entire open pancreas into a defunctionalized jejunal loop. A side-to-side procedure may be used, or an invagination in which the pancreas is placed into the jejunal loop.
   b. **Distal pancreatectomy** is used to treat a distal ductal obstruction.
   c. **Duval operation.** A proximal ductal obstruction is usually treated by amputating the tail of the pancreas and draining the pancreas retrogradely into a defunctionalized jejunal loop.
   d. For a patient with severe pain and a fibrotic, nondilated duct, possible surgical procedures include:
      (1) **Child operation,** which is a 95% pancreatectomy
      (2) **Splanchnicectomy,** either abdominal or thoracic
         (a) This merely divides the splanchnic nerves and serves only to relieve the pain of pancreatitis with no direct effect on the underlying disorder.
         (b) It should be noted that a splanchnicectomy also eradicates the pain from appendicitis and other intra-abdominal problems, which may lead to the delayed diagnosis of an abdominal emergency.

E. **Pseudocyst** is a late complication of pancreatitis.

1. **Pathologic findings**
   a. The pseudocyst begins as a lesser sac collection and forms as a result of fibrosis, thickening, and organization of the organs bordering the collection.
   b. The pseudocyst is not lined by epithelium and consists only of the inflammatory response of the neighboring organs.
   c. The organs forming the walls are the stomach, duodenum, colon, and transverse mesocolon. The major organ involved is generally the stomach, which forms the anterior surface of the pseudocyst.
   d. Maturation of the pseudocyst takes 3–5 weeks. It is not truly formed until the walls are sufficiently organized to become firm anatomic structures.
   e. The natural history of the pseudocyst depends on its size. Small pseudocysts may resolve; large pseudocysts with mature organized walls generally do not resolve.

2. **Clinical presentation**
   a. During the maturation phase, the patient recovers from a bout of pancreatitis but develops a persistent elevation of amylase, a low-grade fever, a minimally elevated white blood cell count, and chronic pain.

b. Continuous minor bleeding into the pseudocyst tends to cause a gradual decrease in hemoglobin and hematocrit.

c. Pseudocysts are usually diagnosed by ultrasound or CT scan.

3. Treatment

a. The goal is to allow the maturation phase to continue until the walls of the pseudocyst have matured.

    (1) The patient is generally treated with total parenteral nutrition or an elemental diet for 3–4 weeks, until maturation has occurred. Prematurely starting the patient on a full diet is likely to cause an exacerbation of the pancreatitis.

    (2) Maturation-phase treatment sometimes must be cut short due to sepsis or to hemorrhage within the pseudocyst.

    (3) Small pseudocysts may resolve with medical treatment.

b. Mature pseudocysts are treated surgically by:

    (1) Internal drainage, if possible.

        (a) The best approach is through the anterior wall of the stomach to locate the firm connection that usually exists between the posterior stomach and the pseudocyst.

            (i) An opening is made between the stomach and the pseudocyst, and the wall of the opening is sutured for hemostasis.

            (ii) The pseudocyst then drains into the stomach and generally resolves.

        (b) If the pseudocyst is not fixed to an organ that lends itself to internal drainage, a defunctionalized loop of jejunum may be sutured to the pseudocyst wall to establish internal drainage.

    (2) External drainage, which is used if the pseudocyst is not found to be mature and if suturing of the pseudocyst wall is not safe. The external drainage results in a pancreatic fistula, which usually will heal with continued parenteral nutrition.

    (3) Excision of a pseudocyst, which is rarely done; however, this may be indicated if the pseudocyst is small and is located distally in the tail of the pancreas.

III. PANCREATIC MALIGNANCIES

A. Pancreatic adenocarcinoma

1. The incidence of pancreatic adenocarcinoma is rapidly increasing, especially in men.

a. It is now the fourth commonest cause of cancer death for men in the United States.

b. It accounts for approximately 25,000 annual fatalities, according to the American Cancer Society estimate for 1985.

c. The rising incidence may be associated with tobacco and coffee use, diabetes, or asbestos exposure.

d. The tumor occurs most often between ages 50 and 70.

2. Clinical presentation

a. Early symptoms are usually vague, such as epigastric pain, weight loss, backache, and depression.

b. Thrombophlebitis may be the initial presentation. It is migratory and ultimately develops in as many as 10% of the patients.

c. The **symptoms at the time of presentation** are related to the **location of the tumor** within the pancreas.

    (1) The head of the pancreas is the commonest site. Tumors in this site produce weight loss and obstructive jaundice in 75% of the patients.

        (a) The jaundice is painless, although back pain or vague abdominal discomfort may be present in up to 25% of patients at this stage.

        (b) Because of the retroperitoneal location of the pancreas, tumors must be very large or metastatic to become evident on physical examination. However, an upper abdominal mass may be palpable.

            (i) It represents the tumor mass in as many as 20% of patients, indicating incurability.

            (ii) If the mass represents an enlarged, nontender gallbladder **(Courvoisier gallbladder),** the cause is most commonly an obstructing pancreatic neoplasm, but the gallbladder is palpable in fewer than 50% of the patients.

    (2) Carcinomas of the body or tail of the pancreas are less common and generally present at a more advanced stage because only about 10% produce obstructive jaundice.

3. **Diagnosis.** Screening for early pancreatic cancer is not likely to be useful because even tumors as small as 2–3 cm are not usually curable.
   a. **Noninvasive imaging techniques**
      (1) CT scan and ultrasonography are the most useful tests in diagnosing pancreatic cancer. Tumors 2–3 cm in size can often be detected by these techniques.
      (2) Upper gastrointestinal radiographs can detect pancreatic tumors after they are large enough to distort the duodenum, a late finding.
   b. **Invasive diagnostic techniques**
      (1) Percutaneous fine-needle aspiration uses ultrasound or CT to direct a small-bore needle to a mass, a highly reliable technique to diagnose a malignancy. A cytologic specimen is obtained with virtually no risk of complication.
      (2) ERCP uses a flexible duodenoscope to cannulate the pancreatic duct. Contrast medium is injected and radiographs are taken.
         (a) Small pancreatic cancers can be demonstrated by this technique, and specimens can be collected from the pancreatic duct for cytologic examination.
         (b) Successful cannulation requires a highly skilled endoscopist.
      (3) Percutaneous transhepatic cholangiography (PTC) is useful in the evaluation of patients with obstructive jaundice.
         (a) A long, small-bore needle is inserted, under local anesthesia, through the liver into a dilated hepatic duct, and contrast medium is injected to identify the site of obstruction.
         (b) Jaundice is relieved preoperatively by passing a catheter through the site of obstruction, because very high bilirubin levels may be associated with an increased risk of postoperative complications.
         (c) Potential complications of the procedure are bleeding from the needle tract in the liver and sepsis.

4. **Treatment**
   a. **Pancreaticoduodenectomy,** the **Whipple procedure,** is the standard surgical treatment for adenocarcinoma of the head of the pancreas when the lesion is curable by resection.
      (1) **Resectability** is determined at surgery from several criteria:
         (a) There are no metastases outside the abdomen.
         (b) The tumor has not involved the porta hepatis, the portal vein as it passes behind the body of the pancreas, and the superior mesenteric artery region.
         (c) The tumor has not spread to the liver or other peritoneal structures.
      (2) Histologic **proof of malignancy** is obtained by needle aspiration, either preoperatively or during surgery.
      (3) The **Whipple procedure** (Figure 15-2) involves removal of the head of the pancreas, duodenum, distal common bile duct, gallbladder, and distal stomach.
         (a) The gastrointestinal tract is then reconstructed with creation of a gastrojejunostomy, choledochojejunostomy, and pancreaticojejunostomy.
         (b) The operative mortality rate with this extensive operation can be as high as 15%.
         (c) The complication rate is also considerable, the commonest complications being hemorrhage, abscess, and pancreatic ductal leakage.
   b. Distal pancreatectomy, usually with splenectomy and lymphadenectomy, is the procedure performed for carcinoma of the midbody and tail of the pancreas.
   c. **Total pancreatectomy** has been proposed for the treatment of pancreatic cancer.
      (1) The procedure has two potential advantages:
         (a) Removal of a possible multicentric tumor (present in up to 40% of patients)
         (b) Avoidance of pancreatic duct anastomotic leaks
      (2) However, survival rates are not markedly better, and the operation has not been widely adopted.
      (3) In addition, it has resulted in a particularly brittle type of diabetes, making for an unpleasant postoperative life.
   d. **Palliative procedures** are performed more frequently than curative ones because so many of these tumors are incurable.
      (1) Palliative procedures attempt to relieve biliary obstruction by using either the common bile duct or the gallbladder as a conduit for decompression into the intestinal tract.
      (2) As many as 20% of patients may require further surgery for gastric outlet obstruction if a gastric bypass procedure is not performed initially. Thus, many centers combine a gastrojejunostomy with choledochojejunostomy as the initial procedure.

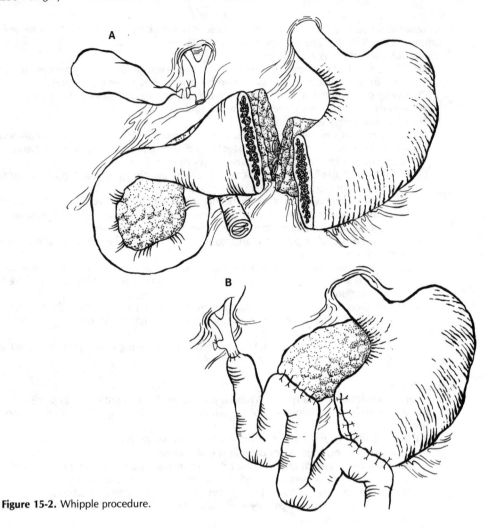

Figure 15-2. Whipple procedure.

(3) Percutaneous transhepatic biliary stents can sometimes be used to provide internal biliary drainage for obstructive jaundice, avoiding a major operative procedure.

e. Chemotherapy has been used in the treatment of pancreatic adenocarcinoma. Multi-drug regimens that include 5-fluorouracil (5-FU) have produced a response (temporary tumor regression or, rarely, cure) in about 20%–25% of the patients with metastases.

f. Combination treatment of pancreatic adenocarcinoma has been used experimentally to improve local control and to prevent metastases. Intraoperative radiotherapy and the interstitial implantation of radioactive "seeds" are being used; results are encouraging with a median survival of 13 months with unresectable disease.

5. Prognosis

a. The prognosis for patients with pancreatic adenocarcinoma is extremely poor.

(1) Overall, the 5-year survival rate is less than 5%, and cures are extremely rare. Most patients die in less than 1 year.

(2) The median length of survival for patients with unresectable tumors is 6 months.

(3) Even for those few patients with resectable tumors, results of surgery are not good. Only about 10% of patients who undergo resection will live 5 years.

b. The poor prognosis is due in part to the difficulty in making a diagnosis while the tumor is at an early stage: Only about 10% of pancreatic adenocarcinomas are resectable at the time of diagnosis.

B. Other pancreatic malignancies are infrequent. They include cystadenocarcinomas (which typically occur in women), nonfunctional islet cell tumors, and peptide-producing tumors, such as insulinomas and Zollinger-Ellison tumors (see Chapter 17 II).

Part IV Gastrointestinal Disorders

STUDY QUESTIONS

Directions: Each question below contains five suggested answers. Choose the **one best** response to each question.

1. A 15-year-old boy is admitted with a history and physical findings consistent with appendicitis. Which of the following findings is most likely to be positive?

(A) Pelvic crepitus
(B) Iliopsoas sign
(C) Murphy's sign
(D) Flank ecchymosis
(E) Periumbilical ecchymosis

2. What is the most reliable method for precisely locating an upper gastrointestinal lesion that is responsible for a bleed?

(A) Upper GI series
(B) Exploratory laparotomy
(C) Upper gastrointestinal endoscopy
(D) Arteriography
(E) Radionuclide scanning

3. The drug most useful for controlling massive bleeding from erosive gastritis is

(A) epinephrine
(B) dopamine
(C) vasopressin
(D) norepinephrine
(E) propranolol

4. Which vessel is most commonly associated with a posterior duodenal ulcer?

(A) Right gastroepiploic artery
(B) Common hepatic artery
(C) Gastroduodenal artery
(D) Superior mesenteric artery
(E) Middle colic artery

5. The commonest cause of massive upper gastrointestinal bleeding is

(A) gastric ulcer
(B) erosive gastritis
(C) gastric carcinoma
(D) Mallory-Weiss tear
(E) duodenal ulcer

6. A 50-year-old man is admitted with massive, bright red rectal bleeding. He recently had a barium enema that demonstrated no diverticular or space-occupying lesion. Nasogastric suction reveals no blood but does produce yellow bile. The patient continues to bleed. What is the next diagnostic step?

(A) Repeat barium enema
(B) Colonoscopy
(C) Upper GI series
(D) Mesenteric angiography
(E) Small bowel follow-through with barium

7. All of the following statements regarding lower gastrointestinal bleeding are true EXCEPT

(A) if bleeding is profuse, angiography may be useful
(B) the mortality rate is about 10%
(C) persistent bleeding is an indication for surgery
(D) only 10%–15% of patients stop bleeding spontaneously
(E) blind total colectomy may be a necessary procedure

8. The lower esophageal sphincter pressure is increased by

(A) glucagon
(B) gastrin
(C) emptying of the stomach
(D) chocolate
(E) acid in the stomach

9. Cricopharyngeal spasm is associated with

(A) increased gastric acidity
(B) Barrett's esophagus
(C) an epiphrenic diverticulum
(D) achalasia
(E) a pharyngoesophageal diverticulum

10. The best treatment for a Zenker's diverticulum is

(A) a Nissen fundoplication
(B) cricopharyngeal myotomy and excision or resuspension of the diverticulum
(C) excision of the diverticulum
(D) long myotomy with plication of the diverticulum
(E) esophageal resection

11. All of the following statements regarding achalasia are true EXCEPT

(A) there is a high incidence of carcinoma in patients with achalasia
(B) both manometry and esophagoscopy are required for diagnosis
(C) there is hypertension of the lower esophageal sphincter
(D) nonsurgical treatment consists of pneumatic dilations
(E) a Nissen fundoplication is recommended for all surgical candidates with achalasia

12. All of the following statements regarding diffuse esophageal spasm are correct EXCEPT

(A) radiologically, it resembles advanced achalasia
(B) it is treated surgically by a long esophagomyotomy
(C) it is associated with esophageal diverticula
(D) it cannot be diagnosed by 24-hour pH testing
(E) calcium channel blockers may be beneficial in this disease

13. Gastroesophageal reflux is best characterized by which of the following statements?

(A) It is synonymous with hiatal hernia
(B) It results from a higher than normal lower esophageal sphincter pressure
(C) It may be associated with increased gastrin production
(D) It is diagnosed by manometry and 24-hour monitoring of pH in the lower esophagus
(E) It is a relative contraindication to esophagoscopy

14. A leiomyoma of the esophagus is best characterized by which of the following statements?

(A) It should be biopsied during endoscopy for diagnosis
(B) It should be treated surgically by enucleation
(C) It is a rare tumor of the esophagus
(D) It is best diagnosed by 24-hour pH testing
(E) It can be diagnosed by manometry

15. The typical carcinoma that develops in association with Barrett's esophagus is

(A) epidermoid
(B) mucoepidermoid
(C) small cell
(D) adenocarcinoma
(E) squamous cell

16. The 5-year survival rate for patients with esophageal carcinoma who have been treated surgically is

(A) 60%
(B) 45%
(C) 30%
(D) 20%
(E) 10%

17. The correct surgical treatment for a Mallory-Weiss tear of the esophagus is

(A) transthoracic ligation of varices
(B) transthoracic antireflux procedure
(C) laparotomy, gastrotomy, and oversewing the bleeding vessel
(D) laparotomy and resection of the gastroesophageal junction
(E) antibiotics and observation

18. The blood supply to the stomach and duodenum arises from all of the following arteries EXCEPT

(A) gastroepiploic artery
(B) common hepatic artery
(C) splenic artery
(D) superior mesenteric artery
(E) inferior mesenteric artery

19. What substance is secreted by the G cells?

(A) Gastrin
(B) Pepsin
(C) Pepsinogen
(D) Gastric acid
(E) Glucagon

20. Gastric acid production is altered by all of the following hormones or actions EXCEPT

(A) cholecystokinin
(B) gastrin
(C) vagal stimulation
(D) secretin
(E) glucagon

21. The development of peptic ulcer disease has been associated with all of the following substances or syndromes EXCEPT

(A) Mallory-Weiss syndrome
(B) caffeine
(C) alcohol
(D) Zollinger-Ellison syndrome
(E) aspirin

22. Which of the following statements concerning tumors of the duodenum is true?

(A) Tumors of the duodenum, both benign and malignant, are common disorders

(B) The commonest malignant tumor of the duodenum is a malignant lymphoma

(C) Benign duodenal tumors are usually fibromas

(D) Treatment of resectable malignant lesions usually requires pancreaticoduodenectomy (Whipple's procedure)

(E) Benign tumors of the duodenum require vagotomy with antrectomy

23. All of the following statements regarding gastric carcinoma are true EXCEPT

(A) the incidence is decreasing

(B) surgery offers the best chance at cure for favorable lesions

(C) the outlook is improving with newer treatment options

(D) most patients with gastric carcinoma present with advanced disease

(E) pain is a common presenting symptom

24. Massive upper gastrointestinal bleeding occurs in an otherwise asymptomatic, normal man following a violent episode of retching and vomiting without blood. The most likely cause of this man's bleeding is

(A) hiatal hernia

(B) Mallory-Weiss tear

(C) carcinoma of the stomach

(D) duodenal ulcer

(E) gastritis

25. Which of the following statements regarding the small bowel is true?

(A) The entire small bowel is intraperitoneal

(B) The jejunum is longer in length, larger in diameter, and thinner-walled than the ileum

(C) The muscularis, the muscle layer, provides the strength for the placement of sutures or staples for the creation of a bowel anastomosis

(D) Peyer's patches are most prominent in the distal ileum

(E) The marginal artery of Drummond provides the blood supply to the duodenum

26. Which of the following conditions is a cause of fat malabsorption?

(A) Pancreatic insufficiency

(B) Cholelithiasis

(C) Resection of the distal half of the small bowel and the right colon for Crohn's disease

(D) Duodenal diverticulum

(E) Deficiency of vitamin A or vitamin E

27. After absorption, all of the following nutrients are transported across the mucosal cells into the portal venous system EXCEPT

(A) saccharides

(B) amino acids

(C) vitamin C

(D) triglycerides

(E) bipeptides

28. Which of the following tumors of the small intestine have malignant potential?

(A) Adenomatous polyps

(B) Hamartomatous polyps

(C) Juvenile (retention) polyps

(D) Leiomyomas

(E) Fibromas

29. The commonest small bowel malignancy is

(A) adenoma

(B) adenocarcinoma

(C) carcinoid tumor

(D) lymphoma

(E) leiomyosarcoma

30. Which treatment method is most appropriate for a patient with acute perirectal pain and with a tender, fluctuant perirectal area?

(A) Abdominoperineal resection

(B) Abdominal transsacral rectal resection

(C) Removal of an anal fissure

(D) Drainage of an abscess

(E) Antibiotic therapy alone

31. Familial polyposis of the colon is most often associated with which of the following conditions?

(A) Carcinoma of the pancreas

(B) Carcinoma of the colon

(C) Granulomatous disease of the colon

(D) Pneumatosis cystoides intestinalis

(E) Sigmoid volvulus

32. Pathology reveals a poorly differentiated adenocarcinoma, extending into the muscularis propria with 3 of 22 lymph nodes positive for metastatic cancer. The Astler-Coller modification of Duke's stage is

(A) B_1

(B) B_2

(C) C_1

(D) C_2

(E) D

Questions 33 and 34

A 63-year-old white man presents with a 3-day history of increasing crampy abdominal pain, constipation, and intermittent vomiting. He continues to pass gas. Other than the present complaints, he has been healthy. Examination reveals a distended abdomen with high-pitched bowel sounds. There is no localized tenderness. There are no rectal masses. The stool is heme-positive.

33. Diagnostically, the first steps should be to perform

(A) total colonoscopy
(B) mesenteric angiography
(C) flat plate and erect abdominal x-rays
(D) upper gastrointestinal x-rays with small bowel follow-through
(E) barium enema

34. Therapeutically, the first steps should be

(A) a Fleet enema, clear liquids by mouth, and careful observation
(B) emergency colonoscopy for colonic decompression
(C) intravenous fluids, nasogastric suction, and careful observation
(D) colonoscopic decompression with use of a rectal tube if necessary
(E) immediate exploratory laparotomy

(end of group question)

35. Upon abdominal exploration, a patient is found to have a nonobstructing carcinoma of the transverse colon and apparent liver metastases. The best treatment is to

(A) biopsy the liver nodules, then close the abdomen
(B) close the abdomen
(C) resect the colon lesion only
(D) resect the colon lesion and biopsy the liver lesion
(E) perform a colostomy

36. What has been found to be an acceptable screening technique for detecting recurrent colon cancer?

(A) Screening sigmoidoscopy
(B) Screening the stool for occult blood
(C) Stool cytology
(D) Measurement of carcinoembryonic antigen levels
(E) Colonoscopy

37. In which of the following disorders is there an increased risk of carcinoma of the colon?

(A) Granulomatous disease of the colon
(B) Perianal fistula and abscess
(C) Chronic ulcerative colitis
(D) Chronic diverticulitis
(E) Peutz-Jeghers syndrome

38. Sigmoidoscopy will reveal what typical finding in a patient with Crohn's disease involving the rectum?

(A) Fungating mass
(B) Mucosal ulcers and fissures adjacent to normal-appearing mucosa
(C) Pseudopolyps
(D) Sheets of white blood cells with inflamed mucosa
(E) Edema

39. The most acceptable method of treatment for the first episode of uncomplicated acute colonic diverticulitis is

(A) diverting transverse colostomy
(B) primary resection and reanastomosis
(C) bowel rest and parenteral antibiotics
(D) Mikulicz resection
(E) antibiotic enemas

40. All of the following statements regarding liver anatomy are true EXCEPT

(A) the remnant of the umbilical vein lies along the leading edge of the falciform ligament
(B) the portal vein is the most posterior structure in the normal porta hepatis
(C) although the hepatic artery carries only 25% of liver blood flow, it supplies 50% of the oxygen used by the liver
(D) the adrenal veins are not part of the portal system
(E) the falciform ligament on the surface of the liver marks the main boundary fissure between the right and left hepatic lobes

41. All of the following statements about post-traumatic hemobilia are true EXCEPT

(A) optimal treatment is common bile duct exploration and resection of the lesion
(B) patients generally present more than 1 month after injury
(C) patients may present with symptoms of either gastrointestinal bleeding or common bile duct obstruction
(D) hemobilia is due to the formation of connections between the arterial and biliary trees
(E) arteriography is useful in the diagnosis

42. All of the following disorders are pre- or intra-hepatic (sinusoidal) causes of portal hypertension EXCEPT

(A) alcoholic cirrhosis

(B) hemochromatosis

(C) schistosomiasis

(D) Budd-Chiari syndrome

(E) postnecrotic cirrhosis

43. All of the following problems commonly occur with the use of balloon tamponade for control of variceal bleeding EXCEPT

(A) pneumonia

(B) aspiration of nasopharyngeal secretions

(C) rebleeding following removal of the tube

(D) gastritis

(E) esophageal ulceration or perforation

44. The commonest cause of death in patients with alcoholic cirrhosis following portosystemic shunting is

(A) bleeding esophageal varices

(B) hepatic failure with encephalopathy

(C) malnutrition

(D) hepatocellular carcinoma

(E) cardiac failure with peripheral edema and ascites

45. Of the factors listed, which most determines long-term survival following a shunting procedure in an alcoholic patient with cirrhosis of the liver?

(A) A low-protein diet

(B) Control of ascites

(C) A low-salt intake

(D) Abstinence from alcohol

(E) Use of lactulose

46. What characteristic radiographic finding would be seen in a patient with a gallstone that has eroded into the duodenum?

(A) A widened duodenal C-loop

(B) Gallbladder calcification

(C) Evidence of gas-forming organisms in the retroperitoneum

(D) Air in the biliary tree

(E) A filling defect in the rectosigmoid colon

47. Common duct stones are present in what percentage of patients undergoing cholecystectomy?

(A) 0 to 5%

(B) 10%–20%

(C) 40%–50%

(D) 60%–70%

(E) greater than 70%

48. Which of the following findings in acute pancreatitis is not well visualized with ultrasonography?

(A) Cullen's sign

(B) Biliary obstruction

(C) Pancreatic pseudocyst

(D) Pancreatic abscess

(E) Pancreatic calcification

49. All of the following findings are useful in determining the prognosis in acute pancreatitis EXCEPT

(A) a white blood cell count over 20,000

(B) a serum calcium level less than 8 mg/dl

(C) hypoxia

(D) a serum amylase level greater than 1000 Somogyi units

(E) patient's age greater than 55 years

50. A patient with the first episode of acute pancreatitis may manifest all of the following clinical findings EXCEPT

(A) hypotension

(B) Grey-Turner's sign (flank ecchymosis)

(C) "reversed 3" sign on plain x-ray of the abdomen

(D) "string" sign on barium study of the colon

(E) tachycardia

51. The most accepted surgical procedure used to treat a chronic pancreatic pseudocyst is

(A) percutaneous drainage

(B) internal drainage to the gastrointestinal tract

(C) pancreatectomy

(D) excision of the pseudocyst

(E) excision of the tail of the pancreas with subsequent pancreatic duct anastomosis to the bowel

52. A patient with obstructive jaundice due to pancreatic carcinoma might have all of the following clinical findings EXCEPT

(A) a palpable gallbladder

(B) pain early in the course of the disease

(C) pulmonary metastases

(D) thrombophlebitis

(E) a mass in the head of the pancreas

Directions: Each question below contains four suggested answers of which **one or more** is correct. Choose the answer

    A if **1, 2, and 3** are correct
    B if **1 and 3** are correct
    C if **2 and 4** are correct
    D if **4** is correct
    E if **1, 2, 3, and 4** are correct

53. An 18-year-old girl is admitted to the hospital with acute abdominal pain. She gives a history of intermittent abdominal pain and anorexia with vomiting. Examination of the abdomen reveals fullness in the right lower quadrant with localized tenderness. The differential diagnosis in this patient should include

(1) ruptured ovarian cyst
(2) ectopic pregnancy
(3) ovarian tumor
(4) perforated appendicitis with abscess

54. Air within the biliary tree on a plain abdominal x-ray usually is associated with which of the following?

(1) Perforated gastric ulcer
(2) Choledochoduodenostomy
(3) Intestinal obstruction
(4) Cholangitis with a gas-forming organism

55. A 50-year-old man who ate a large meal at a company banquet ended up in the emergency room with excruciating left upper abdominal pain radiating through to his back. The history reveals that his pain followed an episode of severe retching and vomiting. Which of the following studies should be ordered to provide the diagnosis?

(1) Chest x-ray
(2) Splenic radionuclide scan
(3) Gastrografin swallow
(4) Celiac arteriogram

56. Causes for intestinal obstruction include

(1) congenital lesions
(2) inflammatory lesions
(3) extrinsic lesions
(4) radiation injury

57. A 40-year-old man with a history of alcohol abuse is admitted to the emergency room with a history of hematemesis following several episodes of vomiting. At endoscopy, a 2-cm tear is seen near the gastroesophageal junction on the lesser curve of the stomach. No active bleeding is noted. Large varices are seen that are not bleeding. The history and findings are most consistent with a diagnosis of

(1) peptic ulcer disease
(2) bleeding esophageal varices
(3) gastritis
(4) Mallory-Weiss syndrome

58. A previously healthy 55-year-old man is admitted to the hospital with a history of a massive lower gastrointestinal bleed. He is no longer actively bleeding at the time of admission. His hemoglobin was 9 and his blood pressure, 120/60. Initial studies should include

(1) nasogastric tube
(2) rectal examination
(3) sigmoidoscopy
(4) laparotomy

59. True statements regarding Barrett's esophagus include which of the following?

(1) It may reveal gastric columnar epithelium on biopsy
(2) It is almost always a malignant lesion
(3) It most commonly affects the distal esophagus
(4) It is treated by pneumatic dilation

60. True statements concerning duodenal ulcers include which of the following?

(1) Most duodenal ulcers are located in the first portion of the duodenum
(2) Most patients present with a history of epigastric pain, which may radiate to the back and which is frequently relieved by food
(3) Most duodenal ulcers can be diagnosed by an upper GI series
(4) The preferred treatment of uncomplicated duodenal ulcer is simple surgical excision

61. Superior mesenteric artery syndrome has which of the following characteristics?

(1) It occurs in young, thin females
(2) It is an obstruction of the duodenum by the superior mesenteric artery
(3) Typical symptoms are vomiting and postprandial pain
(4) It sometimes can be treated by weight gain

62. A patient who had a gastrectomy has developed the dumping syndrome. Which of the following statements might this patient's surgeon make about this syndrome?

(1) It can cause epigastric pain due to small bowel distention
(2) It causes nausea, dizziness, and palpitations
(3) It occurs because rapid emptying of the stomach causes jejunal distention from fluid accumulation
(4) It can be controlled by dietary modifications

63. True statements concerning the afferent loop syndrome include which of the following?

(1) The syndrome causes postprandial distention, pain, and nausea that are relieved by vomiting bilious materal not mixed with food
(2) It occurs frequently in patients with a Billroth I gastrojejunostomy
(3) Treatment consists of providing good drainage of the afferent limb, usually by conversion of a gastrojejunostomy to a Roux-en-Y anastomosis
(4) The syndrome is difficult to correct and recurs frequently after operative revision

64. Which of the following nutrients must be replaced parenterally after resection of the terminal ileum in a patient with Crohn's disease?

(1) Vitamin E
(2) Iron
(3) Bile salts
(4) Vitamin B_{12}

65. Common signs and symptoms of Crohn's disease include

(1) abdominal mass
(2) enterovesical fistula
(3) anemia
(4) bloody diarrhea

66. Characteristics of the short bowel syndrome include which of the following?

(1) Most patients require long-term total parenteral nutrition
(2) It is a commonly occurring syndrome after colectomy
(3) Caloric intake must be reduced significantly
(4) Absorption of water is poor

67. True statements concerning radiation injury to the small bowel (chronic radiation enteritis) include which of the following?

(1) The 5-year survival rate is less than 50%
(2) The signs and symptoms of chronic radiation injury are similar to those of tumor recurrence
(3) Gastrointestinal bleeding may be caused by a fistula between a major artery and the bowel
(4) The manifestations of chronic injury appear within 1 month of radiation therapy

68. Which of the following hepatic neoplasms commonly present with rupture into the free peritoneal space?

(1) Hepatic adenoma
(2) Hemangioma
(3) Hepatocellular carcinoma
(4) Infantile hemangioendothelioma

69. An association has been found between hepatocellular carcinoma and a number of prior diseases and environmental factors. Which of the following would belong in that category?

(1) Chronic alcohol abuse
(2) Hepatitis B surface antigen
(3) Aflatoxins
(4) Oral contraceptives

70. True statements regarding metastatic hepatic tumors include which of the following?

(1) Solitary, slow-growing hepatic metastasis from colon carcinoma has a 20%–30% 5-year survival rate after surgical resection
(2) Multiple metastatic liver tumors have not been greatly responsive to chemotherapy
(3) Colorectal cancer metastatic to the liver often is associated with an elevated level of carcinoembryonic antigen
(4) Hepatic metastatic tumors are less common than primary hepatic tumors

---

SUMMARY OF DIRECTIONS

A	B	C	D	E
1, 2, 3 only	1, 3 only	2, 4 only	4 only	All are correct

---

71. True statements about hepatic abscesses include

(1) the commonest hepatic abscess in the United States is of bacterial origin
(2) amebic abscess is the commonest hepatic abscess in third-world countries
(3) endocarditis can cause a hepatic abscess
(4) standard treatment for a solitary bacterial hepatic abscess is broad-spectrum antibiotic treatment alone

72. True statements regarding the distal splenorenal (Warren) shunt include which of the following?

(1) It selectively decreases the elevated venous pressure in the splenic bed
(2) It maintains good portal venous perfusion to the liver
(3) This procedure is commonly followed by ascites
(4) It is usually associated with more encephalopathy when compared to a portocaval shunt

Directions: The groups of questions below consist of lettered choices followed by several numbered items. For each numbered item, select the **one** lettered choice with which it is **most closely** associated. Each lettered choice may be used once, more than once, or not at all.

Questions 73–77

The commonest manifestations of ulcer disease are gastric ulcers and duodenal ulcers. These share certain characteristics but are dissimilar in other ways. For each phrase describing a characteristic of ulcer disease, select the most appropriate response.

(A) Gastric ulcer
(B) Duodenal ulcer
(C) Both
(D) Neither

73. The major cause is hypersecretion of gastric acid

74. Degeneration into cancer may occur

75. Complications include bleeding and perforation

76. Smoking and aspirin use are associated with an increased incidence

77. Surgery is the treatment of choice

Questions 78–82

For each type of secretion below, select the cell type that secretes it.

(A) Chief cells
(B) Parietal cells
(C) Brunner's gland cells
(D) G cells
(E) Argentaffin cells

78. Hormone

79. Hydrochloric acid

80. Mucus

81. Intrinsic factor

82. Pepsinogen

ANSWERS AND EXPLANATIONS

1. The answer is B. [*Chapter 9 I C 6 b*] The iliopsoas sign is pain in the lower abdomen and psoas region that is elicited when the thigh is flexed against resistance. It suggests an inflammatory process, such as appendicitis. Crepitus suggests a rapidly spreading gas-forming infection. Murphy's sign is elicited by palpating the right upper quadrant during inspiration and suggests acute cholecystitis. Flank and periumbilical ecchymoses suggest retroperitoneal hemorrhage.

2. The answer is C. [*Chapter 9 III E 1*] Upper gastrointestinal endoscopy is the most versatile, reliable, and rapidly performed examination for precisely locating the site of upper gastrointestinal bleeding. Endoscopy can be used in most situations except when bleeding is massive, and it is useful when more than one type of pathology is present, which is often the case. An upper GI series, arteriography and radionuclide scanning are helpful but only in selected cases. Exploratory laparotomy is most useful as a diagnostic procedure only when the bleeding is so rapid that exsanguination is imminent.

3. The answer is C. [*Chapter 9 III F 1 d*] The only drug proven to reduce massive bleeding from erosive gastritis is vasopressin. It is contraindicated in the presence of coronary artery disease. It is effective both intravenously and by selective intra-arterial mesenteric infusion, but it often is only a temporary measure.

4. The answer is C. [*Chapter 9 III F 2 c (5) (a)*] Duodenal ulcers that penetrate posteriorly usually have the gastroduodenal artery or one of its branches at the base of the ulcer. Although ulcers have the potential to erode into the right gastroepiploic, common hepatic, superior mesenteric, or middle colic artery, this is less common. Giant gastric ulcers also can penetrate into nearby arteries, especially the middle colic artery and the left gastric artery.

5. The answer is E. [*Chapter 9 Table 9-1*] Massive upper gastrointestinal bleeding is usually due to a posterior duodenal ulcer that erodes into the gastroduodenal artery. Gastritis, gastric ulcer, Mallory-Weiss tear, and gastric carcinoma are less common causes of massive upper gastrointestinal bleeding.

6. The answer is D. [*Chapter 9 IV C 2 b (1)*] The most likely cause of massive lower gastrointestinal bleeding in the absence of diverticula is an angiodysplastic lesion of the colon, particularly the right colon. An upper GI series and small bowel studies should only be done after an exhaustive colonic workup has failed to demonstrate the source of bleeding. Colonoscopy in the face of massive bleeding is unreliable and difficult and carries the risk of colonic perforation. In addition, it will not usually demonstrate an angiodysplastic lesion. A repeat barium enema is also unlikely to help. The most helpful study in this patient would be selective mesenteric angiography.

7. The answer is D. [*Chapter 9 IV C, D*] In lower gastrointestinal bleeding, about 75% of patients spontaneously stop bleeding without further intervention. If bleeding continues, angiography and radionuclide scanning are useful to identify the source. Persistent bleeding is an indication for surgery. Occasionally, the precise bleeding point cannot be identified, and a "blind" total colectomy may be necessary. Mortality rate for lower gastrointestinal bleeding is about 10%.

8. The answer is B. [*Chapter 10 I D 3 a, b*] The lower esophageal sphincter is under both neural and hormonal control. Gastrin is one of the hormones that increases lower esophageal sphincter tone.

9. The answer is E. [*Chapter 10 II A 1 a, b*] A pharyngoesophageal diverticulum (Zenker's diverticulum) is caused by an incoordination of the cricopharyngeus muscle during swallowing. An epiphrenic diverticulum is associated with muscular incoordination at the gastroesophageal junction. Barrett's esophagus is columnar epithelium in the esophagus, and achalasia results from lack of neural cells in the myenteric plexus of the esophageal wall.

10. The answer is B. [*Chapter 10 II A 4 a, b*] Myotomy and excision or resuspension is the treatment of choice for a Zenker's diverticulum. Excision without myotomy can result in a higher incidence of recurrence. The Nissen fundoplication is used for gastroesophageal reflux. The Heller procedure of a long myotomy is used for diffuse esophageal spasm.

11. The answer is E. [*Chapter 10 II B 1 a, c, 3 a, b, 4 a, b*] Achalasia is a disease characterized by the abnormal peristalsis in the body of the esophagus, a high resting pressure in the lower esophageal sphincter, and failure of the lower esophagus to relax appropriately during swallowing. Manometry and esophagoscopy are used in making the diagnosis of achalasia. Although surgery (myotomy) seems to afford better results than nonsurgical treatment, patients who are poor-risk surgical candidates can be treated by pneumatic dilation. A Nissen fundoplication is not indicated.

12. The answer is A. [*Chapter 10 II C 3 a, b, 4 a, b*] Diffuse esophageal spasm is a disease characterized by incoordinated contractions of the esophagus. On a barium swallow, achalasia resembles a tube with a distal tapering in it. This is distinctly different from the barium swallow of a patient with diffuse esophageal spasm. Epiphrenic diverticula are associated with diffuse esophageal spasm. The diagnosis of diffuse esophageal spasm is made by manometry. It can be treated medically with calcium channel blockers or surgically by a long esophagomyotomy. Twenty-four–hour pH testing is used to identify patients with gastroesophageal reflux.

13. The answer is D. [*Chapter 10 II D 1 a, c, 3 a–c*] Esophagoscopy is frequently used in the diagnosis of gastroesophageal reflux and in staging the amount of esophagitis that is present. Gastrin production is often decreased in patients with gastroesophageal reflux. Twenty-four–hour pH testing is useful in confirming gastroesophageal reflux, and manometry reveals decreased lower esophageal sphincter pressure.

14. The answer is B. [*Chapter 10 IV A 1 b, c*] A leiomyoma is the commonest benign tumor of the esophagus. These tumors are usually diagnosed by barium swallow, and if endoscopy is performed, a biopsy of the mucosa should not be performed. The leiomyoma is located submucosally, and a biopsy may interfere with definitive treatment by surgical enucleation. Twenty-four–hour pH testing is used to identify patients with gastroesophageal reflux. Manometry is helpful in identifying motility disorders of the esophagus.

15. The answer is D. [*Chapter 10 IV B 3 a (2)*] Barrett's esophagus is associated with a change in the squamous lining of the esophagus to a columnar epithelium. This is thought to be an acquired condition and is associated with the development of adenocarcinoma of the esophagus.

16. The answer is E. [*Chapter 10 IV B 5 a (3)*] Carcinoma of the esophagus remains a disease with a dismal 5-year survival rate. The inability to diagnose the disease in its early stages certainly contributes to the poor prognosis. There are presently protocols using preoperative chemotherapy and radiation therapy, which, hopefully, will allow survival in these patients to improve.

17. The answer is C. [*Chapter 10 VI C 1, 2*] Most patients with Mallory-Weiss tears of the esophagus stop bleeding spontaneously. If there is continued bleeding, the surgical treatment includes laparotomy, a high gastrotomy, and oversewing the bleeding vessel.

18. The answer is E. [*Chapter 11 I A 3 a, B 2 a*] The left and right gastroepiploic arteries supply blood to the greater curvature of the stomach. The right gastric artery arises from the common hepatic artery. The short gastric vessels derive from the splenic artery. The inferior pancreaticoduodenal arcade comes from the superior mesenteric artery. The inferior mesenteric artery, however, supplies blood to the left side of the colon, not to the stomach or duodenum.

19. The answer is A. [*Chapter 11 I A 4 b (3) (b)*] The G cells secrete the hormone gastrin. Gastrin, in turn, causes the secretion of gastric acid by the parietal (oxyntic) cells and pepsinogen by the zygomatic (chief) cells. Pepsinogen is the precursor of pepsin, an enzyme active in protein digestion. Chief cells are also stimulated by cholinergic impulses and by secretin. Glucagon is a hormone secreted from the wall of the stomach and duodenum and by alpha cells in the pancreas; it has a hyperglycemic effect.

20. The answer is E. [*Chapter 11 I C 1–4*] Gastrin and vagal stimulation are potent promoters of hydrochloric acid production by the stomach. Cholecystokinin is a weak stimulator of acid production. Secretin release from the duodenum inhibits gastrin production, thereby decreasing gastric acid output. Glucagon is not involved in the regulation of acid output.

21. The answer is A. [*Chapter 11 II B 2, 3; VI A*] Aspirin, alcohol, and caffeine have all been linked to the development of ulcers. The Zollinger-Ellison syndrome is an ulcer diasthesis due to a pancreatic tumor. The Mallory-Weiss syndrome refers to a linear mucosal tear of the gastroesophageal junction, which is unrelated to ulcer disease.

22. The answer is D. [*Chapter 11 IV B 1*] Both malignant and benign duodenal tumors are rare. The commonest malignant tumor of the duodenum is adenocarcinoma. These lesions are usually advanced on presentation and, if resectable, usually require a pancreaticoduodenectomy. Benign tumors found in the duodenum include lipomas, leiomyomas, and adenomas. These usually can be treated by local excision.

23. The answer is C. [*Chapter 11 IV A 1 a (1), (2), (5), (7)*] Despite a decreasing incidence of gastric carcinoma, the prognosis remains unchanged. For early disease, surgery offers the best chance of cure, but most patients present with nodal disease or distant metastases. Pain and weight loss are frequent symptoms of gastric carcinoma.

24. The answer is B. [*Chapter 10 VI A; Chapter 11 VI A*] Massive upper gastrointestinal bleeding in an otherwise normal person following an episode of violent vomiting is a classic history for a patient with Mallory-Weiss tear of the esophagus. The forceful vomiting tears the esophageal mucosa at the gastro-esophageal junction, resulting in bleeding. Hiatal hernia, gastric carcinoma, duodenal ulcer, and gastritis are possible but less likely causes of massive bleeding when the blood appears after a bout of vomiting.

25. The answer is D. [*Chapter 12 I A 1–4*] Peyer's patches are agglomerations of lymphoid tissue in the submucosa, which are most prominent in the more distal ileum. The duodenum is retroperitoneal, and the jejunum and ileum are intraperitoneal. The jejunum is the same length but has thicker walls than the ileum. The submucosa, not the muscularis, provides the strength to hold sutures or staples for surgical anastomoses. The marginal artery of Drummond represents the collaterals between the superior mesenteric and inferior mesenteric artery adjacent to the wall of the left colon.

26. The answer is A. [*Chapter 12 I B 2 c*] Fat absorption depends upon the presence of bile acids, micelles for solubilization, pancreatic lipases for metabolism, and the proximal bowel (duodenal and jejunal) mucosa for absorption. Thus, pancreatic insufficiency is a cause of fat malabsorption. Cholelithiasis (stones in the gallbladder) alone does not cause biliary obstruction and has no effect on fat absorption. Duodenal diverticula generally do not cause obstruction of the pancreatic or common bile duct, and hence do not effect fat absorption. Deficiencies of vitamins A and E may occur in the *presence* of fat malabsorption but are not causes of it.

27. The answer is D. [*Chapter 12 I B 2 c–f*] Monoglycerides and fatty acids are absorbed in the mucosal cells, then synthesized into triglycerides, and transported into the intestinal lymphatics as chylomicrons. All other nutrients, including starch, amino acids, vitamin C, and peptides, are transported across the mucosal cells into the portal venous system.

28. The answer is A. [*Chapter 12 II A 1 a, b*] The adenomatous polyps found in familial polyposis syndromes are premalignant lesions. The hamartomatous polyps found in patients with Peutz-Jeghers syndrome, leiomyomas, and fibromas have no malignant potential. Juvenile (retention) polyps are benign hamartomas, not true neoplasms, which usually autoamputate.

29. The answer is B. [*Chapter 12 II A 2 a–e*] Malignant tumors constitute 75% of symptomatic small bowel tumors and usually present with bleeding, perforation, or obstruction. Common primary small bowel malignancies in descending order of frequency are: adenocarcinomas (40%), carcinoid tumors (30%), lymphomas (20%), and sarcomas. Adenomas are benign epithelial tumors. Leiomyosarcomas are the commonest sarcoma of the small bowel but not the commonest malignancy.

30. The answer is D. [*Chapter 13 VI C 2 a*] The patient described in the question with perirectal pain has a perirectal abscess, which should be drained. Antibiotic therapy alone will not cure an abscess; adequate drainage is essential. Whether to drain a perirectal abscess in an outpatient setting or in the operating room is a matter of clinical judgment. Factors that must be considered are the extent of the disease process and the immune competence of the patient.

31. The answer is B. [*Chapter 13 VII E 1*] Total colectomy is recommended for patients with familial polyposis of the colon because *all* untreated patients will develop cancer. The resection should be done as soon after the diagnosis as is convenient because all patients will develop cancer by 40 years of age.

32. The answer is C. [*Chapter 13 VIII A 4 a, 7 d*] The most widely accepted pathologic staging system for colorectal cancer is the Astler-Coller modification of Duke's classification. A poorly differentiated adenocarcinoma that extends into the muscularis propria with positive nodal involvement is stage C_1.

33. The answer is C. [*Chapter 13 VIII A 6; XIV B 3*] Flat plate and erect films of the abdomen should be performed first. Further studies may be performed based on the results of this initial survey.

34. The answer is C. [*Chapter 13 XV A 3 a*] As with all partial bowel obstruction, the initial treatment involves nasogastric suction, intravenous fluids, and often antibiotics.

35. The answer is D. [*Chapter 13 VIII A 10 b (1), (4)*] The colonic lesion should be resected if possible to prevent bleeding, obstruction, and control local disease. A liver biopsy is recommended for tissue diagnosis of metastatic disease.

36. The answer is D. [*Chapter 13 VIII A 10 a*] Carcinoembryonic antigen (CEA) levels drop after a successful resection of colorectal cancer, and a later rise in the CEA level signals a recurrence. The measurement of CEA levels is reliable enough to be accepted as a screening test for recurrent colorectal cancer. Examining the stool for occult blood is the technique that is applied to large populations as a screening test for colonic cancer but has not been used to determine recurrent disease.

37. The answer is C. [*Chapter 13 X B 6 d*] Chronic ulcerative colitis shows a predictable increase in the incidence of carcinoma of the colon with each additional year of active colitis. The cancers are often multicentric and frequently behave more malignantly than other colonic cancers.

38. The answer is B. [*Chapter 13 X A 1 b*] Crohn's disease of the colon results in serpiginous ulcers of the mucosa and adjacent mucosal edema. One endoscopic finding that helps to differentiate Crohn's colitis from ulcerative colitis is the presence of skip areas of normal mucosa; these are absent in ulcerative colitis. Pseudopolyps are hallmarks of ulcerative colitis, and sheets of white blood cells generally occur in pseudomembranous colitis, which is caused by *Clostridium difficile.*

39. The answer is C. [*Chapter 13 XII H 1*] Most episodes of acute diverticulitis will resolve with medical management. This includes bowel rest and administering parenteral fluids and broad-spectrum antibiotics. Surgery is indicated for recurrent episodes as well as for complications of the disease.

40. The answer is E. [*Chapter 14 I A 1 a–c*] The falciform ligament marks the segmental fissure between medial and lateral segments of the left lobe. The surface landmarks of the main boundary fissures are the inferior vena cava posteriorly and the gallbladder fossa anteriorly. All of the other statements listed in the question are correct.

41. The answer is A. [*Chapter 14 I G 4 e*] Hemobilia is an occasional complication after liver trauma. Patients present late with either gastrointestinal bleeding or symptoms of biliary obstruction. Diagnosis is best made by arteriography, and optimal treatment is angiographic embolization of the involved artery.

42. The answer is D. [*Chapter 14 II C 1–3*] The Budd-Chiari syndrome is a posthepatic cause of portal hypertension, not a pre- or intrahepatic cause. It is a syndrome characterized by hepatic venous thrombosis, resulting in marked hepatic congestion and hepatomegaly. The commonest etiologic factors in this disorder are oral contraceptives, tumors, trauma, and hematologic disorders associated with increased thrombogenicity. The Budd-Chiari syndrome is a rare cause of portal hypertension. By far, the commonest cause is cirrhosis of the liver: It is the etiology in 85% of portal hypertension cases in the United States.

43. The answer is D. [*Chapter 14 II E 3 c (1)–(4)*] Gastritis is not a common problem associated with balloon tamponade and is not related to the use of the tube. Gastric ulceration can occasionally occur where the gastric balloon is inflated. Pneumonia, aspiration of nasopharyngeal secretions, rebleeding following removal of the tube, and esophageal ulceration or perforation are common problems with balloon tamponade and can be minimized by keeping the balloon inflated for the briefest amount of time and by careful attention to removing secretions above the tube.

44. The answer is B. [*Chapter 14 II H 2, 3*] Hepatic failure is the commonest cause of death following a nonselective portosystemic shunting procedure. It is related to a deprivation of portal blood in the liver. Portal blood appears to be necessary in the maintenance of hepatocellular function, and nonselective shunting always results in hepatofugal flow. A repeat of variceal hemorrhage following shunting is unusual if the shunt remains patent. Another common cause of death in individuals with cirrhosis is infection, such as pneumonia or primary peritonitis. Malnutrition, hepatic carcinoma, and cardiac failure are less common causes of death in individuals with cirrhosis undergoing shunting procedures.

45. The answer is D. [*Chapter 14 II I*] Whether or not a patient with alcoholic cirrhosis continues to abuse alcohol is the most important factor in determining survival. A low-protein diet, control of ascites, a low-salt intake, and the use of lactulose are types of therapy that are indicative of the severity of liver failure.

46. The answer is D. [*Chapter 14 III D 4 d (4) (b)*] Any abnormal communication between the biliary tree and the intestinal tract will produce air in the biliary tract. When a gallstone erodes into the intestinal tract, it is usually a large gallstone that slowly erodes into the duodenum, forming a scarred, well-established tract without gas-forming organisms. If a filling defect is present, it is usually in the terminal ileum, secondary to the large gallstone's obstruction of the lumen.

47. The answer is B. [*Chapter 14 III F 1*] Some 10%–20% of patients with gallstones develop choledocholithiasis. Often the choledocholithiasis is "silent" and is discovered only on the operative cholangiogram.

48. The answer is A. [*Chapter 15 II B 3 c (2)*] Cullen's sign is periumbilical ecchymosis secondary to hemorrhagic pancreatitis with blood dissection up the falciform ligament. Ultrasonography would not be used to identify this sign. However, ultrasonography is a very useful procedure in the diagnosis of pancreatitis as well as its complications.

49. The answer is D. [*Chapter 15 II B 4 a, b, 5*] The serum amylase level may indicate the presence of biliary tract disease with pancreatitis; it is not a prognostic indicator in acute pancreatitis. Any factor that reflects pancreatic necrosis, hemorrhage, infection, or continued third-space loss indicates a poor prognosis.

50. The answer is D. [*Chapter 15 II B 3 e (1), 4 c (1) (f), (2) (b)*] Patients with acute pancreatitis are often critically ill and may even demonstrate blood dissection into the peritoneum, causing flank ecchymosis. The bowel may have an ileus near the pancreas, causing "reversed 3" roentgenographic findings. In severe cases, retroperitoneal hemorrhage can lead to large third-space fluid losses, hypovolemia, hypotension, and tachycardia. Barium studies may demonstrate the "pad sign," a smoothing out of the duodenal mucosal folds by the edematous pancreas.

51. The answer is B. [*Chapter 15 II E 3*] Internal drainage is the preferred method of treatment for a pancreatic pseudocyst. The pseudocyst must be well formed and mature enough to allow sutures to hold within the tissue. Generally, a cystogastrostomy is the simplest procedure to perform.

52. The answer is B. [*Chapter 15 III A 2*] Migratory phlebitis is present in about 10% of patients with pancreatic cancer. The commonest site of pancreatic cancer is the pancreatic head, which often does not produce symptoms until late in the disease, thus delaying the diagnosis.

53. The answer is E (all). [*Chapter 9 I C 4*] While the case presented in the question of the 18-year-old girl with acute abdominal pain is consistent with a diagnosis of perforated appendicitis, all of the other disorders listed (i.e., ruptured ovarian cyst, ectopic pregnancy, and ovarian tumor) must be included in the differential. A thorough gynecologic examination should be performed in all women with abdominal pain.

54. The answer is C (2, 4). [*Chapter 9 I F 1 c (5)*] Any abnormal communication between the bile duct and the gastrointestinal tract may allow air to enter the bile duct. This communication can be secondary to surgery (e.g., choledochoduodenostomy) or can result from an inflammatory process, such as erosion of a gallstone into the duodenum. Cholangitis can also cause air in the bile ducts when the biliary obstruction is complicated by a gas-forming organism. This represents a surgical emergency, resulting in death if the biliary tree is not promptly drained.

55. The answer is B (1, 3). [*Chapter 9 I F 2 b, c*] The patient has a classic history of Boerhaave's syndrome. In this disease, severe retching and vomiting of large amounts of food cause perforation of the intrathoracic esophagus, resulting in a left pleural effusion. A Gastrografin swallow will confirm the diagnois of pleural effusion.

56. The answer is E (all). [*Chapter 9 II A 2*] Intrinsic lesions (e.g., congenital webs), inflammatory lesions (e.g., Crohn's disease), extrinsic lesions (e.g., abscesses), and radiation injury have all been shown to cause small bowel obstruction. Treatment of these conditions depends on the cause.

57. The answer is D (4). [*Chapter 9 III E 1 a (4)*] Mallory-Weiss syndrome consists of upper gastrointestinal bleeding with linear nonperforating laceration, usually of the proximal gastric mucosa. A Mallory-Weiss tear accounts for about 10% of all upper gastrointestinal bleeds. The condition is usually self-limited, and medical therapy, including antacids, is usually adequate. Rebleeding is uncommon (1%–2% of cases).

58. The answer is A (1, 2, 3). [*Chapter 9 IV B 1–3*] In the management of lower gastrointestinal hemorrhage, the initial workup includes an anorectal examination to rule out an anorectal lesion, a nasogastric tube to rule out bleeding from the upper gastrointestinal tract, and a sigmoidoscopy to evaluate the distal colon. Angiography or radionuclide scanning may be necessary. Persistent bleeding is the principal indication for surgery.

59. The answer is B (1, 3). [*Chapter 10 II D 4 b (1) (b)*] Barrett's esophagus involves replacement of the distal esophageal mucosa by columnar epithelium, of either the intestinal or gastric type. Gastric acid reflux is felt to be the usual etiology, and in many cases control of reflux, either by H_2-receptor blocking agents or by an antireflux procedure, will result in reversion back to normal mucosa. If the abnormal mucosa persists despite optimal therapy, adenocarcinoma develops in 10% of cases.

60. The answer is A (1, 2, 3). [*Chapter 11 II B 1 a, 4 a, b, 5*] Duodenal ulcers commonly are in the first portion of the duodenum. Duodenal ulcer patients frequently are found to have increased acid production. The history is characteristic and consists of epigastric pain radiating to the back, which is frequently relieved by food. Most ulcers are diagnosed by an upper gastrointestinal series. Endoscopy may be done; however, since the incidence of carcinoma is small in duodenal ulcers, endoscopy is not necessary on a routine basis. The initial treatment of duodenal ulcer is medical management consisting of H_2-receptor antagonists, often combined with antacid therapy. Surgical therapy is usually reserved for complications of duodenal ulcer disease.

61. The answer is E (all). [*Chapter 11 V C 1, 2*] The superior mesenteric artery takes a sharp origin from the aorta and courses over the duodenum. In thin patients, this can occasionally cause compression of the duodenum manifested by vomiting and postprandial pain. Patients who are immobile for a long period of time, such as patients in body casts, may also develop the syndrome as retroperitoneal fat is progressively lost. Gaining weight may lift the artery off the duodenum and, thus, relieve the symptoms. The condition can be treated surgically by releasing the ligament of Treitz, thereby removing the duodenum from beneath the superior mesenteric artery.

62. The answer is E (all). [*Chapter 11 VII C 1, 2*] Dumping syndrome is a complication of gastrectomy. It is characterized by epigastric fullness or pain, nausea, tachyarrhythmia, and diarrhea. These occur because premature gastric emptying ("dumping") releases hypertonic chyme into the small bowel, with consequent jejunal distention from the rapid accumulation of fluid. Dumping syndrome affects most postgastrectomy patients to a mild degree and can usually be managed by dietary control.

63. The answer is B (1, 3). [*Chapter 11 VII B 1, 2*] The afferent loop syndrome is caused by intermittent mechanical obstruction of the afferent loop of a Billroth II gastrojejunostomy. This obstruction causes discomfort as the afferent loop contracts and becomes distended. As the force of contraction empties the afferent loop, the symptoms are relieved. The symptoms of the afferent loop syndrome can be ameliorated by converting the Billroth II gastrojejunostomy to a Roux-en-Y type of anastomosis. Relief usually is complete after revision, and, if done properly, recurrence of symptoms is very unusual.

64. The answer is D (4). [*Chapter 12 II B, E 3 f*] Vitamin B_{12} is the only nutrient absorbed exclusively in the terminal ileum; therefore, parenteral replacement is necessary after resection of this area. Although bile salts are also absorbed primarily in the terminal ileum, they usually do not require replacement either enterally or parenterally.

65. The answer is A (1, 2, 3). [*Chapter 12 II B 2 b*] Signs and symptoms of Crohn's disease include an abdominal mass, anemia, diarrhea (usually not bloody), abdominal pain, lethargy, fever, weight loss, and anorectal disease. Complications of the disease include intestinal obstruction, usually due to stricture and inflammation, intra- or retroperitoneal abscesses, and fistulas that form from bowel to skin, bladder, vagina, urethra, or to other loops of bowel.

66. The answer is D (4). [*Chapter 12 II E 1*] With short bowel syndrome, absorption of all nutrients, including water, is poor. While all patients require total parenteral nutrition immediately after the loss of most of their bowel, eventually most patients can be weaned from parenteral nutrition gradually. As a total colectomy leaves the entire small bowel intact (approximately 20 feet in length), it does not cause short bowel syndrome. Caloric intake must increase because of malabsorption.

67. The answer is A (1, 2, 3). [*Chapter 12 II F*] Chronic radiation enteritis generally becomes evident months to years after the conclusion of radiation therapy to the small bowel. At that time, the possibility of tumor recurrence must be excluded as the signs and symptoms are similar. Due to the breakdown of tissues that occurs, fistulas may form between the bowel and major arteries (enteroarterial fistula); at times, these fistulas cause severe gastrointestinal hemorrhage. The overall prognosis for severe radiation enteritis is poor; the 5-year survival is less than 50%.

68. The answer is B (1, 3). [*Chapter 14 I C 1 a, 2 a (2), 4 a, D 1 c (3)*] Both hepatocellular carcinoma and hepatic adenomas frequently present with rupture through the capsule and hemorrhage into the free peritoneal space. This is not typical of other hepatic tumors, including hemangioma. Hemangiomas typically produce symptoms by enlarging and either causing pain or compressing adjacent structures.

69. The answer is A (1, 2, 3). [*Chapter 14 I D 1 b (1), (2), (5) (b)*] Chronic alcohol abuse, hepatitis B surface antigen, and aflatoxins are clearly associated with the development of hepatocellular carcinoma. Oral contraceptives, by contrast, have shown an association with hepatocellular adenoma but not carcinoma.

70. The answer is A (1, 2, 3). [*Chapter 14 I E 1, 2 a (2), 3 a, d (2)*] The commonest tumor of the liver is a metastatic tumor. Results of treatment for colorectal carcinoma metastatic to the liver have been very disappointing, with fluorouracil (5-FU) as the principal drug being tested. The only bright spot in this disease is the fact that a solitary colon metastasis to the liver can be cured by surgery. Such a lesion should, therefore, be actively sought, and the patient should be referred to a center specializing in liver resections. Testing for carcinoembryonic antigen (CEA) is often positive in metastatic colon cancer, although CEA is not specific for colon cancer.

71. The answer is A (1, 2, 3). [*Chapter 14 I F 2 a (2), c, 3*] In the Western world, most hepatic abscesses are bacterial in origin. The primary source may be abdominal, but seeding from a distant focus of infection, such as a subacute bacterial endocarditis, can also be the cause. Amebic abscesses, caused by *Entamoeba histolytica,* are commoner than bacterial abscesses in third-world countries. The standard treatment for a bacterial hepatic abscess is primarily surgical drainage. Besides removing infectious and necrotic matter, drainage allows identification of the infecting organism and, thus, more appropriate antibiotic therapy. Ultrasonically guided catheter drainage may also be effective if minimal necrotic debris is present.

72. The answer is A (1, 2, 3). [*Chapter 14 II H 4 a–e*] The Warren shunt selectively decompresses the splenic venous bed while maintaining excellent hepatic portal perfusion. Maintaining this perfusion may decrease the incidence of encephalopathy when compared to a portocaval shunt. At the same time, the portal pressure within the mesenteric system is maintained, making ascites a common problem following this procedure.

73–77. The answers are: 73-B, 74-D, 75-C, 76-C, 77-D. [*Chapter 11 II A 1–8, B 1–6*] The etiology of gastric ulcers is multifactorial, but damage to the gastric mucosal barrier appears to be the key. Reflux of bile into the stomach is thought to change the mucosal barrier, allowing gastric acid to enter the mucosa and injure it. Drugs, such as ethanol, indomethacin, and aspirin, can alter the mucosal barrier, and the combination of smoking and aspirin ingestion is strongly implicated in the development of gastric ulcers. Patients with gastric ulcers seem to have lower than normal rates of acid secretion. Although evidence suggests that gastric ulcer does not degenerate into carcinoma, gastric cancer will ulcerate in 25% of cases; thus, it is mandatory that nonhealing ulcers be examined histologically for signs of malignancy. Initial medical therapy is indicated for gastric ulcers; however, surgery is recommended if malignancy cannot be ruled out, if perforation or hemorrhage occurs, or if medical therapy fails.

The major cause of duodenal ulcers is increased acid production. Smoking, caffeine ingestion, and aspirin use are all associated with an increased incidence of duodenal ulcer, but they have not proven to be causative. In the absence of complications, such as perforation, hemorrhage, or obstruction, medical management of duodenal ulcer is usually successful. Although stomach cancers can ulcerate and mimic ulcers, there is no evidence to suggest that benign ulcers can degenerate into cancer.

78–82. The answers are: 78-D, 79-B, 80-C, 81-B, 82-A. [*Chapter 11 I A 4 b (2), B 3 b*] G cells, in the gastric antrum, secrete the hormone gastrin, which stimulates secretion of hydrochloric acid and pepsinogen. The parietal, or oxyntic, cells, located in the gastric fundus and body, produce hydrochloric acid and intrinsic factor. Brunner's glands are located in the proximal duodenum, where they produce an alkaline mucus that presumably protects the mucosa. The chief or zygomatic cells, found deep in the fundic glands of the gastric mucosa, secrete pepsinogen, the precursor of pepsin, which is the protein-digesting enzyme. Argentaffin cells are found throughout the stomach; their function is unknown.

Part V
Endocrine Disorders

16
Thyroid, Adrenal, Parathyroid, and Thymus Glands

John S. Radomski
Herbert E. Cohn

I. THYROID GLAND. Indications for operations on the thyroid gland have varied since excision was first described by Kocher in the late 1800s. In early years, operations on the thyroid were done primarily to relieve the pressure symptoms of large iodine-deficiency goiter, to control hyperthyroidism, or to remove thyroid neoplasms. With the advent of iodized salt, iodine-deficiency goiters have been almost eliminated, and hyperthyroidism is now controlled mainly by nonoperative means. However, surgery remains the mainstay of treatment for thyroid neoplasms and, in many instances, is important in their diagnosis.

A. Vasculature of the thyroid gland

1. Arterial supply

a. The superior thyroid artery, which is the first branch of the external carotid artery, supplies the superior pole of the thyroid.

b. The inferior thyroid artery, which arises from the thyrocervical trunk as a branch of the subclavian artery, supplies the lower pole of the gland.

c. A thyroidea ima artery occasionally arises from the aortic arch and connects to the thyroid isthmus inferiorly.

2. Venous drainage of the thyroid is an interconnecting system of veins without valves.

a. The superior thyroid veins drain along the course of the superior thyroid arteries into the internal jugular vein.

b. The middle thyroid vein drains directly into the internal jugular vein.

c. The inferior thyroid veins drain from the lower pole and isthmus either directly into the internal jugular vein or into the innominate vein.

3. Lymphatic drainage

a. The thyroid gland always drains to the ipsilateral lymph nodes in either the anterior or posterior triangle of the neck, along the course of the internal jugular vein to the nodes in the tracheoesophageal groove or to the antero- or paratracheal nodes in the mediastinum.

b. The **nodes in the tracheoesophageal groove** are most important in the spread of thyroid malignancies, since involvement of these nodes may cause tumor extension into the underlying recurrent nerve, trachea, or esophagus.

B. Innervation of the thyroid gland

1. Recurrent (inferior) laryngeal nerve

a. Course. The recurrent laryngeal nerve runs in the tracheoesophageal groove in intimate relationship to the posteromedial aspect of the thyroid gland.

(1) On the right, the nerve recurs around the subclavian artery and runs an oblique course from lateral to medial, crossing the inferior thyroid artery before entering the tracheoesophageal groove.

(2) On the left, the nerve recurs around the ligamentum arteriosum in the mediastinum and runs a course parallel to the tracheoesophageal groove throughout its course in the neck.

b. Branches. The nerve divides into an external branch, which is sensory to the larynx, and an internal branch, which supplies the intrinsic muscles of the larynx.

c. Injury to the recurrent laryngeal nerve most commonly occurs where the nerve crosses the inferior thyroid artery or where it penetrates the cricothyroid membrane, but injury can occur anywhere along its course [see I D 2 e (4) (d)]. Injury can be avoided by visualizing the nerve throughout its course during operations requiring complete thyroid lobectomy.

2. Superior laryngeal nerve
   a. Course. The nerve is intimately intertwined with the branches of the superior thyroid artery.
   b. Branches. The superior laryngeal nerve has an external branch, which is sensory to the larynx, and an internal branch, which is motor to the cricothyroid muscle.
   c. Injury. The superior laryngeal nerve can be injured during mobilization of the upper pole of the thyroid, especially when the lobe is enlarged.
      (1) Injury results in voice weakness, which is especially noticeable in singers or orators.
      (2) Injury can be avoided by ligation of the branches of the superior thyroid artery at their junction with the gland rather than along the course of the artery in the neck.

3. Parathyroid glands (see III)
   a. Course
      (1) The superior parathyroids are located at the junction of the upper and middle third of the thyroid on the posteromedial aspect.
      (2) The inferior parathyroids are located in relationship to the lower pole of the thyroid, either on the surface of the gland or within a 3-cm circle, the center of which is formed by the junction of the inferior thyroid artery and the recurrent laryngeal nerve.
   b. Injury to the parathyroids during thyroid surgery usually occurs during total lobectomy or total thyroidectomy and results from disruption of the blood supply to the parathyroids. If this occurs, the consequence is either temporary or permanent hypoparathyroidism, unless the parathyroids can be successfully reimplanted (see III A).

C. Abnormalities of thyroid descent (see Chapter 18 III B)

1. Route of descent
   a. Normal descent. The thyroid migrates downward from its point of origin at the foramen cecum at the base of the tongue. It descends to assume its normal position on either side of the trachea at the level of the thyroid and cricoid cartilages.
   b. Abnormal descent of the thyroid may result in ectopic placement of thyroid tissue in the tongue, in the midline of the neck, or in the mediastinum.

2. Glottic (lingual) thyroid
   a. Location. Glottic (lingual) thyroid occurs when the thyroid fails to descend into the neck and remains at the base of the tongue. It may be the only functioning thyroid tissue in the individual.
   b. Symptoms of obstruction or difficulty with speech are usually related to goiter formation in the lingual mass.
   c. Diagnosis is by inspection or indirect laryngoscopy. A radioiodine thyroid scan should be done to identify the mass as thyroid tissue.
   d. Management
      (1) Suppression of thyroid-stimulating hormone (TSH) with thyroxine should be the first step in management, since glottic thyroid tissue is usually hypofunctioning.
      (2) Surgical removal should be considered when a patient has obstructive symptoms, especially if hormonal therapy is ineffective.

3. Ectopic midline thyroid tissue
   a. Location. A diagnosis of ectopic midline thyroid tissue should be considered when a midline mass is encountered below the hyoid bone.
   b. Diagnosis. If there is no thyroid gland in the neck, the ectopic thyroid should be confirmed by radioiodine scan, since removal of the ectopic tissue would leave the patient without functioning thyroid tissue.

4. Mediastinal thyroid
   a. Location. Most aberrant thyroids in the mediastinum are located in the anterior–superior mediastinum. They may represent **substernal extensions** from an enlarged thyroid or **normal thyroid tissue**, resulting from aberrant embryologic descent of the thyroid into the mediastinum.
      (1) Normal functioning thyroid tissue will take up radioiodine and, thus, can be confirmed by a radioiodine scan of the mediastinum.

(2) Many substernal extensions of the thyroid (i.e., **substernal goiters**) result from adenomatous hyperplasia and, as a result, do not take up radioiodine.
  (a) Substernal goiters usually occur in older age-groups.
  (b) They usually result in tracheoesophageal compression.
  (c) They do not respond to nonoperative attempts to relieve pressure symptoms by
      suppressing TSH with thyroxine.
  b. Management. Operation is usually advised to relieve pressure symptoms or to diagnose
     an otherwise undiagnosed mediastinal mass. Substernal goiters can be removed through
     a cervical incision without the need for sternotomy, since their blood supply is derived
     from the neck.

5. Thyroglossal duct cysts and sinuses
  a. Location. Thyroglossal duct cysts usually present as midline masses located between
     the hyoid bone and the thyroid isthmus. They are always connected to the base of the
     tongue, traversing the center of the hyoid bone.
  b. Signs or symptoms
    (1) They may be solid or cystic and may communicate with the skin, forming a sinus.
    (2) These lesions may present at any age, but most are seen in children.
    (3) A history of redness and inflammation from infection in the cyst is present in one-
       third of the cases.
  c. Management. Treatment involves radical excision, including a portion of the hyoid
     bone and the proximal duct extending to the base of the tongue (Sistrunk procedure).

D. Thyroid dysfunction requiring surgery

1. Normal thyroid function
  a. Triiodothyronine and thyroxine. The **follicular cells** of the thyroid are derived primari-
     ly from the floor of the foregut. These cells produce the thyroid hormones triiodothyro-
     nine (T_3) and thyroxine (T_4; tetraiodothyronine).
    (1) Hormone synthesis and release
      (a) Iodine and tyrosine combine to form T_3 and T_4.
      (b) Both of these hormones bind with thyroglobulin and are stored in the gland until
         released into the bloodstream.
      (c) Release is under the control of TSH from the pituitary and thyrotropin-releasing
         hormone (TRH) from the hypothalamus.
      (d) A feedback mechanism regulating T_3 and T_4 release is related to the level of cir-
         culating T_3 and T_4.
    (2) Hormonal action
      (a) The thyroid hormones activate energy-producing respiratory processes, result-
         ing in an increase in the metabolic rate and an increase in oxygen consumption.
      (b) Increased glycogenolysis results in a rise in blood sugar.
      (c) The thyroid hormones also enhance metabolic, circulatory, and somatic neuro-
         muscular actions of catecholamines.
         (i) The result is an increase in the pulse rate, cardiac output, and blood flow.
         (ii) Nervousness, irritability, muscular tremors, and muscle wasting can also oc-
            cur.
         (iii) These effects can be blocked by the use of β-blockers, such as propranolol.
  b. Thyrocalcitonin. The **parafollicular,** or **C cells,** are derived from the ultimobranchial
     body. These cells are part of the amine precursor uptake and decarboxylation (APUD)
     cell system (see Chapter 17 II) and produce thyrocalcitonin.

2. Graves' disease (diffuse toxic non-nodular goiter)
  a. Pathogenesis. Graves' disease is thought to be an autoimmune disease, resulting from a
     defect in cell-mediated immunity.
    (1) A substance known as **long-acting thyroid stimulator (LATS)** is produced, which in-
       creases the size of the thyroid and its production of thyroid hormone.
    (2) A clinical syndrome of hypermetabolism with associated abnormal eye signs and an
       unusual form of pretibial edema results.
  b. Clinical presentation
    (1) Hypermetabolic state
      (a) Symptoms include palpitations, sweating and intolerance to heat, irritability, in-
         somnia, nervousness, weight loss, and fatigue.
      (b) Signs include an audible bruit over the gland, tremors of the hands and tongue,
         cardiac arrhythmias, and a widening of the palpebral fissure of the eye.

(2) **Abnormal deposition of mucopolysaccharide and round cell infiltration** in the tissues is characterized by exophthalmos, edema of the eyelids, chemosis, and pretibial edema.

c. **Diagnosis**
   (1) Graves' disease is confirmed by the presence of an elevated total serum T_4, an increase in the T_3 resin uptake (T_3RU), and an increase in T_3 by radioimmunoassay.
   (2) An elevation of the free thyroxine index (the T_3RU value times the total serum T_4) and an increase in radioiodine uptake distinguish this form of thyrotoxicosis from thyrotoxicosis without hyperthyroidism (caused by thyroiditis, factitious thyrotoxicosis, or struma ovarii).
   (3) A thyroid scan shows an enlarged thyroid with uniform uptake throughout.
   (4) The serum cholesterol level is decreased, and the blood sugar and alkaline phosphatase are increased.

d. **Medical treatment.** The preferred method of treatment is medical, since the disease has a tendency to remit spontaneously after 1–2 years in adults or after 3–6 months in children.
   (1) **Radioiodine (^{131}I)** administered orally is simple, safe, and inexpensive.
      (a) It obviates the need for surgery and apparently does not increase the risk of carcinoma.
      (b) It has, however, several disadvantages.
         (i) It may produce chromosomal abnormalities in the fetus if administered during pregnancy.
         (ii) It may cause an increase in germ cell chromosomal abnormalities in later life if administered during childhood or early adulthood.
         (iii) Because of its slow onset of effectiveness, concomitant use of antithyroid drugs may be necessary if the patient is severely symptomatic.
   (2) **Antithyroid drugs** are effective in about 50% of patients, especially those with symptoms of short duration and with a small gland. They are rapidly effective and can reverse symptoms in a short period of time.
      (a) These drugs act by altering various stages of iodine metabolism.
         (i) Propylthiouracil and methimazole act through competitive inhibition of peroxidase, blocking the oxidation of iodide to elemental iodine. Propylthiouracil also interferes with the peripheral conversion of T_4 to T_3.
         (ii) Iodine in high concentrations blocks the release of thyroid hormones by inhibiting proteolysis. However, glands treated with iodine suppression escape this therapeutic effect after 10–14 days of therapy.
         (iii) Propranolol, a β-adrenergic blocker, reduces the secondary effects of hypermetabolism, such as tachycardia, without affecting the production of T_3 or T_4.
      (b) Their main disadvantage is that the incidence of recurrence is high if the drugs are stopped, so that prolonged therapy is required.
      (c) Their use must be stopped if drug toxicity occurs, manifested by fever, rash, arthralgia, a lupus-like syndrome, and agranulocytosis.

e. **Surgical treatment.** The preferred operation for Graves' disease is bilateral subtotal thyroidectomy.
   (1) **Indications.** Thyroidectomy is indicated for Graves' disease under the following circumstances.
      (a) When medical therapy has failed because remission has not occurred after treatment for 1 year in adults or for 3 months in children, because the patient refuses to take the medication, or because the patient develops an allergic reaction to the antithyroid drugs
      (b) When radioiodine therapy is not advisable because the patient is a woman in her childbearing years for whom radioiodine is contraindicated because of its possible carcinogenic or teratogenic effects, or because the patient is a child for whom radioiodine is contraindicated because of its unknown late carcinogenic or teratogenic effects
   (2) **Objectives** of surgery are to remove enough thyroid tissue to correct the hyperthyroidism, while leaving enough tissue to prevent hypothyroidism (usually 10–20 g) with a minimum of perioperative complications. Despite this, the incidence of postoperative hypothyroidism may be as high as 40%.
   (3) **Preoperative preparation.** To minimize the risk of thyroid storm [see I D 2 e (4) (a)], the patient should be euthyroid prior to operation.

(a) **Antithyroid drugs** are usually given until the patient is euthyroid, and then Lugol's solution or saturated potassium iodide is given for 7–10 days before surgery.

　(i) This reduces the risk of thyroid storm both during and after surgery. It also reduces the size and vascularity of the thyroid gland, which increases the technical ease of surgery.

　(ii) However, it takes several weeks or longer to achieve the euthyroid state. Moreover, in a pregnant woman, thyroid drugs can cross the placenta and can cause fetal goiter.

(b) **Propranolol** can be given in conjunction with Lugol's solution if patients have had adverse reactions to antithyroid drugs.

　(i) This is rapidly effective in restoring the euthyroid state and in reducing thyroid size and vascularity. Moreover, it is not known to cause any fetal abnormalities should the patient be pregnant.

　(ii) Propranolol must be given for 4–5 days postoperatively to prevent thyroid storm, since the half-life of circulating thyroid hormone is 5–10 days.

(4) Complications of thyroidectomy

(a) **Thyroid storm** is a severe hypermetabolic state that causes hyperpyrexia and tachyarrhythmias due to uncontrolled hyperthyroidism.

　(i) Thyroid storm is rarely seen when the patient is adequately prepared preoperatively. It occurs most often when a patient has undiagnosed hyperthyroidism and is operated on for some unrelated emergency.

　(ii) Treatment is with large doses of antithyroid drugs, iodine, and propranolol.

(b) **Hemorrhage** is possible due to the increased vascularity of the hyperactive thyroid.

　(i) Postoperative hemorrhage can cause airway obstruction due to tracheal compression and laryngeal edema.

　(ii) Treatment is by opening the wounds, evacuating the clot, and controlling the bleeding.

(c) **Hypoparathyroidism** usually develops within the first 24 hours following surgery and results in a subnormal serum calcium concentration.

　(i) Symptoms of hypocalcemia include numbness and tingling circumorally or in the fingers and toes, nervousness, and anxiety. Increased neuromuscular transmission is evidenced by positive Chvostek's and Trousseau's signs.

　(ii) Treatment is with intravenous calcium gluconate, followed by oral calcium therapy after several days if hypocalcemia persists.

　(iii) Serum calcium levels should be checked daily for at least 3 days after thyroidectomy.

(d) **Recurrent laryngeal nerve injury** produces vocal cord paralysis.

　(i) Unilateral injury is usually manifested by hoarseness. If the nerve is intact, the patient usually recovers a normal voice in 3 weeks to 3 months, postoperatively.

　(ii) If the injury is bilateral, airway obstruction results, due to paralysis of the vocal cords in the midline adducted position. This requires emergency intubation or tracheostomy. If the nerve is intact and the injury is temporary, recovery usually occurs in 3–6 months. If the injury is permanent, it will require either a permanent tracheostomy or lateral fixation of the arytenoid cartilages with Teflon injections into the cord.

3. Plummer's disease (toxic nodular goiter) is a hyperthyroid state caused by either an autonomously hyperfunctioning nodule in an otherwise normal gland, or several hyperfunctioning nodules in a multinodular gland. This disorder is most commonly seen in women over 50 years of age and is usually associated with a history of preexisting nontoxic multinodular goiter.

a. Clinical presentation

(1) Symptoms are not those of the classic hyperthyroidism seen with Graves' disease but are usually related to cardiac arrhythmias, such as palpitations.

(a) Muscle weakness may be seen but is rarely profound.

(b) Hypermetabolic symptoms are infrequent.

(2) Signs suggesting Plummer's disease are arrhythmias, occasional muscle wasting, and the presence of a multinodular goiter.

b. Laboratory studies

(1) T_3 and T_4 are elevated.

(2) Radioiodine uptake is increased in the hyperfunctioning nodules.

(3) The nodules will not be suppressed by exogenously administered T_4 (thyroxine).

c. Surgical treatment

(1) Since the hyperthyroidism of Plummer's disease results from an abnormality within the thyroid gland itself, thyroidectomy is the preferred form of treatment.

(2) Preoperative preparation and perioperative management are the same as for Graves' disease [see I D 2 e (1)–(3)].

E. Enlargements of the thyroid (goiters)

1. **Overview.** Enlargements in the thyroid gland have been collectively referred to as **goiters**. Goiters may be **diffuse** or **focal** and may be either smooth or nodular. They may be associated with normal thyroid function or with thyroid hyperfunction or hypofunction.

   a. Diffuse non-nodular goiters with normal or decreased function are due to benign causes.

   b. Focal or nodular goiters with normal function may be due to thyroid neoplasms.

2. **Diffuse thyroid enlargements**

   a. Colloid and iodine-deficiency goiters

   (1) Incidence. They occur infrequently in the United States.

   (2) Clinical presentation. These are large, bulky, soft enlargements of the thyroid, which may grow to sizable proportions. They occasionally produce compressive symptoms.

   (3) Treatment

   (a) Compressive symptoms may require surgery, but more often than not they are removed for cosmetic reasons.

   (b) Other treatment is medical and depends on the cause of the goiter.

   b. Thyroiditis. Inflammations of the thyroid can be acute, subacute, or chronic.

   (1) Acute thyroiditis is an uncommon disorder caused by the hematogenous spread of microorganisms into the thyroid gland.

   (a) Clinical presentation

   (i) The clinical picture is that of acute inflammation with pain and tenderness, swelling, and redness over one or both lobes.

   (ii) The condition may occur in an immunocompromised patient.

   (iii) Staphylococci and streptococci have been incriminated, but any organism can be causative.

   (b) Diagnosis is established by needle aspiration with appropriate bacteriologic studies.

   (c) Treatment is by open drainage or localized resection with administration of appropriate antibiotics.

   (2) Subacute thyroiditis (giant cell, granulomatous, or de Quervain's thyroiditis) is thought to be viral in origin and is often preceded by an upper respiratory infection.

   (a) Clinical presentation

   (i) It is characterized by sore throat, enlargement of the gland (which may be asymmetrical), and tenderness and induration over the gland.

   (ii) Patients may have symptoms of hyperthyroidism due to the release of thyroid hormone from the gland secondary to the inflammation, but the radioiodine uptake is always decreased, distinguishing it from Graves' disease.

   (iii) The disorder is self-limited, usually lasting from 2–6 months.

   (iv) Occasionally, subacute thyroiditis is painless, causing hyperthyroidism without symptoms of inflammation in the gland, so that it may resemble Graves' disease clinically. This form is also distinguished from Graves' disease by the low radioiodine uptake. Painless thyroiditis not infrequently occurs during the postpartum period.

   (b) Treatment. Symptoms are controlled with either aspirin or corticosteroids.

   (i) Beta-adrenergic blockade may be used to relieve the symptoms of hyperthyroidism.

   (ii) Antithyroid drugs are ineffective, since the hyperthyroidism is not caused by increased thyroid hormone synthesis.

   (3) Chronic thyroiditis occurs in two major forms, Hashimoto's and Riedel's.

   (a) Hashimoto's thyroiditis (struma lymphomatosa) is a relatively common autoimmune disorder that occurs predominantly in women. It is considered to be autoimmune since it coexists with other autoimmune conditions and is associated with the presence of antithyroid antibodies in the serum.

   (i) Clinical presentation. Because Hashimoto's thyroiditis is a rather common form of thyroid enlargement today, it should be considered in any woman who has a goiter and hypothyroidism. It is usually unassociated with any other symptoms. The enlargement in the thyroid is most commonly diffuse and less commonly nodular or asymmetrical. There does not appear to be a predilection for thyroid cancer, but thyroid cancer should be suspected when the thyroiditis is associated with one or more nodules. Needle biopsy is helpful in confirming the diagnosis.

   (ii) Diagnosis. Thyroid function studies are usually normal. Radioiodine uptake and scans show decreased uptake with patchy distribution.

   (iii) Treatment. This form of thyroiditis is usually treated with long-term thyroxine therapy. The gland will usually regress in size unless there is considerable fibrosis. Surgery is indicated when a dominant mass is not suppressed by thyroxine therapy; when the gland continues to enlarge despite thyroxine therapy; and when the history and physical findings or the needle biopsy are suggestive of thyroid malignancy.

  (b) Riedel's (fibrous) thyroiditis is a relatively rare form of thyroiditis in which the thyroid parenchyma is almost completely replaced with dense fibrous tissue.

   (i) Clinical presentation. Riedel's thyroiditis usually occurs in middle age and may cause pressure symptoms, such as cough, dyspnea, or dysphagia. Because the gland is usually stony hard, the condition is difficult to distinguish from thyroid malignancy.

   (ii) Treatment. Surgery, namely resection of the isthmus, is needed both to confirm the diagnosis and to relieve the symptoms.

  3. Nodular thyroid enlargements. Diffuse multinodular goiter is the commonest form of thyroid enlargement. It is the cause of a palpable nodule in the thyroid in as many as 10% of the adult population.

   a. Clinical presentation. These goiters are caused by adenomatous hyperplasia of the thyroid gland.

   (1) The thyroid enlargement is thought to be due to long-standing stimulation of the thyroid by TSH during a period of suboptimal thyroid hormone production.

   (2) The progression to multinodularity occurs through a process of cyclic changes of hyperplasia and colloid formation.

   (3) Despite the relatively high incidence of adenomatous hyperplasia, the presence of biologically active thyroid cancer in multinodular goiters without clinical evidence of malignancy occurs in fewer than 1% of cases.

   b. Pathogenesis. The nodules in the glands show a wide variety of pathologic findings.

   (1) Some are filled with colloid, while others show evidence of cystic degeneration.

   (2) There may be focal calcification, hemorrhage, or scarring.

   c. Diagnosis

   (1) Most patients are asymptomatic, and the nodularity is detected on routine physical examination.

   (2) Occasionally, attention may be drawn to the nodules because of pain, difficulty in swallowing, or dyspnea if the nodules enlarge either spontaneously or due to hemorrhage.

   (3) Thyroid function studies are normal, as are thyroid antibodies. Radioiodine uptake is normal but scanning shows variegated uptake of the radioiodine in the areas of multinodularity.

   d. Treatment

   (1) If there are no clinical signs of malignancy and the gland is not symptomatic, no treatment is necessary, and simple observation is appropriate.

   (2) If the gland is cosmetically objectionable or if pressure symptoms develop, then exogenous thyroid hormone should be given. The purpose of thyroxine therapy is to suppress endogenous TSH stimulation of the gland and allow the gland to shrink. Lifelong suppressive therapy with thyroxine should be given to minimize recurrence.

   (3) Subtotal thyroidectomy is advisable if the glands are large enough to produce compressive symptoms and do not regress with thyroxine therapy.

   (4) If patients develop clinical signs of malignancy, this should be confirmed by needle aspiration biopsy, and appropriate surgery should be performed.

F. Thyroid neoplasms

1. **Overview.** The commonest reason for thyroid surgery today is to diagnose or treat a suspected thyroid neoplasm that cannot be diagnosed by conventional means. Not infrequently, a solitary or prominent thyroid nodule is detected on physical examination in an asymptomatic patient. The concern is that the nodule will be malignant, although most solitary thyroid nodules are benign. **Clinical pathologic classification** of primary thyroid malignancies is shown in Table 16-1.

2. **Assessment of thyroid nodules**
   a. **Patient's age**
      (1) In children, 50% of thyroid nodules are malignant.
      (2) During the childbearing years, most nodules are benign.
      (3) The incidence of cancer in nodules increases by about 10% a decade after age 40 years.
   b. **Patient's sex**
      (1) Thyroid cancer is commoner in women than in men.
      (2) Benign thyroid nodules are also commoner in women.
      (3) The likelihood that a nodule will prove to be malignant is greater in men than in women.
   c. **Family history of thyroid malignancy.** Medullary carcinoma of the thyroid may be transmitted as a mendelian dominant trait, but other thyroid cancers are not transmitted genetically.
   d. **History of radiation exposure**
      (1) Exposure of the head or neck region to therapeutic x-rays has been found to increase the incidence of thyroid cancer 5- to 10-fold.
         (a) The radiation exposure has been as low as 50 rads and as high as 6000 rads.
         (b) The radiation has been given for a variety of disorders, such as an enlarged thymus in infancy, enlarged tonsils and adenoids during childhood, congenital hemangiomas of the head or neck region, acne vulgaris, and Hodgkin's disease.
      (2) Thyroid cancers from radiation exposure are no different from those that occur without a prior history of radiation, but the latent interval from the time of radiation exposure until the development of thyroid cancer varies with the age at which the radiation exposure occurred.
         (a) When the thyroid is irradiated during infancy, the mean interval until development of thyroid cancer is 10–12 years.
         (b) When the thyroid is irradiated during adolescence, the mean interval until development of thyroid cancer is 20–25 years.
         (c) When the thyroid is irradiated during adulthood, the mean interval until development of thyroid cancer is 30 years.
   e. **Characteristics of the nodule**
      (1) **Consistency**
         (a) Nodules that are firm in consistency suggest malignancy; however, malignant nodules may undergo cystic degeneration so that they may be somewhat soft to palpation.
         (b) Soft nodules are likely to be benign; however, long-standing adenomatous hyperplasia may be associated with calcification in the nodule.
      (2) **Infiltration** of the nodule into the surrounding thyroid or overlying structures, such as the strap muscles or trachea, suggests malignancy. However, malignant nodules may have no sign of infiltration and may mimic benign nodules.
      (3) **Nodulation. Solitary nodules** have a 20% chance of being malignant. **Multiple nodules** are present in as many as 40% of proven cases of thyroid malignancy.
      (4) **Growth patterns.** Nodules that suddenly appear or suddenly increase in size should be suspected of being thyroid neoplasms. Hemorrhage into a preexisting nodule, such as adenomatous hyperplasia, can cause a sudden increase in the size of the nodule, but this is frequently associated with pain.
   f. **Ipsilateral lymph node enlargement** suggests thyroid malignancy. In children, as many as 50% of thyroid cancers are first detected because of cervical lymph node enlargement.
   g. **Mobility of the vocal cords** should be assessed preoperatively in all patients undergoing thyroid operations.
      (1) Ipsilateral vocal cord paralysis in a patient with a thyroid nodule is almost always diagnostic of a thyroid malignancy that has infiltrated the recurrent laryngeal nerve.

Table 16-1. Clinical Pathologic Classification of Primary Thyroid Malignant Lesions

Pathologic Variety	Local Invasion by Primary Lesion	Multicentric Thyroid	Regional Lymph Node Metastases	Distant Metastases
Carcinoma				
Well-differentiated				
Papillary*	Uncommon	Common	Common	Uncommon
Follicular*				
Low-grade, encapsulated	Rare	Rare	Uncommon	Occasional
High-grade, angioinvasive	Common	Occasional	Common	Common
Hürthle cell tumors	Uncommon	Common	Common	Occasional
Sclerosing ("occult" or minimal)	Uncommon	Rare	Occasional	Rare
Medullary (parafollicular C-cell origin)	Common	Constant in familial Occasional in sporadic	Common	Common
Anaplastic	Always	Common	Common	Common
Lymphoma	Involves entire gland	Involves entire gland	Systemic disease usual but not constant	

*Associated foci of anaplastic carcinoma convert this to virulence of anaplastic variety. (Reprinted with permission from Block MA, Cerny JC: Endocrine system. In *General Surgery—Therapy Update Service.* Edited by Beahrs OH and Beart RW Jr., Media, PA, Harwal Medical Publications, 1984, p 2-7.)

(2) Since vocal cord paralysis may not be associated with voice changes, the cords should be examined by either indirect or direct laryngoscopy or by nasal pharyngoscopy.

(3) Examination should be repeated postoperatively if voice abnormalities occur.

3. **Diagnostic studies.** Although clinical evaluation is the mainstay in distinguishing benign from malignant thyroid nodules, alone it may be insufficient, and other diagnostic studies may be needed.

   a. Thyroid function tests are of little value in diagnosing thyroid cancer. Nearly all thyroid cancers are nonfunctioning, as are the nodules of adenomatous hyperplasia. Therefore, fewer than 1% of all thyroid malignancies will be associated with hyperfunction.

   b. Antithyroid antibodies may be elevated in patients with Hashimoto's thyroiditis, but thyroid cancer may coexist with thyroiditis; thus, a positive antibody test does not preclude the diagnosis of thyroid cancer.

   c. Thyrocalcitonin assay will be elevated in patients with medullary carcinoma of the thyroid.

   d. Radioisotope scanning of the thyroid may be done with radioiodine or with technetium-99m (^{99m}Tc) pertechnetate.

   (1) Isotope tracers are taken up by normally functioning thyroid tissue, which appears as a "hot" area on a thyroid scan; nodules that do not take up the tracers appear as "cold" areas.

   (a) Approximately 20% of cold nodules will be malignant, and approximately 40% of thyroid cancers will take up the radioisotope tracer to some degree.

   (b) Radioisotope scanning may exclude nodules that are not malignant if they appear "hot" but does not discriminate benign "cold" nodules from malignant ones.

   (2) Iodine-123 (^{123}I) and -125 (^{125}I) give less radiation exposure than iodine-131 (^{131}I) because they have shorter half-lives than ^{131}I. They do not provide any better discrimination than ^{131}I between benign and malignant thyroid nodules.

   (3) ^{99m}Tc pertechnetate is trapped but, in contrast to radioiodine, is not organified by the thyroid gland.

   (a) Nodules that are "cold" to radioiodine will also be "cold" to ^{99m}Tc.

   (b) Tumors of the thyroid may take up ^{99m}Tc and appear "hot" on the scan due to the vascularity of the tumor. Thus, all nodules that are "hot" on a ^{99m}Tc scan should be scanned with radioiodine to determine their function.

   (c) ^{99m}Tc delivers only a fraction of the radiation that is delivered by ^{131}I. It does not discriminate any better than does ^{131}I between benign and malignant thyroid nodules.

   e. Ultrasonography

   (1) Using an ultrasound probe, an image of the size and shape of the thyroid gland and the nodules that it contains can be mapped. Thyroid nodules, thus, can be identified as either cystic, solid, or complex (i.e., a mixture of solid and cystic components).

   (2) While ultrasonography is able to distinguish pure cysts of the thyroid, which are rarely malignant, from complex or solid masses, it cannot distinguish benign from malignant complex or solid masses.

   (3) Ultrasonography is helpful in identifying thyroid nodules that are not clinically palpable and in directing a needle to a nonpalpable nodule for biopsy.

   f. Needle biopsy of the thyroid is designed to obtain cells for histopathologic or cytopathologic examination as an aid in the diagnosis of thyroid nodules and the planning of therapy. Needle biopsy is the most useful diagnostic tool, aside from surgery, for distinguishing benign from malignant thyroid nodules. The combination of core biopsy or large-needle biopsy with fine-needle aspiration is considered the best method for diagnosing or excluding malignancy in a thyroid nodule. However, none of these biopsy techniques, which are discussed below, can distinguish benign from malignant follicular neoplasms.

   (1) Core biopsy

   (a) Using a 14-gauge, specially designed needle (Vim-Silverman or Tru-Cut), this biopsy technique obtains from the thyroid nodule a cylinder of tissue that is then fixed and stained for histopathologic analysis.

   (b) It is the most accurate method of assessing the histologic nature of a thyroid nodule.

(c) Because of the large size of the needle, it is unsuitable for biopsying small nodules.

(d) The incidence of complications is relatively high.

(2) Large-needle biopsy

(a) A plug of tissue is aspirated from the nodule by applying suction to a syringe attached to an 18- or 20-gauge needle that is inserted into the nodule. Fragments of tissue are obtained in this way for histopathologic preparation as well as cells for cytopathologic preparation.

(b) This technique has the same advantages as core biopsy and has a lower rate of complications.

(3) Fine-needle aspiration

(a) This technique obtains a specimen for cytopathologic examination.

(b) In contrast to the other techniques, which provide a core of tissue, fine-needle aspiration allows individual cells and clusters of cells to be examined.

(c) The technique requires interpretation by a well-trained thyroid cytopathologist.

(d) It has a good degree of accuracy and specificity in diagnosing thyroid malignant lesions and, due to the small size of the needle, is associated with virtually no complications.

(e) Its main disadvantage is that it obtains only cells for evaluation.

4. Operative approach to the thyroid nodule

a. Overview. Operative removal is the mainstay of treatment for thyroid carcinoma.

(1) The extent of the operation will depend upon the:

(a) Type of thyroid cancer

(b) Extent of the tumor as determined from the preoperative assessment and the operative findings. For a solitary nodule confined to one lobe, the minimal operation is total removal of that lobe and the isthmus and removal of the anterior portion of the opposite lobe.

(c) Biologic aggressiveness of the tumor (see I F 4 b)

(2) A frozen section of the resected tissue must always be obtained to determine whether the nodule is benign or malignant.

(a) If the lesion is grossly benign in appearance and the frozen section reports a benign lesion, but the permanent sections reveal it to be papillary or follicular carcinoma, the extent of further surgery is determined by the biologic aggressiveness of the lesion.

(b) If the lesion grossly appears to be malignant and is confined to one lobe without invasion of surrounding tissues, then total removal of that lobe and the isthmus, and near-total removal of the opposite lobe are appropriate therapy.

(c) If the lesion grossly appears malignant and extends beyond the thyroid or involves both lobes, then total thyroidectomy is indicated.

(3) Lymph node resection is indicated when nodes appear to be grossly involved.

(a) The resection should generally concentrate on nodes in the interjugular location.

(b) Prophylactic removal of uninvolved lymph nodes is of no proven benefit.

(4) The parathyroid glands and the recurrent laryngeal nerve should be identified in all operations. The parathyroid glands should be reimplanted in an appropriate skeletal muscle site if their blood supply is compromised during thyroidectomy.

(5) The complication rate following total thyroidectomy, and especially the incidence of permanent hypoparathyroidism, is significantly greater than the rate following near-total thyroidectomy. Therefore, total thyroidectomy should not be done unless it is of proven clinical benefit.

b. Biologic aggressiveness of thyroid cancers. Three risk groups have been defined for patients with well-differentiated thyroid cancer, based on an analysis by the Lahey Clinic.

(1) Low-risk group. This group consists of women under 50 years of age and men under 40 years of age with papillary thyroid carcinoma.

(a) Unless both lobes are grossly involved with tumor, patients in this group do as well with near-total thyroidectomy as with total thyroidectomy. The remaining thyroid remnant is ablated postoperatively with [131]I.

(b) After surgery, patients should receive exogenous thyroid hormone for life to suppress endogenous TSH production.

(c) With comparable treatment, the recurrence rate and death rate in this group were found to be significantly lower than in the high-risk group.

(2) Medium-risk group. This group consists of women under 50 years of age and men under 40 years of age with follicular carcinoma.

(a) In this group, there is a higher incidence of recurrence after near-total thyroidectomy than in the low-risk group. Therefore, total thyroidectomy is indicated as the primary treatment.

(b) Radioiodine is administered postoperatively if there is any uptake in the neck on a scan after surgery.

(c) Patients should receive exogenous thyroid hormone for life to suppress endogenous TSH production.

(3) **High-risk group.** This group consists of women over 50 years of age and men over 40 years of age with *either* papillary or follicular carcinoma.

(a) In this age-group, the tumors are much more aggressive and require a more aggressive initial approach, since local recurrences are more difficult to treat and the mortality rate is significantly greater. Thus, total thyroidectomy is indicated in these patients.

(b) Lymph node dissection of palpable nodes should be more extensive than in the low-risk groups.

(c) As in the medium-risk group, radioiodine ablation of any tissue demonstrating radioiodine uptake postoperatively should be carried out, and exogenous thyroid hormone should be administered to suppress TSH production.

5. **Types of thyroid malignancy**
   a. **Papillary carcinoma**
   (1) **Incidence**
      (a) Papillary carcinoma accounts for 80% of all thyroid cancers in children and 60% in adults.
      (b) It affects women twice as often as men and is the commonest histologic type seen in patients with a prior history of radiation exposure.
   (2) **Characteristics**
      (a) The tumor is characterized by a slow rate of growth with spread to regional lymphatics in 50% of the cases. It spreads by way of the bloodstream in fewer than 5% of cases.
      (b) Tumors range in size from occult (less than 1.5 cm in diameter) to tumors that involve an entire lobe or both lobes.
      (c) In 40% of cases, the tumor is multicentric in origin.
         (i) Microscopic multicentric lesions rarely develop into clinical carcinoma.
         (ii) Macroscopic multicentric lesions will usually behave biologically like papillary cancer.
      (d) Some tumors are well encapsulated with minimal invasion of adjacent normal thyroid. Others are poorly encapsulated with invasion to perithyroidal structures.
   (3) **Prognosis**
      (a) Prognosis is excellent with occult or well-encapsulated intrathyroidal carcinoma. Patients with these tumors have a 20-year survival rate of better than 90%.
      (b) Prognosis is poor when the tumor is poorly encapsulated and extends by extrathyroidal invasion. The 20-year survival rate is less than 50%.
      (c) Prognosis is also poor as the patient's age increases beyond 40 years.
      (d) Survival does not appear to be adversely affected by lymphatic spread.
   b. **Follicular carcinoma**
   (1) **Incidence**
      (a) Follicular carcinoma accounts for approximately 20% of all thyroid malignancies. It is commoner in areas of the world where iodine-deficiency goiter is in evidence.
      (b) It also affects women twice as often as men.
      (c) Its relative frequency increases after age 40.
   (2) **Characteristics**
      (a) Follicular carcinoma spreads primarily through the bloodstream by way of angioinvasion. It rarely spreads to regional lymph nodes except for locally invasive nodules that extend into the perithyroidal tissue.
      (b) The tumor is slow-growing and usually unifocal.
      (c) When found cytologically to be combined with papillary elements, its biologic behavior is similar to that of papillary carcinoma.
   (3) **Prognosis**
      (a) Prognosis is good when there is minimal vascular invasion with a better than 80% 20-year survival rate.

(b) Prognosis is poor when there is gross invasion with a less than 20% 20-year survival rate.

c. Medullary carcinoma

(1) Incidence

    (a) Medullary carcinoma of the thyroid accounts for fewer than 10% of all thyroid cancers.

    (b) It occurs at all ages without predilection for either sex.

    (c) It most commonly occurs sporadically but also can be genetically transmitted.

        (i) When it occurs sporadically, it usually appears as a solitary lesion.

        (ii) When transmitted genetically, it may occur as a solitary lesion or may be a part of multiple endocrine adenomatosis (MEA) syndrome type II (Sipple's syndrome; see Chapter 17 I B 2, C 2, D 2).

(2) Characteristics

    (a) Early spread to the lymphatics is characteristic, and spread by way of the bloodstream is also common.

    (b) There are two types of medullary carcinoma, which are indistinguishable histologically:

        (i) Those characterized by aggressive, rapid growth, rapid spread, and early metastasis

        (ii) Those characterized by slow growth and a prolonged course despite metastasis

    (c) Since these tumors arise from the C cells of the thyroid, they produce thyrocalcitonin.

        (i) This hormone can be detected by radioimmunoassay in early stages of tumor development.

        (ii) In patients with hereditary MEA type II, the disease can be detected in this way prior to the development of clinically evident malignancy.

(3) Prognosis is poorer than for papillary or follicular carcinoma and is related to the stage of the tumor at the time of its initial diagnosis.

    (a) Stage I medullary carcinoma has a 50% 20-year survival rate.

    (b) Stage II has a less than 10% 20-year survival rate.

    (c) Death results from generalized metastasis.

    (d) Hereditary MEA syndrome is totally curable by total thyroidectomy if detected and treated prior to the development of clinically evident malignancy.

d. Anaplastic carcinoma

(1) Incidence

    (a) This tumor accounts for fewer than 10% of all thyroid cancers.

    (b) It is commonest between the ages of 50 and 70 years and shows no predilection for either sex.

(2) Characteristics

    (a) Anaplastic carcinomas are characterized by small cells, giant cells, or spindle cells.

    (b) They usually arise from a preexisting, well-differentiated thyroid neoplasm, such as a follicular lesion.

    (c) They grow rapidly into local structures, such as the trachea and esophagus, and metastasize early by way of the lymphatics and the bloodstream, so that they are usually incurable at the time of initial presentation.

(3) Prognosis

    (a) Prognosis is poor with a fatal outcome in almost all instances, regardless of the type of treatment.

    (b) When treatment appears successful, the lesion may well have been a lymphoma instead of a small cell anaplastic carcinoma, and the histologic nature of the neoplasm should be confirmed by electron microscopy.

e. Lymphosarcoma (lymphoma)

(1) Incidence. This tumor accounts for fewer than 1% of all thyroid malignancies and affects mostly women 50–70 years of age.

(2) Characteristics

    (a) Pathologically, these are usually small-cell tumors and may be difficult to distinguish from small cell anaplastic carcinoma except by electron microscopy.

    (b) The lesion may occur primarily in the thyroid gland as an extranodal growth, or it may be part of a generalized lymphomatous process.

(c) The focal type is best treated by radiation therapy, whereas the diffuse type will probably require systemic multidrug chemotherapy.

(3) **Prognosis** is variable and depends on the cell type and whether the tumor is focal or diffused.

II. ADRENAL GLAND

A. **Introduction.** The adrenal glands are important to the surgeon primarily because they are the source of several tumors, benign and malignant, and of hyperplasias, primary and secondary. Some of these lesions produce syndromes due to the overproduction of normal adrenal hormones, including Cushing's syndrome, Conn's syndrome, and pheochromocytomas. The diagnosis and treatment of these disease states require a thorough knowledge of the production, action, and metabolism of the adrenal hormones.

1. **Embryology.** The adrenal gland consists of two distinct parts, the **cortex** and the **medulla**, each of which has a different embryologic origin.

   a. **The adrenal medulla** originates from ectodermal cells of neural crest origin.

   (1) These cells migrate from the sympathetic ganglion and combine to form the medulla, which is surrounded by mesodermal cortex.

   (2) Additional **collections of adrenal medullary tissue** can form. These are most frequently found in the paraganglia, in the organ of Zuckerkandl just below the origin of the inferior mesenteric artery, and in the mediastinum.

   b. **The adrenal cortex** is derived from mesodermal cells near the genital ridge.

   (1) These cells coalesce to form a complete layer around the ectodermal cells that will form the adrenal medulla.

   (2) Occasionally, these cells become separated from the main cortex and form **adrenocortical rests**. These are most commonly found in the ovary or testis and near the adrenal glands and kidneys.

2. **Anatomy.** There are two adrenal glands, each one lying on the medial aspect of the superior pole of a kidney. The normal combined weight of the two glands is about 10 g.

   a. **Histology.** Three distinct areas can be recognized in the cortex.

   (1) The **zona glomerulosa** is the outer zone where the production of **aldosterone** takes place.

   (2) The **zona fasciculata** is the intermediate zone where cortisol and the other **glucocorticoids** are produced.

   (3) The **zona reticularis** is the inner zone where **androgens** and **estrogens** are made.

   b. **Vasculature of the adrenal glands**

   (1) **Arterial supply** to the adrenals varies but arises from three primary sources, that is, the phrenic artery, aorta, and renal artery.

   (2) **Venous drainage** is more constant. There is usually a large single vein on each side of the body. The right adrenal vein drains into the vena cava, and the left adrenal vein empties into the left renal vein. Small accessory veins can occur.

   (3) **Adrenal portal system.** Venous blood from the cortex, containing high levels of glucocorticoids, drains into the medulla, helping to induce the enzyme phenylethanolamine-*N*-methyltransferase. This enzyme methylates norepinephrine to form epinephrine.

B. **Adrenal hormones and catecholamines**

1. **Steroid hormones.** The **adrenal cortex** produces three main classes of steroid hormones: the **glucocorticoids**, the **mineralocorticoids**, and the **sex steroids—androgens** and **estrogens**.

   a. **Glucocorticoids.** The most important glucocorticoid physiologically is **cortisol**. Production of cortisol takes place primarily in the **zona fasciculata**. There is a diurnal variation with the highest levels occurring around 6:00 A.M.

   (1) **Regulation**

   (a) **Adrenocorticotropic hormone (ACTH; corticotropin)** is produced by the anterior pituitary gland. ACTH stimulates the production of cortisol by the adrenal. **Cortisol**, in turn, exerts a negative feedback on ACTH production at the hypothalamic–pituitary level.

   (b) **Corticotropin-releasing factor (CRF)** is produced by the hypothalamus and stimulates the release of ACTH from the pituitary.

      (c) Free cortisol is the active hormone. Normally, most circulating cortisol is bound to **corticosteroid-binding globulin (CBG)**. When large amounts of cortisol are produced, the binding sites become saturated and the levels of free hormone will rise.

    (2) Metabolism. Cortisol is metabolized in the liver by conjugation with glucuronide. This renders it water-soluble for urinary excretion. The level of urinary 17-hydroxy-corticosteroids reflects glucocorticoid production and metabolism. However, in states of hypercortisolism, the urinary free cortisol is more accurate.

  b. Mineralocorticoids. The major mineralocorticoid produced by the adrenal gland is **aldosterone**, which is produced in the **zona glomerulosa** of the adrenal cortex.

    (1) Regulation

      (a) Aldosterone production is regulated chiefly by the **renin–angiotensin system**.

        (i) Renin is released by the juxtaglomerular cells of the kidney in response to a fall in blood pressure.

        (ii) Renin converts **angiotensinogen** (made in the liver) to **angiotensin I**.

        (iii) Angiotensin I is converted to **angiotensin II** by **angiotensin-converting enzyme**, which is produced by endothelial cells.

        (iv) Angiotensin II stimulates the adrenal cortex to release **aldosterone**.

      (b) Aldosterone production is minimally controlled by ACTH.

      (c) The sympathetic nervous system can also stimulate the release of aldosterone.

    (2) Metabolism. Aldosterone is metabolized in a similar manner to cortisol. It is excreted in the urine in small quantities and can be measured by radioimmunoassay.

  c. Sex steroids. Androgens and **estrogens** are produced in the **zona reticularis** of the adrenal cortex. The urinary level of 17-ketosteroids reflects the androgen production. Estrogens can also be measured in the urine.

2. Catecholamines. The **adrenal medulla** is the site of catecholamine production, including dopamine, norepinephrine, and epinephrine.

  a. Regulation. Catecholamine production is under the control of the sympathetic nervous system.

  b. Metabolism

    (1) The pathways of catecholamine production and metabolism in the adrenal medulla are summarized in Figure 16-1. Dopamine can also be metabolized by an alternate pathway to homovanillic acid (HVA).

    (2) The levels of metanephrine, normetanephrine, vanillylmandelic acid (VMA), and the individual catecholamines can be measured in the urine to evaluate the function of adrenal tumors.

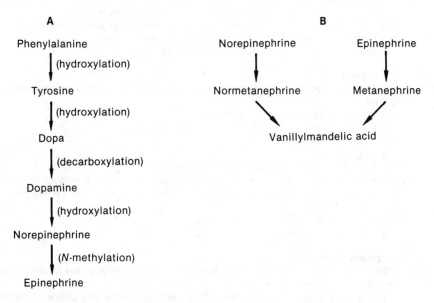

Figure 16-1. Pathways of (*A*) catecholamine production and (*B*) metabolism.

C. Congenital virilizing adrenal hyperplasia

1. Pathogenesis

a. If an adrenocortical hormone or an enzyme is missing from the pathway of cortisol production, the consequent shortage of cortisol will cause an increase in ACTH activity, and adrenal hyperplasia will result. The cortisol precursors will then be shunted into the production of androgens.

b. Although several different enzymes can be congenitally absent, the commonest defect is a block in hydroxylation at C-21 of the cortisol molecule.

2. Clinical presentation

a. Virilization results from the hormonal defect. In the female, this produces **pseudohermaphroditism**, and in the male, **macrogenitosomia precox**.

b. In a minority of cases, the block is more complete, and a severe salt-losing state with vascular collapse results from the aldosterone deficiency.

3. Diagnosis.
The diagnosis can be suspected from the characteristic virilization and the excess levels of 17-ketosteroids in the urine.

4. Treatment

a. The metabolic deficiency is treated with steroid replacement.

b. In females, plastic surgical procedures are often necessary to correct the genital deformities.

c. An accurate sex assignment must be made in female pseudohermaphrodites by means of karyotyping and Barr body analysis.

D. Adrenocortical insufficiency (Addison's disease).
This condition is important to the practicing surgeon because patients with Addison's disease are not capable of undergoing the stress of surgery without receiving corticosteroid support.

1. Types.
Addison's disease may be primary or secondary.

a. **Primary adrenocortical insufficiency** results in diminished or absent function of the adrenal cortex because of adrenal pathology. **Causes** include:

(1) An autoimmune attack on the adrenal gland

(2) Bilateral adrenal tuberculosis

(3) Adrenal fungal infections

(4) Bilateral adrenal hemorrhage, which can occur:

(a) Secondary to meningococcal septicemia

(b) Postpartum

(c) In patients on anticoagulant therapy

b. **Secondary adrenocortical insufficiency** is due to atrophy of the adrenal cortex secondary to a decreased pituitary production of ACTH. **Causes** include:

(1) ACTH suppression by corticosteroid drugs. This is the commonest cause of adrenal insufficiency encountered in the surgical patient.

(2) Primary pituitary pathology is a less common cause.

2. Clinical presentation

a. **Cortisol deficiency**, which occurs in both the primary and secondary forms, is manifested by:

(1) Anorexia, malaise, and weight loss

(2) Poor tolerance of stress

(3) Hypoglycemia

(4) Hypotension

(5) Occasionally, hyperpigmentation of the skin

b. **Aldosterone deficiency** occurs only in the primary form, since aldosterone production is not primarily under feedback control via ACTH. It causes a tendency for:

(1) Volume depletion

(2) Hyponatremia and hyperkalemia

(3) Azotemia and acidosis

3. Preparation for surgery

a. After a patient discontinues steroid therapy, it can take up to a year for the hypothalamic–pituitary–adrenal axis to return to normal function.

(1) Usually, a patient who has taken steroids regularly for any period during the past year is assumed to have inadequate adrenal reserve.

(2) If there is time, an ACTH stimulation test may be performed to assess the patient's adrenocortical reserve.

b. Perioperative steroid replacement is handled on an individual basis and depends on how long the patient was taking steroids, the dose that was taken, and the magnitude of the planned procedure. The following is a general **guideline** for a patient undergoing a major operation who is a **chronic steroid user:**

(1) Hydrocortisone (300 mg) is given on the day of surgery (100 mg before surgery, 100 mg during, and 100 mg after).

(2) The steroid dose is tapered off over the next 3–5 days, until the patient is back on his or her preoperative oral dose.

E. Hyperadrenocorticalism (Cushing's syndrome)

1. Types. Cushing's syndrome results from the effects of chronically elevated cortisol levels. Different mechanisms cause three types of Cushing's syndrome.

a. Adrenal Cushing's syndrome accounts for about 15% of the cases.

(1) It is caused by an excess of cortisol that is produced autonomously by the adrenal cortex. This can be due to an adenoma, a carcinoma, or bilateral nodular dysplasia.

(2) The remaining adrenocortical tissue atrophies, and ACTH levels are low because of suppression by the excess cortisol.

b. Ectopic Cushing's syndrome also represents about 15% of the cases.

(1) In this form, ACTH is produced by an extra-adrenal, extrapituitary neoplasm. The result is a hyperplasia of the adrenocortical tissue with consequent hypercortisolism.

(2) The cause is most commonly an oat cell carcinoma of the lung, but the syndrome can also occur with bronchial carcinoids, thymomas, and tumors of the pancreas and liver.

c. Pituitary Cushing's syndrome, or **Cushing's disease**, accounts for about 70% of the cases of Cushing's syndrome.

(1) It results from an overproduction of ACTH by the pituitary, which results in bilateral adrenal hyperplasia.

(2) The source of the excess ACTH has been debated.

(a) Pituitary tumors, either chromophobic or basophilic adenomas, probably account for the majority of cases. Some autopsy series have shown pituitary tumors in at least 60% of patients with Cushing's disease.

(b) However, in the remaining patients no tumor was found. This raises the possibility of an abnormality in the hypothalamic–pituitary axis, resulting in increased ACTH secretion.

2. Clinical presentation. The presentation of Cushing's syndrome is extremely variable and consists of any combination of various features. The commonest manifestations are listed in Table 16-2.

3. Diagnosis. No one test is conclusive for Cushing's syndrome. However, the normal **diurnal rhythm** of cortisol secretion is usually lost in Cushing's syndrome. The laboratory test results and the clinical presentation must be considered together to make an accurate diagnosis.

a. Plasma total cortisol is the most direct measurement, since Cushing's syndrome is a state of hypercortisolism.

(1) The accuracy of this determination is increased by measuring morning and afternoon samples, as well as a morning sample after a suppressing dose of dexamethasone the night before.

Table 16-2. Common Manifestations of Cushing's Syndrome

Hypertension	Peripheral muscle wasting
Diabetes	Striae
Hypokalemic alkalosis	Easy bruisability
Osteoporosis	Hirsutism
Buffalo hump	Acne
Truncal obesity	Menstrual irregularities
Muscle weakness	Emotional lability

(2) Plasma cortisol levels are suggestive of Cushing's syndrome if they exceed 30 μg/dl at 8:00 A.M. and 15 μg/dl at 5:00 P.M., or 10 μg/dl at 8:00 A.M., following a midnight dose of 1 mg dexamethasone, especially if these results are reproducible on several different days.

(3) The overnight dexamethasone suppression test is not fully reliable, as both false-positives and false-negatives occur. Adjusting the dose of dexamethasone on the basis of the patient's weight may reduce the number of false-positive and false-negative results.

b. Urinary free cortisol is the most reliable urinary index of hypercortisolism due to the increased renal clearance of unmetabolized cortisol, if further confirmation is needed.

4. Pathogenesis. Once the diagnosis of Cushing's syndrome has been made, the underlying pathophysiologic mechanism (see II E 1) must be identified.

a. The plasma ACTH level gives a good indication of the type of Cushing's syndrome.

(1) Extremely low values are seen with adrenal Cushing's syndrome due to the suppressive effects of cortisol.

(2) Very high levels occur with ectopic Cushing's syndrome due to the autonomous ACTH production.

(3) In pituitary Cushing's syndrome, the values are normal in 50% of the cases but are elevated in the other 50%.

b. Differentiating ectopic from pituitary Cushing's syndrome when the ACTH level is in the intermediate range can be difficult. Three methods are helpful in making this distinction:

(1) High-dose dexamethasone suppression test. After the diagnosis of Cushing's syndrome has been made, the patient is given dexamethasone, 8 mg/day for 2 days, and the urine is collected for measurement of 17-hydroxycorticosteroids. In pituitary Cushing's syndrome, the 17-hydroxycorticosteroid levels will usually drop below 50% of normal, whereas they will show no suppression in the ectopic syndrome. However, there have been enough recorded exceptions in both cases to make this test of questionable value.

(2) Jugular versus peripheral ACTH levels. Samples of venous blood are drawn from a peripheral site and, by catheterization, from the inferior petrosal sinus. Ratios of petrosal to peripheral ACTH greater than 2.0 have correlated with a pituitary source for the Cushing's syndrome, and ratios less than 1.5, with an ectopic source.

(3) Plasma lipotropic hormone (LPH, lipotropin) concentration. This tends to be higher than the ACTH concentration with ectopic Cushing's syndrome, while the opposite holds true for pituitary Cushing's syndrome.

5. Localization of the tumor

a. Pituitary Cushing's syndrome. Polytomography of the sella turcica has localized some pituitary tumors, but computed tomography (CT) and magnetic resonance imaging (MRI) are more sensitive and are specific for detecting small adenomas.

b. Ectopic Cushing's syndrome. A chest film usually shows the offending neoplasm; however, a technique such as CT or MRI may be needed to detect pancreatic or hepatic tumors.

c. Adrenal Cushing's syndrome. Several techniques are available.

(1) CT or MRI can correctly identify over 90% of adrenal lesions, including adenomas larger than 1 cm in diameter, carcinomas, and bilateral hyperplasia.

(2) Radioisotope scanning

(a) Radioiodine-labeled 19-iodocholesterol can successfully localize functioning adrenocortical tumors; however, the radiation dose is in the millicurie range, and several days are needed before enough of the isotopic label accumulates to provide an image.

(b) A new radiocholesterol analogue, NP-59, may offer quicker images with less radiation.

(3) Arteriography can localize adrenal tumors and is helpful in assessing the arterial supply of a neoplasm before its surgical removal.

(4) Retrograde adrenal venography can also localize adrenal tumors and allows for bilateral cortisol measurements. However, there is a 5% risk of adrenal hemorrhage and possible infarction.

(5) Venacavography is helpful, if a malignancy is suspected, to assess the intravenous extension of the tumor.

6. **Treatment**
  a. **Curative therapy**
    (1) **Ectopic Cushing's syndrome.** Treatment is directed toward the underlying neoplasm secreting ACTH. Removal of the tumor is curative. However, because of the diffuse nature of oat cell lung cancers, often only palliative therapy can be offered.
    (2) **Adrenal Cushing's syndrome.** Treatment involves total adrenalectomy of the gland affected by adenoma or carcinoma. Even if all of the malignant tissue cannot be removed, palliative therapy is easier if as much tumor as possible is resected.
    (3) **Pituitary Cushing's syndrome.** Treatment depends on the cause.
      (a) **Transsphenoidal resection** of the tumor is the procedure of choice if a pituitary adenoma is localized.
      (b) **Pituitary irradiation** from an external source has been effective in up to 80% of children. However, the cure rate is only about 15%–20% for adults.
        (i) Implantation of yttrium-90 may improve results, but this requires a separate operation for implantation and may cause progressive hypopituitarism.
        (ii) There is a lag period with radiation therapy of up to 18 months before effects are seen.
      (c) **Bilateral total adrenalectomy**
        (i) With the advent of effective transsphenoidal removal of pituitary adenomas, bilateral adrenalectomy is now reserved for cases where no pituitary adenoma is found, where radiation has failed, or where the patient is too sick to tolerate the prolonged radiation process or to await its ultimate effect.
        (ii) The advantage of bilateral adrenalectomy is its immediate and complete control of the cushingoid state.
        (iii) The disadvantages are the increased morbidity and mortality secondary to the operative procedure. It produces a permanent addisonian state, and in at least 15% of the cases, an ACTH-secreting pituitary tumor develops (**Nelson's syndrome**). Therefore, all patients treated for Cushing's disease with bilateral total adrenalectomy must be monitored yearly with visual field examination and sellar tomography.
  b. **Palliative chemotherapy** can be offered to those patients with unresectable or incompletely resected malignancies and, during the lag phase, to those undergoing radiation treatment. Remissions can be obtained in about 60% of the cases, but relapse is rapid after drug cessation. Two groups of drugs exist with differing sites of action.
    (1) Drugs acting on the adrenal cortex, inhibiting steroid synthesis, include mitotane (formerly called o,p'-DDD), metyrapone, trilostane, and aminoglutethimide.
    (2) Centrally acting drugs appear to be fast-acting and less toxic. They apparently act by affecting the hypothalamic release of CRF and, therefore, pituitary ACTH production. These drugs include cyproheptadine (a serotonin antagonist) and bromocriptine (a dopamine agonist).

F. **Primary hyperaldosteronism (Conn's syndrome)**

  1. **Overview.** Conn's syndrome is due to the excess secretion of aldosterone by the adrenal cortex as a result of a unilateral adenoma of the adrenal gland in 85% of the cases and to bilateral adenomas in fewer than 5%. Bilateral hyperplasia causes about 10% of the cases. Rarely, the syndrome is due to an adrenocortical carcinoma.

  2. **Types.** It is important to **distinguish primary from secondary hyperaldosteronism**. It is also important to distinguish hyperaldosteronism due to an adenoma from that due to hyperplasia, since surgical excision is curative for most cases of adenoma, but the response is not as good in hyperplasia.
    a. **In the primary form**, plasma renin levels are normal or low.
    b. **In the secondary form**, there is an increase in plasma renin and, subsequently, in aldosterone. This results from a decrease in pressure on the juxtaglomerular cells of the kidney. Common causes include renal artery stenosis, malignant hypertension, and edematous states, such as congestive heart failure, cirrhosis, and the nephrotic syndrome.

  3. **Signs and symptoms.** The increased secretion of aldosterone leads to hypertension, muscle weakness and fatigue, polyuria and polydipsia, and headaches.

  4. **Diagnosis.** Most of the laboratory abnormalities follow from the hypersecretion of aldosterone.

    a. Plasma electrolytes. Frequently, the potassium level is low, and the sodium level is high-normal. The carbon dioxide content may be elevated due to alkalosis.

    b. Sodium loading. Hypokalemia and a significant increase in urinary potassium may be induced (or will persist if already present) by giving the patient a high-sodium diet (200 mEq/day).

    c. Plasma and urinary aldosterone levels

        (1) One of the commonest causes of a missed diagnosis is the measurement of aldosterone before potassium repletion.

        (2) After potassium repletion, the serum and urinary aldosterone levels are markedly elevated in most patients with Conn's syndrome.

    d. Plasma renin activity. This helps to distinguish primary from secondary hyperaldosteronism. The activity is very high in the secondary form but low, even undetectable, in the primary disease.

    e. Postural response of aldosterone. The response of aldosterone production to 4 hours of upright posture is helpful in distinguishing hyperaldosteronism due to an adenoma from that due to hyperplasia. In patients with an adenoma, there is no change or a decrease in aldosterone production. With hyperplasia, there is an increase in aldosterone levels.

  5. Localization of adenomas

    a. Selective sampling of the adrenal venous blood to determine aldosterone concentration is the most accurate means of identifying an adenoma.

    b. CT and MRI have been shown to be at least 80% accurate in detecting adrenal adenomas and are much less invasive than adrenal venous sampling, which can be performed should CT and MRI fail to reveal a lesion.

    c. Iodocholesterol scanning [see II E 5 c (2)] can be used to localize aldosterone-producing adenomas.

  6. Treatment

    a. Surgical treatment

        (1) For patients with primary hyperaldosteronism due to an adrenocortical adenoma, the treatment of choice is total adrenalectomy of the involved gland.

        (2) It is important to restore potassium levels to normal prior to surgery.

    b. Medical management

        (1) Spironolactone, a direct antagonist to aldosterone at the kidney tubule, gradually leads to a reduction in blood pressure and a return to normal potassium levels.

        (2) Spironolactone is used in patients with primary hyperaldosteronism caused by adrenal hyperplasia, since the results of surgery have been disappointing in these patients.

        (3) Spironolactone is also used in the preoperative restoration of normal serum potassium levels in patients with adenomas.

G. Pheochromocytoma

  1. Overview. Pheochromocytomas are functionally active tumors, which arise from the neural crest–derived chromaffin tissue.

    a. Pheochromocytomas produce excess amounts of catecholamines, particularly norepinephrine and epinephrine.

    b. Most of these tumors (about 90%) are benign, but some (10%) are found to be malignant. There is a higher incidence of malignancy with extra-adrenal tumors.

        (1) Histologic examination is not an accurate means of determining the malignancy of a pheochromocytoma.

        (2) Malignancy is determined by the presence of metastases or direct invasion by the tumor.

    c. Pheochromocytomas can occur as part of the syndrome of multiple endocrine adenomatosis type II (Sipple's syndrome—see Chapter 17 I B 2). The adrenal medullary abnormality is bilateral in up to 80% of these cases.

  2. Location

    a. About 90% of all pheochromocytomas are found in the adrenal medulla. Approximately 10% of these are bilateral.

    b. Of the extra-adrenal 10%, most are found in the organs of Zuckerkandl, the extra-adrenal paraganglia, the urinary bladder, and the mediastinum.

3. Signs and symptoms
  a. Hypertension results from the excessive production of catecholamines.
    (1) The hypertension is sustained in about half the patients and intermittent in the others.
    (2) However, patients with the sustained variety can have paroxysms of more severe hypertension superimposed.
  b. Other findings include attacks of headaches, sweating, palpitations, tremor, nervousness, weight loss, fatigue, abdominal or chest pains, polydipsia and polyuria, and convulsions.

4. Diagnosis
  a. Urinary levels of metanephrine and VMA are the most reliable diagnostic screening tests. These are elevated in 90%–95% of the cases.
  b. Fractionated plasma and urinary catecholamine levels can increase the accuracy of the diagnosis to virtually 100%.
  c. The need for potentially hazardous provocative tests, using histamine, tyramine, and glucagon, has been greatly reduced. These tests are used only in the rare patient with equivocal biochemical findings.

5. Localization of the tumor
  a. CT and MRI have emerged as the most accurate, minimally invasive means of localizing pheochromocytomas. They are accurate in over 95% of cases.
  b. Arteriography should be used only after adequate α-adrenergic blockade, since it can precipitate a hypertensive crisis.
  c. Scintigraphy with radioiodine-labeled *m*-iodobenzylguanidine (MIBG), which structurally resembles norepinephrine, has been helpful in cases where CT has failed to localize the tumor, especially with small extra-adrenal tumors.
  d. Vena cava sampling. If the pheochromocytoma still has not been localized, samples of blood can be taken by catheter from different parts of the vena cava and other veins for hormonal analysis.

6. Surgical treatment
  a. Preparation for surgery should include adrenergic blockade with both α- and β-blockers.
    (1) Adrenergic blockade is helpful for three reasons.
      (a) It provides preoperative control of hypertension.
      (b) It reduces the risk of dramatic swings in blood pressure during surgery.
      (c) It provides vasodilation, allowing restoration of a normal blood volume (blood volume can be about 15% below normal in patients with pheochromocytomas).
    (2) Alpha-blockade is achieved first. Phenoxybenzamine therapy is begun 2 weeks prior to surgery, starting with 40 mg/day and adjusting the dose until hypertension and associated symptoms are controlled.
    (3) Beta-blockade is then obtained with propranolol, starting about 3 days before surgery, to control tachycardia. A starting dose of 40 mg/day may need adjustment if tachycardia persists.
  b. Operation
    (1) The patient should be monitored with an arterial and a central venous pressure line because of the potential for wide blood pressure changes and the large fluid requirements. A Swan-Ganz catheter should be used in elderly patients and in those with cardiac disease.
    (2) The approach should be transabdominal in all cases because of the high incidence of multiple and extra-adrenal tumors.
    (3) Total adrenalectomy is the procedure of choice for pheochromocytomas.
  c. Special situations
    (1) Malignant pheochromocytomas are treated by surgical excision of the tumor. If this cannot be accomplished, then as much tumor as possible is resected, and pharmacologic control of the catecholamine excess is started. Chemotherapy can be used for extensive metastatic disease.
    (2) When pheochromocytoma is a component of **multiple endocrine adenomatosis**, a bilateral total adrenalectomy should be performed. If only one gland is removed, there is a high incidence of recurrence on the other side.

H. Adrenal cysts and other adrenal tumors

1. **Adrenal cysts** occur infrequently, showing up in fewer than 0.1% of autopsies.
   a. **Types.** Most adrenal cysts are either endothelial cysts (lymphangiomatous or angiomatous) or pseudocysts, resulting from hemorrhage into normal adrenal tissue or into an adrenal neoplasm. Rarely, are they retention cysts or cystic adenomas.
   b. **Symptoms.** A large cyst can present as a palpable mass and can cause dull aching or gastrointestinal symptoms due to pressure. With cystic neoplasms, symptoms are those of the underlying process.
   c. **Diagnosis.** CT and MRI are the best methods available for diagnosing adrenal cysts.
   d. **Treatment.** Since a neoplasm cannot be excluded, these cysts should be surgically excised.

2. **Virilizing tumors of the adrenal cortex** are either adenomas or carcinomas of the adrenal cortex.
   a. **Symptoms**
      (1) **In females**, hirsutism, amenorrhea, and an enlarged clitoris are characteristic. In female patients, it is important to exclude other causes of virilization, particularly congenital virilizing hyperplasia in the young and an arrhenoblastoma of the ovary in older patients.
      (2) **In males**, pseudoprecocious puberty occurs.
      (3) **In all patients**, some of the features of Cushing's syndrome may be evident. The urinary 17-ketosteroids are increased.
   b. **Diagnosis.** CT or MRI provide the best localization of the tumor.
   c. **Treatment** consists of complete surgical excision. Mitotane is used for metastatic disease.

3. **Feminizing tumors of the adrenal cortex** are either adenomas or carcinomas of the adrenal cortex.
   a. **Symptoms.** In females, the tumor causes rapid premature sexual development. In males, there will be gynecomastia, decreased libido, and testicular atrophy.
   b. **Diagnosis.** Localization is by CT or MRI.
   c. **Treatment.** Complete surgical excision offers the only hope for cure. Mitotane is used for metastatic disease.

4. **Nonfunctioning adrenal masses** have been discovered at autopsy in up to 9% of patients. With the growing use of CT and MRI scanning, an increased number of these are being discovered during life.
   a. Although adenomas cannot be distinguished from carcinomas except by excision and inspection, carcinomas are rare when lesions are nonfunctional and smaller than 3 cm in diameter.
   b. These patients should probably be followed up with a repeat CT or MRI in 3 months. However, if a nonfunctioning mass is larger than 3 cm or is enlarging, surgical excision is the safest course to take.
   c. A CT-directed needle biopsy of nonfunctional tumors less than 3 cm in diameter may help to distinguish benign cortical adenomas from early cortical carcinomas.

III. PARATHYROID GLANDS

A. **Introduction.** The parathyroid glands are important to surgeons for two reasons. First, because surgeons treat patients with symptomatic hyperparathyroidism, they must know the cause and management of various hyperparathyroid conditions, and second, during operations in the neck, it is imperative that the integrity of the parathyroids be preserved to avoid injury, the consequence of which can be permanent hypoparathyroidism. There is no satisfactory replacement for endogenously produced parathyroid hormone, and the patient with hypoparathyroidism is doomed to a lifelong process of episodic, symptomatic hypocalcemia despite calcium and vitamin D therapy.

1. **Embryology.** In most individuals, there are two superior and two inferior parathyroid glands, which differ in their embryologic origin.
   a. **Superior parathyroid glands**
      (1) The superior parathyroid glands arise from the fourth branchial pouch in close proximity to the origin of the thyroid (the floor of the foregut) and descend into the neck.

    (2) Because of the embryologic origin, abnormal parathyroid locations may be either intrathyroidal or within the posterior mediastinum near the tracheoesophageal groove or the esophagus.

  b. Inferior parathyroid glands

    (1) The inferior parathyroids arise from the third branchial pouch in relationship to the thymic anlage. They cross the superior glands in their descent into the neck.

    (2) Not infrequently, they are associated with the thymus gland in the anterior–superior mediastinum.

2. Anatomy

  a. Clinical presentation. Some 85%–95% of individuals have four parathyroid glands, but as few as three glands and as many as five have been identified in 10%–15% of the population. The average parathyroid gland weighs from 40–70 mg.

  b. Location

    (1) The superior parathyroid glands usually lie at the junction of the upper and middle third of the thyroid gland on its posteromedial surface and in the tracheoesophageal groove.

      (a) They usually lie posteriorly to the recurrent laryngeal nerve and are in close proximity to the thyroid gland.

      (b) Occasionally, they may even be intrathyroidal.

    (2) The inferior parathyroid glands lie within a circle with a 3-cm diameter, the center of which is the point where the recurrent laryngeal nerve crosses the inferior thyroid artery.

      (a) The inferior parathyroids usually lie in a plane anteriorly to the recurrent laryngeal nerve.

      (b) They frequently are in close proximity to or within the cervical limb of the thymus gland.

  c. Vasculature

    (1) Arterial supply

      (a) The arterial supply is derived mainly from the inferior thyroid artery, arising from the thyrocervical trunk.

      (b) Since the superior parathyroid glands have been reported to receive their blood supply from the superior thyroid artery in 10% of autopsies, this artery should always be left intact when the superior parathyroid glands are exposed, so that their blood supply is not disrupted.

    (2) Venous drainage from the parathyroid glands is into the superior, middle, and inferior thyroid veins. These veins can be cannulated to provide blood specimens for parathyroid hormone analysis as a means of localizing sources of increased parathyroid hormone production.

  d. Histopathology

    (1) The normal parathyroid gland has a significant amount of fat interspersed with chief and oxyphil cells.

    (2) Hypercellular glands, seen in hyperparathyroid states, have a paucity of fat. The hypercellularity is mostly oxyphil-cell hyperplasia, but occasionally chief-cell hyperplasia may also be noted.

    (3) Histologically, one cannot distinguish the hypercellularity of a hyperplastic gland from that of a gland harboring an adenoma.

B. Parathyroid hormone (parathormone, PTH)

  1. Calcium metabolism regulation. PTH is a major regulator of calcium metabolism.

    a. It acts in conjunction with calcitonin and activated vitamin D_3 to regulate the plasma concentration of the ionized form of calcium. There is normally a reciprocal relationship between the serum calcium concentration and PTH secretion.

    (1) As serum calcium falls, the secretion of PTH increases.

    (2) As serum calcium rises, the secretion of PTH decreases.

    b. PTH exerts its biologic effect on bone, intestine, and kidney.

    (1) It increases the mobilization of calcium and phosphate from bone by stimulating osteoclastic and osteolytic activity.

    (2) It acts synergistically with 1,25-dihydroxyvitamin D_3 to increase the absorption of calcium and phosphorus from the gut.

(3) Renal effects
  (a) PTH raises the renal threshold for calcium by promoting the active reabsorption of calcium in the distal nephron.
  (b) It also lowers the renal threshold for phosphate by inhibiting phosphate reabsorption in the proximal tubule.
  (c) PTH secretion and phosphate depletion stimulate the activation of 1,25-dihydroxyvitamin D_3 via the activation of 1α-hydroxylase.

2. Increased, unopposed PTH secretion has the following clinical effects on bone, intestine, and kidney:
  a. Hypercalcemia
  b. Altered calcium excretion
    (1) Initially, hypocalciuria occurs due to increased calcium reabsorption.
    (2) This reverts to hypercalciuria in chronic hyperparathyroid states when the hypercalcemia exceeds the renal threshold for calcium.
  c. Hypophosphatemia
  d. Hyperphosphaturia

3. Laboratory tests. Serum PTH levels can be measured by radioimmunoassay. Normal values vary from laboratory to laboratory, depending in part upon whether the C or N terminal of the PTH molecule is used in the assay.

C. Hyperparathyroidism

1. Primary hyperparathyroidism
  a. Incidence. Primary hyperparathyroidism is a relatively common disorder, accounting for 1 in every 800 hospital admissions. It most commonly occurs sporadically but may occur as:
    (1) Part of a multiple endocrine adenomatosis syndrome (see Chapter 17 I)
    (2) Familial hyperparathyroidism
    (3) Ectopic or pseudohyperparathyroidism due to the production of a PTH-like substance from an extraparathyroidal tumor.
  b. Etiology and pathology
    (1) Fully 90% of primary hyperparathyroidism cases are due to a solitary adenoma of one of the four glands.
    (2) About 8%–10% are due to four-gland hyperplasia. The hyperplasia may be asymmetrical with one or two glands grossly enlarged. Microscopically, however, all glands show hypercellularity.
    (3) Parathyroid carcinoma accounts for 1% of primary hyperparathyroidism cases.
    (4) About 0.4% of cases are due to multiple adenomas involving more than one gland.
    (5) Microscopically, the glands have a paucity of fat and appear hypercellular (see III A 2 d).
  c. Clinical presentation
    (1) Most patients with primary hyperparathyroidism are asymptomatic, and the altered state is discovered only because an elevated serum calcium level is noted on routine multichannel biochemical screening.
    (2) When patients are symptomatic, the symptoms follow the mnemonic "**stones, bones, moans, and abdominal groans.**"
      (a) Stones. Renal lithiasis occurs in 50% of patients with symptomatic primary hyperparathyroidism (although primary hyperparathyroidism occurs in fewer than 10% of all patients who have renal lithiasis).
      (b) Bones. Osteitis fibrosa cystica (von Recklinghausen's disease of bone) is seen mostly in patients with secondary and tertiary hyperparathyroidism, which are due to chronic renal disease (see III C 2, 3).
      (c) Moans. Psychiatric manifestations—personality disorders or frank psychoses—may accompany primary hyperparathyroidism but are relatively uncommon.
      (d) Abdominal groans
        (i) The incidence of peptic ulcer disease is increased in primary hyperparathyroidism, usually associated with hypergastrinemia that results from the hypercalcemia.
        (ii) Cholelithiasis or pancreatitis may also occur, accounting for abdominal symptoms.

(3) Most patients have nonspecific symptoms, such as weakness, easy fatigability, lethargy, constipation, and arthralgia.

d. Diagnosis

(1) Laboratory studies

(a) An elevated serum calcium level is the cornerstone of diagnosis.

(i) This should be demonstrated on at least three blood specimens, drawn on three different occasions.

(ii) While primary hyperparathyroidism is a relatively common cause of hypercalcemia, other causes must be excluded, such as metastatic bone disease, myeloma, sarcoidosis, the use of thiazide diuretics, milk–alkali syndrome, hypervitaminosis, thyrotoxicosis, and Addison's disease.

(b) A serum PTH level that is disproportionately high for the serum calcium level (measured concomitantly) is diagnostic for primary hyperparathyroidism (Figure 16-2).

(i) In patients with metastatic bone disease, hypercalcemia occurs without a disproportionate elevation of PTH.

(ii) In patients with secondary hyperparathyroidism, the serum PTH level is elevated and the serum calcium is low.

(iii) In patients with hypoparathyroidism, the serum calcium and serum PTH are both low.

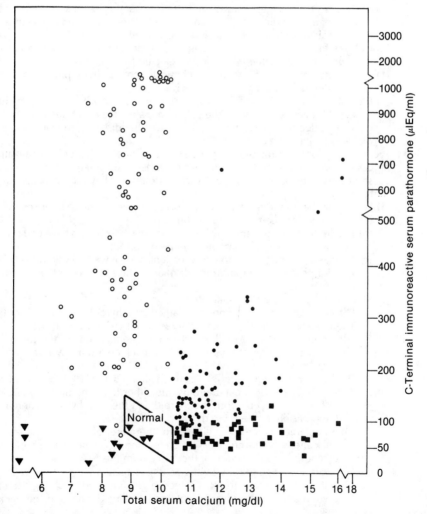

Figure 16-2. The relationship between serum calcium and serum parathormone levels in primary hyperparathyroidism surgically proven (●), secondary hyperparathyroidism (○), hypoparathyroidism (▼), and hypercalcemia due to metastatic bone disease (■).

        (iv) The serum PTH level can also be elevated in patients with **pseudohyper-parathyroidism,** a disorder characterized by an extraparathyroidal source of PTH. For example, tumors arising from the APUD cell system (see Chapter 17 II A 2) may produce a PTH-like substance that is indistinguishable from PTH by normal laboratory means.
    (c) The serum phosphorus level is decreased and the serum chloride:phosphorus ratio usually exceeds 33:1.
    (d) The tubular reabsorption of phosphorus is less than 80%, resulting in hyperphosphaturia.
    (e) Measurement of urinary cyclic adenosine monophosphate (cyclic AMP) demonstrates elevated levels.
    (f) Urinary calcium excretion is increased when the patient is on a calcium-restricted diet.
  (2) Radiographic studies
    (a) X-rays of the skull may show a "ground-glass" appearance in the outer two-thirds of the skull. Skull x-rays are also obtained to search for enlargement of the sella turcica due to a pituitary tumor, which may connote multiple endocrine adenomatosis.
    (b) X-rays of the proximal ends of the long bones may demonstrate bony reabsorption or brown tumors of the bone.
    (c) X-rays of the fingers may demonstrate subperiosteal absorption on the radial side of the middle phalanges and in the tufts of the terminal phalanges. Abnormal calcification in the digital vessels may also be seen.
e. Indications for surgery. Once the diagnosis of primary hyperparathyroidism is confirmed biochemically, patients should be selected for operation.
  (1) All symptomatic patients with biochemically proven hyperparathyroidism should be considered for surgery.
  (2) Operation is also advised for an asymptomatic patient whose serum calcium levels exceed 11 mg/dl, especially if the patient has a decrease in bone density, hypercalciuria, or a decrease in renal function due to other diseases, such as hypertension or diabetes mellitus.
f. Preoperative localization of the parathyroid glands. In general, localization techniques should be reserved for patients who are being considered for re-exploration because of persistent or recurrent hyperparathyroidism following unsuccessful parathyroid surgery.
  (1) Localizing the abnormal parathyroids preoperatively is helpful for several reasons.
    (a) It helps to reduce the operating time.
    (b) It helps to define the anatomy of the neck in patients who have had prior surgery in whom the normal anatomy may be distorted.
    (c) It helps to define the pathology in patients who have had prior unsuccessful surgery for primary hyperparathyroidism and who still have either persistent or recurrent hypercalcemia.
  (2) Methods of preoperative localization
    (a) Ultrasonography will define an enlarged parathyroid in 70%–80% of the cases. The ultrasound criteria for an enlarged parathyroid gland include:
      (i) A hypoechoic area in close proximity to either pole of the thyroid gland
      (ii) The presence of internal echoes that exclude a pure cyst or vascular structure
    (b) Dual-tracer imaging, using ^{99m}Tc and thallium-201 (^{201}Tl), is helpful in localizing 70%–80% of enlarged parathyroids due either to adenoma or hyperplasia.
      (i) ^{201}Tl is taken up by both the thyroid and the parathyroid, whereas ^{99m}Tc is trapped only in the thyroid.
      (ii) An enlarged parathyroid gland can, therefore, be localized by scanning the neck after administering ^{201}Tl, then rescanning the neck with ^{99m}Tc, followed by computer subtraction of the ^{99m}Tc from the ^{201}Tl image.
    (c) Thyrocervical angiography by the Seldinger technique
      (i) If the thyrocervical trunk is selectively cannulated, and angiograms of the thyroid and parathyroid are obtained, enlarged glands in the neck can be seen.
      (ii) If the internal mammary artery is selectively cannulated, enlarged parathyroids in the mediastinum can be seen.

      (iii) Stroke has been reported as a complication of thyrocervical angiography; therefore, this technique should not be used indiscriminately.

      (iv) It is reserved primarily for patients who have previously been operated upon unsuccessfully, who develop recurrent hyperparathyroidism after operation, or who have had no success with other localization techniques.

    (d) Selective venous sampling and PTH assay. The Seldinger technique can be used in the venous system to obtain blood samples from different venous sites for PTH assay. Because the study is costly and time-consuming, it is reserved only for patients in whom initial surgery was unsuccessful or who had a recurrence of hyperparathyroidism after initial successful treatment.

      (i) Retrograde injection of the thyroid veins is performed, and each of the draining thyroid veins is selectively cannulated.

      (ii) A disproportionately high PTH level in one or more of the venous samples helps to localize the lesion to one side of the neck or the other.

      (iii) Significant elevation in samples obtained from veins on both sides of the neck suggests four-gland hyperplasia.

    (e) CT and MRI

      (i) CT is particularly successful in localizing enlarged parathyroids in the mediastinum. In addition, it allows visualization of parathyroids that may not be visible by ultrasound or dual-tracer imaging.

      (ii) MRI seems to be as successful as CT in localizing parathyroids. It reveals enlarged parathyroids in the T_2 weighted image.

      (iii) Used alone or in combination, CT and MRI are the most accurate of the noninvasive localization studies but are also the most expensive.

g. Surgical treatment

  (1) Successful surgery requires a thorough knowledge of the anatomy of the normal parathyroids and their abnormal locations. When possible, all four parathyroid glands should be identified at surgery.

  (2) When a solitary adenoma is present, it should be removed and at least one other parathyroid gland should be biopsied. Biopsy of the gland will demonstrate its normal cellularity and exclude the possibility of asymmetrical hyperplasia.

  (3) Management of four-gland hyperplasia. Two options are currently available.

    (a) Subtotal parathyroidectomy, leaving a well-vascularized remnant (100 mg of parathyroid tissue in the adult and 150 mg in the child) to provide for normal parathyroid function. There is a 5% recurrence rate after subtotal parathyroidectomy.

    (b) Total parathyroidectomy with autotransplantation of minced parathyroid tissue into a well-vascularized, accessible forearm muscle so that recurrence can be treated without reoperation on the neck. There is a real danger of permanent hypoparathyroidism after total parathyroidectomy and reimplantation if the autotransplant does not survive.

h. Postoperative management. Postoperative hypocalcemia usually develops after successful therapy.

  (1) Asymptomatic postoperative hypocalcemia requires no treatment.

  (2) Symptomatic hypocalcemia always requires treatment.

    (a) In severely symptomatic patients, treatment should begin with intravenous calcium gluconate.

    (b) Mildly symptomatic patients may be given oral calcium in the form of calcium lactate, calcium carbonate, or calcium gluconate. Doses ranging from 4–20 g a day may be required.

  (3) If hypocalcemia remains symptomatic despite calcium supplementation, additional therapy with vitamin D may be needed. Supplemental calcium and vitamin D therapy should be continued until serum calcium levels return to normal.

  (4) Patients with significant bone disease will require prolonged calcium therapy to permit remineralization of the calcium-depleted skeleton.

2. Secondary hyperparathyroidism

a. Etiology and pathology

  (1) Secondary hyperparathyroidism is seen in patients with chronic renal failure. These patients are unable to synthesize the active form of vitamin D, and, therefore, they develop chronic hypocalcemia, hyperphosphatemia, and impaired calcium absorption.

(2) If untreated, secondary hyperparathyroidism may result in symptomatic bone demineralization, metastatic calcification in soft tissues, and accelerated vascular calcification. It occasionally can cause severe pruritus and painful skin ulcerations.

b. Treatment

(1) Medical treatment. Initial treatment is with:

(a) Dialysis with a high-calcium bath

(b) Phosphate-binding antacids

(c) Calcium supplements plus the active form of vitamin D

(2) Surgical treatment. In patients who are refractory to medical therapy, subtotal parathyroidectomy is indicated, since secondary hyperparathyroidism is always associated with four-gland hyperplasia.

3. Tertiary hyperparathyroidism

a. Etiology. This term refers to the hyperparathyroidism that persists in patients with chronic renal disease despite a successful renal transplant.

(1) Apparently, the parathyroid hyperplasia of long-standing renal disease becomes autonomous despite the return of serum calcium levels to normal.

(2) Patients are often hypercalcemic, hypophosphatemic, and hypercalciuric.

(3) Tertiary hyperparathyroidism may produce the same symptoms as those seen in secondary hyperparathyroidism.

b. Surgical treatment. When persistent, tertiary hyperthyroidism is treated by subtotal parathyroidectomy.

IV. THYMUS GLAND

A. Introduction. The thymus is important to the surgeon because it is the origin of a variety of tumors and because it is significantly involved in the development of cellular immunity and, as such, has been implicated in a variety of disease states.

1. Embryology

a. The thymus arises from the third branchial pouch and descends into the anterosuperior mediastinum.

b. It is a multilobulated structure with many fibrous septa. Each lobule has a **cortex** and a **medulla**.

(1) The cortex consists primarily of lymphocytes, which appear to migrate to the medulla and then emigrate from the thymus.

(2) The medulla also contains Hassall's corpuscles, which are composed of concentric layers of epithelial cells. Their function is unknown.

2. Anatomy

a. Development

(1) Because of the bilateral origin of the thymus gland, it develops two lobes and a roughly **H**-shaped configuration.

(2) Two limbs of the thymus extend into the neck and are often associated with the inferior parathyroid glands.

(3) The inferior limbs extend along the surface of the pericardium and abut the pleura.

(4) The thymus reaches maximal size shortly after birth and then begins to involute during adolescence and early adult life.

b. Functions

(1) Cellular immunity. The thymus is essential for the development of cellular immunity, which controls such processes as delayed hypersensitivity reactions and transplant rejection.

(a) The thymic-dependent portion of the immune system consists principally of the thymus and a circulating pool of small lymphocytes that produce cell-mediated immune reactions.

(i) While removal of the neonatal thymus in certain strains of mice leads to significant impairment in immunologic capacity, it has no such effect in the human newborn.

(ii) However, impaired thymic development may be associated with immunologic deficiency disorders.

(b) The thymus is the first organ to manufacture lymphocytes during fetal life, but most of the cells produced in the thymus die there.

(2) Immune system function and thymic lesions. Histologic abnormalities in the thymus, such as lymphoid hyperplasia or thymic tumors, are frequently seen in association with certain autoimmune diseases, suggesting a relationship between thymic function and immune system disorders. The autoimmune diseases are:

(a) Myasthenia gravis (see IV C)

(b) Systemic (disseminated) lupus erythematosus

(c) Erythroid agenesis

(d) Hypogammaglobulinemia

(e) Rheumatoid arthritis

(f) Dermatomyositis

c. Vasculature

(1) Arterial supply to the thymus is derived from small branches of the internal mammary or pericardiophrenic arteries.

(2) Venous drainage is primarily to a single thymic vein that drains into the left innominate vein.

B. Thymic tumors

1. Incidence. Thymic tumors (**thymomas**) are among the commonest tumors of the anterior–superior mediastinum in the adult.

a. While thymic tumors can occur at any age, they are commonest in the fifth and sixth decades of life.

b. Males and females are equally affected.

c. Some 40%–50% of patients with thymomas have associated myasthenia gravis.

2. Pathology

a. While thymic tumors have been described according to their cell of origin as lymphoid, epithelial, spindle cell, or mixed, it is almost impossible to distinguish benign from malignant thymic tumors microscopically.

(1) Two-thirds of thymic tumors are considered benign, and of these, 10% are simple cysts (see Chapter 18 III A 1).

(2) Spindle cell thymomas appear to have a better prognosis than epithelial thymomas, which have a poor prognosis.

b. The best index of the benign or malignant nature of the tumor is its tendency to invade contiguous structures.

(1) Benign tumors are well encapsulated.

(2) Malignant tumors are invasive, spreading by direct invasion of contiguous structures and onto adjacent pleural surfaces. Distant spread is extremely rare.

3. Diagnosis

a. Most patients with thymomas are asymptomatic, and the tumor is discovered incidentally on a routine chest x-ray. Symptoms, when present, are related to invasion by malignant thymomas and consist of chest pain, dyspnea, or superior vena cava syndrome.

b. The existence of a thymoma is suggested by either:

(1) An abnormality on chest x-ray, CT scan, or MRI (Figure 16-3)

(2) The presence of myasthenia gravis

(a) This condition should prompt a search of the mediastinum for a thymic tumor.

(b) A lateral chest x-ray is most helpful, since small tumors may be obscured by the great vessels in standard posterior–anterior chest x-rays.

c. Recently, CT and MRI have been helpful in identifying the degree of invasion of thymic tumors.

4. Surgical treatment. Most thymic tumors are removed through a sternal-splitting median sternotomy.

a. Thymic tumors that are not associated with myasthenia gravis or another clinical syndrome require mediastinal exploration and total removal of the tumor.

(1) Benign tumors can be removed by local excision.

(2) Malignant tumors

(a) If possible, all areas of invasion should be removed.

(b) When invasive thymic tumors are nonresectable or cannot be removed completely, postoperative radiation may be valuable. Chemotherapy and immunotherapy have not been clinically useful.

b. Thymic tumors that are associated with myasthenia gravis or other clinical syndromes should be removed, including the entire remaining thymus gland.

A

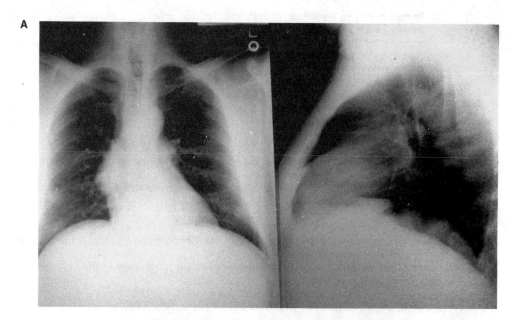

B

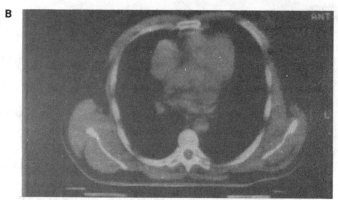

Figure 16-3. *A*, Posterior–anterior and lateral chest x-ray, showing an anterior mediastinal mass in the right hemithorax in a patient with a thymoma. *B*, CT scan from the same patient, showing an anterior mediastinal mass without fixation to the underlying pericardium.

C. Myasthenia gravis

1. **Overview.** Myasthenia gravis is an autoimmune disease of neuromuscular transmission that causes skeletal muscle weakness. It is characterized by spontaneous remissions and by exacerbations that are often precipitated by an upper respiratory infection. The commonest symptoms are ptosis, double vision, dysarthria, dysphagia, nasal speech, and weakness of the arms and legs.

2. **Pathophysiology**
   a. **Normal neuromuscular transmission**
      (1) The neurotransmitter acetylcholine is produced at the nerve terminal of the myoneural junction.
      (2) The acetylcholine binds to receptor sites on the muscle end plates.
      (3) This action triggers muscle contraction.
   b. **Neuromuscular transmission in myasthenia gravis.** It appears that antibodies to acetylcholine receptors develop, which decrease the available number of receptor sites on the muscle end plates, resulting in reduced muscle contraction.

3. Treatment

    a. Medical treatment. Patients with myasthenia gravis respond to drugs that stimulate the neuromuscular junction, such as neostigmine and pyridostigmine.

    b. Surgical treatment

        (1) In patients with thymic tumors, surgical removal of the tumor is advised, although the effect on the myasthenia is unpredictable. However, even in patients without thymic tumors, thymectomy appears to be the treatment of choice for all forms of myasthenia except purely ocular myasthenia. Thymectomy seems to:

            (a) Increase the percentage of permanent remissions

            (b) Decrease the morbidity and mortality of the disease

            (c) Improve the response to medication in patients who do not undergo complete remission

        (2) **Pre- and postoperative management** have significantly reduced the morbidity and mortality rates of surgery.

            (a) Surgery in patients with myasthenia gravis creates several problems.

                (i) The sternal-splitting incision reduces the ability of patients with impaired muscle strength to ventilate properly and to mobilize secretions.

                (ii) The use of parasympathomimetic drugs improves muscle strength but also increases pharyngeal and tracheobronchial secretions.

            (b) Preoperative plasmapheresis has been used to good effect.

                (i) It eliminates the need for parasympathomimetic drugs and eliminates circulating acetylcholine receptor antibodies.

                (ii) This produces significant improvement in perioperative muscle strength and virtually eliminates the need for prolonged ventilatory support.

    c. Results of medical and surgical treatment

        (1) Without surgery, spontaneous remissions occur in 18% of patients with myasthenia gravis, whereas thymectomy induces complete remission in approximately 38% of patients.

        (2) Sustained improvement is achieved with medication in only 33% of patients without surgery and in 85% of patients following thymectomy.

        (3) The best results from thymectomy are usually seen in young patients with myasthenia of relatively short duration who have become increasingly refractory to medication.

17

Multiple Endocrine Adenomatosis and Tumors of the Endocrine Pancreas

John S. Radomski
Herbert E. Cohn

I. MULTIPLE ENDOCRINE ADENOMATOSIS

A. Overview. Multiple endocrine adenomatosis (MEA) syndromes, or **multiple endocrine neo-plasia (MEN)** syndromes, are characteristic patterns of endocrine hyperfunction inherited as autosomal dominant traits.

1. Many of the endocrine cell types involved originate from the neuroectoderm and have the ability to secrete peptide hormones, amines, or both, but no unifying molecular defect is currently known.

2. Certain features are present in all MEA syndromes.
    a. All are autosomal dominant traits with significant phenotypic variability.
    b. The involved endocrine glands develop either hyperplasia, adenoma, or carcinoma.
    c. The neoplasias in the involved glands can develop simultaneously or at different times.
    d. Ectopic hormone production is common.

B. Types. Three types of MEA have been identified.

1. **Type I (Wermer's syndrome)** involves the parathyroid glands, pancreatic islets, and pituitary gland.
    a. Hyperparathyroidism (see Chapter 16 III C) is present in 90% or more of the patients with over one-half having hyperplasia of multiple parathyroid glands.
    b. Pancreatic tumors are present in 80% of patients.
        (1) These are usually non-beta islet cell tumors, which usually cause the Zollinger-Ellison syndrome (see II C).
        (2) However, other syndromes can occur (see II and Chapter 15 III).
    c. Pituitary tumors are present in 65% of cases. These are usually chromophobe adenomas, which produce acromegaly, galactorrhea, amenorrhea, or Cushing's syndrome.
    d. Approximately 90% of patients present with hypercalcemia, hypoglycemia, peptic ulcer, or complaints secondary to a pituitary mass.

2. **Type II (Sipple's syndrome)** comprises medullary carcinoma of the thyroid, pheochromocytoma, and parathyroid hyperplasia.
    a. Medullary thyroid carcinoma (see Chapter 16 I F 5 c) occurs in all patients.
        (1) It is usually multifocal and is often preceded by nonmalignant hyperplasia of the parafollicular C cells.
        (2) Serum calcitonin levels are elevated, although in the premalignant state, stimulation with calcium or pentagastrin may be necessary to identify this.
    b. Pheochromocytomas (see Chapter 16 II G) occur in approximately 40% of patients.
        (1) They are usually bilateral and occasionally are malignant.
        (2) They often present later than the medullary thyroid cancer.
    c. Parathyroid hyperplasia, with consequent hyperparathyroidism, develops in 60% of patients and resembles that of type I.

3. **Type III (mucosal neuroma syndrome)** is considered a variant of type II and is sometimes labeled **type IIb**; Sipple's syndrome then becomes **type IIa**.
    a. As in type II, patients develop medullary thyroid carcinoma and pheochromocytoma.
    b. However, the features most characteristic of type III are a distorted body habitus and the development of multiple neuromatous mucosal nodules.
    c. In addition, type III presents at a much earlier age, usually in the first or second decade of life, and assumes a much more aggressive course.

C. Diagnosis

1. MEA type I (Wermer's syndrome)

a. Most patients with MEA type I present with symptoms of peptic ulceration related to the pancreatic gastrinoma (see II C 1 b) or with symptoms related to the pituitary tumor (see I B 1 c).

b. The hyperparathyroidism is usually asymptomatic and is usually detected by an elevated serum calcium level.

2. MEA type II (Sipple's syndrome) [also known as MEA IIa]

a. The diagnosis is suspected in all kindred of any patient with **medullary carcinoma of the thyroid**.

(1) The inherited trait can be diagnosed in the premalignant stage, when **C-cell hyperplasia** is present before the medullary carcinoma develops.

(2) Finding an elevated serum thyrocalcitonin level leads to the diagnosis. Infusion of calcium and pentagastrin helps to stimulate an abnormal thyrocalcitonemia in those with C-cell hyperplasia or occult medullary carcinoma before either is clinically detectable.

b. Hyperparathyroidism is usually detected by elevations in the serum calcium and parathyroid hormone levels.

c. Pheochromocytomas or **adrenal medullary hyperplasia** may be asymptomatic but should be detectable by biochemical screening for elevated serum and urine catecholamines.

3. MEA type III (mucosal neuroma syndrome) [also known as MEA IIb]

a. Because MEA type III assumes so aggressive a course, early diagnosis is important so that effective treatment can begin promptly.

b. The diagnosis is similar to that for type II. The early appearance of mucosal neuromas and the body habitus should help in making the diagnosis.

D. Treatment

1. MEA type I

a. If only the pancreatic and parathyroid components of this syndrome are present, the **hyperparathyroidism** is treated first. This may reduce the production of gastrin and relieve the peptic ulceration.

(1) Subtotal parathyroidectomy is required, since the parathyroid disorder is usually four-gland hyperplasia.

(2) If the hypergastrinemia and peptic ulceration persist, treatment is directed towards the **Zollinger-Ellison syndrome** (see II C 5). This involves removal of the gastrin-producing tumor, if possible, and removal of the end-organ (i.e., total gastrectomy) if the tumor cannot be removed and if the use of histamine$_2$- (H$_2$-) receptor antagonists does not control the ulceration.

b. Pituitary tumors are usually treated by stereotactic transsphenoidal hypophysectomy, using an operating microscope to minimize the risk of injury to the posterior pituitary.

2. MEA type II

a. Medullary carcinoma should be treated in the premalignant stage, when only C-cell hyperplasia is present, at which time total thyroidectomy is curative.

b. Pheochromocytoma or adrenal medullary hyperplasia, if present, should be treated prior to thyroidectomy, since these hormone-producing disorders can lead to hypertensive crises during thyroidectomy.

c. Hyperparathyroidism can be treated at the time of total thyroidectomy by the protocol described in Chapter 16 III C 1, 2.

3. MEA type III is treated similarly to type II. Because type III assumes so aggressive a course, prompt and effective treatment is important.

II. TUMORS OF THE ENDOCRINE PANCREAS

A. Pathophysiology

1. The pancreatic islet cells and the endocrine cells of the gut (labeled **APUD cells,** standing for **a**mine **p**recursor **u**ptake and **d**ecarboxylation) originate from embryonic cells that have certain cytochemical properties in common.

a. They have a high amine content.
b. They have the ability for amine precursor uptake.
c. They produce the enzyme amino acid decarboxylase.

2. Tumors that arise from these APUD cells are termed **apudomas**. The various kinds of apudomas arising in the pancreas include:
   a. Insulinomas
   b. Gastrinomas (Zollinger-Ellison syndrome)
   c. Glucagonomas
   d. Vipomas (for vasoactive intestinal peptide, or **VIP**)
   e. Somatostatinomas

B. Insulinomas

1. **Overview.** An insulinoma is a tumor originating in the beta cells of the pancreatic islets that releases abnormally high amounts of insulin.
   a. Approximately 80%–90% of insulinomas are solitary, benign adenomas.
   b. About 10% are malignant with the potential to metastasize.
   c. The remainder are islet cell hyperplasia (termed **nesidioblastosis** in children).

2. **Clinical presentation.** The abnormally elevated insulin levels and the resultant hypoglycemia produce the following clinical picture.
   a. Bizarre behavior; unconscious episodes
   b. Palpitations, nervousness, and other symptoms of sympathetic discharge
   c. Whipple's triad:
      (1) Episodes of illness precipitated by fasting
      (2) Hypoglycemia during the episodes usually with blood glucose levels below 60 mg/dl
      (3) Relief of hypoglycemic symptoms by oral or intravenous administration of glucose

3. **Diagnosis.** Once suspected, the diagnosis must be confirmed by documenting the abnormal circulating insulin levels.
   a. Measurement of fasting insulin and glucose levels. An effective screening test is to have the patient fast for 72 hours or until symptoms of hypoglycemia appear, and then to test the insulin and glucose levels. An elevated insulin level in the presence of a low glucose level (insulin:glucose ratio greater than 0.25) effectively confirms an insulinoma.
      (1) Essentially all patients with insulinomas will become hypoglycemic within 72 hours.
      (2) As many as 40% will develop symptoms within 2 hours of beginning the fast.
   b. Comparing insulin and proinsulin levels can be helpful.
      (1) Proinsulin is the single-chain intracellular precursor that is cleaved, prior to secretion, into insulin and C peptide.
      (2) Normally, less than 20% of the total circulating immunoreactive insulin is proinsulin.
      (3) In patients with insulinoma, proinsulin levels frequently represent more than 20% of the total circulating insulin.
   c. Provocative tests may be necessary to prove the diagnosis.
      (1) Tolbutamide or glucagon may be infused intravenously: An elevated insulin level is diagnostic of insulinoma.
      (2) Fish insulin may be infused: Endogenous insulin levels will be suppressed in the normal individual but not in the insulinoma patient. (Fish insulin is not immunoreactive with human insulin.)
      (3) Calcium may be infused: This will cause the release of insulin and proinsulin in insulinoma patients, resulting in symptoms of hypoglycemia.

4. **Treatment**
   a. Surgical treatment
      (1) Surgical management is based on preoperative localization of the tumor.
         (a) Over 75% of all insulinomas are smaller than 1.5 cm, so that arteriography, computed tomography (CT), and magnetic resonance imaging (MRI) are less sensitive for detecting insulinomas than for larger tumors. Selective arteriography may detect 50% of these tumors.
         (b) Percutaneous catheterization of the portal vein with serial insulin measurements can also help to localize the area of the tumor.
      (2) Exploration of the entire pancreas for a palpable mass is undertaken first.
         (a) If the tumor is palpable or is visible as a reddish-brown discoloration, it should be either enucleated or removed as part of a distal pancreatectomy.

(b) If lymph nodes adjacent to the tumor are firm and enlarged, suggesting carcinoma, or if the tumor feels malignant (i.e., firm and infiltrative), then a standard form of resectional therapy should be performed, such as pancreaticoduodenectomy or total pancreatectomy with lymphadenectomy.

(3) If no lesion is palpable (as occurs about 10%–20% of the time) but preoperative tests have clearly documented hyperinsulinism but not the tumor location, then intraoperative ultrasonography may help to locate the insulinomas. If the tumor is not localized, then the management is debatable.

   (a) The classic procedure is to resect the tail of the pancreas and examine the specimen pathologically. If a tumor is still not found, all of the pancreas but the head and the uncinate process is removed, and the operation is terminated.

   (b) The surgeon may proceed to total pancreatectomy if the tumor is not found in the tail of the pancreas.

   (c) The surgeon may resect only 80%–90% of the pancreas and then observe the patient for hyperinsulinism postoperatively. If medical measures then fail to control the patient's symptoms, a total pancreatectomy may be necessary.

(4) When islet cell hyperplasia is present, an 80%–90% subtotal pancreatectomy will usually control the symptoms.

(5) Blood glucose levels should be monitored in the operating room to prevent hypoglycemia.

  b. Medical treatment is limited to patients who are incurable operatively or who have malignant disease.

5. Prognosis

  a. Approximately 65% of patients are cured by surgery.

  b. The operative mortality rate is 10%.

  c. Patients with malignant insulinomas have a 60% 2-year survival rate.

C. Gastrinomas (Zollinger-Ellison syndrome)

1. Pathogenesis

  a. Symptoms in this disorder result from oversecretion of gastrin, the consequence of which is peptic ulceration because of high gastric acid secretion.

  b. The cause is usually a non-beta islet cell tumor of the pancreas (i.e., a D-cell or A-cell tumor).

  c. Zollinger-Ellison syndrome may be a component of MEA type I.

2. Clinical presentation

  a. Abdominal pain secondary to the peptic ulceration is present in over 90% of the patients.

  b. Diarrhea is common, resulting from:

   (1) Gastric hypersecretion, which creates a low duodenal pH and inactivates pancreatic enzymes, resulting in steatorrhea

   (2) Gastrin-stimulated intestinal motility, which impairs fluid and electrolyte absorption

  c. Gastrointestinal hemorrhage from the peptic ulceration occurs in up to 40% of patients.

  d. Ulcer perforation and gastric outlet obstruction also occur.

  e. Profound dehydration and malnutrition may be present.

3. Diagnosis

  a. The following conditions should alert the physician to the possibility of Zollinger-Ellison syndrome:

   (1) Recurrent ulcer symptoms

   (2) Recurrent ulcer, following a standard surgical procedure for peptic ulcer disease

   (3) An ulcer that is refractory to intensive treatment with antacids or H_2-receptor blockers

  b. **Laboratory findings** provide the diagnosis.

   (1) **Gastric acid hypersecretion** is present in 70%–80% of patients. It is manifested by:

    (a) A 12-hour overnight basal acid output (BAO) of over 100 mmol of hydrochloric acid

    (b) A 1-hour BAO of more than 15 mmol

    (c) Little or no increase in gastric acid secretion after stimulation by pentagastrin or betazole

     (i) This test demonstrates that the parietal cells are under maximal stimulation.

     (ii) Results are expressed as the ratio of basal:maximal acid output (BAO:MAO), which usually exceeds 0.6 in patients with Zollinger-Ellison syndrome.

(2) **Elevated levels of serum gastrin** are the key to the diagnosis.
(a) Gastrin levels are determined by radioimmunoassay, which measures both the heptadecapeptide itself and its precursor form, G-34 or "big gastrin."
(b) Most patients with Zollinger-Ellison syndrome have a fasting serum gastrin level of 500 pg/ml or more (the normal level is 20–150 pg/ml).
(c) Some patients have an intermediate serum gastrin level of 200–500 pg/ml. A gastrin stimulation test may then aid in the diagnosis.
(i) In Zollinger-Ellison syndrome, an infusion of calcium will raise the gastrin level by more than 300 pg/ml and an infusion of secretin will raise it by 100 pg/ml or more.
(ii) Peptic ulcer patients and normal persons will not show this response.
(d) Extremely high gastrin levels (over 5000 pg/ml) or the presence of α-chain human chorionic gonadotropin in the serum strongly suggests a malignant gastrinoma.
(e) Serum gastrin levels also may be elevated by pathologic processes other than non-beta islet cell carcinoma of the pancreas, including:
(i) Non-beta islet cell adenomas
(ii) Antral G-cell hyperplasia
(iii) Gastric outlet obstruction
(iv) A retained gastric antrum, following incomplete antrectomy for peptic ulcer disease
(v) Conditions that cause gastric hypoacidity (which is a stimulus for gastrin production), including pernicious anemia, atrophic gastritis, and gastric carcinoma
(f) Another innovative technique combines selective injection of secretin into mesentery arteries with simultaneous measurement of gastrin.
c. **X-ray films** will usually show upper gastrointestinal ulceration.
(1) Frequently, multiple ulcers are seen.
(2) Ulcers are sometimes seen in the distal duodenum and jejunum.

4. **Localization of the tumor.** Localization studies are the same as described for insulinomas. Arteriography is less accurate for gastrinomas since these tumors are less vascular than insulinomas.

5. **Treatment** of Zollinger-Ellison syndrome is centered around removal of the causative tumor plus control of the end-organ (gastric mucosal) response.
a. The tumor should be removed if possible because approximately 60% are malignant.
(1) Unfortunately, the tumor is frequently multifocal or difficult to identify at laparotomy.
(2) Only about 20% are resectable.
(3) Lesions in the wall of the duodenum (present in fewer than 5% of cases) and in the tail of the pancreas are the commonest types of resectable tumors.
b. The end-organ response, namely gastric hypersecretion, and the complications it causes may be treated either by surgical means or by the use of H_2-receptor blockers.
(1) Total gastrectomy is the classic treatment of choice.
(a) It should be done even in the presence of metastasis because of the slow-growing nature of the tumor.
(b) It results in control of the severe gastrointestinal hypersecretion and ulceration, and it is well tolerated by most patients.
(2) Prolonged H_2-receptor blockade with cimetidine may control the gastrointestinal manifestations of Zollinger-Ellison syndrome, but the failure rate is as high as 15%.

6. **Prognosis** for the Zollinger-Ellison syndrome is good if the gastrointestinal hyperacidity can be controlled by surgical or medical measures. Although two-thirds of the causative tumors are malignant, they are very slow-growing, and patients may live a long time.

D. **Pancreatic cholera** is a syndrome of severe diarrhea associated with hypersecretion of a pancreatic non-beta islet cell tumor.

1. **Symptoms.** The syndrome has been called **WDHA syndrome** because of the following symptoms.
a. **W**atery diarrhea
b. **H**ypokalemia and a resultant profound muscular weakness due to the high potassium content in the stool
c. **A**chlorhydria

2. **Pathogenesis.** The probable cause is an increase in the secretion of VIP due to a pancreatic tumor.

   a. The tumor is solitary in 80% of cases and is usually localized to the body or tail of the pancreas.

   b. One-half of the tumors are malignant and frequently have metastasized by the time of surgery.

3. **Treatment** is surgical excision when possible. If not, ''debulking'' the tumor may improve the diarrhea.

4. **Prognosis** is poor. The average length of survival after surgery is 1 year.

E. **Glucagonomas** are tumors of the pancreatic $alpha_2$ islet cells that cause hypersecretion of glucagon.

   1. The patient is usually diabetic and has weight loss, dermatitis, anemia, and stomatitis.

   2. Sixty-five to seventy percent of these tumors are malignant.

Part V Endocrine Disorders

STUDY QUESTIONS

Directions: Each question below contains five suggested answers. Choose the **one best** response to each question.

1. All of the following statements about substernal goiters are correct EXCEPT

(A) they are usually seen in older age-groups
(B) they may result in tracheoesophageal compression
(C) they infrequently take up radioiodine
(D) they frequently respond to thyroid suppressive therapy, eliminating the need for operative removal
(E) they frequently result from adenomatous hyperplasia

2. Signs and symptoms of hyperthyroidism are commonly produced by all of the following conditions EXCEPT

(A) Graves' disease
(B) toxic nodular goiter
(C) subacute thyroiditis
(D) Hashimoto's thyroiditis
(E) silent thyroiditis

3. A 40-year-old man had a subtotal thyroidectomy. Several hours later he complained of difficulty breathing. On examination, he had stridor and a markedly swollen, tense neck wound. A first step in the management of this patient should be to

(A) intubate with an endotracheal tube
(B) perform a tracheostomy
(C) control the bleeding site in the operating room
(D) open the wound to evacuate the hematoma
(E) aspirate the hematoma

4. Injury to both recurrent laryngeal nerves, a potential complication of thyroidectomy, results in all of the following EXCEPT

(A) voice fatigue and hoarseness
(B) bilateral vocal cord paralysis
(C) airway compromise
(D) midline, adducted vocal cord position (on laryngoscopy)
(E) the need for an urgent tracheostomy

5. A 50-year-old patient who presents with an asymptomatic diffuse multinodular goiter should be treated initially with

(A) radioiodine
(B) propylthiouracil
(C) observation
(D) subtotal thyroidectomy
(E) suppressive doses of thyroid hormone

6. A first-degree relative of a patient with medullary thyroid cancer has an elevated thyrocalcitonin level on screening. Her neck examination is completely normal, and she is asymptomatic. Proper therapy would involve

(A) frequent follow-up examinations to detect thyroid nodules
(B) lifelong thyroid suppression with thyroxine
(C) ablation of the thyroid gland with ^{131}I
(D) total thyroidectomy
(E) fine-needle aspiration of each lobe of the thyroid

7. The commonest cause of Addison's disease (adrenocortical insufficiency) seen today is

(A) postpartum adrenal hemorrhage
(B) exogenous steroid use
(C) tuberculosis
(D) metastatic tumor replacement of the adrenal glands
(E) autoimmune disease

8. The commonest cause of Cushing's syndrome is

(A) adrenal adenoma
(B) adrenal carcinoma
(C) pituitary adenoma
(D) ectopic ACTH
(E) nodular hyperplasia

9. All of the following statements are true concerning radiation therapy as a primary treatment for pituitary Cushing's syndrome EXCEPT

(A) better results are obtained in children
(B) it may result in progressive hypopituitarism
(C) implantation of yttrium-90 may improve results over external beam therapy
(D) there is a long lag period (up to 18 months) before results are seen
(E) there is a cure rate of approximately 40%–50% in adults

10. Treatment with spironolactone would be indicated as definitive treatment in a hypertensive patient with elevated serum aldosterone levels and

(A) unilateral adrenal adenoma
(B) bilateral adrenal adenomas
(C) bilateral adrenal hyperplasia
(D) unilateral adrenal carcinoma
(E) secondary hyperaldosteronism

11. One of the commonest causes of a missed diagnosis in patients with an aldosterone-producing adenoma of the adrenal gland (Conn's syndrome) is

(A) failure to measure the postural response of serum aldosterone
(B) measurement of serum aldosterone before potassium repletion
(C) measurement of serum potassium after sodium loading
(D) failure to visualize a tumor on CT
(E) failure to visualize a tumor on iodocholesterol scanning

12. A 50-year-old hypertensive man has definitive biochemical evidence of a pheochromocytoma. CT and MRI do not reveal any abnormalities, and m-iodobenzylguanidine scanning is not readily available. The next step should be

(A) abdominal exploration
(B) continued clinical observation
(C) mediastinoscopy
(D) selected venous sampling
(E) mediastinal exploration

13. Alpha-receptor blockade (i.e., phenoxybenzamine) preoperatively in a patient with pheochromocytoma accomplishes all of the following actions EXCEPT

(A) control of hypertension
(B) control of arrhythmias
(C) volume repletion
(D) decreased operative morbidity and mortality
(E) decreased episodes of blood pressure fluctuations during surgery

14. In a patient with a confirmed diagnosis of pheochromocytoma, the optimal operative approach should be

(A) thoracicoabdominal
(B) posterior
(C) flank
(D) transabdominal
(E) bilateral posterior

15. Patients with iatrogenic permanent hypoparathyroidism are best treated with

(A) high-calcium diet
(B) oral phosphorous
(C) calcitonin
(D) oral calcium and vitamin D supplements
(E) exogenous parathyroid hormone

16. The superior parathyroid gland is usually located in which direction relative to the recurrent laryngeal nerve?

(A) Superior
(B) Medial
(C) Lateral
(D) Posterior
(E) Anterior

17. Primary hyperparathyroidism is associated with all of the following biochemical abnormalities EXCEPT

(A) hypercalcemia
(B) hypochloremia
(C) hypophosphatemia
(D) hypercalciuria
(E) hyperphosphaturia

18. Most patients with primary hyperparathyroidism initially present with

(A) bone pain
(B) renal stones
(C) psychiatric disturbances
(D) pancreatitis
(E) none of the above

19. Prior to the *initial* exploration for biochemically diagnosed hyperparathyroidism, a surgeon should obtain

(A) an ultrasound
(B) nuclear imaging studies
(C) selective venous sampling
(D) thyrocervical angioplasty
(E) none of the above

20. A dialysis patient begins to complain of occasional pruritus and mild bone pain. Laboratory values show hypocalcemia, hyperphosphatemia, and a parathyroid hormone level three times normal. Management should include all of the following EXCEPT

(A) subtotal parathyroidectomy
(B) high-calcium dialysis bath
(C) oral calcium supplements
(D) phosphate-binding antacids
(E) vitamin D

21. Tumors primary to the thymus gland may be associated with which of the following disorders?

(A) Lupus erythematosus
(B) Scleroderma
(C) Myasthenia gravis
(D) Stricture of the esophagus
(E) Pericarditis

22. Physical examination may be extremely helpful in diagnosing

(A) insulinoma
(B) MEA I
(C) gastrinoma
(D) MEA II (IIa)
(E) MEA III (IIb)

23. A 46-year-old brother of a patient with documented MEA I (Wermer's syndrome) is found on biochemical workup to have elevated serum calcium, parathyroid hormone, and gastrin, as well as an abnormal gastrin response to secretin stimulation. Initial treatment should involve

(A) total gastrectomy
(B) celiotomy and resection of a pancreatic tumor
(C) parietal cell vagotomy
(D) subtotal parathyroidectomy
(E) observation

24. Once a diagnosis of insulinoma is suspected because of the clinical picture, the diagnosis can be established most easily by

(A) tolbutamide provocative test
(B) visceral angiography
(C) measurements of fasting insulin and glucose levels
(D) comparison of proinsulin and insulin levels
(E) percutaneous portal vein catheterization and measurement of insulin

25. Pancreatic cholera, or the WDHA syndrome (watery diarrhea, hypokalemia, and achlorhydria), is believed to be due to a non-beta islet cell tumor of the pancreas that produces an excess of

(A) glucagon
(B) insulin
(C) vasoactive intestinal peptide
(D) gastrin
(E) human pancreatic polypeptide

Directions: Each question below contains four suggested answers of which **one or more** is correct. Choose the answer

A   if **1, 2, and 3** are correct
B   if **1 and 3** are correct
C   if **2 and 4** are correct
D   if **4** is correct
E   if **1, 2, 3, and 4** are correct

26. The normal adrenal gland receives its arterial blood supply from the

(1) aorta
(2) renal artery
(3) phrenic artery
(4) lumbar artery

27. A 55-year-old man has a CT scan of the abdomen performed while he is hospitalized for acute pancreatitis. A 2.5-cm mass is noted in the right adrenal gland. He has no history of diabetes or hypertension, and other than his pancreatitis, which is resolving, he is asymptomatic. Appropriate measures would include

(1) a biochemical workup to determine whether the adrenal mass is functional
(2) follow-up CT scan in 3 months
(3) CT-directed needle biopsy
(4) right adrenalectomy

SUMMARY OF DIRECTIONS

A	B	C	D	E
1, 2, 3 only	1, 3 only	2, 4 only	4 only	All are correct

---

28. Embryologically, the thymus gland is related to the

(1) fourth branchial pouch
(2) inferior parathyroid glands
(3) superior parathyroid glands
(4) third branchial pouch

29. Correct statements about thymic tumors (thymomas) include which of the following?

(1) They are among the commonest mediastinal tumors
(2) They have a female preponderance
(3) Their pathology is best determined at surgical exploration
(4) Most tumors in adults are malignant

30. Recommended treatment for malignant thymomas includes

(1) chemotherapy
(2) radiation therapy
(3) immunotherapy with monoclonal anti–T-cell antibody
(4) resection of the entire tumor, including areas of invasion

31. A 40-year-old woman with generalized myasthenia gravis is being treated with pyridostigmine (Mestinon), a cholinesterase inhibitor. CT scan shows no evidence of a thymoma. The next step in management of this patient should be

(1) continued treatment with pyridostigmine
(2) serial CT scans and thymectomy if a thymoma is detected
(3) high-dose steroid (prednisone) therapy
(4) plasmapheresis followed by thymectomy

32. MEA type I (Wermer's syndrome) includes neoplasias or hyperplasias of which of the following organs?

(1) Thyroid gland
(2) Parathyroid glands
(3) Adrenal glands
(4) Pituitary gland

33. A sibling of a patient with MEA II is found to have a normal baseline calcitonin level but an abnormal calcitonin stimulation test when both calcium and pentagastrin are infused. No thyroid nodules are palpable. Proper treatment of this patient would include

(1) close observation and frequent physical examinations to detect possible thyroid nodules
(2) metabolic screening tests to detect pheochromocytoma
(3) thyroid scan and ultrasound to detect subclinical pathology
(4) total thyroidectomy

Directions: The group of questions below consists of lettered choices followed by several numbered items. For each numbered item select the **one** lettered choice with which it is **most closely** associated. Each lettered choice may be used once, more than once, or not at all.

Questions 34–37

For each diagnostic test listed below, select the condition that it is most likely to detect.

(A) Zollinger-Ellison syndrome
(B) Medullary thyroid disease
(C) Both
(D) Neither

34. Calcium infusion

35. Pentagastrin infusion

36. Tolbutamide test

37. Secretin infusion

ANSWERS AND EXPLANATIONS

1. The answer is D. [*Chapter 16 I C 4 a (2) (a)–(c)*] Substernal goiters usually enlarge as a result of adenomatous hyperplasia and, thus, do not take up radioiodine. They usually occur in older age-groups and usually result in tracheoesophageal compression. They rarely respond to thyroid stimulating hormone suppression and almost always require operative removal both for diagnosis and for the relief of pressure symptoms.

2. The answer is D. [*Chapter 16 I D 2 a (1), c, 3, E 2 b (2) (a), (3) (a) (i)*] Hashimoto's thyroiditis is usually accompanied by hypothyroidism and goiter. Graves' disease and toxic multinodular goiter produce hyperthyroidism because of excess synthesis of thyroid hormone. Subacute thyroiditis and its painless variant are believed to be viral in origin. Symptoms of hyperthyroidism are due to release of hormones from the inflamed gland and not to increased hormone synthesis.

3. The answer is D. [*Chapter 16 I D 2 e (4) (b) (ii)*] Postoperative bleeding following thyroidectomy can cause airway compromise due to tracheal compression. The first step should be to open the wound to evacuate the hematoma, followed by a return to the operating room to control the bleeding site. Attempts to perform either endotracheal intubation or tracheostomy may be difficult until the external compression of the hematoma is relieved.

4. The answer is A. [*Chapter 16 I D 2 e (4) (d)*] Bilateral recurrent laryngeal nerve injury is a devastating complication of thyroidectomy. Both vocal cords are paralyzed in the midline position, resulting in severe airway compromise. This requires an urgent tracheostomy. Hoarseness results from unilateral nerve injury, and voice fatigue is a complication of injury to the external branch of the superior laryngeal nerve.

5. The answer is C. [*Chapter 16 I E 3 d (1)*] A nontoxic multinodular goiter, which produces no symptoms and has no clinical signs of malignancy, should be observed. If the gland is cosmetically bothersome or is producing pressure symptoms, suppressive therapy with thyroxine should be given. Subtotal thyroidectomy would be indicated if symptoms failed to resolve with thyroxine. Antithyroid medications (i.e., propylthiouracil) would not be indicated in this patient.

6. The answer is D. [*Chapter 16 I F 5 c (2) (c), (3) (d)*] The elevated thyrocalcitonin level in a first-degree relative of a patient with medullary thyroid cancer most likely represents C-cell hyperplasia, a premalignant lesion. This is totally curable at this stage by total thyroidectomy. If surgery is postponed until clinical signs of cancer occur, the chance for cure may be lost. Because the parafollicular cells, or C cells, are not responsive to thyroid-stimulating hormone and do not take up radioiodine, thyroxine suppression or ^{131}I ablation are of no clinical use. Blind fine-needle aspirations are not indicated.

7. The answer is B. [*Chapter 16 II D 1 b (1)*] Although postpartum adrenal hemorrhage, tuberculosis, metastases, and autoimmune disease can cause adrenal insufficiency, exogenous steroid use (i.e., prednisone) is the commonest clinical cause of adrenal insufficiency seen today. The exogenous steroids suppress adrenocorticotropic hormone with subsequent atrophy of the adrenal cortex.

8. The answer is C. [*Chapter 16 II E 1 a–c*] Cushing's syndrome can be due to adrenal pathology (15%) [i.e., adenoma, carcinoma, or primary nodular hyperplasia], ectopic adrenocorticotropic hormone (ACTH) production (15%), and adrenal hyperplasia secondary to increased ACTH production from the pituitary gland (70%). Most cases of pituitary Cushing's syndrome are caused by an ACTH-secreting pituitary adenoma.

9. The answer is E. [*Chapter 16 II E 6 a (3) (b)*] Radiation therapy has provided effective treatment in up to 80% of children with pituitary Cushing's syndrome. However, the response in adults has been much lower with cure rates of only 15%–20%. This may be improved with yttrium 90 implants, but progressive hypopituitarism may also occur. The patient also must be in relatively good health to undergo treatment since the beneficial effects often are not seen for 12–18 months.

10. The answer is C. [*Chapter 16 II F 1, 2, 6 b*] Conn's syndrome (primary hyperaldosteronism), which causes hypertension due to an increased secretion of aldosterone, may result from unilateral adrenal adenomas (85%), bilateral hyperplasia (< 10%), bilateral adenomas (< 5%), or adrenocortical carcinoma (rare). Surgery (adrenalectomy) would be the treatment of choice for adenomas (unilateral or bilateral) and carcinomas. Patients with bilateral hyperplasia respond poorly to adrenalectomy and are best treated with spironolactone, an aldosterone antagonist. In secondary hyperaldosteronism, the aldosterone is elevated in response to excess production of renin due to several causes (e.g., renal artery stenosis or malignant hypertension). Treatment should be directed to the underlying condition.

11. The answer is B. [*Chapter 16 II F 4 c (1)*] One of the commonest causes of missed diagnosis of Conn's syndrome is the measurement of plasma aldosterone levels before potassium repletion. Plasma aldosterone levels may not be elevated in the potassium-depleted patient but usually become significantly elevated after potassium and sodium loading. Measuring the serum aldosterone levels after 4 hours of upright posture helps to differentiate primary hyperaldosteronism due to bilateral adrenal cortical hyperplasia from that due to adenoma. CT, MRI, and iodocholesterol scanning are localization studies. Failure to visualize a tumor on these studies would not preclude the diagnosis of primary hyperaldosteronism, since the diagnosis is primarily a biochemical one. Selective adrenal venous sampling could then be used for localization.

12. The answer is D. [*Chapter 16 II G 5 d*] Although 90% of pheochromocytomas are located in the adrenal glands, they can occur in any tissue that is derived from neuroectoderm. When CT and MRI fail to identify a tumor, m-iodobenzylguanidine scanning can be helpful; however, this is not widely available. In the patient described in the question, selective measurements of catecholamines drawn at various levels from the vena cava and its major branches should be done prior to surgical exploration.

13. The answer is B. [*Chapter 16 II G 6 a (2), (3)*] Alpha-receptor blockade is important in the preparation of a patient with pheochromocytoma for surgery because it controls blood pressure and optimizes volume status by decreasing peripheral vasoconstriction. This, in turn, reduces the incidence of blood pressure fluctuations during surgery and operative morbidity and mortality. Propranolol, a β-receptor blocker, can be used to control tachycardia and arrhythmias if present.

14. The answer is D. [*Chapter 16 II G 6 b (2)*] Since pheochromocytoma can be bilateral or multiple in up to 10% of the patients, both adrenal glands and the entire abdomen and retroperitoneum must be explored. This cannot be accomplished through posterior or flank approaches. Although a thoracicoabdominal approach may be necessary at times for exposure, this increases the postoperative morbidity. The ideal approach would be transabdominal.

15. The answer is D. [*Chapter 16 III A*] There is no satisfactory replacement for endogenously produced parathyroid hormone. Calcitonin and phosphorous may be used to lower serum calcium but would have no effect on hypoparathyroidism, and a high-calcium diet would not be sufficient. Thus, patients must take lifelong oral calcium and vitamin D supplements.

16. The answer is D. [*Chapter 16 III A 2 b (1) (a)*] Parathyroid glands can be found in ectopic locations and, when enlarged, can migrate. However, they usually maintain their relationship to the recurrent laryngeal nerve: The superior gland lies posteriorly and the inferior gland lies anteriorly to this structure.

17. The answer is B. [*Chapter 16 III C 1 c, d*] Increased serum calcium occurs in primary hyperparathyroidism, and when the renal threshold for calcium reabsorption is exceeded, hypercalciuria occurs. Increased levels of parathormone result in a decrease in the kidney's tubular reabsorption of phosphate. This leads to hyperphosphaturia and hypophosphatemia. The serum chloride level is usually increased.

18. The answer is E. [*Chapter 16 III C 1 c (1)*] Although bone disease, kidney stones, psychiatric disturbances, and pancreatitis can all be caused by hyperparathyroidism, most patients are asymptomatic when they are diagnosed. The altered state is discovered only because an elevated calcium level is detected on routine multichannel biochemical screening.

19. The answer is E. [*Chapter 16 III C 1 e, f (1), (2)*] Although enlarged parathyroid glands may be found in up to 80% of the cases of biochemically diagnosed hyperthyroidism, the tests listed in the question (i.e., ultrasound, nuclear imaging, venous sampling, and thyrocervical angioplasty) are costly and potentially invasive (particularly angiography). Thus, these studies are generally recommended for re-exploration in patients with persistent or recurrent hyperparathyroidism after previous cervical exploration, which is the most accurate procedure in the hands of an experienced surgeon.

20. The answer is A. [*Chapter 16 III C 2 b (1), (2)*] The patient described in the question has secondary hyperparathyroidism with mild symptoms. Most of these patients can be successfully palliated with calcium supplements, phosphate binders, vitamin D, and a high-calcium dialysis bath. Only if the symptoms are truly refractory or if severe bone pain occurs would subtotal parathyroidectomy be required.

21. The answer is C. [*Chapter 16 IV A 2 b (2) (a)*] Thymic tumors are associated with myasthenia gravis and with immune disorders, such as hypogammaglobulinemia. Thymic tumors secrete a chemical that becomes associated with acetylcholine receptors, stimulating an immune response followed by myasthenia gravis. Many patients with generalized myasthenia gravis improve after a complete thymectomy.

22. The answer is E. [*Chapter 17 I C 3*] Most tumors of the endocrine pancreas and multiple endocrine adenomatosis (MEA) syndromes are diagnosed by biochemical tests. However, MEA III (or IIb) is characterized by multiple mucosal neuromas and a peculiar marfanoid body habitus. Thus, physical examination is very helpful in making the diagnosis.

23. The answer is D. [*Chapter 17 I D 1 a (1)*] A patient with MEA I syndrome with evidence of parathyroid and pancreatic disease should have the hyperparathyroidism treated first. This would entail subtotal parathyroidectomy since the disorder is four-gland hyperplasia. Reduction of serum calcium may reduce serum gastrin. If hypergastrinemia persists, treatment should be directed toward the Zollinger-Ellison component of the syndrome.

24. The answer is C. [*Chapter 17 II B 3 a–c, 4 a (1) (a), (b)*] Once the diagnosis of insulinoma is clinically suspected, it can be confirmed most easily by fasting the patient. Virtually all patients become symptomatic within 72 hours. An inappropriately high insulin level in the presence of hypoglycemia (insulin: glucose ratio over 0.25) effectively confirms an insulinoma. Proinsulin levels and provocative testing may occasionally be needed in equivocal situations. Angiography and portal vein sampling are used to localize the tumor in preparation for surgery *after* the diagnosis has been established.

25. The answer is C. [*Chapter 17 II D 2*] Symptoms of profuse watery diarrhea, hypokalemia, marked muscle weakness, and achlorhydria are believed to be due to a non-beta islet cell tumor that produces an excess of vasoactive intestinal peptide. The tumor is solitary in 80% of cases and is usually localized to the body or tail of the pancreas.

26. The answer is A (1, 2, 3). [*Chapter 16 II A 2 b (1)*] Although the arterial supply to the normal adrenal gland varies, it commonly receives its blood supply directly from the aorta as well as from branches of the phrenic and renal arteries.

27. The answer is A (1, 2, 3). [*Chapter 16 II H 4 a–c*] Nonfunctional adenomas of the adrenal glands are being discovered more frequently with the increased use of imaging studies, such as CT and MRI. Most carcinomas are either functional or larger than 3 cm in diameter. Therefore, a biochemical screen followed by a repeat CT scan in 3 months if it proves to be a nonfunctional adrenal mass is a reasonable approach. However, if the expertise of an interventional radiologist and cytopathologist are available, a CT-directed needle biopsy could also be performed. Immediate adrenalectomy for a nonfunctional adrenal mass less than 3 cm in diameter would not be appropriate unless malignancy was suggested by the biopsy.

28. The answer is C (2, 4). [*Chapter 16 III A 1 b (2); IV A 1 a*] The thymus gland is embryologically derived from the third branchial pouch, as are the inferior parathyroid glands. The inferior parathyroid glands are often found in association with the thymus gland in the anterior–superior mediastinum. The superior parathyroid glands are derived from the fourth branchial pouch and are not associated with the thymus.

29. The answer is B (1, 3). [*Chapter 16 IV B 1, 2*] Thymomas are among the commonest mediastinal tumors and are equally distributed between men and women. It is almost impossible to distinguish benign from malignant thymomas microscopically. The best index of malignancy is its tendency to invade adjacent structures, which is determined at exploration. About two-thirds of thymomas are considered benign.

30. The answer is C (2, 4). [*Chapter 16 IV B 4 a (2)*] Operative therapy for malignant thymomas entails resection of the entire tumor and all contiguous areas of invasion. Postoperative radiation therapy also may be helpful. No benefit has been shown to result from adjuvant chemotherapy or immunotherapy.

31. The answer is D (4). [*Chapter 16 IV C 3 b (1), (2) (b)*] Complete thymectomy appears to be the treatment of choice for all patients with generalized myasthenia gravis. Improvement is achieved in up to 85% of patients following thymectomy as compared to only 35% of patients with continued medical therapy. Good results are also obtained in patients without thymic tumors; therefore, there is no rationale for waiting for radiologic evidence of a thymoma prior to thymectomy. Although steroids can provide symptomatic improvement, they complicate thymectomy by their adverse effects on wound healing and infection. Plasmapheresis eliminates the circulating acetylcholine receptor antibodies and reduces the need for prolonged ventilator support postoperatively.

32. The answer is C (2, 4). [*Chapter 17 I B 1 a–c, 2*] MEA type I, or Wermer's syndrome, involves hyperplasias or neoplasias of the parathyroid glands (90%), islet cell tumors of the pancreas (80%), and pituitary tumors (65%). Medullary carcinoma of the thyroid and pheochromocytoma are associated with MEA II, or Sipple's syndrome.

33. The answer is C (2, 4). [*Chapter 17 I C 2 a (2), D 2 a, b*] The patient described in the question with a normal thyroid examination, a normal baseline calcitonin level, but an abnormal calcitonin stimulation test is likely to have either an early occult medullary thyroid cancer or premalignant C-cell hyperplasia. Total thyroidectomy is curative if medullary carcinoma is treated in the premalignant stage when only C-cell hyperplasia is present. Waiting for clinical abnormalities or evidence of thyroid pathology on ultrasound or scan will allow the disease to progress, adversely affecting the cure rate. All patients with MEA II should be screened for pheochromocytoma; if present, this should be treated prior to the thyroidectomy to avoid hypertensive complications.

34–37. The answers are: 34-C, 35-B, 36-D, 37-A. [*Chapter 17 I C 2 a (2); II B 3 c (1), C 3 b (2) (c) (i), (f)*] Elevated levels of serum gastrin are the key to the diagnosis of Zollinger-Ellison syndrome as most patients have markedly elevated levels (> 500 pg/ml). For patients with intermediate levels (200–500 pg/ml), a stimulation test with either calcium or secretin may aid the diagnosis.

Patients with medullary thyroid disease, either medullary thyroid cancer or the premalignant C-cell hyperplasia, may have an abnormally high baseline calcitonin level. Those with early disease can be diagnosed by stimulation with either calcium or pentagastrin.

Tolbutamide suppression may be helpful in the diagnosis of insulinoma, but it is not useful in the diagnosis of either gastrinoma or medullary thyroid disease.

Part VI
Head and Neck Disorders

18
Benign Lesions of the Head and Neck

Robert T. Sataloff
Joseph R. Spiegel
David A. Zwillenberg

I. INTRODUCTION. Familiarity with the benign conditions reviewed in this chapter is essential to the physician, who must distinguish life-threatening illnesses from those of little consequence, choose appropriate therapy, and avoid injudicious surgery.

A. Overview

1. The commonest neck mass is a reactive node, and these are most often secondary to bacterial or viral infections of the ear, nose, paranasal sinuses, teeth, tonsils, or skin and soft tissues of the head and neck.

2. Most neck masses in children are benign.

3. Most neck masses in adults are malignant.

4. The **"rule of sevens"** is a useful guide:
   a. A mass that has been present for 7 days is inflammatory.
   b. One present for 7 months is malignant.
   c. One present for 7 years is congenital.

B. Workup for acquired lesions (see IV)

1. **The history** should be detailed, especially regarding:
   a. **Family history** of malignancy
   b. **Past malignancy** in the patient
   c. **Risk factors** associated with malignancy, such as:
      (1) Smoking
      (2) Alcohol consumption
      (3) Exposure to radiation, certain fumes, sawdust, or other potential carcinogens
   d. **Recent relevant illness,** such as:
      (1) Upper respiratory infection, sinusitis, or tonsillitis
      (2) Otitis or conjunctivitis
      (3) Dental problems

2. **Physical examination** should include careful inspection and palpation of the scalp, eyes, ears, nose, mouth (including the teeth and tonsils), hypopharynx, and nasopharynx for signs of infection, ulceration, or unsuspected abnormalities.

3. **Laboratory tests** may include:
   a. Complete blood count and differential
   b. Chest x-ray
   c. Tuberculin test for tuberculosis
   d. A heterophil titer ("mono spot" test) for mononucleosis
   e. Thyroid function tests or thyroid scan
   f. Serologic tests for syphilis
   g. Viral titers, especially for Epstein-Barr virus, which is associated with nasopharyngeal carcinoma and Burkitt's lymphoma

4. **Radiologic studies** may include soft-tissue x-rays of the neck, xeroradiograms, a barium swallow, a complete gastrointestinal (GI) series, or scanning procedures, such as computed tomography (CT), magnetic resonance imaging (MRI), bone scan, or other radioisotope scans.

5. **Endoscopy** is indicated to search for the tumor if a primary neoplasm is suspected. Endoscopic biopsy and radiologic studies should precede any incision in the neck (see Chapter 19 II B).

6. **Treatment** depends on the findings during the workup.
   a. Antibiotics should be administered if a bacterial infection is present.
   b. Antituberculosis drugs may be needed.
   c. Consultation with a specialist in another field may be helpful.
      (1) A dental consultation may be useful if the teeth seem to be the source of a problem.
      (2) If dandruff, scabies, or another dermatologic condition is noted, a dermatology consultation is indicated.
   d. Should a mass not shrink significantly or disappear within a reasonable period of time, usually 6 weeks, then surgical treatment or biopsy may be indicated.
      (1) If cervical adenopathy persists, then:
         (a) The presence of enlarged or cryptic tonsils is believed by many to be an indication for tonsillectomy.
         (b) Equivocal dental findings are an indication for dental treatment.
      (2) If neither tonsils nor teeth are implicated, then persistent cervical adenopathy is an indication for excisional biopsy after a complete evaluation for malignancy.
      (3) A neck mass biopsy is the last step in a proper workup.

II. NECK ABSCESSES

A. **Overview.** A patient presenting with fever and a fluctuant neck mass most probably has an abscess.

1. The source of infection should be identified, and drainage should be carried out.

2. Due to the danger to the carotid artery, airway, and cranial nerves, deep neck abscesses should be treated only by those knowledgeable in the standard techniques and anatomy of the area. They should be treated on an emergency basis.

B. **Types of abscesses**

1. **Bezold's abscesses** are neck abscesses arising from the ear.

2. **Ludwig's angina** is an abscess occupying sublingual space.
   a. It generally arises from a dental source.
   b. It can cause death from airway obstruction and, thus, frequently requires tracheostomy.

3. **Parapharyngeal abscesses** arise from the posterior teeth or tonsils and involve the carotid sheath. They can cause mediastinitis and carotid "blowout" (erosion of the artery wall leading to massive hemorrhage).

4. **Retropharyngeal abscesses** can cause mediastinitis.

5. **Peritonsillar abscesses (quinsy)** arise as a complication of acute tonsillitis.
   a. They present with ipsilateral palatal edema, contralateral deviation of the uvula, "hot potato" voice, trismus, and dysphagia. The patient may have only a low-grade fever or be afebrile.
   b. They are the commonest abscesses in the peripharyngeal space.

III. CONGENITAL MASSES

A. **Parenchymal cysts**

1. **Thymic cysts**
   a. **Embryology.** The thymus arises from the third pharyngeal pouch and migrates caudally and medially to descend into the superior mediastinum.
      (1) During this descent, an attachment may be left in the neck.
      (2) Thymic tissues may present in the neck as separate nodules of mature thymus or may occur in association with ciliated or columnar epithelial remnants of the pharyngeal outpouching.
      (3) Thymic cysts may occur anywhere on a line from the mandibular angle to the suprasternal notch.

    b. Characteristics
- **(1)** Some 95% of thymic cysts are unilateral, and 90% of thymic ectopias are cystic.
- **(2)** They are generally found in children, and there is a male predominance.
- **(3)** They may be uni- or multilocular.
- **(4)** Loculated cysts generally contain amber to brown fluid, which may be clear or turbid.

    c. Complications
- **(1)** Cysts are often asymptomatic but may be painful if infected or if they grow suddenly.
- **(2)** Midline cysts may cause dysphagia.
- **(3)** Both benign and malignant hyperplasia have been reported in these cysts.
- **(4)** Myasthenia gravis is not found in association with cervical thymic cysts.

    d. Differential diagnosis
- **(1)** Branchial cleft cysts seldom extend inferiorly to the clavicle and often present with signs of acute inflammation.
- **(2)** Cystic hygromas are lateral, spongy, and more diffuse. They are generally seen in infants.

    e. Treatment. Surgery is the treatment of choice.

2. Parathyroid cysts
    a. Characteristics
- **(1)** These unusual cysts generally present in adults between the ages 30 and 50 as a solitary mass at either inferior pole of the thyroid gland.
- **(2)** Tracheal deviation is usual and causes a variable degree of respiratory obstruction.
- **(3)** Hoarseness may occur due to pressure on the recurrent laryngeal nerve.

    b. Treatment consists of surgical excision.

B. Lesions of thyroid origin

1. Overview. The thyroid gland originates at the foramen cecum and descends centrally to the thyroid and cricoid cartilages.
    a. The thyroglossal duct may pass in front of, through, or behind the hyoid bone. It is generally obliterated but may persist.
    b. Elements of thyroidal primordium may remain at any site in its passage.
- **(1)** These may give rise not only to cysts and fistulas but also to accessory thyroid tissue and neoplasms.
- **(2)** Most cystic remnants occur in the midline around the hyoid bone.
- **(3)** Solid tumors of thyroglossal duct origin occur almost exclusively within the tongue and above the hyoid bone.

2. Thyroid rests
    a. Characteristics
- **(1)** Thyroid rests may be lingual or may occur in the neck.
- **(2)** Endotracheal ectopias may occur.
- **(3)** Palpation of the normal position of the thyroid often reveals easily palpable tracheal rings in patients with these rests.

    b. Treatment is dictated by the degree of obstruction present and the presence of other thyroid tissue.
- **(1)** A thyroid scan should be performed prior to the removal of lesions suspected of being thyroid rests to ensure that there is functional thyroid tissue in the usual location.
- **(2)** Some 70%–80% of patients have no other functional thyroid.

3. Thyroglossal cysts, sinuses, and fistulas
    a. Anatomy
- **(1)** These occur in the midline unless previous surgery has produced distortion.
- **(2)** About 20% are suprahyoid, 15% occur at the hyoid, and 65% are infrahyoid.

    b. Characteristics
- **(1)** **Fistulas** are almost always the result of infection with spontaneous or surgical drainage. Fistulas can drain internally, externally, or both (**complete fistulas**).
- **(2)** **Thyroglossal duct cysts** present by age 10 in 50% of cases.
  - **(a)** There is no sexual predominance, but there is a racial predominance; the cysts occur more often in whites.
  - **(b)** Cysts usually measure 2–4 cm in diameter and gradually increase in size, although the size may fluctuate.
  - **(c)** They rise and fall with the larynx during swallowing.

    c. Treatment is total surgical excision (Cistrunk procedure), including the:
      (1) Cyst and sinus to the base of the tongue
      (2) Whole fistula if one is present
      (3) Middle third of the hyoid bone

C. Cutaneous branchiogenic cysts are extremely rare asymptomatic nodules, which are noted soon after birth and gradually increase in size.

  1. Anatomy. They are located in the suprasternal notch.

  2. Treatment is by local surgical excision.

D. Teratomas are growths composed of multiple tissues foreign to the part of the body in which they arise.

  1. Types
    a. Epidermoid cysts, the commonest type, are lined by squamous epithelium and are without adnexa.
    b. Dermoid cysts are epithelium-lined cavities, containing skin appendages (e.g., hair, glandular tissue, and follicles).
    c. Teratoid cysts are lined with simple stratified squamous epithelium or respiratory epithelium and contain cheesy keratinous material. They are rare in the head and neck.

  2. Cervical teratomas are most commonly present at birth. Appearance after age 1 year is rare.
    a. Characteristics
      (1) The lesions are usually 5–12 cm in their long axis and are semicystic, although they may be solid. They are usually unilateral.
      (2) Infants with cervical dermoids usually have stridor, apnea, or cyanosis due to tracheal compression or deviation. Dysphagia may also be present.
      (3) Some infants are asymptomatic at birth but become symptomatic within weeks or months.
    b. Associated anomalies. There is an increased incidence of maternal hydramnios, but affected infants show no increase in associated anomalies.
    c. Treatment. Early excision in infants is mandatory.

  3. Malignant teratomas of the neck are rare and occur exclusively in adults. Prognosis is very poor.

  4. Nasal dermoids are often apparent shortly after birth.
    a. Anatomy. The nasal dorsum is the commonest site, but they may occur in the tip of the nose or the columella.
    b. Characteristics
      (1) They show a male predominance of 2:1.
      (2) They must be differentiated from encephaloceles and gliomas.
    c. Treatment. Early removal is important. Recurrences secondary to incomplete removal are common.

E. Vascular tumors (see Chapter 26 II B 3 a)

  1. Hemangiomas constitute the commonest tumors of the head and neck in children. Girls are more often affected than boys, and the lesions are usually solitary.
    a. Types
      (1) Capillary hemangiomas, such as nevus flammeus (port-wine stain) and strawberry nevus are characteristically found in the dermis.
        (a) They rarely appear in adults.
        (b) They have an early period of evolution, then may develop suddenly and get quite large, after which they often regress.
      (2) Cavernous hemangiomas are more permanent. Spontaneous regression is more likely in those present at birth than in those appearing afterwards.
      (3) Arteriovenous hemangiomas occur almost exclusively in adults and have a predilection for the lips and perioral skin.
      (4) Invasive hemangiomas occur in the deep subcutaneous tissues, deep fascial layers, and muscles.

             (a) These hemangiomas present as neck masses, predominantly in children.

             (b) They tend to recur long after excision but do not metastasize.

             (c) The masseter and trapezius are the muscles most commonly involved in the head and neck.

             (d) **Intramuscular hemangiomas** most commonly present in young adults as palpable, mobile, noncompressible masses.

                 (i) They generally are without thrills, pulsations, or bruits.

                 (ii) Pain secondary to compression of other structures is usually present.

        (5) **Subglottic hemangiomas** are usually capillary in type. Due to their location they often present, at birth or soon thereafter, with stridor and usually with cutaneous involvement as well.

    b. Treatment

        (1) Congenital **cutaneous hemangiomas** are generally treated expectantly, at least initially.

             (a) When patients reach school age, cosmetically deforming lesions may be excised.

             (b) Steroids may be used to slow a rapid growth phase if necessary.

             (c) Tunable dye and copper vapor lasers have shown promise in the treatment of cutaneous lesions.

        (2) **Subglottic lesions** may require tracheotomy, steroids, and, in some cases, laser excision.

        (3) Surgery may be needed for extensive lesions.

        (4) Radiation therapy has been used to suppress tumor growth. However, radiation alone will not effect a cure, and its use in these lesions is controversial.

2. Cystic hygromas are found predominantly in the neck and are usually noted at birth or soon thereafter.

    a. Anatomy. They are commoner in the posterior triangle.

        (1) They may reach up into the cheek or parotid region and down into the mediastinum or axilla.

        (2) Large masses extend past the sternocleidomastoid muscle into the anterior compartment and may cross the midline.

        (3) They may involve the floor of the mouth and the base of the tongue.

    b. Symptoms and signs may include:

        (1) Difficulty in nursing

        (2) Facial or neck distortion

        (3) Respiratory distress

        (4) Brachial plexus compression with pain or hyperesthesia

        (5) A sudden increase in size secondary to spontaneous hemorrhage, which can be fatal.

    c. Characteristics

        (1) There is no predilection for either sex or for either side of the body.

        (2) The hygromas can be progressive, static, or regressive.

        (3) Small lesions are unilocular and firm.

        (4) Large tumors are loculated, shiftable, and compressible.

        (5) The hygromas generally display transillumination.

        (6) The cyst walls are usually tense, and since the loculi tend to communicate, rupture of one locule can cause a partial collapse of all of them.

    d. Treatment. Surgery is the mainstay of treatment.

        (1) Recurrences are common because the cysts insinuate themselves into adjacent structures, so that resection is often incomplete.

        (2) The greater the lymphangiomatous component of a hygroma, the more likely it is to recur.

3. Oral and perioral lymphangiomas are relatively common lesions that are usually found at birth or soon thereafter. They behave very much like cystic hygromas.

F. Branchial cleft anomalies

   1. Embryology

    a. In the fourth week of gestation, five ridges appear on the ventrolateral surface of the embryonic head with a groove between each. These form the branchial arches and clefts, respectively.

    b. The pharyngeal pouches develop internally at the same level as the external grooves.

   2. Types

    a. A **sinus,** or **incomplete fistula,** has either an internal or an external opening.

    b. A **complete fistula** has both an internal and an external opening.
    c. A **cyst** has neither an internal nor an external opening
    d. **Combinations** of any of the above types can occur.

3. Anatomy. Branchial cleft anomalies are located along the anterior border of the sternocleido-mastoid muscle or deep to it. They can occur anywhere between the external auditory canal and the clavicle.

    a. **First branchial cleft anomalies** are always superior to the hyoid bone.
        (1) If a fistula is present, it courses superiorly to end near the external auditory canal.
        (2) The cyst and tract may lie in the parotid gland with a variable relationship to the facial nerve.

    b. **Second cleft anomalies** are the commonest type.
        (1) An external opening, when present, is about two-thirds of the way down the sterno-cleidomastoid anteriorly.
        (2) The fistula, if present, ascends with the carotid sheath and crosses over the hypoglossal and glossopharyngeal nerves and between the external and internal carotid arteries to end at the tonsillar fossa. This is the **commonest branchial anomaly**.

    c. **Third cleft anomalies** are rare.
        (1) The external opening occurs in the same position as in a second cleft fistula.
        (2) The tract ascends along the carotid sheath posteriorly to the internal carotid artery, over the hypoglossal nerve, under the glossopharyngeal nerve, and over the vagus nerve to open in the pyriform sinus.

    d. **Fourth branchial cleft anomalies** have never been seen in their entirety.
        (1) Theoretically, they would have an external opening anterior to the sternocleidomastoid muscle in the lower neck.
        (2) They would descend along the carotid sheath into the chest, passing under the subclavian artery on the right and the aortic arch on the left, ascend into the neck to cross the hypoglossal nerve, then descend to open into the esophagus.

4. Characteristics
    a. Branchial cleft cysts are generally smooth, round, nontender masses.
    b. An increase in size during upper respiratory infections is common.
    c. An infected branchial cleft cyst may abscess or rupture spontaneously to form a sinus.
    d. The size and the location of a branchial cleft anomaly determine the symptoms.
        (1) Large cysts may cause dysphagia, stridor, and dyspnea.
        (2) Small cysts are often not discovered until adulthood because of their slow rate of growth and minimal symptoms.

5. Treatment
    a. Complete excision without damage to the surrounding vital structures is the definitive treatment. Antibiotics are given if the lesion is infected.
    b. Incision and drainage are avoided, if possible, since these will make subsequent excision more difficult.

G. Encephaloceles are congenital brain herniations, which may be confused with nasal dermoids or polyps. Meningitis or cerebrospinal fluid leaks are not uncommon, particularly with manipulation.

1. Anatomy
    a. They are usually discovered early in life. About 75% are occipital, 15% are sincipital, and 10% enter the nose or nasopharynx.
    b. These lesions may or may not communicate centrally. **Communicating** lesions will increase in size and tension when the infant cries; **noncommunicating** ones generally do not.

2. Treatment should include total removal. The lesions need not be treated as emergencies if there is no imminent threat of meningitis.

IV. ACQUIRED LESIONS

A. Leukoplakia and **keratosis** are white lesions, occurring on the mucosa of the mouth, pharynx, or larynx. **Erythroplakia** is a similar red patch.

1. **Etiology.** These lesions are associated with repeated trauma (from poorly fitting dentures, decayed teeth, and so forth), smoking, or use of alcohol. There is little correlation between the clinical appearance of the lesions and their histology, although erythroplakia is somewhat more likely to be carcinoma.

2. **Diagnosis. Biopsy,** to rule out squamous cell carcimona, should be performed:
   a. In high-risk patients (smokers and drinkers)
   b. If the lesion persists after the removal of an irritative focus

3. **Treatment.** Benign leukoplakic lesions require no treatment but do require continued observation.

B. Papillomas

1. **Squamous papillomas** of the oral cavity usually occur singly but may be multiple.
   a. They are usually pedunculated and cauliflower-like in appearance.
   b. Recurrence is rare after excision.

2. **Nasal vestibular papillomas** are **warts** that are similar in appearance and behavior to cutaneous warts elsewhere on the body.

3. **Inverted papillomas**
   a. Anatomy
      (1) The lesions typically arise from the lateral nasal wall and can invade the sinuses and orbits.
      (2) Grossly, the lesions appear bulky and deep red to grey in color; they vary in consistency.
      (3) Unlike nasal polyps of allergic origin (see IV C), they are unilateral.
   b. Characteristics
      (1) Patients generally present with nasal obstruction, a postnasal drip, and headaches. A few have epistaxis. These lesions occur mainly in men aged 30–50.
      (2) The reported incidence of malignant transformation ranges from 2%–15%.
   c. Treatment is complete excision. Recurrence is common because excision is often incomplete.

4. **Laryngeal papillomas** are the commonest laryngeal tumors of childhood and may be found at any age.
   a. Juvenile type. This type occurs predominantly in childhood and tends to involute at puberty.
      (1) Etiology. The etiology is believed to be viral.
      (2) Characteristics
         (a) Multiple papillomas are commonest and may involve the airway from the epiglottis to the bronchi.
         (b) Hoarseness is an early sign and obstruction is a later one.
      (3) Treatment
         (a) A tracheotomy may be necessary but should be avoided if possible because it predisposes to tracheal seeding of the papillomas.
         (b) Laryngoscopic removal, often by the use of a carbon dioxide laser, is the mainstay of therapy.
         (c) Interferon therapy has not proven as useful as early reports predicted.
         (d) Recurrence and spread are common.
   b. Adult type. In this form, the papilloma is generally single.
      (1) As in the juvenile form, the papilloma tends to recur following excision.
      (2) Recurrent lesions can undergo malignant transformation, particularly in patients exposed to radiation.

C. Nasal polyps are very rare before age 5 and occur predominantly in men.

1. **Etiology.** Nasal polyps are believed to be an allergic response, but this has not been clearly established.
   a. They may be associated with asthma and an idiosyncratic reaction to aspirin.
   b. In children, the presence of nasal polyps should prompt a sweat test to rule out cystic fibrosis.

2. **Characteristics**
   a. Polyps may recur frequently.
   b. Involvement of the paranasal sinuses is common.

3. Treatment. Ethmoid or maxillary sinus surgery may be necessary to afford the patient an adequate nasal airway and relief of symptoms.

D. Fibrous lesions

1. **Nodular (proliferative) fasciitis** presents as a rapidly growing, discrete soft-tissue mass.
   a. **Etiology**
      (1) Most probably a reactive, non-neoplastic response to injury, it may occur at any time from childhood to age 70.
      (2) The lesions may be mistaken for sarcoma.
   b. **Characteristics.** Fascia is the primary tissue involved.
   c. **Treatment.** The lesions generally do not recur after excision.

2. **Proliferative myositis** occurs in adults and appears to be post-traumatic in origin.
   a. **Characteristics**
      (1) Like nodular fasciitis, it can be confused with sarcoma.
      (2) The lesion involves muscle diffusely.
      (3) Occasionally, spontaneous regression occurs.
   b. **Treatment.** Lesions do not recur after excision.

3. **Traumatic myositis ossificans,** bony deposits in muscle due to trauma, generally presents as a painful mass in the muscle 1–4 weeks after a single severe trauma.
   a. **Characteristics**
      (1) In the head and neck, the masseter or sternocleidomastoid is generally involved.
      (2) X-ray reveals feathery opacities or irregular radiodensities.
      (3) The condition must be differentiated from **myositis ossificans progressiva,** which is a progressive, systemic illness.
   b. **Treatment.** Persistent painful masses are excised. Local recurrence is common.

4. **Desmoid tumors** are benign, locally invasive, encapsulated tumors.
   a. **Etiology**
      (1) They arise from the muscular fasciae and are often associated with prior trauma.
      (2) These tumors are uncommon in the head and neck but, when found, usually arise from the sternocleidomastoid muscle.
   b. **Treatment.** Complete surgical excision is the treatment of choice.

E. Tumors of skeletal muscle

1. **Characteristics**
   a. Extracardiac **rhabdomyomas** have a predilection for the head and neck.
   b. They show a slight male predominance.
   c. Signs and symptoms depend on the site and size of the tumor.

2. **Treatment.** Rhabdomyomas tend to recur if incompletely excised.

F. Tumors of peripheral nerves (see Chapter 26 II B 6)

1. **Schwannomas** are solitary, encapsulated tumors attached to or surrounded by a nerve. They are primarily located centrifugally and are often painful and tender. They are not associated with von Recklinghausen's disease or with malignant change, in contrast to neurofibromas.

2. **Acoustic neuromas** are a type of schwannoma.
   a. **Etiology.** They arise from the eighth cranial nerve, usually start within the internal auditory canal, and can involve the cerebellopontine angle.
   b. **Characteristics.** Signs and symptoms may include hearing loss, tinnitus, imbalance, and vertigo.
   c. **Treatment.** Early discovery is important as it will result in earlier resection with a consequent decrease in morbidity and mortality.

3. **Neurofibromas** are usually multiple and unencapsulated.
   a. **Etiology.** The lesions generally occur as a component of von Recklinghausen's disease but may occur as solitary lesions or, rarely, as multiple lesions that are not a part of von Recklinghausen's disease.

   b. Characteristics
   - **(1)** Neurites (axons) pass through the tumor.
   - **(2)** In 8% of patients, neurofibromas undergo malignant changes.
   - **(3)** Usually these lesions are located centripetally and are characteristically asymptomatic.
   - **(4)** Café-au-lait spots, vitiligo, gliomas, osseous changes, meningitis, spina bifida, syndactyly, hemangiomas, or retinal and visceral manifestations may be present.

   4. Traumatic neuromas are reactive hyperplasias due to a nerve's attempts at regeneration following injury. They are generally oval or oblong, gray, firm, and unencapsulated, and persistent hyperesthesia and tenderness are the usual signs.

   5. Most neurogenous tumors of the head and neck can be excised safely without sacrificing nerves. If an important nerve must be cut, it should be reanastomosed or a nerve graft interposed.

G. Granular cell tumors

   1. Congenital epulis occurs on the gum pads of newborns in the region of the future incisors. The lesion can be quite large, does not recur after excision, and may spontaneously regress. The female:male ratio is 8:1.

   2. Nonepulis form of granular cell tumors occurs mainly in young adults, especially in blacks.

H. Paragangliomas (chemodectomas) can occur in the head or neck (see Chapter 19 XII A).

I. Nondental lesions of the jaw

   1. Giant cell granuloma
   - **a. Types.** This jaw lesion can occur in two forms:
     - **(1) Central granulomas** occur within the jaw.
     - **(2) Peripheral granulomas,** occurring on the gingival or alveolar mucosa, are four times commoner.
   - **b. Characteristics.** The mucosa is generally intact, but x-rays of the central lesions show radiolucent areas.
   - **c. Treatment.** Excision or curettage is the treatment of choice.

   2. Fibrous dysplasia of the jaw is noted early in life.
   - **a. Characteristics**
     - **(1)** It shows active growth in childhood and stabilization in adulthood.
     - **(2)** Swelling of the bone is the commonest sign and may be either minor or significant enough to cause obvious facial asymmetry.
     - **(3)** The maxilla is more commonly involved than the mandible.
     - **(4)** X-rays reveal sclerosis, lytic lesions, or unilocular lesions.
   - **b. Treatment**
     - **(1)** Obvious deformity, pain, or interference with function suggests the need for surgery.
     - **(2)** Malignant transformation is possible but uncommon, and conservative resection appears to be the best treatment.

   3. Torus is a benign bony growth, occurring at the midline of the palate (**maxillary torus**) or bilaterally lingual to the bicuspid (**mandibular torus**). Tori are slow-growing and generally of no significance except that they may interfere with the fitting of dentures.

   4. Osteomas are slow-growing benign tumors in the sinuses, the jaws, or the external ear canals. They may require excision if they produce headache or occlusion of drainage.

J. Laryngeal lesions

   1. Laryngocele is a dilatation of the laryngeal saccule, producing an air sac that communicates with the laryngeal ventricle. Anything that increases intralaryngeal pressure will increase the size of a laryngocele (e.g., coughing, straining, playing a wind instrument). A **laryngopyocele** is an infected laryngocele. It can be fatal if it results in asphyxia or if the purulent contents drain into the tracheobronchial tree.
   - **a. Anatomy.** Laryngoceles may be unilateral or bilateral. They may also be **internal** (within the larynx), **external** (presenting in the neck), or both (combined).
     - **(1)** An internal laryngocele causes bulging of the false cord and aryepiglottic fold.

(2) The external type appears as a neck swelling at about the level of the hyoid bone and anterior to the sternocleidomastoid.
   b. Characteristics
   (1) Internal laryngoceles cause hoarseness, breathlessness, and stridor on enlargement.
   (2) External laryngoceles increase in size with coughing or the Valsalva maneuver.
      (a) They are tympanic to percussion.
      (b) A hissing may be heard as the laryngocele empties air into the larynx when the air pressure is reduced.
   c. Diagnosis
   (1) Plain films may show cystic spaces that contain air.
   (2) Tomograms may help to demonstrate the continuity between the internal and external components.
   (3) CT and MRI scanning show these lesions well.
   d. Treatment
   (1) Symptomatic laryngoceles are treated by surgical excision.
   (2) Laryngopyoceles should be treated by incision, drainage, and subsequent excision.

2. Laryngeal webs
   a. Characteristics
   (1) They may be congenital or may follow bilateral vocal fold disruption.
   (2) When extensive, they present with stridor, weak phonation, and feeding problems.
   b. Treatment. Laser excision is now generally the preferred treatment, and placement of a stent or keel is often required.

3. Vocal nodules
   a. Anatomy. Vocal nodules are bilateral benign masses that usually occur at the junction of the anterior and middle thirds of the true vocal cords.
   b. Etiology. They are associated with vocal abuse.
   c. Treatment
   (1) Vocal nodules are best treated by modifying the patient's speaking or singing technique.
   (2) Surgery is rarely necessary and is generally performed only after a trial of speech therapy.

4. Vocal polyps
   a. Characteristics. Vocal polyps are usually unilateral and often do not regress with speech therapy—two important points in distinguishing the polyps from vocal nodules.
   b. Treatment
   (1) The recommended therapy is careful excision with microscopic visualization and avoidance of injury to the underlying lamina propria.
   (2) In selected cases, the laser may be helpful.

5. Laryngeal granulomas
   a. Anatomy. Laryngeal granulomas occur over the vocal processes of the arytenoid cartilages.
   b. Etiology. They are generally the result of trauma, usually from an endotracheal tube.
   c. Treatment
   (1) Antireflux therapy is often helpful.
   (2) They are best treated by excision after a period of observation.

6. Arytenoid dislocation
   a. Etiology. Arytenoid dislocation generally is the result of endotracheal tube or external trauma.
   b. Characteristics. A soft, breathy voice after extubation should arouse suspicion.
   c. Treatment. Prompt reduction is essential; otherwise, the arytenoid will usually become fixed in the dislocated position.

7. Contact ulcers
   a. Anatomy. Contact ulcers are mucosal disruptions usually located posteriorly on the vocal cords.
   b. Etiology. They sometimes result from trauma (e.g., from intubation), occasionally from vocal abuse, and often from gastric reflux esophagitis or heavy coughing.
   c. Treatment. Elevation of the head of the bed; avoidance of caffeine, chocolate, late-night snacks, and fried or fatty foods; and antacid therapy will usually result in prompt resolution of the ulcers.

V. INFECTIONS OF THE HEAD AND NECK

A. Common head and neck infections (otitis media, mastoiditis, and sinusitis) are now controlled with antibiotics, which must be given at high doses and over long periods for these sequestered spaces.

B. Tonsillar and adenoidal hypertrophy and infection. Tonsillectomy with adenoidectomy was once the commonest operation in the United States. It remains quite prevalent, but is now performed for specific **indications:**

1. **Obstructive hypertrophy**
    a. Patients benefiting from tonsillectomy with adenoidectomy are those with airway obstruction, sleep apnea, cor pulmonale, dysphagia, or failure to thrive.
    b. **Adenoidectomy** is performed in children with chronic nasal obstruction, especially when they also demonstrate chronic serous otitis media or orthodontic problems.

2. **Recurrent infection.** Patients with documented recurrent adenotonsillitis are improved after tonsillectomy with adenoidectomy. A history of 3–6 episodes yearly is a relative indication.

3. Most authors suggest tonsillectomy after treatment for **peritonsillar abscess** in patients with a history of previous tonsillitis.

C. Atypical mycobacterial infection presents as an inflamed mass or draining sinus in the head and neck. It is commonest in children and adolescents.

1. Pulmonary involvement is very rare.

2. It commonly is associated with the parotid or submandibular glands, but it is not isolated to these sites.

3. Fixation of overlying skin and sinus formation are common. Biopsy can lead to a chronically draining sinus tract.

4. Treatment is by surgical excision or curettage and drainage. Antimycobacterial drug therapy is not indicated.

19
Malignant Lesions of the Head and Neck

Robert T. Sataloff
Joseph R. Spiegel
David A. Zwillenberg

I. OVERVIEW

A. Epidemiology

1. Primary malignant neoplasms of the head and neck account for 5% of new cancers every year in the United States, excluding skin cancer.

2. The male:female ratio is 3:1 to 4:1, and most lesions occur in patients over 40 years of age.

3. Approximately 80% of primary head and neck malignancies are squamous cell carcinomas. The remainder are thyroid cancers, salivary neoplasms, and other rare tumors.

4. The number of patients with a second primary malignancy at the time of initial presentation has been reported to be as high as 17%.

B. Risk factors

1. Cigarette smoking, snuff dipping, alcohol consumption, and exposure to radiation are etiologic factors in most squamous cell carcinomas of the head and neck.

2. Some 85% of patients with head or neck cancer presently smoke or formerly smoked cigarettes.

C. Evaluation of the patient starts with a careful history and physical examination.

1. **History.** The patient should be questioned about:
   a. Exposure to etiologic agents (tobacco, alcohol, and irradiation)
   b. Associated symptoms, including hoarseness or sore throat of more than 3 weeks' duration, dysphagia, dyspnea, nonhealing ulcers, hemoptysis, and neck mass
   c. Any history of head or neck malignancy
   d. Nutritional status, family history, and psychosocial status. The patient's nutritional status is a prime concern in choosing therapy.
      (1) Many patients are malnourished, either because of alcoholism or from an obstructive tumor.
      (2) Treatment is sometimes delayed because of the need for hyperalimentation. In most patients, this can be accomplished with nutritional supplements or tube feedings into the stomach, but parenteral nutrition is sometimes required.

2. **Physical examination** must include inspection of all the skin and mucosal surfaces of the head and neck.
   a. An intranasal examination and indirect mirror examination of the nasopharynx and hypopharynx are included.
   b. A careful palpation of the oral cavity, base of the tongue, and oropharynx is mandatory.
   c. Fiberoptic examination is performed whenever indirect mirror examination is inadequate.

D. Treatment is based on the site and pathology of the primary cancer and the extent of the local, regional, and distant disease.

1. **Surgery** is the indicated treatment for many patients with head and neck cancer. Treatment time is short, and careful pathologic examination of the tissue removed is possible. In addition, the effects of radiation are avoided, and radiation can be saved for recurrent disease or other primaries. The choice of surgery can be influenced by many factors.

a. Malnourishment can increase the perioperative risk of morbidity and mortality.
b. The patient may have a coexistent systemic disease (i.e., diabetes, chronic obstructive pulmonary disease, or coronary artery disease), which increases the surgical risk.
c. The necessary procedures can be disfiguring and can leave the patient with severe functional deficits. Thus, the patient may refuse recommended surgery.
  (1) Resection of the larynx, for example, alters communication.
  (2) Surgery on the tongue, oropharynx, hypopharynx, or mandible can alter or prevent swallowing.
d. Surgery should be performed in institutions that have professionals trained to provide the intensive perioperative care and the rehabilitation that are needed.
e. Surgery is contraindicated in patients with distant metastases.

2. Radiation therapy
  a. Radiation alone is adequate treatment for many early lesions.
    (1) It can provide cures without the functional or cosmetic deficits associated with surgery.
    (2) It can treat multiple primary lesions simultaneously.
    (3) It can prophylactically treat regional nodes that are clinically negative.
  b. Surgery and postoperative radiation can significantly increase survival rates in advanced lesions.
  c. **Complications of radiotherapy** include mucositis, xerostomia, loss of taste, dermal and soft tissue fibrosis, dental caries, and bone and soft tissue necrosis. Dental examination is required prior to radiotherapy. Dental treatment during or for up to 2 years after radiotherapy can be extremely hazardous due to decreased vascularity and consequent delayed healing.

3. Chemotherapy is currently used palliatively for advanced, inoperable tumors. It is also being tested in adjuvant therapy protocols. Cisplatin is the most effective agent. Methotrexate, bleomycin, 5-fluorouracil, and other agents have been used successfully as well.
  a. Most **palliative regimens** use single agents or cisplatin-based multidrug combinations with response rates ranging from 25%–70%.
  b. Pre- and postoperative **adjuvant protocols,** using chemotherapy, are currently being evaluated. Results are encouraging because tumor response rates are high; however, studies have yet to show a significant impact on survival.
  c. Chemotherapy can be delivered by intra-arterial infusion with an indwelling pump system via the external carotid artery.
  d. Patients on chemotherapy should be monitored for signs of toxicity, including hearing loss.

E. Rehabilitation should be planned at the same time as treatment.

  1. Cosmetic and functional defects are reconstructed at the time of the cancer resection whenever possible. The use of **surgical flaps** (see Chapter 26 I D) has greatly facilitated reconstruction. The flaps may be:
    a. Local flaps (nasolabial, forehead)
    b. Distant pedicled skin flaps (deltopectoral, omocervical)
    c. Pedicled myocutaneous flaps (pectoralis major, latissimus dorsi, trapezius)
    d. Free microvascular flaps

  2. Prosthetic rehabilitation is necessary when portions of the maxilla, mandible, or palate are resected.

  3. When the larynx is removed, intensive rehabilitation is required to re-establish the voice.
    a. Initially, patients are taught to speak with an electric larynx applied in the mouth, on the neck, or in the dentures.
    b. Later, they learn to speak with regurgitated air (esophageal speech) or with a Blohm-Singer prosthesis (a one-way valve) placed in a surgically created tracheoesophageal fistula.

  4. Many patients who undergo partial laryngectomy, pharyngectomy, or glossectomy require training to facilitate swallowing and to avoid aspiration.

II. CANCER OF THE NECK

A. Anatomy

  1. Divisions. The neck is divided into anterior and posterior triangles.

    a. The anterior triangle is bounded by the midline of the neck, the inferior border of the mandible, and the anterior border of the sternocleidomastoid muscle. It can be further subdivided into submandibular, submental, superior carotid, and inferior carotid triangles.

    b. The posterior triangle is bounded by the posterior border of the sternocleidomastoid muscle, the anterior border of the trapezius, and the clavicle. It is further divided into supraclavicular and occipital triangles.

2. Lymphatic drainage

    a. Fascial planes of the neck enclose the lymphatic system.

      (1) The **superficial fascia** is subcutaneous and envelops the platysma.

      (2) The **deep fascia** has three parts:

        (a) Superficial layer, which invests the sternocleidomastoid and trapezius muscles

        (b) Pretracheal fascia (middle)

        (c) Prevertebral fascia (deep)

    b. Lymph nodes on each side of the neck number approximately 75.

      (1) Most lie within the deep jugular and spinal accessory chains.

      (2) The jugular chain is divided into superior, middle, and inferior groups.

      (3) Other nodal groups are the submental, submandibular, superficial cervical, retropharyngeal, paratracheal, anterior scalene, and supraclavicular.

B. Evaluation of a neck mass. A workup for malignancy should be undertaken in all adults with a persistent neck mass.

1. History and physical examination. A careful history is taken, and the head and neck are examined for evidence of a possible primary cancer (see I C).

2. Diagnosis. If the primary cancer is not identified on the initial examination, then a **workup** includes:

    a. A chest x-ray, barium swallow, and films of the sinuses

    b. A gastrointestinal (GI) series, intravenous pyelography, and other x-ray studies, if warranted by findings on the history and physical examination

    c. Panendoscopy (direct laryngoscopy, esophagoscopy, bronchoscopy, and nasopharyngoscopy)

    d. If the endoscopic survey is negative, random **biopsies** of the nasopharynx (right, middle, and left) are performed. A random biopsy of the tongue base or a tonsillectomy may also be worthwhile.

    e. If all biopsies are negative, the next step is to proceed with open neck biopsy and frozen section.

C. Staging of metastatic neck disease

1. Stage N0: No clinically positive node

2. Stage N1: A single clinically positive node homolateral to the primary tumor and 3 cm or less in its greatest diameter

3. Stage N2a: A single clinically positive homolateral node larger than 3 cm but less than 6 cm in its greatest diameter

4. Stage N2b: Multiple clinically positive homolateral nodes with none larger than 6 cm in greatest diameter

5. Stage N3a: Multiple clinically positive homolateral nodes with at least one larger than 6 cm in greatest diameter

6. Stage N3b: Bilateral clinically positive nodes

7. State N3c: Only contralateral clinically positive nodes

D. Treatment. If a primary cancer is identified and confirmed with biopsy, the metastatic neck disease is treated in conjunction with the primary.

1. Types of neck dissection

    a. Radical neck dissection is an en bloc dissection of the cervical lymphatics.

      (1) It includes the removal of the sternocleidomastoid muscle, internal jugular vein, and spinal accessory nerve.

(2) It is performed when squamous cell carcinoma is found in a neck mass with an unknown primary cancer or in conjunction with excision of the primary tumor.

b. Modified (functional, conservative) neck dissection removes the cervical lymphatics within their fascial compartments.

(1) It spares the sternocleidomastoid muscle, internal jugular vein, and spinal accessory nerve.

(2) Indications include:

(a) Elective neck dissections

(b) A single node less than 3 cm in diameter that is to be treated postoperatively with radiation

(c) Differentiated thyroid cancers with neck metastases

(d) Simultaneous bilateral neck dissections

2. Elective neck dissection refers to surgical treatment of N0 disease.

a. There is controversy about when and if to use elective neck dissections, since radiation therapy can provide prophylaxis for metastatic neck disease in many cases.

b. The choice between surgery or radiation usually depends on the treatment of the primary tumor.

c. In general, when elective neck dissection is performed, it is done for a primary cancer that has a 30% or greater rate of occult metastasis.

III. CANCER OF THE NASAL CAVITY AND PARANASAL SINUSES

A. Anatomy

1. Basic structure

a. All sinuses come in pairs, and all are contiguous with the nasal cavity through their natural ostia.

b. The nose and sinuses are lined with a respiratory mucosa, which is pseudocolumnar with goblet cells and cilia.

2. Lymphatic drainage is to the parapharyngeal or retropharyngeal nodes. Secondary lymphatics are the subdigastric nodes of the internal jugular chain.

B. Classification

1. Most tumors (59%) are in the maxillary sinus, 24% are in the nasal cavity, 16% in the ethmoid sinuses, and 1% in the frontal and sphenoid sinuses.

2. Some 80% of the malignancies are squamous cell carcinoma.

a. Tumors that arise anteriorly tend to be well differentiated.

b. Those arising from the posterior nasal cavity and ethmoids are generally poorly differentiated.

c. Nasal and sinus cancers are locally invasive. Nodal metastases are unusual and tend to occur late, even with extensive local disease.

3. About 10%–14% of the malignancies are adenocarcinomas, including adenoid cystic carcinoma.

4. Inverted papilloma (see Chapter 18 IV B 3) has a 12%–15% incidence of associated squamous cell carcinoma.

C. Clinical evaluation

1. Presenting symptoms can include nasal obstruction; epistaxis; localized pain; tooth pain; cranial nerve deficits; a mass in the face, palate, or maxillary alveolus; proptosis; and trismus.

2. Diagnosis. The **extent of the disease** is determined by physical examination and radiographic studies.

a. Computed tomography (CT scan) is particularly useful for identifying bony erosions and orbital or intracranial extension.

b. Arteriography is rarely needed.

c. Most biopsies can be performed under local anesthesia.

D. Staging is available for maxillary sinus cancer.

1. **Stage TX:** Cannot be assessed

2. **Stage T0:** No evidence of a primary cancer

3. **Stage T1:** Tumor confined to the inferior antrum without bone erosion

4. **Stage T2:** Tumor confined to the superior antrum without bone erosion of the inferior or medial walls

5. **Stage T3:** Extensive tumor involving the skin of the cheek, the orbit, the anterior ethmoids, or the pterygoid muscles

6. **Stage T4:** Massive tumor involving the cribriform plate, posterior ethmoids, sphenoid, naso-pharynx, pterygoid plates, or base of the skull

E. Treatment

1. **Maxillary sinus cancer**
   a. T1 and T2 tumors are treated with subtotal or radical maxillectomy. Radiation is used when cancer may have been left at the surgical margins and for recurrences.
   b. T3 and T4 tumors receive radiotherapy followed by re-evaluation for surgical resection. Orbital exenteration and skin resection are performed when necessary.

2. **Ethmoid sinus or nasal cavity tumors** are usually treated with radiation therapy followed by surgery for residual disease.

3. **Extensive cancers** are treated with combined craniofacial resection for selected patients.

4. **Inverted papillomas** are treated by en bloc resection that includes the lateral nasal wall and ethmoid sinus.

5. **Cervical lymph node metastases** are treated with radiotherapy followed by radical neck dis-section for residual disease.

F. Prognosis

1. There is an overall cure rate of approximately 30%–35%.

2. The 5-year survival rate for patients with T1 and T2 lesions is 70%.

3. The 5-year survival rate for patients with T3 and T4 lesions is 15%–20%.

IV. CANCER OF THE NASOPHARYNX

A. Anatomy

1. **Basic structure.** The nasopharynx is the most cephalad portion of the pharynx.
   a. Its **roof** is formed by the basioccipital and sphenoid bones, and its **posterior wall** is formed by the atlas.
      (1) These walls are covered by mucosa, and the adenoid tissue is embedded within.
      (2) The lateral wall contains the orifice of the eustachian tube, and, just posterior to that, the fossa of Rosenmüller.
   b. The choanae define the **anterior limit,** and the free edge of the soft palate provides the **inferior limit.**

2. **Lymphatic drainage** is to the lateral retropharyngeal, jugulodigastric (tonsillar), and high spinal accessory nodes.

B. Epidemiology and classification

1. There is a high incidence of nasopharyngeal cancer among persons from the Kwan Tung province of China.

2. There is a high incidence of elevated Epstein-Barr virus titers among persons with cancer of the nasopharynx.

3. Nasopharyngeal cancer occurs at younger ages than do most solid head and neck tumors.

4. Some 85% of nasopharyngeal tumors are epithelial; 7.5% are lymphomas. Epithelial tumors commonly arise in the fossa of Rosenmüller.

C. Clinical evaluation

1. **Presenting symptoms** are anterior or posterior epistaxis, cervical adenopathy, serous otitis media, and nasal obstruction. Headache, diplopia, facial numbness, trismus, ptosis, and hoarseness may also be present. At presentation, 60%–70% of patients will have nodal disease, and 38% will have cranial nerve involvement.

2. **Diagnosis**
   a. Nasopharyngeal cancer can best be evaluated and monitored with CT and magnetic resonance imaging (MRI).
   b. When a patient presents with an elevated Epstein-Barr virus titer, these titers can be monitored and can be expected to fall with successful treatment and to rise with recurrences.

D. Staging

1. **Stage TIS:** Carcinoma in situ

2. **Stage T1:** Tumor is confined to one site, or no tumor is visible but random biopsy is positive.

3. **Stage T2:** Tumor involves two sites (posterosuperior and lateral walls).

4. **Stage T3:** Tumor has extended to the oropharynx or nasal cavity.

5. **Stage T4:** Tumor has invaded the skull or a cranial nerve.

E. Treatment

1. Radiation is the primary treatment for all epithelial nasopharyngeal tumors. The dose, usually 6500–7500 rads, is delivered to the nasopharynx and to both sides of the neck.

2. Radical neck dissection is performed for residual nodes if the primary tumor is controlled.

F. Prognosis. The 5-year survival rate is 40% in patients without positive nodes and 20% in patients with positive nodes.

V. CANCER OF THE ORAL CAVITY

A. Anatomy

1. **Basic structure.** The oral cavity extends from the lip anteriorly to the faucial arches posteriorly. It includes the lips, the buccal mucosa, the gingivae, the retromolar trigones, the hard palate, the anterior two-thirds of the tongue (the oral tongue), and the floor of the mouth.

2. **Lymphatic drainage** is to the submental, submandibular, and deep jugular nodes.

B. Etiology

1. Approximately 90% of patients are heavy smokers or snuff-dippers.

2. Approximately 80% of patients are heavy drinkers.

3. Syphilis accounts for a small number of cases.

4. Herpesvirus type 1 is currently under investigation as a cause.

C. Clinical evaluation

1. **Presenting symptoms** can include loose teeth, painful or nonhealing ulcers, odynophagia, otalgia (with posterior lesions), and cervical adenopathy. The lip is the commonest site of oral cavity carcinoma, followed by the oral tongue, and the floor of the mouth.

2. **Diagnosis**
   a. Mandibular x-rays should be taken to assess bony involvement by adjacent tumors.
   b. Pain is often a late symptom, occurring after ulceration develops and frequently delaying the diagnosis.

(1) Nodal metastases (up to 30% of them occult, microscopic metastatic disease) are found in 50% of patients with squamous cell carcinoma of the anterior tongue and in 58% of patients with cancer of the floor of the mouth (occult metastases in up to 12% of the cases).

(2) Metastases are uncommon and usually occur late in cancer of the lip or the buccal mucosa.

D. Staging

1. Stage T1: Tumor less than 2 cm in its greatest diameter

2. Stage T2: Tumor 2–4 cm in its greatest diameter

3. Stage T3: Tumor more than 4 cm in its greatest diameter

4. Stage T4: Massive tumor with involvement of the mandible pterygoid muscles, antrum, root of the tongue, or skin.

E. Treatment

1. Stage T1, N0 tumors can be treated with either local excision or radiotherapy.

2. Stage T2 or larger lesions should be treated with combined surgery and radiation.
   a. Surgery involves an en bloc resection of the tumor and radical neck dissection.
   b. Either a partial mandibulectomy is included or else the tumor is "pulled through" medially to the mandible into the neck (i.e., the tumor is removed en bloc with the radical neck specimen, leaving the mandible intact).

3. Tumors attached to the mandible may be removed with a partial thickness of mandible (i.e., the lingual plate or alveolar process). The mandibular arch is kept intact when possible.

4. Tumors demonstrating bony erosion in the mandible are removed with a full-thickness portion of bone.

F. Prognosis

1. The overall 5-year survival rate for cancer of all oral cavity sites is approximately 65%.

2. For lip cancer, 5-year survival rates as high as 90% have been reported.

3. The prognosis for tongue lesions is worse if the lesion is posterior. Posterior lesions involving the tongue base can invade the pre-epiglottic space, necessitating laryngectomy.

VI. CANCER OF THE OROPHARYNX

A. Anatomy

1. Basic structure
   a. The oropharynx is bounded by the free edge of the soft palate superiorly, the tip of the epiglottis inferiorly, and the anterior tonsillar pillar anteriorly.
   b. It contains the soft palate, the tonsillar fossae and faucial tonsils, the lateral and posterior pharyngeal walls, and the base of the tongue.
   c. The parapharyngeal space lies directly lateral to the oropharynx.
      (1) It contains the glossopharyngeal, lingual, and inferior alveolar nerves, the pterygoid muscles, the internal maxillary artery, and the carotid sheath.
      (2) It is a site of early extension of an oropharyngeal tumor.
      (3) It also provides a pathway for the tumor to spread to the base of the skull.

2. Lymphatic drainage is primarily to the jugulodigastric (tonsillar) nodes.
   a. Tumors of the soft palate, lateral wall, and tongue base also spread to the retropharyngeal and parapharyngeal nodes.
   b. Retromolar trigone lesions can drain to submaxillary nodes.

B. Etiology

1. Alcohol and tobacco use are commonly found together in patients with oropharyngeal cancer. There appears to be a synergistic effect of the two substances, but it has not been defined.

2. Local mucosal irritation, malnutrition, and immune defects have also been implicated.

C. Clinical evaluation

1. Presenting symptoms

a. The commonest presenting symptom is persistent sore throat.

   (1) This is frequently accompanied by ipsilateral otalgia (referred pain via the tympanic branch of the glossopharyngeal nerve).

   (2) A vague sensation of throat irritation, restriction of tongue motion ("hot potato voice"), odynophagia, and bleeding may also be noted.

   (3) Most patients, especially those with large lesions, are significantly malnourished.

b. Many patients present with cervical adenopathy.

   (1) Nodal metastases are found in 76% of patients with cancer of the base of the tongue and in 60% of patients with tonsillar cancer.

   (2) Most such nodes are palpable.

2. Initial examination must include careful palpation of the tonsils and base of the tongue. Many small tumors are difficult to see but may be easily palpated.

3. Diagnosis is often made late in the course.

a. Many patients are asymptomatic until tumors are quite large and ulcerated.

b. Others are treated conservatively for incorrectly diagnosed lesions.

c. All lesions should be evaluated by endoscopy under general anesthesia before treatment is chosen.

D. Staging (Table 19-1)

1. Stage TIS: Carcinoma in situ

2. Stage T1: Lesion of 2 cm or less in greatest diameter

3. Stage T2: Lesion larger than 2 cm but less than 4 cm in greatest diameter

4. Stage T3: Lesion larger than 4 cm in greatest diameter

5. Stage T4: Lesion larger than 4 cm, with invasion of bone or of soft tissues of the neck or the root of the tongue.

E. Treatment

1. T1 and T2 lesions are treated with radiotherapy.

2. Combined therapy offers improved survival rates for most large lesions and is indicated when nodal metastasis is present.

3. Composite resection (the "jaw-neck" or "commando" procedure) is the **commonest surgical procedure.**

a. It involves a radical neck dissection and partial mandibulectomy in continuity with excision of the tumor.

b. A tracheotomy is routine.

c. A laryngectomy is performed when either:

   (1) The tumor invades the pre-epiglottic space through the vallecula epiglottica

   (2) The entire tongue base and both hypoglossal nerves are removed.

Table 19-1. International College of Surgeons Staging of Oropharyngeal Cancer

Stage I	T1	N0	M0
Stage II	T2	N0	M0
Stage III	T3	N0	M0
	T4	N0	M0
	Any T	N1	M0
	Any T	N2	M0
Stage IV	Any T	N3	M0
	Any T	Any N	M1

    d. Occasionally, the larynx is spared after total glossectomy in young and otherwise healthy patients.

F. Prognosis. The poor prognosis of oropharyngeal cancers is directly related to their late diagnosis.

   1. In tonsillar cancers, 5-year survival rates range from 63% for patients with T1 tumors to 21% for those with T4 disease.

   2. Patients with tumors of the base of the tongue have 5-year survival rates of 40%–60% for T1 disease, and 10%–20% for T4 disease. A high incidence of late presentation is reflected in the large number of T4 patients.

   3. For patients with tumors of the palatal arch, the 5-year survival rates range from 77% for T1 disease to 20% for T4 disease.

   4. The presence of nodal metastases reduces the 5-year survival rate significantly: for N0 it is 75%; for N1, 25%.

VII. CANCER OF THE HYPOPHARYNX AND CERVICAL ESOPHAGUS

A. Anatomy

   1. Basic structure
    a. The hypopharynx extends from the pharyngoepiglottic fold to the inferior border of the cricoid, excluding the larynx.
    b. It includes the pyriform sinuses, the postcricoid area, and the posterior pharyngeal wall.

   2. Lymphatic drainage. There is a rich lymphatic network.
    a. The pyriform sinuses drain to jugulocarotid and midjugular nodes.
    b. The posterior pharyngeal wall drains primarily to retropharyngeal nodes.
    c. Lower hypopharyngeal areas drain to paratracheal and low jugular nodes.
    d. The cervical esophagus additionally is drained by mediastinal nodes.

B. Classification and etiology

   1. Ninety-five percent of the tumors in this region are epithelial cancers.

   2. About 60%–75% arise in the pyriform sinuses and 20%–25% on the posterior pharyngeal wall; rarely, tumors arise in the postcricoid area.

   3. As with other head and neck tumors, the tumors are related to heavy alcohol intake and tobacco use.

C. Clinical evaluation

   1. Presenting symptoms. The triad of throat pain, referred otalgia, and dysphagia is present in more than 50% of patients.
    a. Hoarseness and airway obstruction signal laryngeal involvement.
    b. Small postcricoid tumors often present with mild symptoms of sore throat, a "lump in the throat," and throat clearing.
    c. Cervical metastases (41% of them occult) are found in 75% of patients with pyriform sinus cancers and in 83% of pharyngeal wall tumors (66% occult).

   2. Diagnosis. A barium swallow and endoscopy with biopsy complete the workup.

D. Staging

   1. Stage TIS: Carcinoma in situ

   2. Stage T1: Carcinoma confined to the site of origin

   3. Stage T2: Extension of the tumor to an adjacent site without fixation of the hemilarynx (vocal cord)

   4. Stage T3: Extension of the tumor to an adjacent site with fixation of the hemilarynx

   5. Stage T4: Massive tumor with invasion of bone, cartilage, or the soft tissues of the neck

E. Treatment

1. Laryngopharyngectomy and radical neck dissection, followed by radiotherapy, are necessary for most T3 and T4 lesions.
   a. If the tumor is T1 or T2 and spares the apex of the pyriform sinus, a supraglottic laryngectomy can be considered.
   b. Some small T1 tumors can be treated by radiation therapy alone or by surgical resection via a lateral pharyngotomy.
   c. Cancers of the cervical esophagus can require removal of the pharynx, esophagus, and larynx.

2. Reconstruction of circumferential defects of the hypopharynx and cervical esophagus can be accomplished by multiple methods. The ideal procedure to reconstruct swallowing function and reduce operative morbidity is chosen on an individual basis. The following types of reconstruction are available for consideration:
   a. Regional skin flaps, such as deltopectoral or cervical (this requires multiple stages)
   b. Pedicled myocutaneous flaps (pectoralis major, latissimus dorsi)
   c. Esophagectomy, followed by gastric "pull-up" (raising the stomach into the chest or neck to replace the esophagus)
   d. Colon interposition
   e. A free intestinal graft or soft tissue flap with microvascular anastomosis

F. Prognosis is poor because of extensive submucosal spread and the high incidence of cervical metastasis.

1. The overall 5-year survival rate is approximately 30% for patients with hypopharyngeal tumors.

2. It rises to 50% for those who qualify for supraglottic laryngectomy.

VIII. CANCER OF THE LARYNX

A. Anatomy

1. **Divisions.** The larynx is divided into three regions.
   a. **The supraglottis** extends from the tip of the epiglottis to include the false vocal cords and roof of the ventricle.
   b. **The glottis** extends from the depth of the ventricle to 1 cm below the free edge of the true vocal cord.
   c. **The subglottis** extends from 1 cm below the free edge of the true vocal cord to the inferior border of the cricoid cartilage.

2. **Lymphatic drainage**
   a. The supraglottis has a rich network that crosses the midline and drains to the deep jugular nodes.
   b. The glottis has poorly developed, sparse lymphatics.
   c. The subglottis drains through the cricothyroid membrane to the prelaryngeal (delphian) and pretracheal nodes.

B. Classification and etiology

1. Over 90% of patients have a significant smoking history.

2. Heavy alcohol consumption is common, but not a definite etiologic factor.

3. Some 95%–98% of the tumors are squamous cell carcinomas.

4. Verrucous carcinoma is a variant of squamous cell carcinoma that is locally invasive but almost never metastasizes. It can undergo malignant transformation to a more aggressive malignancy, especially after radiotherapy.

C. Clinical evaluation

1. **Presenting symptoms**
   a. The commonest symptom is hoarseness.
   b. Stridor, cough, hemoptysis, dysphagia, and aspiration also occur.

    c. Neck masses are uncommon at the time of presentation in glottic tumors.

  2. Diagnosis
    a. All patients require direct laryngoscopy and biopsy.
    b. Laryngograms, a barium swallow, stroboscopic laryngoscopy, and CT scan may be helpful.

D. Staging

  1. Stage TIS: Carcinoma in situ

  2. Stage T1: Tumor confined to the site of origin

  3. Stage T2: Tumor spread to an adjacent laryngeal site

  4. Stage T3: Tumor confined to the larynx with fixation of the hemilarynx

  5. Stage T4: Tumor with cartilage destruction or extension beyond the larynx

E. Treatment

  1. Carcinoma in situ is treated by excision of the involved vocal cord mucosa, and is then closely monitored.

  2. Most T1 lesions are treated with radiation because the resulting voice is usually of better quality than after surgical excision. However, surgery is still indicated for many patients.
    a. Removal of the vocal cord by traditional techniques or by using a carbon dioxide laser is recommended by some authors, but partial cordectomy by laser is still controversial.
    b. Some glottic lesions that involve the anterior commissure may be treated by hemilaryngectomy (vertical laryngectomy) because of the increased risk of cartilage involvement.
    c. Some small lesions of the tip of the epiglottis can also be treated with limited surgical resection.

  3. Supraglottic (horizontal) laryngectomy is the treatment for large supraglottic tumors.
    a. This procedure removes the epiglottis, aryepiglottic folds, and false vocal cords, sparing the true vocal cords.
    b. For transglottic tumors (supraglottic tumors that spread to a true vocal cord), a suprahemilaryngectomy may be considered.
    c. Radical neck dissection, radiation, or both, is often necessary, since nodal metastases (30% of which are occult) are found in 55% of supraglottic cancers.

  4. All T3 and T4 lesions require total laryngectomy, often combined with radical neck dissection. Postoperative radiotherapy is usually indicated.

  5. Verrucous carcinoma is treated surgically, using a conservative laryngectomy when possible. There is no need for elective radical neck dissection, and radiotherapy has been implicated in the causation of anaplastic transformation.

F. Prognosis is better in laryngeal cancer than with other head and neck sites. Five-year survival rates by stage are as follows:

  1. Stage T1: 85%–90% with surgery or radiation

  2. Stage T2: 80%–85%

  3. Stage T3: 75%

  4. Stage T4: 30%

IX. CANCER OF THE EAR

A. Anatomy

  1. Basic structure. The **tympanic membrane** separates the external canal from the middle ear. The portions of the ear susceptible to tumors include the external ear (pinna), external auditory canal, and middle ear.

  2. Lymphatic drainage of the external ear and canal is anterior through the parotid, posterior to the mastoid nodes, and deep to the jugulodigastric nodes.

B. Classification and etiology. Cancer of the ear is rare.

1. The **etiology** has been related to thermal burns, chronic suppurative infection, and exposure to radium. Cancer of the pinna may come from actinic radiation.

2. About 86% are epithelial cancers. Basal cell carcinomas comprise 8%, melanoma and adeno-carcinoma comprise 2% each, and rhabdomyosarcoma and spindle cell sarcoma comprise 1% each. Other malignancies, such as osteogenic sarcoma, are extremely rare.

3. Approximately 80% of ear cancers arise on the auricle, 15% in the external canal, and 5% in the middle ear.

4. **Lytic lesions** deep in the temporal bone should be worked up as possible metastases and may be from an adenocarcinoma, hypernephroma, melanoma, or other primary tumor.

C. Clinical evaluation

1. **Presenting symptoms**
   a. Most ear tumors present as an infected, painful, chronically draining ear.
   b. If a mass is present in the external canal, it is usually friable.
   c. Vertigo and facial paralysis are ominous signs.

2. **Diagnosis**
   a. When cancer is suspected, the mass is biopsied under controlled conditions. Significant hemorrhage may occur.
   b. CT and MRI scanning are necessary in most cases to evaluate the extent of tumor invasion.

D. Treatment

1. Cancers of the auricle can usually be treated with wedge excision.

2. In deeper, more advanced cancers, radical surgery provides the best chance for cure.
   a. Tumors of the canal that are at least 5 mm lateral to the eardrum can be treated by excision of the external canal.
   b. Cancers that impinge on the tympanic membrane without middle ear invasion are treated with partial (lateral) temporal bone resection. This removes the external canal, eardrum, incus, and malleus, while sparing the facial nerve.
   c. Cancers that involve the middle ear or pneumatized spaces are probably best treated by total en bloc temporal bone resection.

3. Radiation therapy has not produced satisfactory cure rates and is used best to treat recurrent or residual disease.

4. Combined therapy may be indicated in some cases.

E. Prognosis. Results are difficult to evaluate because of the small number of cases reported.

1. For patients requiring temporal bone resection, 5-year survival rates range from 25%–35%. However, many of these operations transgressed the tumor, leaving gross tumor behind. Newly described en bloc procedures should improve these statistics.

2. For lesions confined to the pinna, an 80% cure rate can be expected after treatment.

X. CANCER OF THE SKIN (see Chapter 26 II C–F). Cancers of the skin account for 25% of all cancers, and fully 90% of skin cancers occur on the head and neck.

A. Basal and squamous cell carcinomas. Basal cell carcinoma accounts for 60% of skin cancers, and squamous cell carcinoma for 30%.

1. **Etiology**
   a. Sunlight
   b. Radiation
   c. Arsenic
   d. Burns, scars
   e. Genetic disorders (xeroderma pigmentosa, basal-cell nevus syndrome, albinism)

2. Clinical evaluation

  a. Skin cancers usually present as slowly enlarging cutaneous or subcutaneous lesions. Some form nonhealing ulcers.

  b. Nodal metastasis is uncommon.

3. Treatment. Therapy includes electrodesiccation, curettage, cryosurgery, excision, Mohs' surgery, radiation, and topical fluorouracil.

  a. Surgical excision is preferred for squamous cell carcinoma because it allows removal of a margin.

  b. Basal cell carcinomas of the nasolabial folds, medial and lateral canthi, or postauricular regions are especially aggressive. They can invade multiple tissue planes, and, therefore, require an extensive surgical resection.

  c. Mohs' surgery involves the precise mapping and frozen-section control of the entire resection bed. It is especially useful for cancers in areas known for aggressive patterns of spread and recurrence. It allows for early reconstruction because of reliable surgical margins.

  d. Radiation therapy is usually reserved for advanced lesions in areas where surgical excision leaves a cosmetically unacceptable defect (the nose, eyelid, lip).

    (1) Radiation probably should not be employed when tumors invade bone or cartilage.

    (2) These cases require radical excision.

  e. All positive nodes should be treated with radical neck dissection or radiotherapy.

B. Malignant melanoma

1. Epidemiology

  a. Malignant melanoma accounts for 1% of all cancers.

  b. Some 20%–30% of all melanomas arise in the head and neck.

  c. Melanoma occurs predominantly in whites. It commonly occurs in persons aged 30–60 and is rare in children.

2. Etiology

  a. Sunlight and heredity

  b. Melanomas may arise from **junctional nevi** (see Chapter 26 II D 2 a).

    (1) These are usually present from birth.

    (2) Nevi which undergo malignant transformation are usually in an irritated or exposed area.

    (3) Melanomas can also arise on the mucosal surfaces of the head and neck.

3. Pathologic variants include:

  a. Lentigo maligna melanoma

  b. Superficial spreading melanoma

  c. Nodular melanoma

4. Staging is by depth of invasion.

  a. Stage T1: Up to 0.75 mm deep

  b. Stage T2: 0.76 to 1.5 mm

  c. Stage T3: 1.51–3.0 mm

  d. Stage T4: More than 3.0 mm

5. Treatment is by wide excision of the melanoma.

  a. A radical neck dissection is performed for positive nodes.

    (1) A parotidectomy is added to the radical dissection for lesions of the anterior scalp, eyelids, auricle, and cheek because the first-level lymphatic drainage is to the periparotid nodes.

    (2) Elective radical neck dissection is usually performed on patients with T3 and T4 tumors.

  b. Radiation therapy is usually reserved for palliative treatment of recurrent disease.

  c. Chemotherapy, primarily with dacarbazine (DTIC), is used for disseminated melanoma.

6. Prognosis

  a. This is related to the depth of invasion.

    (1) T1 lesions have a 5-year survival rate of 90%; T4 lesions, 10%.

    (2) N0 lesions have a 5-year survival rate of 90%; N1 and N3 lesions, 10%.

  b. The prognosis in mucosal melanoma is extremely poor.

XI. LYMPHOMA OF THE HEAD AND NECK

A. Epidemiology

1. Some 80% of all malignant lymphomas arise from nodes, many in the head and neck.

2. About 65%–70% of patients with Hodgkin's lymphoma have cervical lymph node involvement.

3. Extranodal presentation is rare in Hodgkin's disease but occurs in 20% of non-Hodgkin's lymphoma cases.

B. Classification

1. Non-Hodgkin's lymphoma is really a group of diseases, which are classified into favorable and unfavorable types on the basis of therapeutic response.
   a. Favorable types include:
   (1) Nodular lymphomas
   (2) Well-differentiated lymphocytic lymphoma
   b. Unfavorable types include:
   (1) Diffuse poorly differentiated lymphocytic lymphoma
   (2) Diffuse histiocytic lymphoma
   (3) Diffuse undifferentiated lymphoma
   (4) Nodular histiocytic lymphoma

2. Hodgkin's lymphoma. The histology of Hodgkin's disease influences prognosis.
   a. Favorable type
   (1) Lymphocyte-predominant
   (2) Nodular sclerosing
   b. Guarded type. Mixed cellular
   c. Unfavorable type. Lymphocyte-depleting

C. Clinical evaluation

1. Presenting symptoms
   a. The usual presentation is of a single enlarged cervical node.
   (1) Initial workup is aimed at discovery of an extranodal primary lesion.
   (2) The enlarged node must be differentiated from squamous cell carcinoma.
   b. Most lymphomatous nodes are firm and rubbery.
   (1) Non-Hodgkin's lymphoma typically presents in upper cervical nodes.
   (2) Hodgkin's disease is discovered in nodes throughout the cervical chain.
   c. The commonest **sites of extranodal involvement** in non-Hodgkin's lymphoma are in the head and neck, particularly in Waldeyer's ring. Other sites include the nasal cavity, paranasal sinuses, orbit, and salivary glands.
   d. About 40% of patients with Hodgkin's lymphoma have systemic symptoms of fever, sweats, weight loss, and malaise.

2. Diagnosis is usually by excisional biopsy of a lymph node.
   a. If a possible extranodal source has been discovered, it should be biopsied first.
   b. Endoscopy should always precede lymph node biopsy to rule out a primary epithelial tumor.
   c. For a node biopsy, one of the largest nodes should be removed in its entirety.
   d. Frozen-section diagnosis is of little value, except to exclude squamous cell carcinoma.

D. Staging is aimed at determining the extent of spread of the lymphoma.

1. After the diagnosis is made, all patients undergo chest x-ray, CT scan of the abdomen, and a bone marrow biopsy.
   a. CT scan of the chest, intravenous pyelography, and lymphangiography are sometimes added, depending on initial findings.
   b. All patients with non-Hodgkin's lymphoma should have a GI series because of the high incidence of gastrointestinal involvement. CT scan of the abdomen occasionally obviates the need for these studies.

2. Staging laparotomy is often necessary for patients with an early stage of lymphoma when treatment with radiotherapy alone is contemplated. Laparoscopy can be substituted when patients also receive chemotherapy.

3. **Stages** are as follows:
   a. **Stage I:** Involvement of a single lymph node region or a single extralymphatic site
   b. **Stage II:** Either of the following:
      (1) Involvement of two or more lymph node regions on the same side of the diaphragm
      (2) Localized involvement of an extranodal site and of one or more lymph node regions on the same side of the diaphragm
   c. **Stage III:** Involvement of lymph node regions or extranodal sites on both sides of the diaphragm
   d. **Stage IV:** Diffuse or disseminated involvement of one or more distant extranodal organs

E. Treatment

1. Patients with stage I or II Hodgkin's disease can be treated with radiotherapy alone.

2. Patients with more advanced stages are treated with **MOPP chemotherapy** [mechlorethamine, vincristine (Oncovin), procarbazine, and prednisone], usually combined with nodal irradiation.

3. Treatment of non-Hodgkin's lymphoma is much less clear-cut.
   a. In general, early stages (I and II) are treated with radiotherapy, and later stages (III and IV), with chemotherapy.
   b. Combined radiation and chemotherapy are usually used for advanced unfavorable lesions.

F. Prognosis

1. **Hodgkin's disease**
   a. **Favorable prognostic factors** include:
      (1) Localized disease
      (2) A limited number of anatomic sites
      (3) Absence of massive disease
      (4) A favorable histology (lymphocyte-predominant and nodular sclerosing)
   b. Stages I and II have 5-year, relapse-free rates of 80%–90%.
      (1) The rate falls to 60%–80% in advanced disease treated with combined therapy.
      (2) Rates as low as 30% have been reported in stage IV lesions.

2. **Non-Hodgkin's lymphoma**
   a. Radiation therapy for stages I and II patients yields 50%–70% cure rates.
   b. With more advanced lesions, patients with a favorable histology can have a 60%–70% 5-year survival rate, and a 30% cure rate.
   c. Patients with an unfavorable histology face a 25%–40% 5-year survival rate with little chance for cure.

XII. UNUSUAL TUMORS

A. Chemodectomas (paragangliomas) arise from chemoreceptor tissue.

1. They are rarely malignant (2%–6% are), but they have the propensity for extensive local invasion.

2. Paragangliomas are often multicentric and associated with other malignancies.

3. They are found in the carotid body, ganglion nodosum of the vagus nerve, aortic arch, jugular bulb, and within the middle ear, orbit, nose, nasopharynx, or larynx. Morbidity and mortality depend on the tumor type and extent.
   a. **Carotid body tumors** usually present as slow-growing, painless neck masses.
      (1) **Characteristics**
         (a) About 2.8% are bilateral. This increases to 26% in patients with a familial tendency for paragangliomas.
         (b) Large tumors can cause dysphagia, airway obstruction, and cranial nerve palsies.
         (c) The mass may be pulsatile and may have a bruit.
      (2) **Diagnosis** is by angiography, which shows a tumor blush at the carotid bifurcation that splays the internal and external carotids.
      (3) **Treatment** is by surgical excision. Large tumors may require carotid bypass.

b. Glomus jugular and glomus tympanicum tumors
   (1) Characteristics
      (a) Glomus jugular tumors arise in the jugular bulb. They can invade the middle ear, the labyrinth, and the cranium. They commonly affect multiple cranial nerves, especially VII, IX, X, XI, and XII.
      (b) Glomus tympanicum tumors arise in the middle ear, along the tympanic nerve. Most patients have pulsatile tinnitus and present with an aural "polyp" or a middle ear mass that can be seen with pneumatic pressure on the tympanic membrane. Hearing loss and vertigo are common.
      (c) Other rare sites of glomus tumor formation are along the vagus nerve in the neck **(glomus vagale),** and in the larynx.
   (2) Evaluation includes angiography, retrograde jugular venography, and CT scan. Biopsy should be avoided.
      (a) Up to 10% of patients with a glomus tumor will have associated bilateral glomus tumor, carotid body tumor, thyroid carcinoma, or other neural crest tumors.
      (b) The tumor is extremely rare in children.
      (c) Four-vessel carotid arteriography should be done.
   (3) Treatment of choice is surgical excision.
      (a) This is easily carried out for small tympanicum tumors but can carry significant morbidity in patients with large tumors because of intracranial extension, hemorrhage, and recurrence.
      (b) Glomus tumors are radiosensitive but not radiocurable.
      (c) New skull-base surgical techniques have rendered essentially all lesions in this area resectable, and radiation should probably be reserved for recurrences, minimal residual disease, and patients physically unfit for surgery.

B. Other rare malignant vascular lesions are found in the head and neck.

1. Angiosarcomas arise from the vascular endothelial cells.
   a. Characteristics. They are fast-growing, extend through the dermis, and frequently metastasize. The commonest site on the head or neck is the scalp.
   b. Treatment. The only chance for cure is complete excision.

2. Hemangiopericytoma arises from the pericytes of Zimmerman around capillaries.
   a. Characteristics. Approximately 25% are found in the head and neck. They are locally invasive and display an inconsistent malignant potential. Distant metastasis is not uncommon, but nodal spread is rare.
   b. Treatment is by surgical excision. Local recurrence is common.

3. Kaposi's sarcoma (see Chapter 26 II G 2 d) is a rare tumor that arises in the skin and presents as a bluish-red macule.
   a. It is receiving recent attention because a large percentage of patients with acquired immune deficiency syndrome (AIDS) present with Kaposi's sarcoma.
   b. Treatment. Head and neck neoplasms in these patients tend to be multiple and have usually been treated with radiotherapy.

C. Esthesioneuroblastoma (olfactory neuroblastoma) is a rare neurogenic lesion that arises from the olfactory mucosa at the roof of the nose.

1. Presenting symptoms
   a. It presents as a nasal mass with the usual symptoms of epistaxis and obstruction.
   b. Involvement of the cribriform plate is routine, and intracranial extension is common.

2. Diagnosis. Pathologic diagnosis can be difficult. Workup includes CT scan and occasionally angiography.

3. Treatment is with combined intracranial and intranasal resection and radiotherapy in selected cases.
   a. Local recurrence rates are high (50%), but metastasis is uncommon (20%).
   b. The 5-year survival rate is about 50%.
   c. However, since most of the literature predates the current mode of therapy, recurrence and survival statistics should improve.

D. Tumors of bone and soft tissue

   1. Osteogenic sarcoma
      a. Characteristics. It is the commonest malignant tumor of bone. It occurs rarely in the head and neck. The commonest site in the head and neck is the jaws. Only about a dozen cases have been reported that were primary to the temporal bone.
      b. Etiology. Previous bone disease and prior irradiation have been implicated as etiologic factors.
      c. Treatment is by radical excision.
         (1) The efficacy of adjuvant radiation therapy is controversial.
         (2) The most recent literature suggests that chemotherapy should be reserved for metastatic disease but this is also controversial.
      d. Prognosis. The 5-year survival rate is extremely poor.

   2. Ewing's sarcoma
      a. Characteristics. It occurs in the skull and facial bones in about 9% of the cases. It is usually a painful, swollen lesion.
      b. Treatment is with radiation and adjuvant chemotherapy.
      c. Prognosis. The 5-year survival rate is about 50%.

   3. Ameloblastoma is a locally invasive tumor arising from the odontogenic apparatus.
      a. Presenting symptoms. It usually presents as a painless swelling and is much commoner in the mandible than in the maxilla.
      b. Treatment is by conservative local excision. Radiation can be used for the rare malignant case.

   4. Rhabdomyosarcoma (see Chapter 26 II G 2 c) is primarily a disease of children.
      a. Characteristics. It can occur in the orbit, oral cavity, pharynx, face, neck, ear, paranasal sinuses, or salivary glands.
      b. Treatment. It is treated with radiation and chemotherapy.
      c. Prognosis. Except for tumors in the orbit, which have an 80% 2-year survival rate, the prognosis is poor.

   5. Soft tissue sarcomas [fibro-, lipo-, and chondrosarcomas (see Chapter 26 II G)] are quite rare in the head and neck.
      a. Etiology. They are associated with prior irradiation.
      b. Treatment is with surgery and radiation. Local recurrence rates are high.

   6. Chordoma is a rare tumor arising from the embryonic notochord.
      a. Characteristics. One-half of these tumors occur in the craniocervical region.
      b. Presenting symptoms
         (1) They are slow-growing, locally invasive tumors that cause bone and soft tissue destruction.
         (2) They can present as a nasopharyngeal mass.
      c. Treatment is with surgical excision, radiation therapy, or both. Local recurrence rates are high.

20
Parotid Gland

R. Anthony Carabasi, III

I. INTRODUCTION

A. Anatomy

1. Embryology. The parotid gland is the largest of the salivary glands. The average gland weighs 25 g. It appears in the fourth week of gestation and originates from the epithelium of the oropharynx.

2. Relations

  a. The gland covers the masseter muscle and extends posteriorly beyond the vertical ramus of the mandible and abuts the external auditory meatus.

  b. Enclosing the gland is a dense **fascial sheath**. The tightness of this fascia is responsible for the severe pain that accompanies acute swelling of the gland (**acute parotitis**).

  c. Classically, the parotid gland was thought to have two lobes, superficial and deep. Anatomically, this is probably not the case, but it is useful to think of the gland in this way when discussing the surgical treatment of parotid diseases.

3. Drainage of saliva is via Stensen's duct. This exits anteriorly, pierces the buccinator muscle, and enters the oral cavity opposite the second upper molar. The opening is marked by the parotid papilla, which may be felt by the tongue or a finger.

B. Innervation of the parotid gland (Figure 20-1)

1. The **facial nerve** enters the posterior part of the gland immediately after emerging from the stylomastoid foramen. It divides within the substance of the gland into two trunks, which eventually split into five major **branches**.

  a. Temporal

  b. Zygomatic

  c. Buccal

  d. Mandibular

  e. Cervical

2. The facial nerve and branches separate the superficial and deep portions of the gland.

3. The muscles of expression are supplied by the facial nerve on the ipsilateral side of the face.

II. BENIGN NEOPLASMS.
Approximately 80% of parotid tumors are benign. The commonest presenting feature of these tumors is a painless mass. Many are multicentric and have a high incidence of local recurrence. Facial paralysis is rare. Very careful identification and surgical treatment, comprised of excision that includes a margin of normal gland, is required. Extension into the deep lobe requires total parotidectomy. The facial nerve should be spared, if possible, during surgery for benign parotid neoplasms. The different types of benign tumors are discussed below.

A. Mixed tumors are so named because they contain both stromal and epithelial components.

1. They are the commonest benign salivary tumors and account for 60% of all parotid tumors.

2. They are slow-growing tumors but may be quite large at the time of presentation.

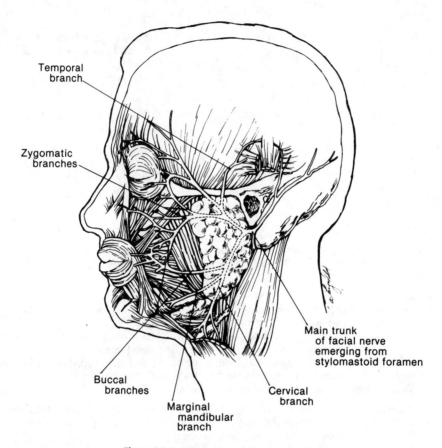

Figure 20-1. Innervation of the parotid gland.

3. At surgery, mixed tumors often seem to "shell out" easily—that is, they seem easy to remove from the surrounding normal tissue. However, this invariably leaves nests of residual tumor, resulting in recurrence that requires re-excision.

4. Radiation therapy has no substantial effect.

B. Papillary adenocystoma (cystadenoma) lymphomatosum (Warthin's tumor)

1. These tumors are composed of both epithelial and lymphoid elements.

2. They are soft (cystic) when palpated.

3. When cut, they are found to contain mucoid material, which appears purulent. However, despite this appearance, the tumors are neoplastic and not inflammatory.

4. Malignant degeneration is rare but may occur in patients who have had prior neck irradiation.

5. This tumor is found in men five times as frequently as in women. It usually occurs between the ages of 40 and 60.

C. Benign lymphoepithelial tumor (Godwin's tumor)

1. This uncommon tumor occurs most frequently in middle-aged or older women.

2. It is characterized by slowly progressive lymphoid infiltration of the gland.

3. Care must be taken not to confuse this lesion with a malignant lymphoma.

4. Occasionally, Godwin's tumor is unencapsulated, and when this occurs, it mimics an inflammatory process.

5. Recurrences may be treated with small doses of radiation.

D. **Oxyphil adenomas** are made up of acidophilic cells called **oncocytes.**

   1. These tumors occur most frequently in elderly patients.

   2. They are slow-growing and do not usually become larger than 5 cm.

E. **Miscellaneous lesions,** such as **hemangiomas** and **lymphangiomas,** also occur. Hemangiomas that do not regress are treated by resection.

III. **MALIGNANT NEOPLASMS.** Malignant tumors comprise 20% of all parotid neoplasms. They are often characterized by pain and facial nerve paralysis, which are features rarely, if ever, found in benign tumors. The different types of malignant neoplasms are discussed below.

A. **Mucoepidermoid carcinoma**

   1. This interesting tumor arises from the ducts of the gland. It is the commonest parotid malignancy and comprises 9% of all parotid tumors.

   2. **Types**
      a. **Low-grade tumors** are the commoner form and are the tumors seen most frequently in childhood.
         (1) They are generally soft to palpation and appear encapsulated at surgery.
         (2) They are treated by excision of the tumor with preservation of those facial nerve branches that are not directly involved by the lesion.
         (3) When low-grade tumors are treated properly, the 5-year survival rate approaches 95%.
      b. **High-grade tumors** are extremely aggressive, unencapsulated tumors, which invade the gland widely.
         (1) Treatment must be radical and includes total parotidectomy, including the facial nerve, plus radical neck dissection (see Chapter 19 II D 1). Neck dissection is done even without palpable nodes because there is a high incidence of microscopic nodal metastasis.
         (2) Surgery is usually supplemented by postoperative radiation.
         (3) The 5-year survival rate is 42% with optimal treatment.

B. **Malignant mixed tumors**

   1. These comprise the second commonest type of malignancy and are responsible for 8% of all parotid tumors.

   2. Treatment is total parotidectomy; a radical neck dissection is also done for either palpable adenopathy or a high-grade tumor.

C. **Squamous cell carcinoma** is a rare tumor in the parotid gland.

   1. It is very hard on palpation and is usually accompanied by pain and nerve paralysis.

   2. It is important to differentiate this lesion from a metastasis arising from a primary tumor elsewhere in the head and neck.

   3. The 5-year survival rate is about 20%.

D. **Other lesions** include **adenocystic carcinoma (cylindroma), acinic cell adenocarcinoma,** and **adenocarcinoma**.

   1. Treatment is total parotidectomy.

   2. Neck dissection is added when obvious nodal disease is present and for high-grade lesions.

   3. High-grade, recurrent, and inoperable tumors should be treated with postoperative radiation.

E. **Malignant lymphoma** may arise as a primary tumor in the gland. The treatment is the same as for other lymphomas (see Chapter 19 XI).

IV. PAROTID TRAUMA

A. Lacerations in the area of the parotid may damage the parenchyma of the gland, Stensen's duct, or the facial nerve.

    1. Parenchymal damage without injury to Stensen's duct usually heals spontaneously.

    2. Stensen's duct. If this duct is lacerated or transected, it should be repaired over a small catheter. This is sutured to the oral mucosa and left in place for 10 days.

    3. Facial nerve injuries
      a. These may recover spontaneously if only a distal branch is transected.
      b. If a main trunk is injured, it will require meticulous repair by primary anastomosis or nerve grafting.
      c. If the injured area is hard to expose, a superficial parotidectomy should be done to facilitate repair.

B. Foreign bodies (e.g., bullets) should be removed.

V. INFLAMMATORY DISORDERS

A. Acute suppurative parotitis is usually found in patients who are debilitated and dehydrated and who have poor oral hygiene. Postoperative patients in this condition are particularly at risk.

    1. The offending organism is usually *Staphylococcus aureus.*
      a. It most likely enters the gland from the mouth via Stensen's duct.
      b. The dehydrated patient whose salivary glands are not secreting actively is prone to rapid growth of the organism in this favorable environment.
      c. The bacterial proliferation leads to an intense inflammatory reaction in the gland with edema and severe pain.

    2. Initial treatment includes hydration, antibiotics, and measures to promote salivation, such as occasional sucking on a lemon.
      a. Cultures from Stensen's duct are taken.
      b. Antibiotics are initially directed against *S. aureus* and are later adjusted as indicated by the results of the cultures.

    3. Surgical drainage is required, if the process is not arrested by the above measures.
      a. An incision is made around the angle of the mandible, and multiple horizontal incisions are made in the parotid fascia.
      b. There are usually multiple abscesses, and each must be drained.
      c. The wound is left open to ensure adequate drainage.

B. Calculous sialadenitis is a condition caused by stones in the salivary ducts. Obstruction of the duct may occur, which causes inflammation and intermittent painful swelling of the gland.

    1. Diagnosis
      a. X-rays may show the stones.
      b. A **sialogram,** in which contrast is injected into the draining duct, will also show areas of obstruction and is useful in cases where the stone is not radiopaque.

    2. Surgery
      a. When the stone is near the end of the duct it can be removed transorally.
      b. If it is deep in the gland, it can be removed by an external incision.
      c. If multiple stones are present and recurrent pain occurs, the entire gland should be removed.

    3. Variants. A variant of sialadenitis can occur in which no stones are found.
      a. If there is a stricture of the duct on the sialogram, it should be dilated.
      b. If symptoms persist, surgery to remove the gland may be necessary.

Part VI Head and Neck Disorders

STUDY QUESTIONS

Directions: Each question below contains four or five suggested answers. Choose the **one best** response to each question.

1. When should a biopsy of a neck mass be performed?

(A) Immediately upon discovery of the mass
(B) Immediately after antibiotic treatment is started
(C) Whenever factors associated with malignancy are present
(D) Whenever a mass presents in infancy
(E) After thorough endoscopic examination of the mouth, larynx, esophagus, and trachea

2. Neck abscesses commonly demand emergency treatment due to the

(A) risk of airway obstruction
(B) high fevers
(C) resistant bacteria that are usually involved
(D) progressive dysphagia that leads to dehydration
(E) pain

3. In a patient with a peritonsillar abscess, common findings include all of the following EXCEPT

(A) fever
(B) muffled voice
(C) infected third molar
(D) asymmetric palatal swelling
(E) trismus

4. A 4-year-old girl presents with a smooth intranasal lesion. True statements about this lesion include which of the following?

(A) If it is unilateral, it should be biopsied
(B) If it is reddish in color, excision should be undertaken immediately
(C) Signs of expansion of the lesion should be sought during straining, crying, or a Valsalva maneuver
(D) It is probably an acquired rather than congenital lesion
(E) If it is bilateral, it can be treated similarly to adult nasal polyps.

5. Allergic nasal polyps are commonly associated with all of the following signs and symptoms EXCEPT

(A) bilateral involvement
(B) epistaxis
(C) aspirin sensitivity
(D) multiple paranasal sinus involvement
(E) asthma

6. A knobby, bone-hard growth at the midline of the palate is discovered during a patient's physical examination. What can be stated about this finding?

(A) Biopsy is necessary
(B) Total excision is the best treatment
(C) Close follow-up is necessary
(D) The lesion is usually related to tobacco use
(E) This is not a malignant lesion

7. A patient with hoarseness is found to have bilateral vocal cord masses at the junction of the anterior and middle thirds. Which of the following statements about this patient's condition is true?

(A) The masses are most likely congenital
(B) The masses are related to trauma
(C) The masses should be biopsied as soon as possible
(D) Laser excision is the treatment of choice
(E) Speech therapy is indicated

8. Indications for removal of the adenoids or tonsils include all of the following EXCEPT

(A) snoring
(B) sleep apnea
(C) recurrent tonsillitis
(D) chronic serous otitis media
(E) peritonsillar abscess

9. All of the following risk factors are associated with the development of a head or neck malignancy EXCEPT

(A) smoking
(B) radiation exposure
(C) alcohol ingestion
(D) drinking nonfluoridated water
(E) malnutrition

Questions 10 and 11

10. A 35-year-old man has right-sided serous otitis media and a right upper neck mass. It is most important to evaluate this patient for

(A) cancer of the right ear
(B) cancer of the right tonsil
(C) cancer of the right maxillary sinus
(D) cancer of the nasopharynx
(E) Hodgkin's lymphoma

11. This patient is next seen 6 months after completing radiation treatment. Which of the following is a poor prognostic sign?

(A) Occasional epistaxis
(B) Persistent sore throat
(C) Persistent serous otitis media
(D) Taste disturbance
(E) Elevated Epstein-Barr virus titers
(end of group question)

Questions 12–14

12. A 62-year-old cachectic man presents with sore throat, muffled voice, weight loss, and a neck mass. He is found to have a 4-cm mass in the base of the tongue with a 2-cm homolateral upper neck mass fixed to the mandible. The most important prognostic factor is

(A) the size of the primary tumor
(B) the presence of the cervical lymph node
(C) the size of the cervical lymph node
(D) involvement of the mandible
(E) poor nutritional status

13. Which of the following additional findings would most affect treatment planning?

(A) X-ray evidence of mandibular erosion
(B) CT evidence of parapharyngeal extension
(C) CT evidence of contralateral nodal enlargement
(D) Multiple lung nodule on chest x-ray
(E) A solitary cold nodule in the thyroid gland

14. The best treatment for this patient's oropharyngeal cancer is

(A) elective neck dissection
(B) modified radical neck dissection
(C) radical neck dissection
(D) bilateral neck dissection
(E) radiation therapy
(end of group question)

15. The commonest presenting symptom of laryngeal cancer is

(A) sore throat
(B) dysphagia
(C) dyspnea
(D) hoarseness
(E) aspiration

Questions 16 and 17

A 65-year-old man is found to have a small invasive squamous cell carcinoma of the right vocal cord. The right vocal cord is paralyzed, and there is a lymph node in the right anterior neck that is 4 cm in diameter.

16. The stage of the tumor is

(A) T2N1
(B) T2N2a
(C) T3N1
(D) T3N2a
(E) T4N3

17. Optimal treatment of the primary tumor should include

(A) total laryngectomy
(B) vertical hemilaryngectomy
(C) supraglottic (horizontal) laryngectomy
(D) right cordectomy
(E) chemotherapy
(end of group question)

18. A 62-year-old man is found to have a 4-cm right pyriform sinus carcinoma with fixation of the right vocal cord. Which of the following findings would most influence planning for surgical resection?

(A) Partial restriction of left vocal cord motion
(B) A 2-cm homolateral neck mass
(C) A 2-cm contralateral neck mass
(D) Circumferential hypopharyngeal involvement
(E) Massive destruction of the thyroid cartilage

19. Treatment of stage T1 laryngeal carcinoma might consist of

(A) supraglottic laryngectomy
(B) total laryngectomy
(C) radiotherapy
(D) chemotherapy
(E) cryotherapy

20. Biopsy of a single enlarged cervical lymph node reveals nodular, non-Hodgkin's lymphoma. Which of the following findings in the subsequent workup would most influence therapeutic planning?

(A) CT evidence of other enlarged homolateral cervical lymph nodes
(B) CT evidence of enlarged contralateral cervical lymph nodes
(C) The presence of a primary lesion in the homolateral tonsil
(D) A lung nodule
(E) Splenomegaly

21. The commonest benign tumor of the parotid gland is

(A) mixed tumor
(B) Warthin's tumor
(C) oxyphil adenoma
(D) hemangioma
(E) lymphangioma

22. The treatment for benign mixed tumors of the parotid gland is

(A) primary irradiation
(B) excision of the gross tumor
(C) radical excision of the parotid gland, including the facial nerve
(D) local excision of the tumor followed by radiation
(E) excision of the tumor with a margin of normal tissue and preservation of the facial nerve

Directions: Each question below contains four suggested answers of which **one or more** is correct. Choose the answer

A   if **1, 2, and 3** are correct
B   if **1 and 3** are correct
C   if **2 and 4** are correct
D   if **4** is correct
E   if **1, 2, 3, and 4** are correct

23. True statements concerning malignant tumors of the parotid gland include which of the following?

(1) Mucoepidermoid carcinoma, occurring in childhood, usually has a good prognosis
(2) Malignant mixed tumors are the commonest malignant parotid tumors
(3) Malignant lymphoma of the parotid gland should be treated in the same way as lymphomas arising elsewhere
(4) Radical neck dissection is routinely performed for all malignant tumors of the parotid gland

24. True statements concerning treatment of traumatic injuries of the parotid gland include which of the following?

(1) Foreign bodies should be removed
(2) Lacerations of Stensen's duct usually heal spontaneously
(3) Transection of the main trunk of the facial nerve should be repaired by primary anastomosis or nerve grafting
(4) Minor damage to the superficial lobe should be treated by superficial parotid lobectomy

ANSWERS AND EXPLANATIONS

1. The answer is E. [*Chapter 18 I B 5, 6 d (3)*] The workup for any head or neck lesion should follow a logical course beginning with a detailed history, a careful physical examination (including a search for signs of infection), appropriate laboratory tests, and relevant radiologic studies. Endoscopy and radiologic studies should precede any incision in the neck. A neck mass biopsy is the last step in a proper workup. The premature biopsy of a squamous cell carcinoma metastatic to the neck from a primary head or neck tumor worsens the overall prognosis by about 20%.

2. The answer is A. [*Chapter 18 II A 2*] The risk of airway obstruction is present in all advanced neck abscesses and in the early stages of some infections. Maintenance of the airway is always the first concern. Fever, pain, and dehydration are common findings but rarely warrant emergency care. Most infections result from mixed bacterial flora that are readily treatable with many standard antibiotics (i.e, penicillin, clindamycin, and cephalosporin).

3. The answer is C. [*Chapter 18 II B 5*] Peritonsillar abscesses commonly present with ipsilateral palatal inflammation, contralateral deviation of the uvula, "hot potato" or muffled voice, trismus, dysphagia, and fever. The source of the infection is acute tonsillitis, not a dental infection.

4. The answer is C. [*Chapter 18 III D 4, G; IV B 2, C*] The lesion in the 4-year-old girl described in the question may be an encephalocele, nasal dermoid, vestibular papilloma, or nasal polyp. In children, the presence of an encephalocele must be ruled out prior to the biopsy of such a lesion. Finding bilateral polyps in a child this young raises the question of cystic fibrosis.

5. The answer is B. [*Chapter 18 IV C 1, 2*] Allergic polyps are usually bilateral. They are commonly associated with generalized allergic rhinitis and asthma and can be involved in a clinical triad with asthma and aspirin sensitivity. Epistaxis is rare. Epistaxis is much commoner in malignant lesions and invasive benign lesions, such as inverted papillomas.

6. The answer is E. [*Chapter 18 IV I 3*] The patient described in the question has a maxillary torus, or torus palatinus. This benign, slow-growing bony mass is of little clinical significance and requires neither biopsy nor follow-up. Tori may interfere with dentures and, in that case, should be excised.

7. The answer is E. [*Chapter 18 IV J 3*] The lesions described in the question are vocal nodules. These masses are caused by vocal abuse and are best treated by speech therapy. Surgery is rarely indicated and, in most cases, should be avoided. There is no risk of malignant transformation, and biopsy is unnecessary.

8. The answer is A. [*Chapter 18 V B 1–3*] All patients with airway obstruction, obstructive sleep apnea, or failure to thrive secondary to adenotonsillar hypertrophy should undergo tonsillectomy with adenoidectomy. Recurrent tonsillitis is currently the commonest indication for tonsillectomy. Chronic serous otitis media is commonly associated with adenoid hypertrophy and is responsive to adenoidectomy. Most authors suggest tonsillectomy after peritonsillar abscess although this in not an absolute indication. Snoring alone is not an indication for tonsillectomy with adenoidectomy. However, snoring is many times associated with sleep apnea, and the upper airways should be fully evaluated in all patients who present with noxious snoring as a major complaint.

9. The answer is D. [*Chapter 19 I B, C 1 d*] Smoking and drinking are significant risk factors in head and neck malignancies. Exposure to radiation is also an etiologic factor. In taking the patient's history, the patient should be questioned about exposure to any of these etiologic agents. As far as is known, dental caries is the only disorder associated with a nonfluoridated water supply.

10. The answer is D. [*Chapter 19 IV C*] The two commonest presenting symptoms of cancer of the nasopharynx are enlarged posterior cervical lymph nodes and unilateral serous otitis media. The other cancers do not generally cause otitis media and usually occur in an older age-group. Hodgkin's lymphoma would only lead to serous otitis media if Waldeyer's ring involvement led to eustachian tube dysfunction, a rare occurrence.

11. The answer is E. [*Chapter 19 IV B 2, C 2 b*] When a nasopharyngeal carcinoma patient presents with elevated Epstein-Barr virus titers, the titers can be followed after treatment as a prognostic sign. The titers will fall with successful treatment and rise with recurrences. All other symptoms mentioned are common side effects of radiation therapy for nasopharyngeal carcinoma.

12. The answer is B. [*Chapter 19 VI F 4*] The single most important factor affecting prognosis in oropharyngeal cancer is the presence of nodal disease. Five-year survival is 75% for patients with N0 disease and 25% for patients with N1 disease. Mandibular involvement and poor nutritional status adversely affect prognosis, but not to the extent that the nodal disease does.

13. The answer is D. [*Chapter 19 I D 1 e*] The presence of distant metastasis is the single most important factor, obviating the consideration of radical therapy for the primary tumor. All other findings are readily resectable extensions of the primary tumor. The thyroid gland is commonly included in radical neck surgery, and the presence of thyroid lesions should not alter surgical planning.

14. The answer is C. [*Chapter 19 II D 1; VI E 3*] Elective neck dissection refers only to surgery in N0 disease. Modified neck dissections are indicated only in N0 or N1 disease. There is no need to address a negative contralateral neck in laryngeal cancer surgically due to the small risk of contralateral lymphatic drainage. Response rates with radiation therapy drop significantly with patients with nodes greater than 3 cm in diameter. Thus, unilateral radical neck dissection is the indicated treatment for this patient.

15. The answer is D. [*Chapter 19 VIII C 1 a*] Hoarseness is by far the commonest presenting symptom of laryngeal cancer. Laryngeal cancer is rarely painful until late in its course. Dyspnea, aspiration, and dysphagia are symptoms of advanced laryngeal cancer, but these are uncommon.

16. The answer is D. [*Chapter 19 II C 3; VIII D 3*] Any carcinoma of the vocal cord that leads to fixation of the cord or of the hemilarynx is at least T3. Massive involvement of surrounding soft tissues would make the tumor stage T4. The presence of a single homolateral lymph node greater than 3 cm but less than 6 cm in diameter makes the stage of the neck N2a. Multiple small lymph nodes on the same side of the neck as the primary tumor is classified as N2a, and lymph nodes involving the opposite side of the neck make the staging N3.

17. The answer is A. [*Chapter 19 VIII E 4*] T3 tumors cannot be adequately treated with partial laryngectomy in most cases; total laryngectomy is required. Radiation is used postoperatively as planned combined treatment in most cases. Chemotherapy is used for inoperable cases or in experimental protocols.

18. The answer is D. [*Chapter 19 VII E 2*] Circumferential hypopharyngeal resection requires specialized reconstruction, either with regional flaps, distant flaps, gastric "pull-up," or a microvascular free flap. Total laryngectomy is required due to the right vocal cord paralysis, and surgery is not affected by involvement of the opposite vocal cord or thyroid cartilage. Either neck mass can be treated with modified or radical neck dissection, which are commonly performed in conjunction with laryngopharyngectomy.

19. The answer is C. [*Chapter 19 VIII E 2*] Equal cure rates are provided with either cordectomy or radiation therapy for T1 laryngeal carcinoma. Cordectomy by laser is recommended by some authorities, but the procedure is still controversial. Vertical hemilaryngectomy may be performed for some glottic lesions that involve the anterior commissure, but total laryngectomy, supraglottic laryngectomy, and chemotherapy are not indicated.

20. The answer is E. [*Chapter 19 XI D 3 c, E 3*] Involvement of sites on both sides of the diaphragm is the criterion of stage III lymphoma. All of the other choices in the question describe stage II disease. Splenic involvement would most influence the decision to use both chemotherapy and radiation instead of either one alone in treatment because it signifies an advanced stage.

21. The answer is A. [*Chapter 20 II A 1*] Mixed tumors account for 60% of all parotid tumors, making them the commonest benign salivary tumors. They are so named because they contain both stromal and epithelial elements. Warthin's tumor contains both epithelial and lymphoid elements and feels like a cyst when palpated. Oxyphil adenoma is composed of acidophilic cells and usually is small. Hemangioma and lymphangioma are uncommon benign parotid tumors.

22. The answer is E. [*Chapter 20 II A 3*] The benign mixed tumor of the parotid gland often seems to "shell out" at surgery. This means that it easily separates from the surrounding normal tissue of the glands. In fact, a resection of normal tissue around the tumor is necessary to prevent recurrence, since nests of tumor cells are left behind by a lesser procedure. The facial nerve should be spared, if possible, during surgery for benign parotid neoplasms.

23. The answer is B (1, 3). [*Chapter 20 III A 2 a, b, B, E*] Mucoepidermoid carcinoma of childhood is usually a favorable lesion, with a 5-year survival rate exceeding 90%. In adults, the prognosis is much less favorable. Malignant lymphoma of the parotid is treated much the same as a lymphoma arising elsewhere. Mucoepidermoid carcinoma is the commonest malignancy of the parotid; malignant mixed tumors are the second commonest. Radical neck dissection is generally performed if a malignant tumor is a high-grade tumor or if nodes are palpable.

24. The answer is B (1, 3). [*Chapter 20 IV A, B*] In the management of parotid gland injuries, bullets and other debris should be removed. Lacerations of Stensen's duct should be repaired over a small catheter, which is brought out into the mouth and sutured to the oral mucosa. Minor damage to the parenchyma alone usually heals spontaneously. Peripheral branches of the nerve may heal spontaneously, but main trunk injuries must be repaired by primary anastomosis or nerve grafting.

Part VII
Special Subjects

21
Trauma and Burns

Jerome J. Vernick
Murray J. Cohen

I. TRAUMA

A. Overview

1. **Incidence.** Trauma is the leading cause of death in people under 35 years of age.
   a. Over 140,000 persons die from trauma every year.
   b. Half of these deaths result from motor vehicle accidents.
   c. Some 10%–15% of traumatized patients have serious multisystem injuries.

2. **Trauma management**
   a. Mortality can be greatly reduced by efficient handling of the injured, which involves three major components:
      (1) **A trauma center** with professional personnel who are trained in delivering rapid care and with facilities capable of handling a number of patients at one time
      (2) **A transportation system** capable of rapid transport to a trauma center
      (3) **Emergency medical technicians** who are capable of maintaining vital functions until the trauma surgeon can take over
   b. The management of trauma requires adherence to an established **order of priority,** ensuring that the most life-threatening injuries will be treated first, but less serious injuries will not be neglected following resuscitation. This order of priority is as follows:
      (1) Initial assessment, including an "AMPLE" history (Table 21-1)
      (2) Provision of airway control and establishment of respiration
      (3) Establishment of venous access and restoration of tissue perfusion
      (4) Diagnosis of immediately life-threatening injuries, followed by rapid treatment
      (5) Reassessment of the patient's status
      (6) Diagnosis of other significant injuries
      (7) Definitive treatment, including surgery, prophylactic antibiotics, and tetanus prophylaxis (see Chapter 2 II).

B. Mechanisms of injury.
Knowing the mechanism of injury allows the physician to anticipate lesions that may otherwise remain undiagnosed and decide on the appropriate management for lesions that may be more extensive than they might at first appear.

1. **Acceleration–deceleration injuries** are typically caused by falls from heights, blunt trauma, or vehicular accidents.
   a. Obvious injuries result from direct contact with the landing site (i.e., the ground or the vehicle).
   b. Subtle injuries result from shearing forces produced by the momentum when heavy organs are suddenly halted or accelerated by a crash.
      (1) Heavy organs include fluid-filled loops of bowel, the blood-filled thoracic aorta, and mobile parenchymal organs, such as the liver and spleen. The momentum of these organs is maintained after the motion of the victim has been stopped.

Table 21-1. Points Covered in the "AMPLE" History

Allergies
Medications
Previous illnesses
Last meal
Events surrounding injury

        (2) Damage occurs because force is exerted on the tethered portion of the viscus by the mobile portion of the viscus, which continues to move.

            (a) The aortic arch shears at the fixed ligamentum arteriosus.

            (b) The small bowel tends to pull away from its mesenteric attachments, creating a "bucket-handle" tear with massive bleeding from mesenteric vessels.

            (c) Avulsion of the spleen at its hilus or peritoneal reflections is common.

            (d) Renal pedicle avulsion is another example of the type of injury that can occur.

2. Missile injuries

    a. Low-velocity missile injuries include most civilian gunshot wounds.

        (1) Missiles fired from handguns have a velocity in the range of 600–1100 feet/sec.

        (2) Wounds from this type of missile are generally restricted to the path and the residual cavity created by the missile as it penetrates tissues, such as blood vessels and organs. However, secondary injuries can occur.

            (a) External articles (buttons or keys) may be driven into the wound by the missile.

            (b) Bone fragments, produced when the missile strikes a large bone, can also cause secondary injury.

    b. High-velocity missile injuries can be recognized by a small entrance wound and a large exit wound with severe underlying tissue damage. These wounds may cause damage remote from the apparent tract of the missile as a large temporary cavity is created when the tissue recoils from the path of the bullet (see I C 5 d).

    c. Shotgun injuries

        (1) Close-range shotgun injuries can be devastating. Large soft tissue defects are created with widespread damage. In addition, these wounds often introduce nonopaque foreign material, which originates from the wadding used in the manufacture of the shotgun shell.

        (2) Long-range shotgun injuries consist of multiple low-velocity pellet injuries. These cause widespread penetration but are generally not severe unless the missile happens to strike a major blood vessel or organ.

    d. The shocking, "knock-down" effect of a missile depends on factors that influence the energy transferred to the victim by the impact.

        (1) Striking energy is directly proportional to the weight of a missile and the square of its velocity.

        (2) Missiles that completely penetrate the victim expend much of their energy on the objects beyond. Maximum energy transfer results from the missile that remains in the victim.

        (3) Penetration is diminished when a bullet is used that expands or tumbles after impact.

    e. Treatment. All missile tracts should be debrided, but missiles need not be removed unless they cause symptoms or are in proximity to a vital structure where body movements or tissue erosion could cause further injury.

C. Management of trauma victims

    1. The initial assessment of the patient's state, performed when the patient arrives in the emergency room, determines the extent of injury and the need for immediate care. Obviously inebriated patients often have serious injuries, but the presence of alcohol does not diminish the trauma team's responsibility to diagnose all injuries properly. The initial assessment can be performed by an experienced physician within seconds. The following three questions should be answered.

    a. Is ventilation adequate?

    b. Is tissue being perfused?

    c. Is significant neurologic injury present?

    2. Airway assessment and control

    a. Assessment

        (1) The mouth and upper airway should be inspected for foreign bodies or other causes of obstruction.

        (2) The patient should be examined for chest wall motion and asymmetry, cyanosis, and evidence of air exchange.

        (3) The chest should be examined for subcutaneous emphysema or fractures and auscultated for breath sounds.

b. Treatment. Rapid measures are necessary to correct unsatisfactory ventilation.

   (1) Early intubation is important, since unstable patients quickly become apneic.

   (a) Oxygen is needed for all severely injured patients. Rapid intubation is necessary in the presence of:

   (i) A decreased level of consciousness

   (ii) Hypotension

   (iii) Major head, face, or neck injury

   (iv) Chest trauma

   (v) Cyanosis

   (b) The neck should not be extended during intubation unless it is definitely known that no cervical spine injury exists. When this is not known, either a nasotracheal tube should be used in spontaneously breathing patients, or a tracheostomy or cricothyroidotomy should be performed.

   (2) Ventilation should be performed with either a hand-held bag or a volume respirator.

   (a) Adequacy of ventilation should be assessed by auscultation of the chest, followed by arterial blood gas measurement. The commonest causes of inadequate ventilation are:

   (i) Incorrect placement of the endotracheal tube into either the esophagus or the right main stem bronchus

   (ii) The presence of a pneumothorax

   (b) Assessment of the thorax is important after ventilation begins.

   (i) After auscultation, if breath sounds are absent in one or both hemithoraces, aspiration with a large-bore needle followed by insertion of a chest tube is an acceptable diagnostic and therapeutic maneuver.

   (ii) A tension pneumothorax produces a high-pressure condition in the pleural space, compressing the pulmonary parenchyma and impairing venous return to the heart. It must be treated rapidly with a chest tube and should not wait for confirmation by chest x-ray.

   (iii) Signs of tension pneumothorax are inadequate ventilation with cyanosis and absent breath sounds, hypotension, a shift of the mediastinum and trachea away from the pneumothorax, and impaired venous return with elevated central venous pressure.

3. Circulatory support. Once adequate ventilation has been established, the physician should rapidly proceed to the next critical stage of resuscitation, namely, establishment of tissue perfusion, or circulatory support.

   a. Cardiac resuscitation

   (1) Closed chest cardiac massage should be performed while fluid resuscitation is begun if the patient is asystolic or demonstrates evidence of poor cardiac function.

   (2) Emergency room thoracotomies are rarely indicated.

   (a) Thoracotomies should be performed only by trained personnel.

   (b) Indications for emergency room thoracotomy are:

   (i) Hypovolemic cardiac arrest despite vigorous blood volume replacement plus closed chest massage and defibrillation

   (ii) Cardiac arrest with penetrating injury to the chest

   (c) Relative contraindications include:

   (i) Major obvious injuries to the central nervous system

   (ii) Failed external cardiac massage lasting more than 10 minutes

   (iii) Major blunt trauma

   b. Assessment of the circulatory status in a patient with a beating heart should include appraisal of:

   (1) Character of the pulse

   (a) A rapid, faint pulse suggests profound hypovolemia in most cases.

   (b) A slow, full pulse may be indicative of severe neurologic injury with increasing intracranial pressure or hypercarbia.

   (2) Peripheral perfusion, as indicated by level of consciousness, rate of capillary refilling, and body temperature

   (3) Blood pressure. The presence of a mild hypotension may be associated with inadequate tissue perfusion.

   (4) Stable vital signs with major injury. The condition of patients with major injury and seemingly stable vital signs is dangerous and deceptive.

     (a) Previously healthy trauma patients, especially if young, are able to maintain pulse and blood pressure, despite a continuing occult hemorrhage, until vasomotor response fails. When this occurs, the patient "crashes," which is manifested by a rapid loss of blood pressure, vomiting, and unconsciousness.

     (b) These patients maintain stable hemodynamic parameters and may remain quietly pale or become excitable with progressive mental deterioration until overt shock develops, at which point they may not respond to further volume replacement.

c. Venous access

     (1) Lines should be inserted by a reliable method with which the physician is comfortable.

       (a) Subclavian catheterization should be learned in controlled settings, not on unstable trauma patients.

       (b) Subclavian lines and a saphenous cut-down are the quickest for venous access.

       (c) The saphenous vein often looks empty and may look pale and tendon-like in a hypovolemic patient. It should be recognized rather than divided.

     (2) Two lines are usually inserted simultaneously.

       (a) It is best to keep one on each side of the diaphragm so that volume replacement is effective in case of vena caval or subclavian venous trauma.

       (b) Shock patients often require four separate lines for volume replacement to raise the blood pressure above 100 mm Hg in under 10 minutes.

       (c) The first intravenous insertion should include the withdrawal of 20 ml of blood for crossmatching and for laboratory studies, including a toxicology profile.

       (d) Femoral artery punctures should be done early for blood gas analyses.

     (3) All resuscitation lines should be replaced in 12–24 hours. The urgent insertion of these lines leaves sterility in question, and catheter sepsis can become a serious problem after 24 hours.

d. Blood components (see Chapter 1 IV). All rapidly infused fluids should be warmed during infusion.

     (1) Plasma

       (a) Pooled plasma carries a relatively high risk of transmitting hepatitis and other viral syndromes.

       (b) Fresh, frozen plasma has a low risk of transmitting viral syndromes.

     (2) Whole blood is generally not available nor indicated.

     (3) Packed red cells

       (a) These are given urgently if the initial hematocrit is less than 25%.

       (b) They are also started if the patient is obviously bleeding vigorously or if volume replacement of more than 1000 ml is required.

       (c) Platelets, 8 units, should be given with each 10 units of red cells.

     (4) Unmatched blood

       (a) Profound shock is an indication for the use of type-specific but uncrossmatched blood cells.

         (i) O-negative blood cells can be used if there is no time even for blood typing.

         (ii) O-positive blood cells are generally safe for young males who have never had a previous blood transfusion. They can be used if O-negative cells are not available.

         (iii) If the patient receives over 4 units of unmatched type O cells, the physician should not revert to the native blood type during resuscitation.

       (b) Legal liability for a transfusion reaction is not a serious problem if the patient faces a 100% mortality risk without red cell replacement.

e. Maintenance of circulating blood volume (see Chapter 1 I). **Fluid replacement** at first is based on judgments made during the initial assessment concerning shock and visible sources of blood loss. Continuing fluid replacement, after an initial 2–3 L of lactated Ringer's solution, is based on the patient's urine output and central venous pressure. Further replacement should be based on continued assessment.

     (1) Urine output. Monitoring the trends in the patient's urine output provides an important guideline to the accuracy of fluid resuscitation and the changing needs of the patient. Renal perfusion disappears early in shock. A urine output in excess of 30 ml/hr implies adequate perfusion to all vital organs and indicates that the patient is not in shock.

     (2) Central venous pressure is usually monitored via a subclavian vein puncture.

    (a) Central venous pressure reflects the available blood volume, which is not necessarily the same as the absolute amount of circulating blood. The available blood volume is decreased if the absolute volume has decreased due to external or internal losses or if the vascular system has dilated so that the normal volume no longer fills it.

    (b) An inadequate circulating volume, as implied by diminished central venous pressure, generally indicates inadequate venous return to the heart. If venous return is inadequate, the cardiac chambers cannot distend to their normal filled volumes and cardiac output, therefore, diminishes.

    (c) The trends in a series of central venous pressure measurements are sometimes more informative than the absolute magnitude on a single reading. Also, in assessing circulating volume, the central venous pressure must be interpreted in conjunction with urine output, pulse rate, and other vital signs.

    (d) Coexisting pulmonary and cardiac derangements can influence central venous pressure readings, and account for the wide variations in initial readings seen in different patients. Because readings are falsely raised by pressure ventilation, it is often advisable to slow the volume replacement when an initially negative central venous pressure reading rises above zero during resuscitation.

(3) **Fluid challenges** can provide valuable guidance in judging the adequacy of volume resuscitation. Examples include:

    (a) Rapid infusion of 200 ml of colloid solution (e.g., albumin, Plasmanate, hydroxyethyl starch) in a patient with progressive tachycardia

        (i) If the central venous pressure rises beyond normal limits (15 cm H_2O), it signifies overload or failure, pericardial tamponade, or tension pneumothorax.

        (ii) If the central venous pressure falls or remains low, it indicates inadequate volume replacement or continued volume loss.

    (b) Infusion of 200 ml of colloid solution in a patient with a slowing pulse rate: If the central venous pressure rises, it indicates adequate or improving volume status.

  f. Control of hemorrhage must accompany fluid resuscitation.

    (1) **External bleeding**

        (a) Applying direct pressure on bleeding wounds with manually held gauze pads is safe and usually effective.

        (b) Proximal and distal digital compression of bleeding superficial vessels may allow visualization of the bleeding point and accurate clamping. Blind clamping is never indicated.

        (c) Pressure dressings may be used to control diffuse bleeding from abrasions and avulsions that involve large areas.

        (d) Temporary packing of missile tracts and stab wounds can slow the blood flow until surgical exposure is obtained.

        (e) Pneumatic splints and medical antishock trousers (MAST) help in tamponading bleeding and increasing peripheral resistance to raise the blood pressure. The antishock trousers provide increased peripheral resistance without the pharmacologic effects of pressor agents.

    (2) **Internal bleeding** requires early diagnosis and prompt treatment by appropriate surgical intervention.

4. Assessment of neurologic injury (see Chapter 27). After adequate ventilation and tissue perfusion have been restored, immediate attention must be given to the patient's neurologic condition.

  a. Head trauma

    (1) **Assessment**

        (a) Loss of consciousness signifies a head injury until such an injury has been ruled out.

        (b) Intracranial trauma cannot be adequately assessed while the patient is in shock.

        (c) If hypotension is present in a patient with a head injury, it is rarely secondary to the head trauma, and the physician must look for another cause of the hypotension.

        (d) The neurologic evaluation should assess the following factors rapidly:

            (i) Level of consciousness. Is the patient alert, lethargic and disoriented, comatose but responsive to pain, or unresponsive?

        (ii) Motor activity and tactile sensation

        (iii) Obvious head trauma, such as a depressed skull fracture, gunshot wound, or leaking cerebrospinal fluid

        (iv) Pupil size and response to light

        (v) Oculocephalic ("doll's eye") reflex. Since testing involves rotating the patient's head, it should only be done after spinal cord injury has been ruled out.

    (e) Evolving hypertension and bradycardia (Cushing's phenomenon) indicate increasing intracranial pressure and a worsening neurologic problem.

  (2) Treatment

    (a) If a neurosurgeon, who is imperative for proper management of patients with head injuries, is not available, then a telephone consultation should be obtained and initial treatment begun, followed by transfer of the patient to a center with a neurosurgeon.

    (b) Initial management includes the following considerations:

        (i) Sterile saline-soaked gauze should be placed over open injuries.

        (ii) Mannitol and other drugs to lower intracranial pressure should be given after consultation with the neurosurgeon.

        (iii) Hypotension and hypoventilation seriously injure brain cells. It is, therefore, important to assess adequately fluid requirements and ventilation.

        (iv) Overhydration increases intracranial pressure and should be avoided once fluid requirements have been met and the patient is stable.

  b. Spinal cord trauma

    (1) Assessment

      (a) Until proven otherwise, the spine should be considered unstable and the cord, therefore, liable to injury in all patients with major blunt trauma.

      (b) The **cervical spine** should be considered unstable in:

        (i) Every unconscious patient

        (ii) Every patient with face and head contusions

        (iii) Every patient with decreased mentation, which precludes adequate neurologic examination

      (c) X-ray films showing all seven cervical vertebrae intact should be obtained before allowing the patient's neck to be extended for any reason. At least three views need to be obtained, including cross-table lateral, anterior–posterior, and odontoid views.

      (d) Evidence of injury to the spinal cord should be sought.

        (i) It should be recognized that the cord may not yet be injured even though the spine is unstable. A negative neurologic examination does not prove the absence of injury to the cervical spine.

        (ii) Appropriate spinal stabilization must be performed until proper studies have been done.

        (iii) Findings, such as absence of motor or sensory function below the injury, loss of muscle tone, and loss of anal sphincter tone, should be sought.

        (iv) Hypotension may be present if there is a loss of vascular tone (arterial and venous) within the affected region.

    (2) Treatment. The required stabilization and reduction of the injury must be done under the supervision of a neurosurgeon or an orthopedic surgeon experienced in treating these injuries.

5. Assessment of other serious injuries. Once the immediate life-threatening crises have been cared for and the patient is stabilized, other injuries can be assessed. Information about events surrounding the injury, allergies of the patient, the patient's medical history, and any medications taken by the patient must be obtained from the patient or others.

  a. Thoracic injuries (see Chapter 4 II)

    (1) Upright chest x-rays should be obtained to:

      (a) Detect fluid collections or a pneumothorax, which may have been missed in the initial assessment

      (b) Search for the presence of great vessel injury, a tracheal shift, or other injuries

    (2) Electrocardiogram and central venous pressure should be monitored for clues regarding cardiac contusions or tamponade, such as elevated ST segments and a rising central venous pressure.

    (3) Bronchography or bronchoscopy to determine if a bronchus is ruptured may be needed urgently if air continues to leak through a chest tube in a patient with a lung that fails to expand with suction.

(4) Contrast esophagography and great vessel aortography to rule out esophageal perforation or aortic injury may be indicated by penetrating wounds that traverse the mediastinum.

(5) Angiography may be needed if the following are found on x-ray:
   (a) Lateral deviation of the nasogastric tube in the esophagus
   (b) A widened mediastinum (greater than 8 cm)
   (c) Loss of visualization of the aortic knob
   (d) Hematoma of the left cervical pleura ("pleural cap")
   (e) A depressed left main stem bronchus
   (f) Right lateral deviation of the trachea
   (g) Forward displacement of the trachea on the lateral chest film
   (h) Fracture of the first or second rib
   (i) Massive chest trauma with multiple rib fractures
   (j) Fracture or dislocation of the thoracic spine
   (k) A major deceleration injury

(6) Surgical treatment
   (a) Thoracic cavity hemorrhage. The patient should undergo urgent thoracotomy in the operating room if more than 1500 ml of blood are found in the chest or if bleeding continues at a rate of 100 ml/hr after the initial hemothorax is evacuated via a chest tube.
   (b) Pericardial tamponade. If a patient with chest trauma develops hypotension with an elevated central venous pressure, pericardial tamponade should be suspected after a tension pneumothorax has been ruled out.
      (i) The principal diagnostic test is a pericardial tap, usually performed by inserting a catheter through the subxiphoid space.
      (ii) If tamponade is present, the catheter should be left in place and the patient taken to the operating room for exploratory thoracotomy.

b. Abdominal injuries
   (1) Overview. These injuries may be subtle or overt. Evidence of trauma may be visible on the abdominal wall or pelvis. Early tense abdominal distention usually indicates severe bleeding. An abdomen that progressively becomes scaphoid suggests herniation of the abdominal contents through a traumatic diaphragmatic hernia. The critical step for the physician is to recognize the presence of an abdominal injury and establish its degree of urgency.
   (2) Peritoneal lavage should be used when the need for abdominal exploration is not clear. It is also useful when physical assessment is not productive; for example, when the patient is unconscious or neurologically impaired. The best technique for peritoneal lavage is the **"open" technique.**
      (a) The bladder is first emptied with a bladder catheter. (The nasogastric tube empties the stomach and provides diagnostic information.) The peritoneal dialysis catheter is inserted through a small incision made in the midline fascia below the umbilicus. One L of crystalloid solution is infused in adults.
      (b) The lavage is positive if gross blood, more than 100,000 red blood cells/ml, vegetable fibers, fecal matter, or bacteria are found.
      (c) It is helpful to leave the dialysis catheter in place after a negative lavage if the patient is to undergo a lengthy orthopedic, neurologic, or thoracic surgical procedure.
         (i) Hypovolemia sometimes occurs during these procedures and may be due to delayed abdominal bleeding.
         (ii) If the peritoneal lavage catheter is in place, lavage can be repeated during the procedure.
   (3) Imaging techniques that aid in the diagnosis of abdominal injury
      (a) Intravenous pyelography
         (i) A unilateral delay or absence of excretion is the major finding noted on a positive emergency intravenous pyelogram.
         (ii) A knowledge of bilateral renal function is essential for the surgeon operating on a patient with multiple, massive intra-abdominal injuries.
      (b) Retrograde pyelography provides morphologic evidence of extravasation of urine or disruption of a ureter or collecting system.

      (c) Cystourethrography is indicated in pelvic fractures when urethral bleeding is evident.

    (4) Surgical treatment

      (a) A generous midline incision has been found to be the most expeditious.

      (b) Hemostasis is the major priority in surgery for abdominal trauma.

        (i) A bleeding aorta can be temporarily clamped for hemostasis while resuscitation is carried out.

        (ii) Rapid methods of temporary hemostasis, such as packing and direct pressure, are applied while fluid resuscitation is carried out.

        (iii) Meticulous exploration and repair should wait until volume replacement is complete and the patient is stable.

      (c) Retroperitoneal hematomas in the pelvis and lower abdominal regions are best not explored unless they are actively expanding or an arterial source has been demonstrated on angiography. Many of these are associated with pelvic fractures and are not controllable by surgical means. However, retroperitoneal hematomas in the upper abdomen, particularly those in proximity to the **duodenum, pancreas,** and **renal pedicles,** should be explored.

        (i) The pancreas and duodenum should be mobilized and then thoroughly palpated to rule out pancreatic disruption.

        (ii) The duodenal disruption can be patched or repaired if the injury is diagnosed early. Delay may cause poor tissue quality that is not safely repaired.

        (iii) Pancreatic transections are best treated by distal resection. Most pancreatic injuries can be handled by simple sump drainage if transection or major duct damage has not occurred.

      (d) Liver injuries should be treated as conservatively as possible.

        (i) Resective debridement of detached or almost detached portions is carried out.

        (ii) Hemostasis is accomplished under direct vision, if possible. Packs can be used for a 24-hour period, and then re-exploration is accomplished when required.

c. Genitourinary injuries (see Chapter 25 V)

  (1) Urethral injury

    (a) Blood at the meatus is an indication for retrograde urethrography. Even gentle insertion of a Foley catheter can disrupt a partially divided urethra.

    (b) Major injuries should be repaired surgically.

  (2) Bladder injuries usually heal spontaneously if adequate urinary drainage is established. (Generally, intraperitoneal bladder ruptures require operative repair.)

  (3) Kidneys are commonly injured organs.

    (a) Most renal injuries can be managed nonoperatively; however, renal pedicle disruption or major parenchymal damage with hemorrhage are the primary indications for surgery.

    (b) Intravenous pyelography provides a good test of renal function, but it is not adequate for determining anatomic continuity of the organ. Extravasated contrast is an indication for drainage of the area where the leakage occurred.

d. Soft tissue injuries (see Chapter 26)

  (1) Debridement is the key to avoiding infection and promoting rapid healing.

    (a) All devitalized tissue must be removed during debridement.

    (b) It is helpful to understand how different tissues respond to injury. The degree of injury often depends on the density of the tissue and its water content.

      (i) The lung, for example, tends to receive relatively minor degrees of damage remote from the missile tract.

      (ii) By contrast, muscle or liver, due to their greater density and water content, develop large temporary cavities and require extensive debridement beyond the apparent missile tract.

  (2) Muscle

    (a) Wide areas of devitalized tissue occur in high-velocity wounds and require debridement.

    (b) Viable muscle tissue visibly contracts when touched with an electrosurgical instrument set on a low power. It also contracts when gently pinched with forceps.

    (c) Muscle that does not react must be removed even though weakness and deformity will result.

(3) Arteries
  (a) Palpable pulses do not rule out arterial injury.
  (b) Grossly injured vascular areas that exhibit intramural bleeding or disruption, require removal. It is not necessary to remove apparently normal areas of arteries.
  (c) Repair should be done with autogenous material if at all possible. There is an increased incidence of infection and failure when prosthetic material is used (see Chapter 7 XI).
  (d) Fasciotomies are almost always required in conjunction with vascular repair. It is far better to do a fasciotomy early in anticipation of swelling and tension in muscle compartments than to wait until tissue loss has occurred.
  (e) Stab wounds and missile tracts in proximity to major vascular structures require either surgical exploration or, at a minimum, emergency arteriography.
(4) Major **veins** should be repaired when injured.
(5) Nerves. It is not necessary to debride nerves that are injured. Exposed nerves should be covered with normal muscle or fat, leaving definitive repair for a future time.
(6) Bone. Contaminated small pieces of bone that are not attached to soft tissue may be removed. Attached bones should generally be left in situ to speed healing.
(7) Lung tissue is usually resistant to remote damage. Because of its spongy nature, the lung absorbs shock without injury, so that a missile tract generally contains all of the injury.
(8) Parenchymal organs, such as the **liver** and **kidney**
  (a) Bleeding is the major problem. Devitalized tissue should be removed with as much functional tissue left as possible.
  (b) An effort should be made to salvage an injured **spleen**, particularly in a child. There is evidence that a small spleen slice, reimplanted in the omentum, will grow and will provide some splenic function.
(9) Genitalia. Very conservative debridement is indicated. Exposed testicular tissue should be covered with scrotal skin or reimplanted under attached skin, if possible.
e. Fractures (see Chapter 28 III B–D)
  (1) A fracture is seldom a major priority in the presence of other, life-threatening injuries.
    (a) Hemorrhage or vascular compromise associated with a fracture gives it a higher priority, as does a threat to the viability of an extremity.
    (b) Bleeding associated with a fracture can account for a large portion of a patient's circulating blood volume, and hypovolemic shock is commonly associated with bilateral femoral fractures.
  (2) Early fractures that are open can be treated in accordance with the associated soft tissue injury.
    (a) Debridement, vascular repair, and other soft tissue surgery should be done prior to stabilization of the fracture.
    (b) However, adequate splinting and stabilization should be accomplished because it decreases the risk of fat embolism syndrome.
    (c) Internal fixation devices are generally hazardous in the presence of extensive soft tissue injury and should be avoided if possible.
  (3) Fractures that are more than 6–8 hours old should be allowed maximal spontaneous recovery before any attempt is made to stabilize them surgically.
f. Tendon injuries require conservative debridement only. Tendons should be covered with normal tissue or they become devitalized and useless.
g. Neck injuries. All penetrating neck injuries and all hematomas in the neck should be surgically explored.
  (1) Arteriography is recommended for penetrating injuries above the angle of the mandible or in the supraclavicular area.
  (2) Bronchoscopy, esophagoscopy, and x-rays with oral diatrizoate meglumine as contrast agent can help to rule out tracheal or esophageal injuries.

II. BURNS

A. Overview. The initial treatment of burns is based on the same principles and priorities as for other forms of trauma [see I A 2 b (1)]. However, one **special priority** is to stop any continuing burn injury caused by smoldering clothes or corrosive chemicals, using neutral solutions to flush away all garments from the injured area. It is also mandatory to assess any concomitant injuries. The management of the burned patient depends on the depth, extent, and location of the burned area. Transfer of the burn patient to a burn center or consultation with the center should be considered for all but minimal burn injuries.

1. **Depth of burns**
   a. **First-degree burns (involvement of epidermis only).** Clinical findings are limited to erythema.
   b. **Second-degree (partial-thickness or intradermal) burns**
      (1) Clinical findings include vesicles, swelling, and a moist surface.
      (2) Partial-thickness burns are painful and are hypersensitive to a light touch or even the movement of air.
      (3) Epithelial remnants (skin appendages) are spared.
      (4) Second-degree burns are categorized into superficial and deep dermal burns.
   c. **Third-degree (full-thickness, entire depth of dermis) burns**
      (1) These burns have a charred, waxen, or leathery appearance and may be white or grayish in color. They usually appear dry. Thrombosed vessels may be evident.
      (2) The burn surface is pain free and is anesthetic to a pinprick or to touch.

2. **Extent of burns.** This is determined by the **"rule of nines"** (Figure 21-1).
   a. Inpatient treatment is required for a patient with either:
      (1) Full-thickness burns extending over 2% or more of the body surface area (BSA)
      (2) Partial-thickness burns extending over 10% or more of the BSA

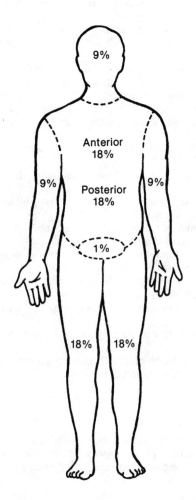

Figure 21-1. *Rule of nines.* The body surface area (BSA) is divided into anatomic areas, each of which is 9% (or a multiple thereof) of the total BSA. This is a simple method of estimating the total burn surface.

b. Intravenous fluid resuscitation is required for all partial- or full-thickness burns extending over 20% or more of the BSA.

3. Location of burns

a. Inpatient treatment is required for second- or third-degree burns of the face, hands, feet, or genitalia.

b. Second- or third-degree burns involving major flexion creases usually require hospital treatment to minimize contractures and other late problems.

B. Airway control and ventilation

1. Airway obstruction may develop rapidly after inhalation injury or may be delayed. **Delayed airway obstruction** is due to progressive swelling and is apt to develop 24–48 hours after the injury. The possibility should be suspected if any of the following conditions are present:

a. A history of being burned in a confined space

b. A facial burn or singed facial hair

c. Charring or carbon particles in the oropharynx

d. Carbonaceous sputum

e. Circumferential burns of the trunk, especially those with a thick eschar (which may require emergency excision—see II D 5)

2. Measurement of arterial blood gases is indicated as well as measurement of carbon monoxide level (carboxyhemoglobin value over 10% is significant) [Rx: F_iO_2 100%].

3. Endotracheal intubation should be done before the patient develops respiratory problems. Intubation is preferable to a tracheostomy in the patient with burns of the face, neck, or respiratory tract, since tracheostomy through a burn carries a high mortality.

C. Circulatory support and fluid resuscitation. Major burns—those involving 20% or more of the BSA—call for fluid resuscitation.

1. Intravenous fluids should be administered through a 14- or 16-gauge intravenous catheter.

a. The catheter may be placed through the burn wound, if required.

b. Intravenous fluids should not be given via a lower extremity, since the site is prone to sepsis and its increased mortality risk.

2. Fluid resuscitation should begin with lactated Ringer's solution.

a. The **volume to be given** is calculated as follows:

(1) For adults:

% BSA burned × kg of body weight × 2–4 ml of electrolyte solution

(2) For children:

% BSA burned × kg of body weight × 3 ml of electrolyte solution

(3) The percentage of the BSA that is burned is estimated by the "rule of nines" (see Figure 21-1).

b. One-half of the calculated amount of fluid is given in the first 8 hours, and the remaining one-half is distributed over the succeeding 16 hours.

c. The volume and rate of fluid administration should be varied, if necessary, depending on the central venous pressure, urine output, and other vital signs.

(1) Optimal urine output is 30–50 ml/hr in adults, and 1 ml/kg of body weight/hr in children.

(2) To aid urine flow and to allow monitoring of output, an indwelling urethral catheter should be inserted early, even in children.

d. Evaporative hypotonic fluid loss is evident after the first 24 hours.

(1) Intravenous fluids at a rate to maintain serum sodium concentration at 140 mEq/L (approximately 4–5 L in a 70-kg patient with 50% burn)

(2) Colloid (controversial) at a rate of 0.3–0.5 ml plasma/kg body weight/% burn

D. Burn wound care

1. Cold compresses may be applied to relieve the pain of partial-thickness burns if the burns cover less than 10% of the BSA. If burns cover a large area, cold compresses or immersion in water will cause an unacceptable lowering of the body temperature with associated problems.

2. Maintenance of body temperature is important, especially in children, who have a high evaporative heat loss and may rapidly become hypothermic.

3. Shielding the burn from air movement by covering it with a clean, warm linen dressing will help to relieve the pain of partial-thickness burns.

4. Topical antimicrobial treatment with agents such as silver nitrate solution is usually recommended for deep second-degree and third-degree burns. However, only specific antibacterial burn wound medications should be applied to the burn.

5. Debridement and escharectomy are best done in specialized centers; however, escharotomy may be urgently required in circumferential extremity wounds, causing distal circulatory impairment, and in circumferential trunk or neck wounds, causing respiratory impairment

E. Other considerations in the care of burn patients

1. Nasogastric intubation is indicated for any patient with nausea or vomiting and for most patients with burns covering 25% or more of the BSA.

2. Analgesia should be confined to conservative use of intravenous narcotics in small, frequent doses.

3. Systemic antibiotics are usually not indicated. However, in some situations, particularly in the early treatment of patients with partial-thickness burns, prophylaxis against β-hemolytic streptococci is warranted.

4. Tetanus toxoid with or without hyperimmune human globulin should be given if the patient's immunization status is not current (according to American College of Surgery guidelines).

5. Chemical burns
   a. Alkali burns are generally deeper and more serious than acid burns.
   b. All chemical burns should be treated by flushing with neutral solutions.
      (1) Immediate drenching in a shower or with a hose is helpful.
      (2) Burns of the eye require extensive flushing over an 8-hour period.

6. Electrical burns are usually deeper and more severe than indicated by the surface appearance.
   a. Muscle and soft tissue injury. Electrical energy is converted to heat as it traverses the body along the path of least resistance (i.e., blood vessels and nerves). Thus, muscles closest to bone, which has a high resistance and, therefore, generates the most heat, incur the most damage.
      (1) Muscle involvement may be markedly underestimated by attention to the surface wounds alone (e.g., fluid requirements are about 50% higher than estimated by surface wounds).
         (a) Brawny edema is characteristic.
         (b) Early escharotomy, fasciotomy, and debridement are often necessary, and repeated explorations at 24–48 hours may be needed.
      (2) Serious **soft tissue injury** results from **high-voltage electrical burns** (generally considered over 1000 volts); **low-voltage electrical burns** (household outlets) cause less soft tissue injury but may cause asystole and apnea.
   b. Surface burns occur at both the entrance and exit points of the current. Unsuspected exit sites, including the scalp, feet, or perineum, should be sought.
   c. Oliguria is common as is **acidosis**.
      (1) Urine output should be maintained at high levels—at least 100 ml/hr in adults. Mannitol administration is usually needed to maintain this level and is mandatory in the presence of myoglobinuria.
      (2) Arterial blood pH should be monitored and maintained with intravenous bicarbonate, given as 50 mEq every half hour until the pH reaches normal levels.
   d. Myocardial infarction (immediate or delayed) is well-described postinjury, thus making continuous cardiac monitoring essential in all patients with electrical burns.
   e. Transverse myelitis and cataracts are long-term sequelae.

22
Spleen
R. Anthony Carabasi, III

I. INTRODUCTION

A. Anatomy

1. Developmental considerations

a. The spleen develops from several masses of mesenchyme in the dorsal mesogastrium. These masses coalesce and move to the left as development progresses. By the end of the third gestational month, the organ is formed. The point at which the spleen remains attached to the dorsal mesogastrium becomes the **gastrosplenic ligament**.

b. The organ itself consists of an outer capsule and trabeculae, which encloses the pulp. The pulp consists of three zones:

(1) The **white pulp** is essentially a lymph node. It contains lymphocytes, macrophages, and plasma cells in a reticular network.

(2) The **red pulp** consists of cords of reticular cells with sinuses in between.

(3) The **marginal zone** is a poorly defined vascular space between the pulps. It contains sequestered foreign material and plasma as well as abnormal cellular elements.

c. The adult spleen weighs between 100 g and 150 g and measures 12 cm x 7 cm x 4 cm.

2. Location. The spleen is located in the left upper quadrant of the abdomen and is protected by the eighth to the eleventh ribs. It is bordered by the left kidney posteriorly, the diaphragm superiorly, and the fundus of the stomach and the splenic flexure of the colon anteriorly.

3. Vasculature

a. The main blood supply to the organ is carried by the **splenic artery,** which is a branch of the celiac axis. It travels along the superior border of the pancreas. At the hilus, it branches into trabecular arteries, which terminate in small vessels to the splenic pulp.

b. The **splenic vein** crosses behind or at the lower border of the pancreas. It joins the superior mesenteric vein to form the portal vein (Figure 22-1).

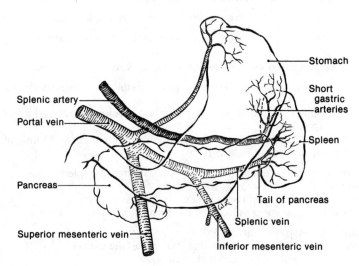

Figure 22-1. Anatomic relationships of the spleen.

B. Physiology. The spleen has multiple functions, some of which remain poorly understood. Its most important functions are its ability to act as a **blood filter** and its role in the **immunologic process** of the body.

1. **Filtering functions. Splenic blood flow** is approximately 350 L of blood a day. Most blood elements pass through rapidly and uneventfully.

   a. **Removal of old or abnormal red blood cells**

      (1) The mechanism by which the spleen, under normal circumstances, removes old or abnormal red blood cells is not known exactly, but it is thought that as the cell ages, its enzyme activity and metabolic capacity decrease. This leads to biophysical changes in the cell, which are accentuated in the substrate-deprived splenic environment.

      (2) The spleen removes about 20 ml of aged or abnormal red cells a day.

      (3) Cells that have immunoglobulin G (IgG) on their surfaces are removed by monocytes in the spleen. This may be the mechanism of increased cell destruction in some diseases, such as idiopathic thrombocytopenia purpura and autoimmune hemolytic anemia.

   b. **Removal of abnormal white cells, normal and abnormal platelets, and cellular debris.** In the splenectomized individual, cells with **inclusion bodies,** such as Howell-Jolly, Pappenheimer, and Heinz bodies, are seen. This is regarded as evidence that the spleen is capable of removing these abnormal cells or inclusion bodies.

2. **Immunologic functions**

   a. **Opsonin production.** The entire reticuloendothelial system is capable of removing well-opsonized bacteria from the circulation, but the spleen, with its highly efficient filtering mechanism, is particularly suited to removing poorly opsonized or encapsulated pathogens.

   b. **Antibody synthesis.** This occurs mainly in the white pulp, where soluble antigens stimulate the production of immunoglobulin M (IgM).

   c. **Protection from infection.** It is now firmly established that splenectomy leaves some patients more prone to infection.

3. **Storage functions.** Approximately one-third of the body's **platelets** are stored in the spleen. In some pathologic states, the percentage is increased.

II. HYPERSPLENISM is an exaggerated destruction or sequestration of circulating blood elements. This can affect red cells, white cells, and platelets.

A. Primary hypersplenism is essentially a diagnosis of exclusion and is made only after possible causes of secondary hypersplenism have been ruled out.

1. It is a rare entity, affecting mainly women.

   a. Any one or all of the formed blood elements may be involved.

   b. The spleen is almost always enlarged.

   c. The hematologic findings may be accompanied by recurring fevers and infections.

2. It may, in some cases, actually be an early manifestation of lymphoma or leukemia.

3. Primary hypersplenism responds to splenectomy. Steroids do not improve the condition.

B. Secondary hypersplenism is caused by an identifiable underlying disease.

1. **Portal hypertension,** which can lead to passive splenic congestion, is the commonest mechanism of secondary hypersplenism.

   a. Although many patients with cirrhosis and portal hypertension develop an enlarged spleen, only 15% develop hypersplenism.

   b. Hypersplenism associated with portal hypertension is usually mild and clinically insignificant; thus, isolated splenectomy is not indicated.

2. **Splenic vein thrombosis** can cause secondary hypersplenism with massive splenomegaly.

   a. Pancreatitis is the usual cause of the thrombosis.

   b. There may be associated bleeding esophageal varices.

   c. The hypersplenism and bleeding varices are cured by splenectomy.

3. **Other causes** of secondary hypersplenism include:

   a. Neoplasms, such as hairy cell leukemia, lymphoma, and metastatic cancer

   b. Myeloproliferative disorders, such as myeloid metaplasia

    c. Disorders causing increased red cell destruction, such as thalassemia major

    d. Disorders of immune response, such as mononucleosis and Felty's syndrome (see IV H)

    e. Diseases that infiltrate the spleen, such as amyloidosis and sarcoidosis

III. ABSOLUTE INDICATIONS FOR SPLENECTOMY

A. Splenic tumors

1. **Primary splenic tumors** are extremely rare.
   a. They include lymphoma, sarcoma, hemangioma, and hamartoma.
   b. Symptoms are caused by the enlarged spleen, and there may be associated hypersplenism.

2. **Metastatic disease.** The spleen is not a frequent site of metastasis, probably due to its efficient immune mechanism. The only exceptions are Hodgkin's and non-Hodgkin's lymphomas, which frequently involve the spleen.

B. Splenic abscess is uncommon, but when present, it has a high mortality rate.

1. **Causes** include the following:
   a. **Infection** of a preexisting lesion, such as a hematoma
   b. **Direct spread** from adjacent structures, such as the pancreas or colon
   c. **Hematogenous seeding** from a remote site (especially in users of intravenous drugs) or during overwhelming bacteremia

2. **Diagnosis** should be suspected if signs of abscess, such as fever and an elevated white blood cell count, occur in association with left upper quadrant fullness or tenderness. It can be confirmed by computed tomography (CT) and scanning with technetium 99m (^{99m}Tc).

C. Hereditary spherocytosis is one of a group of hereditary hemolytic anemias and causes the most severe symptoms. It is transmitted as an autosomal dominant trait.

1. **Characteristics**
   a. It is characterized by a defect of the red cell membrane. This results in loss of red cell surface area, which causes the cell to be spherical (hence the name), small, and more prone to lysis than normal red blood cells.
   b. The cell membrane is thick and rigid, which causes the cells to be held in the splenic pulp, which leads to cell lysis, due to deprivation of glucose and adenosine triphosphate (ATP). This occurs only in the spleen.

2. **Symptoms**
   a. Symptoms of hereditary spherocytosis include malaise, abdominal discomfort, jaundice, anemia, and splenomegaly.
   b. The disease may be complicated by gallstones (rare in patients under the age of 10 years) and by chronic leg ulcers that heal only after splenectomy.

3. **Diagnosis** is based upon the above clinical findings and the results of laboratory studies, which include a demonstration of the following:
   a. Spherocytes and an elevated reticulocyte count on a Wright-stained blood smear
   b. Increased osmotic fragility of the red cells
   c. Chromium 51 (^{51}Cr)-tagged red blood cells, which have a greatly shortened half-life and are sequestered in the spleen

4. **Treatment** is splenectomy.
   a. This cures the anemia and jaundice in all patients. Failure of splenectomy to cure the patient is normally caused by an accessory spleen that has been overlooked during the operation (see VII C 2).
   b. The operation should be delayed until the age of 4 years, if possible, to decrease the chance of postsplenectomy sepsis (see VI D 1 a).
   c. The gallbladder should be removed at the time of splenectomy if gallstones are present.

D. Massive splenic trauma. Irreparable splenic injury may necessitate splenectomy. In lesser injuries, splenic repair is preferable (see V C).

E. Bleeding esophageal varices caused by splenic vein thrombosis (see II B 2) can be cured by splenectomy if the diagnosis is correct.

IV. RELATIVE INDICATIONS FOR SPLENECTOMY

A. Congenital hemolytic anemias (other than hereditary spherocytosis). Although splenectomy is not curative, it reduces the need for multiple transfusions in the following conditions:

1. **Enzyme deficiencies,** such as glucose-6-phosphate dehydrogenase (G6PD) deficiency and pyruvate kinase deficiency

2. **Hereditary elliptocytosis**

3. **Thalassemia major,** transmitted as a dominant trait and characterized by defective hemoglobin synthesis, which causes homozygotes to have severe anemia and hepatosplenomegaly

B. Sickle cell anemia may require splenectomy in the rare cases in which excessive splenic sequestration of red cells is documented. Most patients with the disease "autosplenectomize" due to multiple infarcts caused by stagnation and stasis of the abnormal red blood cells.

C. Idiopathic autoimmune hemolytic anemia occurs most commonly after the age of 50 years and is found in women twice as often as in men.

1. **Clinical presentation**
   a. In this disorder, both warm- and cold-hemolytic antibodies have been described. These presumably shorten the life of the red cells.
   b. The anemia is accompanied by reticulocytosis. There is splenomegaly in 50% of the cases. There may be mild jaundice.

2. **Diagnosis.** The direct Coombs' test is positive. ^{51}Cr-tagged red blood cells may demonstrate sequestration in the spleen.

3. **Treatment.** The disease may run a self-limited course that requires no treatment.
   a. **Steroids and azathioprine** are administered in more persistent cases.
   b. **Splenectomy** is helpful in many patients, especially if they have demonstrated splenic sequestration of ^{51}Cr-tagged red cells, if steroids are ineffective or contraindicated.

D. Idiopathic thrombocytopenic purpura

1. **The etiology** is unknown but is presumed to be immunologic since most patients with chronic disease have platelet-agglutinating antibodies that rapidly destroy transfused platelets.
   a. **The acute form** is commoner in children under 16 years of age. Eighty percent of affected individuals recover spontaneously.
   b. **The chronic form** is commonest in adults, and women predominate in a 3:1 ratio.

2. **Clinical presentation**
   a. This disease is characterized by a decreased platelet count accompanied by increased megakaryocytes in the bone marrow. The spleen is usually not enlarged.
   b. The disease presents as unexplained ecchymoses or petechiae, often accompanied by bleeding from the gums or hematuria.

3. **Treatment**
   a. **Steroids** induce remission in 75% of patients, and about 20% of these have a sustained response.
   b. **Splenectomy** is indicated in individuals who do not respond to steroids or in those who relapse after steroids are tapered off. It is also mandatory if central nervous system bleeding occurs. It produces a sustained remission in 70% of patients.

E. Thrombotic thrombocytopenic purpura is a rapidly progressive and usually fatal disease.

1. **Clinical presentation**
   a. Fever
   b. Thrombocytopenic purpura

        c. Hemolytic anemia
        d. Neurologic disturbances
        e. Renal failure

    2. Diagnosis is confirmed only by biopsy of the purpuric lesion. This shows a characteristic vascular lesion, which consists of occlusion of arterioles and capillaries by a hyaline membrane.

    3. Treatment. The most effective treatment is **splenectomy** and **steroid therapy**. Plasmaphoresis, antiplatelet agents (e.g., dextran), or exchange transfusions with fresh blood have resulted in survival in a small percentage of patients.

    4. Prognosis. The long-term survival rate is less than 10% even with optimal therapy.

F. Primary hypersplenism (see II A)

G. Agnogenic myeloid metaplasia is a mysterious disease that is thought to be related to polycythemia vera and myelogenous leukemia.

    1. Clinical presentation
        a. It is characterized by connective tissue proliferation in the bone marrow, liver, spleen, and lymph nodes, accompanied by proliferation of the hematopoietic tissue of the liver, spleen, and long bones.
        b. The usual symptoms are anemia and splenomegaly, which usually appear in middle-aged or older adults. Secondary hypersplenism may develop, and later in the disease, there may be spontaneous bleeding, spontaneous infections, and splenic infarcts.

    2. Treatment
        a. Primary treatment consists of **alkylating agents** to reduce the size of the spleen and **male hormones** to stimulate failing bone marrow and to treat anemia.
        b. Splenectomy does not change the course of the disease, but it may help to control the hypersplenism. It can reduce the need for transfusions and may also help to control thrombocytopenia.

H. Felty's syndrome

    1. Clinical presentation
        a. Felty's syndrome is a triad consisting of chronic rheumatoid arthritis, splenomegaly, and granulocytopenia.
        b. Spontaneous serious infections can occur due to the neutropenia, and splenectomy is helpful in this group of patients.

    2. Treatment. Splenectomy may also be employed for intractable leg ulcers, severe thrombocytopenia, and anemia.

I. Hodgkin's disease. Advances in therapy have greatly improved chances for the cure or long-term survival of patients with this disease.

    1. Types. There are four histologic types of Hodgkin's disease.
        a. Lymphocyte predominant (best prognosis)
        b. Nodular sclerosing
        c. Mixed cellularity
        d. Lymphocyte depleted (worst prognosis)

    2. Staging. Optimal treatment depends upon accurate staging of the disease. The **Ann Arbor Classification** is listed below. Stages are **subclassified as A (absence)** and **B (presence)** of systemic symptoms (i.e., fever, night sweats, and weight loss of greater than 10%).
        a. Stage 0: No detectable disease following excisional biopsy
        b. Stage I: Disease limited to a single lymph node region
        c. Stage II: Disease limited to two or more lymph node regions on the same side of the diaphragm
        d. Stage III: Disease on both sides of the diaphragm but limited to lymph nodes, spleen, or Waldeyer's ring
        e. Stage IV: Involvement of bone, bone marrow, lung parenchyma, pleura, liver, skin, gastrointestinal tract, central nervous system, kidney, or sites other than lymph nodes, spleen, or Waldeyer's ring

3. Staging laparotomy

a. Staging laparotomy consists of splenectomy, liver biopsy, and complete abdominal exploration with sampling of lymph nodes from multiple areas.

b. Criteria for staging laparotomy in Hodgkin's patients have not been universally accepted.

    (1) Patients with systemic symptoms and clinical stage I or II disease should be considered for laparotomy. It is also important to note that 25% of patients with clinical stage I or II disease are found to have unsuspected disease in the abdomen.

    (2) Laparotomy is not indicated in patients with stage III B or IV in whom chemotherapy is the treatment of choice.

    (3) Approximately 40% of patients who undergo laparotomy have their clinical stage changed as a result of the procedure.

4. Splenectomy is thought to improve tolerance to chemotherapy. Use of the procedure also avoids the injury to the left kidney and lung that occurs if the spleen is irradiated.

J. Non-Hodgkin's lymphoma

1. Staging for non-Hodgkin's lymphoma uses the same classification as for Hodgkin's disease. Careful evaluation will reveal stage III or stage IV disease in most patients.

2. Laparotomy is used infrequently in non-Hodgkin's lymphoma. Percutaneous liver biopsy, laparoscopy, or bone marrow biopsy frequently reveal diffuse disease.

3. Splenectomy may be useful in some of these patients to treat hypersplenism or to relieve symptoms of massive splenomegaly.

V. RUPTURE OF THE SPLEEN may follow either penetrating or nonpenetrating trauma or may occur spontaneously.

A. Traumatic rupture

1. Penetrating trauma. Knife wounds and gunshot wounds are the commonest causes. The resultant wounds are usually obvious. It is very important to realize that the spleen may be injured when the entry wound is in the region of the middle or lower chest as well as when the wounds are in the abdomen.

2. Nonpenetrating trauma. The commonest cause of nonpenetrating trauma is an automobile accident. When the spleen is injured, there is usually profuse bleeding, but in 5% of blunt injuries, the rupture may be delayed.

3. Iatrogenic trauma accounts for 20% of all splenectomies. The trauma results from excessive traction on the splenic attachments or from misplacement of retractors.

4. Delayed rupture

a. Usually, the initial injury is a **subcapsular hematoma**. Eventually, the red cells lyse, and the osmolality of the hematoma increases, causing it to expand. Rupture may be the eventual outcome.

b. About 75% of delayed ruptures occur within 2 weeks of the initial injury and present as acute shock from profuse bleeding.

B. Spontaneous rupture usually occurs because of splenomegaly due to an associated disease, such as mononucleosis, leukemia, or malaria.

C. Treatment. In all cases of isolated splenic injury (with the possible exception of spontaneous rupture), an attempt should be made to salvage the spleen.

1. In minor capsular tears, pressure and application of a topical hemostatic agent will frequently control the bleeding.

2. Deeper lacerations can be treated by splenorrhaphy, using Teflon pledgets, or by partial resection.

3. Massive injuries, especially if there are other injuries that require attention, should be treated by splenectomy.

VI. COMPLICATIONS FOLLOWING SPLENECTOMY

A. Atelectasis of the left lower lung is the commonest complication.

B. Subphrenic abscess may develop and is usually accompanied by a left pleural effusion.

C. Thrombocytosis postoperatively is common. If the platelet count exceeds 1,000,000, anticoagulation may be required to prevent spontaneous thrombosis.

D. Postsplenectomy sepsis

  1. Overview. Some patients are prone to **overwhelming sepsis** following splenectomy. The syndrome begins with nonspecific, mild, influenza-like symptoms and progresses to high fever, shock, and death.

    a. In general, the younger the patient and the more serious the disease requiring the splenectomy, the greater the risk for the development of overwhelming sepsis. The risk is greatest if splenectomy occurs during the first 2–4 years of life, particularly if it is done for a disease of the reticuloendothelial system.

    b. In healthy adults who have the spleen removed for trauma, the incidence of overwhelming sepsis is low (0.5%–0.8%), but it is still higher than that in the normal population (0.01%).

    c. About 80% of septic episodes occur within 2 years after splenectomy.

  2. Treatment

    a. Polyvalent pneumococcal vaccine should be given to all splenectomized patients, which will protect them from 80% of pathogenic pneumococci (the commonest organisms causing the sepsis).

    b. Prophylactic penicillin should probably be given to high-risk patients. Children should receive penicillin until the age of 18. Patients should be instructed to seek medical attention immediately if symptoms begin, and penicillin therapy should be started in an attempt to prevent the full-blown syndrome from developing.

VII. MISCELLANEOUS LESIONS

A. Splenosis is **autotransplantation** of fragments of spleen, which can occur after rupture. It is thought that these fragments can maintain splenic function, including immunocompetence, but this has not been proven.

B. Aneurysms of the splenic artery

  1. The splenic artery is the second commonest site of intra-abdominal aneurysm (the abdominal aorta is commonest).

  2. Aneurysms occur in older patients as a manifestation of generalized atherosclerosis. They also occur in young women, in whom they are usually caused by dysplasia of the splenic artery wall. These are important because they are prone to rupture in the last trimester of pregnancy.

  3. Repair of the aneurysm is indicated if it is enlarging, symptomatic, or found in a woman of childbearing age.

    a. Distal aneurysms require resection and splenectomy.

    b. Proximal aneurysms may be ligated, allowing the spleen to be preserved.

C. Ectopic and accessory spleens

  1. An **ectopic spleen** is caused by a long splenic pedicle, which allows the spleen to "wander" about the abdomen.

  2. Accessory spleens are found in about 10% of autopsies. They are usually located near the hilus or the tail of the pancreas and less frequently in the mesentery. They are only significant if they are overlooked during splenectomy for hematologic disease.

23
Breast

Francis E. Rosato
Anne L. Rosenberg
Bruce E. Jarrell

I. INTRODUCTION

A. Anatomy

1. The parenchyma consists of 15–20 radially arranged segments, each drained by a duct converging at the nipple.

2. Each of these segments or **lobes** is made up of 20–40 **lobules**, each of which consists of 10–100 alveoli.

B. Vasculature

1. Arterial supply of the breast is derived primarily from the internal mammary artery (60%) and the lateral thoracic artery (30%).

2. Venous return is primarily via the axillary vein and the internal mammary veins.

3. Lymphatic drainage. It is clinically significant that the lymphatic vessels drain principally to the axillary lymph node chain. The axillary nodes are arbitrarily divided into three levels based on their relationship to the pectoralis minor muscle (Figure 23-1).

C. Examination of the breast should be done systematically.

1. Visual inspection with the patient sitting may reveal asymmetry, dimpling, ulceration, nodules, and nipple changes. The patient should be asked to raise her arms upward and to press on her hips to effect contraction of the pectoralis major muscle.

2. Palpation
 a. The node-bearing areas (cervical, supraclavicular, infraclavicular, and axillary lymph nodes) should be palpated.
 b. With the patient in the supine position and the ipsilateral arm above the head and a pillow under the ipsilateral shoulder, the breast is then palpated for masses or asymmetric densities.

II. BENIGN CONDITIONS of the breast may present with pain, nipple complaints, or lumps. Although there are many diagnoses in this group of disorders, several are commoner and more important.

A. Fibroadenoma occurs in young women who are usually under 35 years of age and may be multiple in 10%–15% of patients. It is usually a discrete mass 1–4 cm in size that is unattached to surrounding tissue. Treatment is by excisional biopsy, if there is any question at all of the diagnosis. Many young women in their late teens with fibroadenomas may be observed.

B. Cystosarcoma phylloides is a giant fibroadenoma, containing many more cellular components than the usual fibroadenoma. Very rarely does the tumor undergo transformation into a malignant sarcoma. The treatment is wide local excision. If inadequately excised, the tumor has a tendency to recur locally.

C. Chronic cystic mastitis, or **fibrocystic disease of the breast**, is a very common entity characterized by painful multiple bilateral cystic masses that change during the menstrual cycle.

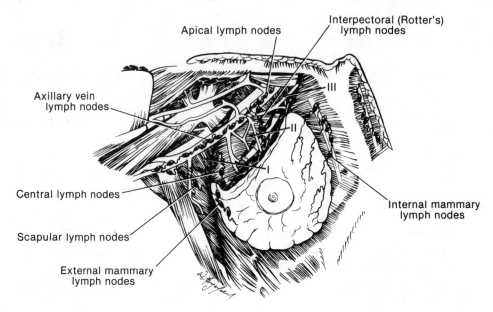

Apical lymph nodes

Interpectoral (Rotter's)
lymph nodes

Axillary vein
lymph nodes

Central lymph nodes

Scapular lymph nodes

External mammary
lymph nodes

Internal mammary
lymph nodes

Figure 23-1. The lymphatic drainage of the breast, showing lymph node groups and levels. *Level I lymph nodes*: lateral to lateral border of pectoralis minor muscle; *level II lymph nodes*: behind pectoralis minor muscle; and *level III lymph nodes*: medial to medial border of pectoralis minor muscle.

    1. The diagnosis is made by breast cyst aspiration and cytologic analysis of the fluid.
      a. Observation is indicated if the mass completely disappears.
      b. Excisional biopsy is indicated:
        (1) If the mass recurs or does not disappear completely
        (2) If the aspirated fluid is bloody or contains suspicious cells

    2. The risk of carcinoma is 3–6 times higher in individuals with this disorder (when there are **atypical cells**) than in the general population. It is 5–15 times higher if there is atypia *and* a family history of breast cancer. Frequent examinations are indicated.

    3. If multiple biopsies have been performed or dense fibrous disease with atypia or a family history of breast cancer is present, a prophylactic simple mastectomy may be justified.

  D. Intraductal papilloma is the number one cause of pathologic nipple discharge, which is spontaneous, serosanguineous, unilateral, and usually from a single duct orifice.

    1. It is a benign lesion, which may or may not be associated with a subareolar mass.

    2. A mammogram should be obtained to rule out other pathology.

    3. Excision of the involved mammary duct is necessary to determine if the lesion is a malignant papillary adenocarcinoma.

  E. Galactocele is a simple, milk-filled cyst. Diagnostic aspiration is curative. Reaspiration may be performed, but surgical resection is rarely necessary.

  F. Ductal ectasia is characterized by dilation of the subareolar ducts. It may be associated with pathologic nipple discharge, a retroareolar mass, nipple retraction, or recurrent mastitis. Treatment consists of local excision of the involved mass.

  G. Intrinsic mastitis (usually related to lactation) **and subareolar recurrent chronic abscesses** are the commonest infections of the breast. Intrinsic mastitis usually responds to antibiotics, while chronic abscesses generally require surgical excision.

  H. Mondor's disease (phlebitis of the thoracoepigastric vein) is a self-limited entity, which needs no treatment.

III. CARCINOMA OF THE FEMALE BREAST

A. Epidemiology

1. **Incidence.** By the age of 70 years, 10% of all women in the United States will have contracted carcinoma of the breast (over 150,000 new cases estimated in 1990).
   a. It is one of the principal causes of cancer deaths in women with an incidence of 75 cases in 100,000 population (over 44,000 new cases estimated in 1990).
   b. The age-adjusted mortality rate and incidence have shown no appreciable change since 1930, which indicates that not only does breast cancer remain a major threat to human life but also that therapy has not improved since that time.
   c. Geographically, carcinoma of the breast has an increased incidence in the north central part of the United States, in the area of the Great Lakes. The incidence is somewhat decreased in the Sun Belt.

2. **Risk factors.** There are multiple factors that increase the risk of developing carcinoma of the breast.
   a. **A family history** positive for breast carcinoma produces a two- to threefold increased risk. This applies only to first-degree relatives, such as a patient's mother, maternal grandmother, maternal aunts, and sisters.
      (1) A first-degree relative of a patient with premenopausal breast carcinoma has a threefold increased risk.
      (2) A first-degree relative of a patient with bilateral breast carcinoma has a fivefold increased risk.
      (3) A first-degree relative of a patient with bilateral premenopausal breast carcinoma has an eightfold increased risk.
   b. **A history of chronic cystic mastitis** with atypical hyperplasia on histology results in a three- to sixfold increased risk of breast carcinoma.
   c. **A previous incidence of contralateral breast cancer** carries a relatively high risk of breast carcinoma occurring in the unaffected breast.
      (1) If an adenocarcinoma was present previously, the risk is increased twofold.
      (2) If the preceding tumor was a lobular carcinoma, there is a 25%–50% likelihood of developing carcinoma in the other breast.
   d. **High socioeconomic status** carries a high risk of developing breast carcinoma.
   e. **Individuals of Western hemisphere extraction** have a greater risk of developing breast carcinoma than do those of Eastern hemisphere extraction; however, the relative "immunity" enjoyed by Easterners is lost after one generation in the Western hemisphere. The difference in risk is not related to the mass of breast tissue.
   f. **Nulliparous women** have a two- to threefold increased risk of breast carcinoma when compared to parous women. The risk is lowest in women who become pregnant prior to the age of 23 years.
   g. **Cerumen.** Women with wet cerumen have a higher risk of breast cancer than do those with dry cerumen.
   h. **Estrogen compounds** have a variable effect in animals on the development of breast carcinoma. Although estradiols and ketones do not produce carcinoma, estratriols do.
      (1) There is no current evidence that breast cancer is caused in humans by exogenous estrogens.
      (2) There is an association, however, with endometrial carcinoma. It is probably prudent to withhold exogenous estrogen from patients who have had breast cancer and from those in high-risk groups since estrogens can support the growth of an already established carcinoma.

B. Symptoms

1. **Breast lumps** are the presenting symptoms in 85%–90% of patients with carcinoma. Approximately 60% of breast lumps are discovered by patients on self-examination.
   a. **Aspiration.** A breast mass may be evaluated by aspiration alone if:
      (1) It is a solitary mass (i.e., there are no other cystic masses).
      (2) There is no evidence of axillary nodal involvement.
      (3) The mass disappears completely and does not recur within 3 months.
      (4) The fluid is not bloody, and the cytology performed on the aspirate is not suspicious for tumor cells.

b. Biopsy. A mass should be biopsied immediately if:
   (1) It is large, hard, or unable to be aspirated.
   (2) There is marked unilateral breast enlargement.
   (3) There is skin dimpling, redness, or edema.
   (4) There is a spontaneous **nipple discharge**.
      (a) Although most nipple discharges are benign and present as serosanguineous drainage from an intraductal papilloma, 10% are malignant.
      (b) Nipple discharge should be evaluated through mammography and cytology of the discharged fluid. When a mass is present in association with the discharge, excision of the mass is indicated.
      (c) When a mass is not present but the quadrant of the breast from which the discharge originated can be localized by local compression, a breast quadrantectomy is indicated.
      (d) When the source of nipple discharge cannot be localized to a specific area of the breast, treatment is controversial. Generally, for patients over 40 years of age, a central duct excision is performed. In young patients, frequent observation may be warranted.
   c. Observation is indicated in select young women in whom nodularity or breast lumps appear to be physiologic. These women may be safely watched through one or two menstrual cycles. Although most are fibroadenomas, well-circumscribed papillary or medullary carcinomas can also be present.

2. Breast pain may be a presenting symptom of carcinoma and should be completely evaluated to eliminate the possibility of malignancy.

3. Metastatic disease may also be the initial symptom, either to a distant organ or to the axillary nodes. In 2% of cases of breast cancer, patients present with axillary node enlargement but no palpable primary breast tumor.
   a. Of all patients presenting with isolated axillary enlargement, one-third to one-half represent occult breast cancer. Hodgkin's disease, lung, ovarian, or pancreatic cancer, and squamous cell carcinoma of the skin must be ruled out.
   b. In this situation, a blind mastectomy (i.e., removal of a breast without evidence of malignancy) is indicated.

4. Asymptomatic patients. Patients may have no symptoms or signs of breast cancer but may be in a high-risk category (i.e., family or personal history of breast cancer) and should be followed closely with mammography, physical examination, and breast self-examination.

C. Diagnosis

1. Self-examination. Over 60% of cancers are discovered by the patients on self-examination (monthly breast self-examination is recommended).

2. Physical examination by a physician is imperative to supplement breast self-examination and radiographic studies since 15% of proven breast carcinomas have negative mammograms. Screening programs, using physical and mammographic examinations of asymptomatic women, have detected many early cancers without axillary node involvement.

3. Mammography (using low-dose radiation) reveals breast architecture.
   a. Suspicious signs of malignancy are asymmetry, skin thickening, irregular masses, or architectural distortions. Clustered irregular microcalcifications are the most ominous finding.
   b. Mammography is useful to support the clinical impression of no evidence of malignancy, to follow patients with a previous history of breast cancer, and to screen for subclinical tumors.
   c. The current recommendation is a baseline mammogram at age 35 and then annual screening for women over 40 years of age and high-risk patients.

4. Ultrasound can be used to determine if a breast mass (palpable and nonpalpable) is solid or cystic.

5. Needle aspiration can confirm the diagnosis of cystic masses, or cytology can be submitted for a solid lesion.

6. Excisional biopsy is the preferred method of diagnosing a breast lesion; however, it is not always possible to perform a biopsy on large masses or on those deeply situated. The biopsy may be done on an outpatient basis, and although definitive treatment may be delayed by weeks, there is no indication that this delay is detrimental to the patient.

   a. Enough tissue should be obtained to submit for estrogen and progesterone receptors (**hormone receptors**). The receptor status affects the overall patient survival. Receptor-positive tumors respond more often to hormonal therapy and have a better prognosis than those that are receptor-negative.

   b. Tissue is also submitted for **flow cytometry** to determine if the tumor is diploid (DNA index = 1.00) or aneuploid (DNA index ≠ 1.00) and to determine the S-phase fraction. Aneuploid tumors with a high S-phase fraction have poor prognoses.

D. Preoperative evaluation of the patient with proven carcinoma of the breast should determine whether spread outside the axilla has occurred, thus indicating inoperability.

  1. Criteria for inoperability as defined by Haagensen:
    a. Extensive edema of the breast
    b. Satellite nodules of carcinoma
    c. Inflammatory carcinoma
    d. A parasternal tumor, indicating spread to the internal mammary nodes
    e. Supraclavicular metastasis
    f. Arm edema
    g. Distant metastasis

  2. Determination of distant metastasis
    a. Extensive examination for distant spread of disease is a preoperative requirement.
      (1) A **bone scan** should be performed if nodes are clinically positive or if nodes are clinically negative but the patient has symptoms of bone pain (all stage II, III, and IV patients).
      (2) Of the **liver function tests**, the alkaline phosphatase is the most sensitive in detecting hepatic metastasis. A liver ultrasound or computed tomography (CT) scan should be performed if the alkaline phosphatase is abnormal or if there is other evidence of distant metastasis.
      (3) A **chest x-ray** detects pulmonary parenchymal or bone metastasis. Chest CT scan should be obtained for stage III patients to evaluate the supraclavicular area and mediastinum.
      (4) A **radioisotope** or **CT scan** of the brain should be done if neurologic signs or symptoms are present.
      (5) A **mammogram** is useful not only to determine additional foci in the involved breast but to determine the presence of metastatic or synchronous disease.
      (6) Although the adrenal glands and ovaries are often involved by metastatic disease, there are no good screening tests for these areas. If warranted, a more extensive evaluation may be performed with an abdominal CT scan.
    b. Pathologic examination. If the presence of metastatic disease seems likely, based on one or more of the screening tests, a pathologic sample of the suspected metastasis must be obtained to prove the diagnosis.
    c. Even if no evidence of metastatic disease is found, there are patients with apparently early disease who later prove to have had **occult dissemination** at the time of initial diagnosis. This figure may approach 25% in some series and represents a very disappointing group to treat.

  3. Pregnancy at the time of diagnosis of carcinoma of the breast is not a contraindication to mastectomy. It is associated with an increased incidence (75%) of positive axillary nodal involvement and, therefore, a worse prognosis. Chemotherapy obviously presents a danger to the fetus and should be avoided. In selected cases, radiation therapy and breast conservation may be considered. Controversy surrounds pregnancy termination, which is the decision of each individual patient.

E. Staging categories are attempts to summate all of the prognostic indicators and relate them to patient survival. Stage I, with no nodal involvement, has the best patient prognosis; stages II and III have an intermediate patient survival rate; and stage IV is characterized by metastatic disease and poor patient prognosis. Below is the staging system of the American Committee on Cancer Staging and End Results Reporting.

1. Tumor, nodes, and metastasis (TNM) classification
   a. Primary tumor (T)
      (1) TIS: carcinoma in situ
      (2) T0: No primary tumor found
      (3) T1: Primary tumor, less than 2 cm in diameter
      (4) T2: Primary tumor, 2–5 cm in diameter
      (5) T3: Primary tumor, greater than 5 cm in diameter
      (6) T4: Extension to chest wall
   b. Nodal involvement (N)
      (1) N1: Mobile axillary nodes with or without tumor
      (2) N2: Fixed axillary nodes
   c. Distant metastasis (M): metastatic disease outside of the breast and axilla

2. Clinical staging is performed with consideration of the TNM classification.
   a. Stage I is characterized by an 85% 5-year survival rate; the tumor is less than 2 cm in diameter. There is no nodal involvement and no distant metastasis.
   b. Stage II is characterized by 66% 5-year survival rate; the tumor is 2–5 cm in diameter. The axillary nodes are palpable and movable. There is no distant metastasis.
   c. Stage III patients have a 41% 5-year survival rate; the tumor is greater than 5 cm in diameter or is characterized by local invasion. Nodes are palpable outside of the axilla. There is no distant metastasis.
   d. Stage IV is characterized by a 10% 5-year survival rate. There is distant metastasis.

3. Cure rates cannot be determined for breast cancer until the occurrence of at least 10 disease-free years.

F. Prognosis of patients with carcinoma of the breast is strongly dependent upon a number of clinical and histologic factors at the time of diagnosis.

1. Histology. The histologic type of carcinoma strongly influences the prognosis. The carcinomas may be categorized by the ability of a cell type to metastasize.
   a. Nonmetastasizing carcinoma is noninvasive and represents 5% of all breast carcinomas. The 5-year survival rate of affected patients is 95%.
      (1) In situ intraductal papillary carcinoma is nonmetastasizing but may develop into invasive ductal carcinoma in up to 50% of cases within 5 years. Treatment, therefore, should be the same as for invasive ductal carcinoma.
      (2) Noninvasive lobular carcinoma is an in situ carcinoma that has a 15%–30% association with the ultimate development of a frank adenocarcinoma within 20 years. The opposite breast is involved by adenocarcinoma as often as the breast containing the noninvasive lobular carcinoma. Either prophylactic **bilateral mastectomy** or close long-term observation is appropriate treatment, since lobular neoplasia (lobular carcinoma in situ) is bilateral in 50% of patients.
   b. Paget's disease of the breast is carcinoma involving the nipple. It may be either invasive or in situ breast carcinoma, which originates from the underlying ducts. Paget's cells infiltrate the epidermis of the nipple, resulting in an eczematous dermatitis. Generally, treatment is similar to that for invasive carcinoma.
   c. Metastasizing carcinoma
      (1) Carcinoma that rarely metastasizes is invasive and represents 15% of all cases of breast carcinoma. The 5-year survival rate for patients with this type of carcinoma is 80%. Examples include:
         (a) Colloid carcinoma, which contains a preponderance of mucin-producing cells
         (b) Medullary carcinoma, which shows lymphocytic infiltration in a sheet-like pattern and has a well-circumscribed margin
         (c) Well-differentiated adenocarcinoma (grade I)
         (d) Tubular carcinoma, which has a low incidence of nodular metastasis and has a good prognosis, even if axillary nodes are involved
         (e) Comedocarcinoma
      (2) Moderately metastasizing carcinoma is highly invasive and spreads early to regional lymph nodes. It represents 65% of all breast carcinomas. The 5-year survival rate for individuals with this type of carcinoma is 60%. Examples include:
         (a) Infiltrating adenocarcinoma of ductal origin, which is the commonest carcinoma of the breast
         (b) Intraductal carcinoma with stromal invasion

(c) Infiltrating lobular carcinoma, which is characterized by small cells infiltrating the lobules

(3) **Highly metastasizing carcinoma** represents fewer than 15% of carcinomas of the breast. It includes any of the previously mentioned tumors that show vascular invasion or are undifferentiated with cells growing in a nonductal or nontubular arrangement. The 5-year survival rate is 55% (grade III and aneuploid tumors).

d. **Inflammatory carcinoma** is any breast carcinoma with local inflammatory signs, including redness, localized warmth, swelling, and pain. Histologically, tumor-plugged subdermal lymphatic vessels are found almost universally. Individuals with inflammatory carcinoma have a very poor prognosis; fewer than 3% survive 5 years.

2. **Size of the primary tumor**, as well as **size, number**, and **location of the involved lymph nodes**, influences patient survival. Most classification systems (see III E) are based on these variables. Classification of breast carcinoma into stages I and II generally indicates operability and, therefore, a better prognosis, whereas classification into stages III and IV indicates inoperability and a worse prognosis.

a. **Primary tumor size**
   (1) Patients with tumors less than 1 cm in diameter have a 10-year survival rate of 80%.
   (2) Patients with tumors 3–4 cm in diameter have a 10-year survival rate of 55%.
   (3) Patients with tumors 5–7.5 cm in diameter have a 10-year survival rate of 45%.

b. **Size and structure of lymph nodes** involved by metastases based on clinical examination
   (1) If no palpable lymph nodes are present, the 10-year survival rate for patients is 60%.
   (2) If palpable, freely movable lymph nodes are present, the 10-year survival rate for patients is 50%.
   (3) If the lymph nodes are fixed to surrounding structures, the 10-year survival rate for patients is 20%.

c. **The number of lymph nodes** involved by metastases may be assigned erroneously if based on clinical evaluation of the axilla. In 25% of the patients whose axillary nodes are not palpable, a tumor is seen microscopically in the nodes. In 25% of patients with palpable nodes, no tumor is found on pathologic examination of the axillary contents. There is a linear relationship between the number of axillary nodes found on pathologic examination and the incidence of recurrence and patient survival.
   (1) Patients with negative axillary nodes have a 10-year survival rate of 65%.
   (2) Patients with one to three positive axillary nodes have a 10-year survival rate of 38%.
   (3) Patients with more than four positive axillary nodes have a 10-year survival rate of 13%.

d. **Location of lymph nodes** involved by metastases
   (1) **Level I axillary nodes** are located low in the axilla and extend between the lateral border of the pectoralis minor muscle and medial border latissimus dorsi muscle. The 5-year survival rate for patients with involvement of this level of lymph nodes is 65%.
   (2) **Level II axillary nodes** are located posteriorly to the pectoralis minor muscle insertion. The 5-year survival rate of patients with involvement of nodes up to this level is 45%.
   (3) **Level III axillary nodes** are located medially to the superior border of the pectoralis minor muscle. The 5-year survival rate of patients with involvement of nodes at this level is 28%.

3. **Other clinical characteristics** of breast carcinoma significantly **worsen the prognosis** and lower the survival rate of patients. These include:
   a. Edema or ulceration of the surrounding skin
   b. Tumor fixation to the chest wall or overlying skin
   c. Satellite skin nodules
   d. Inflammatory carcinoma
   e. Peau d'orange, which is an orange-peel consistency of breast skin due to dermal lymphatic invasion
   f. Skin retraction or dimpling of the breast skin due to shortening of tumor-involved Cooper's ligaments
   g. Involvement of the medial portion of the inner lower quadrant of the breast, which is the least favorable anatomic location for a carcinoma
   h. Arm edema
   i. Evidence of distant metastasis

    4. Estrogen receptor status of tumors (see III H 2) also affects the overall patient survival; that is, if there are hormone receptors in cancer cells, breast cancer may respond to hormonal therapy. Receptor-positive tumors respond more often to hormonal therapy and have a better prognosis than those that are receptor-negative.

G. Treatment for breast carcinoma uses surgery, radiation therapy, and chemotherapy or hormone therapy. Options are determined based on histology and stage of disease (Figure 23-2).

  1. Surgery may be palliative or curative. The choice of procedure is based upon histology, stage, and factors relating to the operative risk of the patient, such as age and concurrent medical illnesses.

    a. Essential components of surgical therapy include the following:

      (1) Removal of all breast tissue in the affected breast is necessary because of the high occurrence of multicentricity of breast lesions. Some 30%–35% of patients have premalignant or malignant lesions in the affected breast in a quadrant other than that in which the tumor has been discovered.

      (2) Removal of axillary nodes to ascertain accurate staging is necessary because of the possible erroneous classification of axillary metastasis based on clinical examination alone. The extent of the axillary dissection differs in the surgical procedures.

    b. Surgical procedures

      (1) Lumpectomy (segmental mastectomy), axillary lymphadenectomy (level I and II), and **postoperative irradiation** are most commonly used for small primary lesions (less than 4 cm), and intraductal carcinomas. Level I and II axillary dissections are over 98% accurate in predicting metastatic disease if the nodes at these levels are not involved.

      (2) Simple mastectomy involves removal of the breast along with the nipple–areola complex. It may be combined with a level I axillary lymph node dissection.

      (3) Modified radical mastectomy (Patey procedure) removes a generous amount of skin, the entire breast, the pectoralis minor muscle, and axillary contents inferior to the axillary vein.

        (a) Several major studies have shown comparable survival rates and patterns of recurrence to the radical mastectomy (Halsted procedure).

        (b) It has a better cosmetic outcome than the radical mastectomy, and breast reconstruction may be achieved by subpectoral placement of a prosthesis.

      (4) Halsted radical mastectomy removes the **pectoralis major muscle** in addition to the tissue removed in a modified radical mastectomy.

        (a) This procedure adequately removes all axillary lymph nodes, the interpectoral fascia nodes (Rotter's nodes), and the primary tumor. The thoracodorsal nerve, which innervates the latissimus dorsi muscle, is also sometimes sacrificed.

        (b) The long thoracic nerve should be carefully preserved to prevent denervation of the serratus anterior muscle, which results in a "winged scapula."

        (c) The Halsted procedure is extremely effective in preventing local recurrence of disease but has the disadvantage of causing an obvious deformity.

      (5) Extended radical mastectomy, which includes removal of the mediastinal lymph nodes, had been advocated for large or medial lesions where there is evidence of

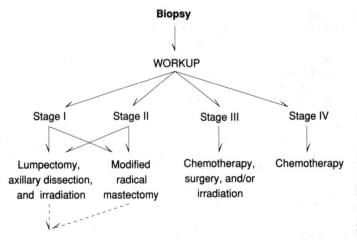

Figure 23-2. Treatment for breast carcinoma, involving surgery, radiation, and chemotherapy, is determined on the basis of histology and stage of disease. Adjuvant chemotherapy is used for node-positive patients and for high-risk node-negative patients. Adjuvant hormone therapy is used for those patients with hormone-sensitive tumors.

internal mammary metastasis. Currently, it is rarely used because of increased surgical morbidity and mortality and unimproved rates of survival when compared to other therapy modalities.

    (6) Reconstruction of the breast following mastectomy (see Chapter 26 I E) may be performed safely without altering survival rates. Reconstruction can be performed immediately, although many surgeons delay the procedure for 3–6 months until wound healing is complete.

c. Postoperative care of the mastectomy patient involves total rehabilitation and observation for tumor recurrence and complications.

    (1) Immediate care includes both mobilization of the arm to prevent limitation of motion and psychological support for the return to normal living. A breast prosthesis should also be supplied.

    (2) Follow-up care should be done for life to detect local and distant recurrences and new primary tumors in the contralateral breast (see III H).

    (3) Edema of the arm occurs in 10%–30% of women following radical mastectomy and interruption of axillary lymphatic vessels. This may occur acutely or chronically and may be aggravated by radiation therapy to the region. All causes of minor trauma (including needle puncture) to the affected arm must be avoided.

        (a) Treatment

            (i) Because each infection increases lymphatic obstruction by obliterating remaining open channels with fibrosis in reaction to the bacteria, even minor skin infections should be treated early with antibiotics.

            (ii) Chronic edema may be treated with a firm, fitted elastic sleeve.

        (b) Complications. Chronic edema of 10 years or longer may lead (although rarely) to the development of lymphangiosarcoma in the affected arm.

2. Radiation therapy may be used for the treatment of primary and metastatic lesions.

    a. Wide removal of the tumor (lumpectomy) with a level I (and II) axillary lymphadenectomy followed by breast irradiation is an alternative primary treatment for selected stage I and II patients with carcinoma of the breast.

    (1) The whole breast is irradiated (4500 rad) with a boost to the tumor site (2000 rad).

    (2) Contraindications are:

        (a) Multicentric lesions

        (b) Tumors greater than 4 cm in diameter

        (c) Retroareolar or nipple lesions (unless the nipple–areola complex is excised)

    (3) Survival results appear comparable to modified radical mastectomy at 8–10-year follow-up for these selected patients.

    (4) There is a 12% recurrence rate in the breast over 5–10 years.

    b. Radiation therapy may be an extremely effective form of palliative therapy in patients with bone or central nervous system metastases, resulting in relief of pain and control of local disease.

    c. Radiation therapy as adjuvant therapy was examined by the *National Surgical Adjuvant Breast Project (NSABP)*, no. 4. The results showed no advantage of adjuvant radiation therapy whether patients demonstrated positive or negative nodal involvement.

3. Chemotherapy or hormone therapy is used in several settings.

    a. Adjuvant therapy is designed to eradicate occult distant metastasis or local residual tumor in stage II or stage III patients with no evidence of distant metastasis. All patients with positive axillary node involvement are felt to be candidates as well as selected high-risk node-negative patients (based upon flow cytometry, tumor size, age, and hormone receptor status).

    (1) Chemotherapy with a triple-drug regimen is the commonest form of adjuvant treatment and involves 6 monthly cycles of cyclophosphamide, methotrexate, and fluorouracil (or cyclophosphamide, adriamycin, and fluorouracil).

        (a) Results show improvement in both the disease-free interval and overall survival of premenopausal women. The results in postmenopausal women are unclear but are probably improved.

        (b) Side effects include:

            (i) Myelosuppression (requiring monitoring of bone marrow function)

            (ii) Carcinogenesis (particularly related to cyclophosphamide, which has been associated with bladder carcinoma and possibly the late onset of leukemia)

    (2) Hormone therapy employs **tamoxifen** (an antiestrogen), in most cases, and is generally used for postmenopausal patients with hormone-positive tumors for 2–5 years. **Oophorectomy** was shown in the *NSABP*, no. 3, to have no effect on long-term survival rates, although it possibly prolonged the disease-free interval prior to recurrence.

b. Chemotherapy or hormone therapy is also used to treat metastatic and recurrent disease.

H. Recurrent disease

1. Types

a. Local recurrence is defined as recurrence of the carcinoma within the operative field. It occurs in up to 15% of patients after radical mastectomy and in more patients with axillary metastasis. A recurrence usually presents within 2 years of surgery and is treated by either local excision, radiation therapy, or both.

b. Second breast carcinoma should be closely examined to determine whether the second lesion is a primary or metastatic lesion. New primary lesions should be treated similarly to any other primary lesion. Metastatic lesions should be treated by lumpectomy only, followed by hormonal therapy or chemotherapy. Determination of the type of lesion is based on several criteria.

(1) Wide histologic disparity favors a second primary tumor.

(2) If nuclear differentiation is greater in the second breast, a second primary tumor is most likely.

(3) If the interposed time between occurrence of the two lesions is greater than 5 years, the tumor is probably a second primary. If the interposed time is less than 5 years, it is more likely to be a metastatic lesion.

(4) Location of the new tumor fully in the breast favors a new primary. Location of the new lesion in the fatty area of the tail of Spence or near the sternum favors a metastatic lesion.

(5) If the lesion is single, a new primary lesion is favored. If it is multiple, it is probably metastatic.

(6) Contiguous in situ changes are usually only seen in a new primary lesion.

c. Distant metastasis occurs most commonly in the bone, liver, or lungs. Other less common sites are the brain, central nervous system, and adrenal glands.

d. Follow-up for breast cancer patients should include:

(1) Frequent physical examinations (every 3–4 months)

(2) Monthly breast self-examination

(3) Annual mammography, bone scan, chest x-ray (or CT scan), and an evaluation of the liver

2. Treatment. Recurrent disease should be proven on biopsy with determination of the estrogen receptor status of the tumor. Treatment should follow by means of either hormonal therapy or chemotherapy.

a. Hormonal therapy is based on the estrogen receptor status of the tumor. Breast tissue normally develops with specific binding sites for control of hormones, including estrogen and progesterone. Fifty percent of tumors have hormone receptors that are sensitive to inhibition by endocrine manipulation, whereas only ten percent of tumors without these receptors respond to similar manipulation.

(1) Sixty-four percent of estrogen receptor–positive tumors respond to hormonal therapy, whereas only four percent of estrogen receptor–negative tumors respond.

(2) In estrogen receptor–positive patients with recurrent disease, a change in the hormonal environment usually affects the tumor size. In premenopausal patients, this change may be accomplished by adrenalectomy or oophorectomy; in postmenopausal patients estrogen therapy is used.

(3) Tamoxifen is an antiestrogen drug and is used in both pre- and postmenopausal patients.

(4) Male hormone therapy may also be useful in the treatment of both pre- and postmenopausal patients.

(5) Patients who respond to one treatment modality generally continue to respond to sequential hormonal therapy, whereas nonresponders do not. Few patients are cured once metastasis occurs, but hormonal therapy is very effective in prolonging survival and in reducing tumor size.

b. Chemotherapy is used in patients with recurrent disease who are estrogen receptor–negative or who do not respond to hormonal therapy. Combinations of cyclophosphamide, methotrexate, fluorouracil, and doxorubicin are usually used in these cases.

Temporary favorable responses, as determined by a measurable decrease in tumor size or the relief of pain, are obtained in 60%–80% of patients with stage IV disease with the initiation of this therapy.

IV. CARCINOMA OF THE MALE BREAST

A. Clinical presentation. Carcinoma of the male breast is uncommon but has a worse **prognosis** than carcinoma of the female breast. Most patients present with a unilateral painless mass. Gynecomastia is the principal differential diagnosis. One must obtain a thorough history regarding drug and hormone intake and alcohol ingestion.

B. Stages. Broken down by stage, not only is the survival rate worse than in women, but the usual case presents at a much later stage. The survival rates are as follows:

1. Stage I disease results in a 38% 10-year survival rate.

2. Stage II disease results in a 10% 10-year survival rate.

3. Stage III and IV disease are uniformly lethal.

C. Treatment is similar to that for carcinoma of the female breast.

1. Radical mastectomy has been the standard treatment.
    a. Modified radical mastectomy may be employed if the pectoralis major muscle is not involved.
    b. Occasionally, a lumpectomy with axillary dissection and postoperative irradiation can be used if the primary tumor is very small and does not involve the nipple–areola complex.

2. Castration is the principal means of endocrine control.

24
Organ Transplantation

Bruce E. Jarrell
Vincent T. Armenti

I. RENAL TRANSPLANTATION

A. Overview. Renal transplantation is a procedure involving the removal of a single kidney from one individual and placing it in another who has markedly impaired renal function. When the operation is successfully performed, patients return to normal lives with the ability to be fully employed, physically active, and unencumbered by dialysis. When successful, it is the best treatment for chronic renal failure, and it significantly debilitates patients only in situations of recurrent rejections if excessive steroid therapy is employed.

1. Classification of renal and other organ transplants depends on the relationship between the donor and the recipient.
   a. Autografts are tissues transferred from one area of the body to another in the same individual (e.g., a skin graft).
   b. Isografts are tissues transferred between genetically identical individuals (e.g., monozygotic twins).
   c. Allografts (homografts) are tissues transferred between genetically dissimilar individuals of the same species (e.g., cadaver renal transplants).
   d. Xenografts (heterografts) are tissues transplanted between species (e.g., porcine skin temporarily grafted on human burn victims).

2. Selection of donors
   a. Living related donors represent approximately one-third of all kidney donors.
   (1) The genotypes of the related donor and recipient are more compatible (see I A 3) than those of an unrelated donor and recipient. There are three potential histocompatibility matches.
      (a) A **perfect histocompatibility (two-haplotype) match** is one in which all antigens are matched. Siblings have a 25% chance of having identical antigens.
      (b) A **half histocompatibility (one-haplotype) match** is one in which 50% of the antigens are matched. Two siblings have a 50% chance of this occurring; however, this match occurs in essentially all parent/child relationships.
      (c) No **histocompatibility match** is present in 25% of siblings. With such a complete mismatch of antigens, the would-be donor is rarely used.
   (2) The living related donor must have a normal history and physical examination. The donor must be free of chronic and acute illnesses, especially infections, malignancies, diabetes mellitus, hypertension, psychiatric disorders, and significant cardiac, renal, pulmonary, and hepatic disease. Renal function must be normal.
   (3) The donor must have an in-hospital evaluation, including intravenous pyelography (IVP) and renal arteriography to demonstrate normal renal and urologic anatomy.
   (4) The mortality rate among donors is extremely low (0.05%) and is principally a result of general anesthesia problems or postoperative pulmonary embolism.
   (5) The donor has rapid compensatory hypertrophy of the remaining kidney. Creatinine clearance equals 70%–80% of the predonation level within 1 year after the donation.
   b. Cadaver donors are the source of kidneys for approximately two-thirds of all transplant recipients.
   (1) The kidneys are from young, previously healthy individuals who sustained irreversible brain injury. The donors must have no evidence of infection, extracranial malignancy, previous renal disease, hypertension, or diabetes. In addition, renal function must have been normal with minimal urinary abnormalities, if any.

    (2) Cadaver donors must fulfill the criteria of brain death as determined clinically by:
      (a) Deep coma with no response to painful stimuli
      (b) Absence of spontaneous respiration in the presence of a high arterial carbon dioxide tension ($PaCO_2$)
      (c) Absence of movement
      (d) Absence of all brain stem and higher reflexes
      (e) Absence of hypothermia and absence of depressant drugs, such as barbiturates in the blood
      (f) No change of these findings over a 24-hour period
      (g) Optionally, isoelectric electroencephalogram, absence of intracranial blood flow, or visual evidence of gross cerebral tissue destruction
    (3) The kidneys are surgically removed from heart-beating, brain-dead cadavers and are rapidly flushed and chilled to 4° C. They are preserved for up to 48 hours by cold storage in ice with no perfusion, using a concentrated potassium solution (i.e., 115 mEq/L), or with pulsatile perfusion, using plasma-type solutions.
  c. **Living unrelated donors** are rarely used in the United States. There is no immunologic advantage to kidneys from these donors over those from cadavers, and there remains the significant risk of the perioperative period.

3. **Immunologic compatibility of the recipient and the donor** determines the outcome of the transplantation for any type of tissue transplant.
  a. **ABO blood group compatibility** must be present. As in blood transfusions, an individual with an O blood type is a universal donor, whereas an individual with an AB blood type may only donate to an AB recipient.
  b. **Crossmatch compatibility** must be present. The recipient's blood is examined for the presence of cytotoxic antibodies specifically directed against antigens on the donor's T lymphocytes. If these antibodies are found, the donor is unacceptable because the recipient's antibodies would immediately attack the new kidney and rapidly destroy it.
  c. **Human leukocyte antigens (HLAs).** Histocompatibility antigen typing is performed. Humans have HLA-A, -B, -C, and -D loci on the immune regulatory gene area of chromosome 6, which is primarily responsible for humoral and cellular immune responses. Attempts to match these antigens between the donor and recipient are made to minimize the genetic dissimilarity between the two.
    (1) **HLA-A and -B loci.** Each locus contains subloci characterized by 30–40 antigenic specificities. These specificities are characterized by specific antisera directed against T-lymphocyte surface antigens. The microcytotoxicity assay uses complement and requires about 6 hours to perform.
      (a) A match between HLA-A and -B indicates an excellent possibility of graft survival when the donor is a living relative.
        (i) There is a 90% graft survival rate at 2 years with a perfect HLA-A and -B match.
        (ii) There is a 65%–85% graft survival rate at 2 years with a 50% HLA-A and -B match.
      (b) Transplantation results are variable when the HLA-A and -B loci of recipients and cadaver donors are matched.
        (i) European studies of HLA-A and -B matches show a significant effect of matching.
        (ii) American results show a weak or no difference between the two groups.
    (2) The **HLA-C locus** is not known to affect the outcome of transplantation.
    (3) The **HLA-D locus** is the locus that determines cellular activity in a mixed lymphocyte reaction.
      (a) Blast cells form in a culture of lymphocytes from both donor and recipient, and the degree of histocompatibility between the two is indicated by the number of blast cells.
      (b) The mixed lymphocyte reaction correlates to the host lymphocytic immune reaction towards the donor cellular antigens in vitro.
      (c) A match of HLA-D loci indicates an excellent possibility of graft survival when the donor is a living relative.
      (d) A match of HLA-D loci is untestable with cadaver donors because of the prolonged (5–7-day) incubation time required to produce results.
    (4) The **DR (D-related) locus** is linked very closely to the HLA-D locus. The DR antigen is detected serologically in a manner similar to the HLA-A and -B locus microcytotoxicity test and in a similar time frame; however, B lymphocytes rather than T lymphocytes are

the target cells because T lymphocytes do not have D-locus antigens upon their surface. A DR-locus perfect match generally results in an improvement in graft survival.

   d. Pretransplantation transfusion

     (1) Random third-party-donor blood transfusions, when given to transplant candidates prior to transplantation, raise the graft survival rate significantly.

       (a) There is a correlation between the number of transfusions given and improvement in graft survival.

       (b) There is an immune response in the form of humoral sensitization after transfusion in approximately 10% of patients. These individuals may create antibodies against the antigens of most of the population, which occasionally prevents transplantation.

       (c) The risk of transmitting hepatitis or other viral illnesses is present as it is with any transfusion.

       (d) The mechanism of graft tolerance after transfusion is unknown. It includes, at least partly, the induction of an active immune blocking phenomenon.

     (2) Donor-specific blood transfusions are used when a recipient and a living related donor have a half histocompatibility (one-haplotype) match for HLA-A, -B, -C, and -DR loci in the presence of a reactive mixed lymphocyte reaction. The recipient is transfused with blood from the potential kidney donor on three separate occasions.

       (a) Donor-specific transfusions sensitize the recipient to that specific donor in 20%–30% of cases; thus, that individual must be eliminated as a donor.

       (b) The transplantation success rate in this group is over 90% at 2 years in comparison to a 65%–85% success rate at 2 years for nontransfused donor/recipient pairs.

   e. Pretransplantation splenectomy may be performed in transplantation candidates with hypersplenism and pancytopenia. Splenectomy reduces the incidence of leukopenia, so that larger amounts of immunosuppressive drugs may be given. In some centers, pretransplantation splenectomy is associated with an increased rate of graft survival. Although the procedure may not increase the short-term risk of infection, the long-term risk is not known.

B. Preoperative management

   1. Transplant candidates. End-stage renal disease patients between the ages of 5 and 70 years who are on maintenance dialysis are candidates for transplantation. Increasing age (above 60 years) is considered high risk because these patients are more susceptible to infectious complications.

   2. Acute or chronic infections, whether bacterial, viral, or fungal, should not be present.

     a. A positive purified protein derivative (PPD) tuberculin test is not necessarily a contraindication to transplantation; if it is positive, isoniazid (INH) should be given for at least the first post-transplantation year. If evidence of active tuberculosis is present, the transplant should be postponed until no active disease is present.

     b. Urine cultures should be negative; if they are positive, a complete urologic examination should be performed. A nephrectomy is performed if the source of infection is renal.

   3. A normal urinary system is ideal, and any urologic problems should be resolved.

     a. Vesicoureteral reflux should be absent; if it is present, a nephrectomy is indicated, particularly with a history of infection.

     b. Vesical outlet obstruction should be relieved prior to transplantation.

     c. A neurogenic bladder may be used as the site for implantation; an ileal loop is rarely necessary.

   4. The recipient's own kidneys are occasionally removed. In addition to infection or reflux, indications for removal include the presence of:

     a. Severe unmanageable hypertension, especially with elevated renin levels

     b. Polycystic kidneys if recurrent cyst hemorrhage or infection occurs. (Polycystic kidneys frequently are associated with a high hematocrit and residual urine output and are best preserved, if possible.)

   5. Autoimmune diseases characterized by glomerular basement membrane antibodies, such as Wegener's granulomatosis, Goodpasture's syndrome, and certain other types of glomerulonephritis (see I F 3 b) should be quiescent prior to transplantation.

   6. Secondary hyperparathyroidism and severe bone disease do not constitute a contraindication to transplantation and usually improve postoperatively.

7. **Significant gastroenterologic disease** should be identified and resolved prior to transplantation.
   a. Active hepatitis should not be present.
   b. Chronic hepatitis should show minimal activity on biopsy (a positive hepatitis surface antigen is not a contraindication in many centers).
   c. Peptic ulcer disease should be identified in older age groups; if present, proof of healing should be obtained. Some centers recommend prophylactic acid-reducing operations because the mortality rate from bleeding or perforated ulcer disease post-transplantation varies from 25%–85%.
   d. Diverticulosis of the colon should be identified in older age groups and in patients with polycystic kidneys. If a patient has extensive diverticula or a previous episode of diverticulitis or diverticular bleeding, a prophylactic colectomy should be considered because of the high mortality rate of these colon complications post-transplantation.

8. **Malignant disease** either currently or in the recent past is a contraindication to immunosuppression and, therefore, to transplantation because of the risk of recurrence.
   a. Low-grade malignancies, especially those of the skin and occurring in the distant past, may be an acceptable risk.
   b. A history of Wilms' tumor in infancy may allow transplantation at an older age. This is because the tumor has a very predictable doubling time, which is defined by the age at tumor presentation plus 9 months. If that amount of time has elapsed since surgical removal of the tumor, and there is no evidence of recurrence, then it is unlikely to recur.

9. **Metabolic diseases,** such as oxalosis, frequently recur rapidly in transplanted kidneys, and good results of the transplantation may be limited.

C. **Operative management**

1. **The surgical procedure** in transplantation involves placing the kidney in either iliac fossa retroperitoneally. The vessels are anastomosed to the iliac artery and vein in adults and occasionally to the aorta and inferior vena cava in small children. The ureter is directly implanted into the bladder (Figure 24-1).

2. **Surgical complications** are not uncommon and are usually treatable if they are recognized at an early stage.
   a. **Vascular complications** include renal artery stenosis or thrombosis and renal vein thrombosis. Patients may present with sudden anuria or severe hypertension postoperatively. Rapid diagnosis may be made by means of a renal flow radioisotope scan, arteriography, or re-exploration.

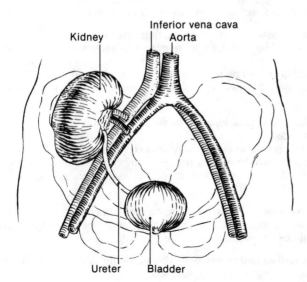

Figure 24-1. Placement of the renal transplant.

    b. Lymphatic complications appear as an acute perinephric lymph collection or lymphocele developing as a result of inadequately ligated lymphatics in the operative field. The lymphocele may present as a mass, as wound drainage, or as acute anuria. The best means of confirming the diagnosis is through ultrasound examination. The lymphocele is drained by either surgical exposure or percutaneous needle aspiration.

    c. Urologic complications in the transplanted patient include urine leakage at the ureter–bladder anastomosis and ureteric obstruction or infarction due to the interruption of ureteric blood supply, which may occur during donor nephrectomy. Arteries leading to the lower pole of the kidney usually vascularize the upper ureter and must be preserved and revascularized. The diagnosis of urologic complications can be confirmed by means of radioisotope scanning, ultrasound examination, or intravenous pyelography. Treatment varies according to each diagnosis.

D. Postoperative management

1. Immunosuppression has significantly changed over the past 5 years with the introduction of cyclosporine. Many centers use cyclosporine as the principal immunosuppressive drug and supplement it with prednisone and azathioprine.

    a. Cyclosporine inhibits antigen recognition and processing by the helper T lymphocyte. This specifically directed mechanism provides potent immunosuppression for organ transplantation, allowing lower doses of other immunosuppressive drugs. This has a net effect of improving graft survival and lowering infectious complications.

      (1) Cyclosporine is a lipid-soluble drug given in a dose ranging from 1–10 mg/kg/day in most patients. The dosage management is based on serum or blood levels measured by either radioimmunoassay or high-pressure liquid chromatography (HPLC). Acceptable levels and the method of measurement vary among centers.

      (2) Cyclosporine has significantly improved graft success in the early follow-up periods (3–4 years), but its long-term effect is not clear at this time.

      (3) Cyclosporine is associated with significant renal toxicity. Administration of cyclosporine at the time of transplantation is associated with an increased incidence of acute tubular necrosis, and long-term administration has been associated with deterioration of renal function, although this effect may be dose-related. Other side effects include:

        (a) Hypertension

        (b) Hirsutism

        (c) Tremor

        (d) Gingival hyperplasia

        (e) Mono- and polyclonal B-cell lymphomas

    b. Orthoclone (OKT-3) is a murine monoclonal antibody produced against human T cells and specifically directed toward the T3 (CD3) antigen. OKT-3 is highly effective in destroying circulating CD3-positive cells. Its principal use is for treating acute rejection, although it is also used during the first 2 weeks following transplantation at some centers. It is associated with pulmonary edema in patients who are fluid overloaded and, therefore, must be administered with caution.

    c. Prednisone is a steroid preparation used in combination with cyclosporine or azathioprine. It has a nonspecific immunosuppressive action on both cell-mediated and humoral immunity.

      (1) High doses (0.5–2 mg/kg body weight/day) are administered early postoperatively, and doses are serially reduced with time.

      (2) Prednisone therapy is associated with very significant complications, especially infections and peptic ulcer disease. The likelihood of these complications occurring is partially dose-related.

    d. Azathioprine (Imuran) inhibits lymphoid differentiation, especially the differentiation of T lymphocytes; however, it operates as a nonspecific immunosuppressant. It is converted to 6-mercaptopurine by the liver.

      (1) Azathioprine is given at a dose of 1–2 mg/kg of body weight and is continued as long as the graft is functional. Up to a 30% dose reduction is necessary if renal function diminishes.

      (2) Therapy is monitored by daily white blood cell and platelet counts.

      (3) Mild to moderate leukopenia develops in some patients.

    e. Antilymphocyte globulin (ALG) is a serum prepared by immunizing nonhuman animals with human lymphatic cells, allowing an immune response to generate antihuman lymphocyte antibodies, which are then collected and purified for human use. It is a specific immunosuppressive agent directed against T lymphocytes and may be monitored by the absolute T-lymphocyte count in the peripheral blood.

(1) Some centers use ALG prophylactically for 14 days postoperatively, and it is used successfully in many centers for acute rejection episodes.

(2) Therapy is associated with an increase in viral infections, especially from cytomegalovirus (CMV). In addition, there is a low risk of anaphylaxis from the foreign serum.

2. **Postoperative renal function** usually returns rapidly to normal in transplanted kidneys from living related donors and in those from most cadavers with a brisk diuresis and a rapid drop in serum creatinine.

a. Cadaver donor transplants are occasionally associated with a 1–10-day episode of acute tubular necrosis. This is usually a temporary condition, resulting from conditions during obtaining or preserving the donor kidney and is followed by a diuresis and normal renal function.

b. The transplanted kidney undergoes compensatory hypertrophy with a final creatinine clearance rate of 70%–80% of normal if rejection does not intervene.

E. **Results of renal transplantation** vary considerably among centers but are still strongly **dependent upon the type of histocompatibility match**. Second and third transplants may be performed safely; the results are generally acceptable and parallel those of earlier transplants.

1. **Living related donor transplants** are the most successful.

a. **Patient survival rates** are 90%–95% at 5 years.

b. **Kidney survival rates** are also excellent.

(1) Perfect matches (two-haplotype matches) result in a 2-year kidney survival rate of 85%–95%.

(2) Half matches (one-haplotype) with low donor/recipient mixed lymphocyte cultures (i.e., with good HLA-D matches) have a kidney survival rate of 70%–85% at 2 years.

(3) Half matches with reactive donor/recipient mixed lymphocyte cultures result in a kidney survival rate of 50%–70% at 2 years.

(4) Half matches with donor-specific transfusions have a kidney survival rate of 90% at 2 years.

2. **Cadaver donor transplants** show much more variable results; however, the results have improved generally because of blood transfusions, better tissue matching, and administration of cyclosporine.

a. **Patient survival rates** over 5 years are 75%–85%.

b. **Kidney survival rates** vary.

(1) Multiple center results suggest that the 1-year graft survival for cyclosporine-treated patients ranges from 70%–90%. After the first year, the rate of kidney loss slowly continues. The rate of loss is exponential with time and has been estimated to have a half-life (i.e., the period of time in which one-half of the kidneys are lost) of 7½ years.

(2) Kidneys that are perfectly matched with the recipient (all HLA-A, -B, and -DR antigens are either completely matched or no antigens are mismatched) may have a modest increase in long-term graft survival. Lesser matches are unlikely to improve graft survival. Prior to cyclosporine use, HLA matching and pretransplant blood transfusion improved graft function, but this is controversial now with the use of cyclosporine.

F. **Complications**

1. **Renal transplant rejection** is an episode of increased immune activity directed towards destruction of the graft.

a. **The incidence of rejection episodes** varies with the type of donor used.

(1) Perfect-match, living related donor transplant recipients experience an episode of rejection in 10%–20% of cases.

(2) Recipients of transplants from cadavers or from non–perfect-match living related donors experience an episode of rejection in 50%–90% of cases.

b. **Four types of rejection** are classified by the time of occurrence in relation to the operation and the type of immune response involved.

(1) **Hyperacute rejection** is associated with preformed antibody and complement deposition on vascular endothelium followed by activation of the coagulation system. It results in a flaccid, cyanotic, anuric, and eventually thrombosed kidney while the patient is still

in the operating room. Histologic examination shows polymorphonuclear leukocytes in peritubular and glomerular capillaries, and endothelial necrosis. Hyperacute rejection is treated by nephrectomy, usually at the time of the transplant operation.

(2) **Accelerated acute rejection** is a rapidly evolving rejection that occurs within the first week of transplantation and is associated with sudden anuria. It is probably a second-set, or anamnestic, immune response, mediated by both humoral and cellular elements. Extensive arteriolar necrosis and vasculitis are revealed by histologic examination. Accelerated rejection is treated by high doses of prednisone but with a poor success rate for both immediate and long-term graft survival.

(3) **Acute rejection** usually occurs within the first 3 months post-transplantation and is the commonest type of rejection. It is characterized by a rising serum creatinine level, increasing proteinuria, oliguria, weight gain, fever, and graft tenderness developing over several days. It is usually diagnosed on clinical grounds or by renal biopsy. There is T-lymphocyte–mediated infiltration of vascular and interstitial renal elements. Traditionally, acute rejection has been treated with high doses of methylprednisolone (i.e., 1–6 g over 1–2 weeks). When this treatment fails, ALG or OKT-3 is used with excellent resolution of the episode in many cases.

(4) **Chronic rejection** is associated with a slow decline in renal function over months or years, usually including a rising serum creatinine level, increasing proteinuria, hypertension, and edema. There is vascular intimal thickening and tubular atrophy. Chronic rejection results from both humoral and cellular destructive events. Although there is no known effective treatment, the process may be slowed by dietary protein restriction.

2. **Infections** are the most dangerous sequelae of immunosuppression and transplantation.
   a. The chance of infection is increased by the use of high doses of steroids to treat rejection episodes. Patients over 45 years of age, diabetics, and patients with advanced disease are most susceptible.
   b. The commonest infection to occur within the first several months post-transplantation is viral, especially CMV. It is not unusual for opportunistic organisms such as *Aspergillus, Cryptococcus,* and *Listeria monocytogenes* to infect the patients.
   c. Administration of immunosuppressive drugs should be stopped or markedly reduced to allow the immune system to eliminate the organism.
   d. There should be aggressive diagnosis so that rapid and appropriate antibiotic treatment can be instituted; when that is accomplished, the patient has an excellent chance of recovery.

3. **Glomerulonephritis** in the transplanted kidney may arise as the recurrence of original disease or de novo.
   a. Glomerulonephritis is diagnosed on renal biopsy. Unfortunately, most of these diseases have no specific treatment other than administration of the immunosuppressive drugs used for the transplant or a return to dialysis.
   b. Recurrent glomerulonephritis is associated with several types of original disease, including:
      (1) Antiglomerular basement membrane disease (e.g., Goodpasture's syndrome, Wegener's granulomatosis)
      (2) Acute immune complex disease
      (3) Membranous glomerulonephritis
      (4) Focal glomerulosclerosis
      (5) Membranoproliferative glomerulonephritis

4. **Long-term complications**
   a. **Cardiovascular disease** continues or worsens post-transplantation in many patients. Any patient with chronic renal failure has a markedly increased risk of death from cardiovascular disease whether he or she is treated by dialysis or transplantation.
      (1) **Hypertension** occurs in up to 83% of patients post-transplantation.
      (2) **Hyperlipidemia** occurs in up to 78% of patients.
      (3) **Coronary heart disease** varies widely in incidence among centers, ranging from 2–25 times the normal risk of death. (Clearly, atherosclerosis continues to progress after the transplantation.)
      (4) **Cerebrovascular disease** is reported to be as much as 300 times commoner than in control populations.
   b. **Cancer.** The incidence of malignant disease is increased in all transplant patients, warranting careful routine long-term screening. Primary cancers develop in 5.6% of all transplant

recipients. This incidence is 100 times greater than that in age-matched controls. It increases with the increasing duration of immunosuppression.

(1) The etiology is related at least in part to an altered immune status with failure of immune tumor surveillance.

(2) Types of malignancy

(a) Skin cancers represent approximately 40% of all primary post-transplant cancers; in areas in which sunlight exposure is high, the frequency approaches 70%.

(b) Non-Hodgkin's lymphomas represent 25% of all primary post-transplant cancers in patients treated long-term with azathioprine and prednisone. This frequency is 350 times the incidence in controls. Commonest are reticulum cell sarcomas, frequently involving the central nervous system.

(c) In cyclosporine-treated patients, non-Hodgkin's lymphoma also occurs but with different characteristics. These tumors tend to occur early post-transplantation. They usually do not involve the central nervous system but rather involve the peripheral lymph nodes, especially nodes of the small bowel. The lymphomas range from benign polyclonal to malignant monoclonal B-cell lymphomas.

(d) Other cancers also occur more commonly in transplant patients than in the general population.

c. **Aseptic necrosis of the hip or knee** occurs in up to 10% of transplant patients long-term, probably as a result of steroid therapy. Frequently, a prosthetic hip replacement is required for relief of pain. The incidence may be minimized by reducing the use of prednisone therapy.

d. **Obesity and cushingoid features** are common in these patients but frequently become less prominent as the daily dose of prednisone is lowered.

e. **Cataracts** occur more commonly in renal transplant recipients than in age-matched controls.

II. HEPATIC TRANSPLANTATION is a procedure involving removal of a diseased liver and replacement by a cadaver donor liver. The procedure itself is difficult due to the presence of portal hypertension, portosystemic collateral connections, coagulopathy, and often a cirrhotic liver. The postoperative course can be smooth or, alternatively, difficult, depending upon the initial state of the patient, the function of the new liver, and any technical problems encountered in the perioperative period. Once recovered, the patient usually returns to health and can look forward to a long life.

A. Recipient selection

1. Patients with end-stage hepatic failure who have a low likelihood for survival past 1–2 years are the commonest candidates for hepatic transplantation. The commonest pathologic processes are:

   a. Primary biliary cirrhosis
   b. Sclerosing cholangitis
   c. Chronic hepatitis (non-A, non-B variety). Hepatitis A rarely requires hepatic transplantation in the United States. Results with hepatitis B are controversial.
   d. Cryptogenic cirrhosis
   e. Alcoholic cirrhosis. Good results, including postoperative rehabilitation, have been obtained in this group of patients, particularly those who abstain from alcohol for a sustained period of time prior to transplantation.
   f. Metabolic diseases, including α_1-antitrypsin deficiency, Wilson's disease, and histiocytosis X
   g. Biliary atresia, usually in children
   h. Congenital hepatic fibrosis
   i. Caroli's disease
   j. Secondary biliary cirrhosis

2. **Controversial indications for transplantation** include:

   a. Primary malignancies of the liver, particularly hepatocellular carcinoma. Insufficient data have been collected to recommend firmly transplant for this disease. Currently, hepatic resection is preferable where feasible.
   b. Fulminant hepatic failure due to hepatitis may result in deep coma, renal failure, and general organ failure. If transplanted before irreversible brain injury occurs, full recovery of the patient can occur. Hepatitis usually recurs histologically, but the clinical manifestations of the disease are significantly altered and improved.

    c. Fulminant hepatic failure due to ingestion of a toxin, such as acetaminophen. If the patient has a significant, severe psychiatric history and this is a suicide attempt, hepatic transplantation may not be indicated. Otherwise excellent results can be obtained.

   3. The commonest clinical events that precipitate the decision to proceed with hepatic transplantation are:

    a. Progressive deterioration of the general status of the patient with muscle wasting, low serum albumin, malnutrition, and generalized malaise

    b. Encephalopathy, whether severe and affecting the level of consciousness, or subtle and affecting higher levels of cognitive activities

    c. Hemorrhage from esophageal varices

    d. Recurrent spontaneous bacterial peritonitis

    e. Ascites that is difficult to manage, requiring dietary restrictions and diuretic therapy

B. Donor selection. Donors are generally similar to donors of other organs. Specific parameters include:

   1. Stable cardiovascular function and absence of infection or malignancy

   2. Liver function that is stable or improving. Laboratory values do not have to be totally normal, and modest elevations in bilirubin, hepatic enzymes, and coagulation function are acceptable if they are acute and potentially reversible.

   3. Age between birth and 60 years

   4. A compatible size of the organ donor, which should be matched to within 10%–20% of the recipient. This is particularly true for pediatric donors, and because of this problem, donors for young children are scarce. Hepatic resections while the organ is stored to reduce liver size have been used to alleviate this problem.

   5. Blood group matching (i.e., an "O" blood group liver into an "O" blood group recipient). No attempt to match organs based on HLA type or crossmatch is currently undertaken.

   6. Viability of the liver for up to 24 hours if preserved in the University of Wisconsin (UW) solution

C. Operative management. The hepatic transplant operation requires 6–12 hours to perform. The steps include:

   1. Removal of the diseased liver. This requires dissection of the porta hepatis structures, the infra- and supra-hepatic vena cavae, and the posterior hepatic structures.

   2. Implantation of the new liver

    a. The blood flow to the diseased liver is interrupted, and the liver is removed, during which time the patient is anhepatic and requires intensive monitoring to maintain normal homeostasis.

    b. The venous return from the lower body torso to the heart is also interrupted, and often an external bypass (the veno-veno bypass) from the femoral and portal veins to the subclavian vein is necessary to maintain cardiac output and prevent lower body edema.

    c. The new liver is sutured into place, including both vena cava connections and the portal vein anastomosis.

   3. Reperfusion of the new liver may be associated with hypotension due to release of substances, such as potassium or acid products, from the preserved liver. Hypothermia may also be a problem. The new liver often functions immediately, resulting in correction of coagulation defects and production of bile.

   4. Maintenance of homeostasis, hepatic arterial reconstruction, and biliary tract reconstruction complete the operation. The bile duct is reconstructed as either a choledochocholedochostomy or a choledochojejunostomy to a Roux-en-Y segment of jejunum.

D. Postoperative management is variable. Specific problems relate to:

   1. Intra-abdominal hematoma due to delayed graft function

   2. Intra-abdominal infection, including opportunistic infections, such as fungal infections

   3. Leakage of the biliary tract reconstruction. This may be due to inadequate biliary duct blood supply, but this has also been associated with hepatic artery thrombosis.

4. Renal failure, usually secondary to either operative hypotension or cyclosporine nephrotoxicity

5. Usual postoperative problems, including pulmonary problems, intravenous catheter sepsis, or ileus

E. Immunosuppression is maintained similarly to renal transplantation (see I D 1).

F. Liver biopsy, which plays an important role in therapeutic decisions, can be performed at the bedside by a percutaneous technique.

G. Long-term survival for most programs is approximately 70% at 1 year; however, survival is a function of the degree of illness of the preoperative patient. Causes for failure, resulting in either death or retransplantation, include:

1. Acute or chronic rejection

2. Infection, including bacterial and fungal sepsis and reactivation of CMV

3. Recurrent or de novo hepatitis

4. Vanishing bile duct syndrome. Pathologically, progressive destruction of the intrahepatic bile ductules in the portal triad is present.

III. PANCREATIC TRANSPLANTATION. The clinical application of pancreatic transplantation has been limited by both technical and immunologic problems. With the use of cyclosporine and both whole organ and segmental grafts, the number of successful transplants has improved. Isolated islet cells, which theoretically could provide physiologic glucose control, have had very limited success.

A. Recipient selection. Pancreas transplantation is generally not performed in selected diabetic patients when moderate to severe secondary complications of diabetes are present. Blood typing and HLA matching are performed.

B. Operative management. Both cadaver whole organ and living related segmental grafts have been used.

1. Cadaver whole pancreas with a segment of duodenum is harvested from a donor. The portal vein, superior mesenteric artery, and celiac axis are included. If a combined liver-pancreas harvest is performed, the splenic artery is taken, and the remainder of the celiac axis is included with the liver harvest.

2. The donor vessels are anastomosed to the recipient's iliac vessels. The duodenum is usually anastomosed to the bladder.

3. Segmental grafts have been taken from living related donors. The vascular anastomoses are managed in the same way. Techniques for duct occlusion as well as enteric drainage have been described in addition to bladder drainage.

C. Postoperative management

1. Protocols for immunosuppression include the use of cyclosporine A and prednisone or triple therapy with the addition of azathioprine.

2. Complications include graft thrombosis, fibrosis, and pancreatic fistula.

3. With improved techniques and immunosuppression, 1-year graft survival is over 50%.

IV. HEART TRANSPLANTATION

A. Recipient selection

1. Patients with end-stage heart disease who are unlikely to survive 1 year may be candidates for heart transplantation.

2. Selected patients with irreversible damage to heart and lungs may be candidates for combined heart–lung transplantation.

   B. Donor selection

   1. Procurement of organs remains an obstacle.

   2. The donor procedure must be timed with the recipient's to keep ischemic time to a minimum.

   3. Donors are matched with recipients for size and blood type.

   C. Immunosuppression. Cyclosporine and prednisone are used as immunosuppressants. Rejection is monitored by frequent endomyocardial biopsies.

   D. Long-term survival. One-year graft survival of about 80% has been reported.

V. SMALL BOWEL TRANSPLANTATION remains an area for the future as it has been complicated by both technical problems and graft-versus-host disease.

25
Urologic Surgery
Demetrius H. Bagley

I. URINARY TRACT INFECTIONS (UTIs) are among the commonest bacterial infections. In evaluating affected individuals, the physician must determine, in addition to the diagnosis and the treatment required for the acute episode, the value of follow-up studies and the need for referral for further evaluation.

A. Clinical presentation

1. **Major symptoms** of urinary tract infection are related to vesical irritation. These include:
   a. Urinary frequency
   b. Urgency
   c. Pain on voiding
   d. Cloudy or foul-smelling urine

2. **Renal infection** may be indicated by the additional symptoms of:
   a. Fever
   b. Chills
   c. Flank pain

B. Diagnosis. Urinary tract infection is usually considered on the basis of clinical findings. The diagnosis is further supported by the finding of pyuria and bacteriuria on urinalysis and is confirmed by culture of the urine.

1. **Urinalysis** is a valuable screening procedure that can be performed in the physician's office.
   a. **Bacteriuria** is strongly indicated by the detection of bacteria on microscopic examination of the urine.
   b. **Pyuria,** the presence of white blood cells in the urine, indicates an inflammatory response within the urinary tract. The number of cells present can be affected by the technique of sample collection, by the handling of the specimen, and by the patient's state of hydration.

2. **Chemical studies.** Attempts have been made to use chemical studies to provide simple rapid screening for the presence of infection.
   a. **Nitrate reduction and urinary esterase detection**
      (1) Nitrate in the urine is reduced to nitrite in the presence of bacteria.
      (2) Leukocytes contain esterases, which can be detected in the urine.
      (3) Both nitrate reduction and urinary esterase can be indicated by a reagent, which changes color, and the two reactions have been combined on a dipstick as a nonspecific indicator of infection.
   b. **Other chemical tests** include:
      (1) Tetrazolium reduction
      (2) Urinary glucose reduction
      (3) Urinary catalase detection

3. **Urine culture** can determine the presence of bacteria in the urine. Standard culture plates or slides coated with agar can be used, and selective media assist in identification of the bacteria present.

4. **Antibiotic sensitivity testing.** Bacteria present in the urine at significant levels should be tested for their sensitivity to antibiotics.
   a. This is determined by culturing known quantities of bacteria on a plate containing disks impregnated with a known amount of antibiotic.

b. The zone of inhibition around these disks is related to both the concentration of the antibiotic and the sensitivity of the organism.

c. In most laboratories, the reported levels of sensitivity are related to serum antibiotic concentrations, which may be considerably less than the urinary concentrations.

C. Treatment of bladder infection consists of the administration of appropriate antibiotics. The duration of therapy has recently been of interest, and 1-day therapy appears to be as effective as therapy lasting 3, 7, or 10 days. In contrast, a longer course of therapy is necessary for renal infections.

II. RENAL INFECTIONS

A. Classification

1. Infections of the parenchyma include:
a. Generalized pyelonephritis
b. Localized forms called lobar nephronia, renal carbuncle, and perirenal phlegmon

2. Abscesses include:
a. Intrarenal abscess
b. Perinephric abscess
c. Infected renal cysts

B. Pyelonephritis usually has an acute onset and affects mainly young women.

1. Clinical presentation. Patients may present with high fever, chills, and flank or midback pain, often with irritative lower tract symptoms.

2. Etiology. The most frequent causative organism is *Escherichia coli.*

3. Diagnosis. Laboratory findings include pyuria and bacteriuria. The urine culture should yield bacteria to substantiate a diagnosis of pyelonephritis, unless the patient has recently taken antibiotics.

4. Treatment. The patient usually responds to antibiotic therapy within 2–5 days.
a. A patient needing a course longer than this should be evaluated further with radiologic studies.
b. Any underlying complications, such as calculus or obstruction, can then be treated appropriately.

C. Acute lobar nephronia describes an acute focal infection with a renal or perirenal mass but without abscess formation.

1. Clinical presentation. This illness is characterized by fever, flank pain, and pyuria, but there may be a more indolent course.

2. Treatment consists of administration of appropriate antibiotics. Patients who do not respond to therapy or who deteriorate clinically should be evaluated further.

D. Abscesses within the perinephric space usually result from rupture of an intrarenal abscess. They are associated with other factors predisposing to the renal abscess, including calculi and diabetes mellitus.

1. Clinical presentation is usually less dramatic than that of pyelonephritis. The fever is usually lower and may persist for several days before diagnosis, and the pain is milder and less frequent.

2. Etiology. *E. coli* and *Proteus mirabilis* are most frequently cultured from these abscesses.

3. Diagnosis. Radiologic studies are often helpful in making the diagnosis.
a. Chest x-ray reveals an effusion or elevation of the diaphragm.
b. An abdominal mass may be detected on excretory urography, but ultrasonography and computed tomography (CT scan) provide the most accurate localization of a perinephric abscess.

4. Treatment consists of drainage, usually with antibiotic administration.

E. Xanthogranulomatous pyelonephritis is a chronic infection of the renal parenchyma and is a pathologic diagnosis.

    1. Clinical presentation
        a. This infection is usually associated with obstruction, and calculi are frequently present.
        b. Women are affected more frequently than men, and the commonest symptoms are fever and flank or abdominal pain.

    2. Etiology. *E. coli* and *P. mirabilis* are the organisms most frequently cultured from this infection.

    3. Diagnosis. Excretory urography may demonstrate a nonfunctioning kidney or the presence of renal calculi. A renal mass can be demonstrated in 60% of patients; it often cannot be distinguished from a renal tumor.

    4. Treatment. If xanthogranulomatous pyelonephritis can be diagnosed preoperatively, it can be treated by partial nephrectomy. Often, it is diagnosed as renal cancer and treated by nephrectomy.

III. PROSTATITIS

A. Overview. Prostatitis, or inflammation of the prostate gland, is often overdiagnosed.

    1. Urinary frequency, urgency, dysuria, and perineal or suprapubic discomfort are symptoms of numerous other disorders, as well as prostatitis.

    2. The various inflammatory and noninflammatory prostatic conditions should be distinguished in patients who have similar symptom complexes; treatment can then be based on an accurate diagnosis.

B. Bacterial prostatitis exists in both acute and chronic forms.

    1. Diagnosis of bacterial prostatitis rests upon:
        a. Finding white blood cells within the prostatic fluid
        b. Detecting a significant number of bacteria in expressed prostatic fluid and distinguishing them from urethral organisms by differential cultures.

    2. Treatment. Patients often respond to a course of antimicrobial therapy, such as sulfamethoxazole–trimethoprim, tetracycline, or cabenicillin.

C. Nonbacterial prostatitis has also been called **prostatosis,** and the diagnosis depends upon finding prostatic fluid containing white blood cells but with cultures negative for bacteria. This diagnosis also includes patients with nonbacterial prostatic infections due to *Mycoplasma* and *Chlamydia* species.

D. Prostatodynia is a term describing symptoms similar to those of prostatitis but without inflammatory cells in the prostatic fluid and with cultures negative for microorganisms.

IV. URINARY CALCULI

A. Phases. The management of patients with urinary calculi within the kidney or ureter can be considered to have two phases.

    1. Acute phase. The patient has symptoms of obstruction or inflammation that result from the presence of the calculus.

    2. Metabolic phase. The metabolic basis for stone formation should be sought so that appropriate treatment prevents the growth or formation of calculi.

B. Clinical presentation

    1. The most frequent acute symptom of upper urinary calculi is pain.
        a. The site of the pain depends on the position of the calculus. The pain may be present in the upper back at the costovertebral angle, in the flank, or in the lower quadrant. It may radiate into the testicle or vulva.

b. Pain results from dilation of the ureter or renal pelvis and can occur with a calculus of any size.

2. Other symptoms include:
  a. Hematuria
  b. Nausea and vomiting
  c. Irritative bladder symptoms
  d. General abdominal discomfort, mimicking gastrointestinal disease

3. Physical examination
  a. Most patients are clearly in severe distress, unable to find any position of comfort.
  b. The abdomen should be examined closely. Bowel sounds may be decreased with a secondary ileus, and the costovertebral area is frequently tender.

C. Diagnosis

1. Urinalysis
  a. Hematuria is usually present, although its absence does not rule out the presence of a calculus.
  b. Crystals may give some indication of the presence and type of calculus.

2. Radiologic findings
  a. Plain radiogram of the abdomen can be very helpful in the evaluation of the patient suspected of having a calculus. Since most calculi are radiopaque, the presence of a calculus may be detected, although its exact identification as a urinary calculus cannot be made on a single plain x-ray.
  b. Excretory urography can usually locate a calculus accurately in the urinary tract. In the presence of obstruction, visualization of the kidney may be delayed, or dilation of the intrarenal collecting system may be apparent.
  c. Other studies are less frequently of value.
    (1) Ultrasonography may define hydronephrosis or demonstrate an acoustic shadow from a calculus.
    (2) Retrograde urography is occasionally valuable to provide contrast within the urinary tract, allowing opacification in the patient who is allergic to contrast medium or has a nonfunctioning kidney.
    (3) CT scan is not very helpful in the diagnosis of urinary calculi, but it has specific benefits in evaluating lucent intraluminal filling defects by differentiating soft tissue lesions from dense calculi.

D. Surgical treatment

1. Indications for surgery
  a. Interventional procedures are not necessary in all patients with calculi or even in all patients with symptomatic calculi. The indications for the removal of calculi or for urinary drainage listed in Table 25-1 are not absolute.
  b. The patient must be actively involved in any decision for intervention. Some patients tolerate pain much better than others and may prefer to wait for a ureteral calculus to pass by itself. Others may find that any delay interferes with their life-style and may demand early intervention.

2. Surgical procedures
  a. Any renal or ureteral calculus can be removed by open surgical procedures. However, there has been a strong movement away from such procedures to endourologic and endoscopic techniques.
  b. Percutaneous nephrostomy can approach calculi throughout the kidney and in the ureter.

Table 25-1. Indications for Removal of Urinary Calculi

Severe pain
Infection
Severe obstruction
Growth of calculus
Nonprogression
Interference with life-style

(1) Large calculi can be fragmented, using ultrasonic, electrohydraulic, or laser lithotriptors, and small calculi can be withdrawn intact.

(2) The percutaneous approach has been more effective for simple renal calculi, and less successful for branched renal calculi or for ureteral calculi.

3. Transurethral procedures

a. Ureteral calculi that originated in the renal collecting system become symptomatic as they pass into the ureter and cause obstruction.

b. Most ureteral calculi pass spontaneously.

(1) Those measuring less than 4 mm in diameter and located in the distal ureter are the most likely (90%) to pass.

(2) This probability declines to 50% as the calculus increases from 4–5.9 mm in diameter.

(3) It drops to 20% for calculi greater than 6 mm.

(4) Proximal ureteral calculi are less likely to pass, but the frequency is also related to the size of the calculus.

c. **Surgical removal**

(1) Calculi below the pelvic rim can be manipulated with a **"basket"** (a catheter with wires to trap the stone) from the level of the bladder.

(2) Success has been achieved by visualizing the calculus with a **ureteroscope** passed directly into the ureter. Calculi can then be retrieved with various grasping instruments or fragmented for removal.

4. Shock wave lithotripsy

a. This procedure consists of an external energy source, which is focused to provide a high-pressure zone that can be directed to fragment a calculus within the body.

(1) Spark gap, piezoelectric, and electromagnetic energy sources have been employed.

(2) Stone localization has been by either fluoroscopy or sonography.

(3) The energy source is coupled to the patient with a water bath or a water-filled pliable cushion.

b. The fragments must pass through the ureter.

c. The success has been highest for small intrarenal calculi, but ureteral calculi have also been treated. Stones greater than 2.5 cm in diameter and branched calculi are best treated by combination therapy with percutaneous debulking.

d. Complications requiring additional procedures, such as percutaneous nephrostomy or ureteroscopy, occur in 10%–30% of cases.

E. Metabolic evaluation and prophylaxis. It is important to know the composition of any calculi removed from or passed by a patient to direct appropriate metabolic study and eventual therapy. Table 25-2 lists the chemical types of calculi in descending order of occurrence.

1. Calcium-containing calculi. Most calculi contain calcium in the form of calcium oxalate, calcium phosphate, or both. The frequency of calculi containing calcium is three times greater in men than in women.

a. All patients who form a calcium calculus should be screened with a blood count, urinalysis, serum chemistry evaluation, excretory urography, and analysis of a 24-hour urine sample to check for calcium, phosphate, uric acid, creatinine, oxalate, and citrate.

b. Young women with a single calculus, men with a second calculus, and patients with calculi that are increasing in number or size should have a full metabolic evaluation, which can be performed as an outpatient procedure before and after calcium loading to distinguish patients with **renal hypercalciuria, absorptive hypercalciuria, hyperparathyroidism,** or **normocalciuric stone formation.**

Table 25-2. Composition of Urinary Calculi

Descending Frequency of Occurrence
Calcium oxalate and calcium phosphate
Calcium oxalate
Struvite (magnesium ammonium phosphate)
Calcium phosphate
Uric acid
Cystine

    c. Treatment is tailored to the patient and may include:
      (1) Thiazide diuretics
      (2) Orthophosphates
      (3) Dietary calcium restriction
      (4) Potassium citrate
      (5) Hydration to maintain a urine output of 3–4 L/day (in all patients)
    d. Conditions other than those listed in IV E 1 b, resulting in calcium stone formation, include:
      (1) Sarcoidosis
      (2) Renal tubular acidosis (type 1, distal renal tubular acidosis)
      (3) Hyperoxaluria

2. Infection-related calculi
    a. Struvite (magnesium ammonium phosphate) stones are associated with urinary tract infections and occur in women more often than in men.
      (1) Formation of struvite stones requires the presence of urea-splitting bacteria, which maintain a low pH with increased concentrations of bicarbonate and ammonium ions.
      (2) *Proteus* species are the commonest organisms causing stone formation.
    b. Treatment includes removal of the calculus and eradication of the urinary tract infection.
      (1) Antibiotic therapy pre- and postoperatively is essential.
      (2) Urease inhibitors have also been of value.

3. Uric acid calculi constitute only 5%–10% of stones in the United States.
    a. Uric acid is insoluble in water, but the urate salt can be formed by alkalization of the urine.
      (1) The pK_a of uric acid is 5.75, and, therefore, calculi can be dissolved and their formation prevented by maintaining the urinary pH at 6.5–7.0.
      (2) Allopurinol, which is a xanthine oxidase inhibitor, prevents the formation of uric acid and, thus, lowers the serum and urinary concentrations.
    b. Uric acid calculi are radiolucent and, therefore, must be demonstrated by x-ray studies using contrast medium or by other studies, such as ultrasonography or CT.

4. Cystine calculi
    a. Cystinuria is an uncommon autosomal recessive disorder that results in decreased reabsorption of dibasic amino acids from the renal tubule. **Cystine calculi** form only because of the low solubility of cystine in urine with a pH of up to 7.0.
    b. Fluid diuresis and alkalization to a peak pH of 7.5 is the most important **therapeutic measure**. Cystine-binding drugs, such as D-penicillamine or α-mercaptopropionylglycine, have also been used in patients with recurrent calculi.

V. GENITOURINARY INJURIES (see Chapter 21 1 C 5 c). Injuries to the genitalia and urinary tract are often associated with other injuries, and a high index of suspicion for genitourinary injuries in the patient with multiple trauma should be maintained to avoid a potentially disastrous situation.

A. Scrotal and testicular injury. Although the scrotum and its contents are mobile, they are subject to blunt and penetrating injuries.

1. Clinical presentation. The patient's only complaint may be local pain, and physical examination may be difficult if a large hematoma is present.

2. Diagnosis. Ultrasonography can be useful in examining the testicles.

3. Treatment
    a. Conservative treatment is sufficient if the testicles are palpably normal or if there is a nonexpanding hematoma.
    b. Surgical exploration
      (1) This should be undertaken in the following situations:
        (a) If a hematoma is enlarging
        (b) If the testicle has been fractured
        (c) If injury to the scrotum penetrates deeper than the dartos muscle
      (2) Appropriate repair of the scrotal contents can be undertaken, and the wound can be closed with drainage.

B. Urethral injury. The urethra is prone to damage when a "straddle" injury (e.g., from trauma while riding a bicycle) or pelvic fracture has occurred. The diagnosis rests upon proper evaluation of the patient in whom there is a suspicion of injury.

 1. Clinical presentation. The **classic signs of urethral damage** include:
  a. Blood at the urethral meatus
  b. Perineal ecchymosis or swelling
  c. Inability to void
  d. Palpable lower abdominal mass
  e. Associated pelvic fracture

 2. Diagnosis. Retrograde urethrography is the most valuable technique for the diagnosis of urethral injury. Contrast medium is injected into the urethra to fill the full length of the lumen.

 3. Treatment. If a urethral injury is demonstrated, **cystotomy drainage** should be performed.

C. Bladder injury

 1. Clinical presentation
  a. Injury to the bladder must be suspected in any patient with pelvic fracture or a history of lower abdominal trauma.
  b. Local or generalized abdominal pain and tenderness may be present on physical examination.

 2. Diagnosis. X-ray may demonstrate an associated pelvic fracture, while **cystography** is the most definitive test for **bladder rupture**.
  a. The bladder should be filled to capacity with 300 ml of contrast medium.
  b. Films should be obtained with the bladder full and again after drainage in an attempt to detect leakage of contrast from the ruptured bladder.

 3. Treatment. A ruptured bladder is treated by catheter drainage. Surgical repair is necessary as well in the case of intraperitoneal rupture.

D. Renal injury

 1. Clinical presentation. Renal injury should be suspected in patients with abdominal or lower thoracic trauma. Patients may have localized flank pain or may be free of symptoms. A **local flank contusion** should increase the suspicion of injury. **Hematuria** supports the diagnosis, but its absence does not rule out renal injury.

 2. Classification. Renal injuries can be grouped according to severity, and treatment can be tailored to the injury.
  a. Minor injuries
   (1) Renal contusions or **ecchymoses** constitute approximately 85% of renal trauma.
   (2) Minor injuries also include **subcapsular hematomas** and **superficial cortical lacerations**.
   (3) Surgical exploration is not necessary.
  b. Major injuries
   (1) Major renal trauma includes **deep lacerations of the kidney,** extending into the collecting system. The value of immediate surgical exploration versus conservative treatment is controversial.
   (2) Multiple lacerations and **fragmentation of the kidney** are also considered major injuries and require early surgical intervention.
  c. Vascular injuries constitute only approximately 1% of blunt renal trauma.
   (1) The patient may **present** with massive bleeding or may be stable with the kidney showing lack of perfusion upon excretory urography.
   (2) Prompt diagnosis and treatment are required in any attempt to save the kidney.

 3. Diagnosis
  a. Excretory urography has been used most frequently and should be performed very early in the patient with multiple trauma.
  b. Arteriography can accurately define the renal injury and has been essential for diagnosis of renal pedicle damage.
  c. CT scan can accurately define parenchymal injuries.

VI. UROLOGIC CANCER

A. **Overview.** Diagnosis and treatment of neoplasms constitute a large portion of urologic practice. There have been dramatic advances in the treatment of certain neoplasms, such as testicular tumors and superficial bladder tumors, over the past 10 years. However, some lesions, such as renal carcinoma, remain poorly responsive, amenable only to surgical extirpation. Knowledge of urologic cancer must include familiarity with the natural history and alternative forms of therapy of the major urologic neoplasms.

B. **Renal cell carcinoma**

1. **Epidemiology**
   a. Renal cell carcinoma, also known as **renal adenocarcinoma** or **hypernephroma,** is the third commonest urologic cancer and is by far the **commonest malignant tumor of the kidney.**
   b. It occurs more frequently in men than women in a ratio of 3:1, and it achieves its peak incidence in the fifth and sixth decades of life.

2. **Etiology.** Although the etiology of this lesion is not known, environmental chemicals, smoking, exogenous hormones, and viruses have been associated with the occurrence of the tumor.

3. **Clinical presentation**
   a. The classic triad consisting of **flank mass, gross hematuria,** and **flank** or **abdominal pain** is a late manifestation of renal tumors and occurs in only 5% of patients.
   b. Hematuria is the most frequent finding, occurring in more than 38% of patients.
   c. Fever, anemia, erythrocytosis, as well as evidence of metastases may be the presenting symptoms of this tumor.

4. **Diagnosis**
   a. **Excretory urography with nephrotomography** is usually the first study obtained to indicate the presence of a renal tumor presenting as a renal mass. The pattern of the mass may be characteristic of a renal tumor, or the presence of calcification may suggest the diagnosis.
   b. Frequently, other studies are needed to differentiate among various renal masses.
      (1) **Ultrasonography** is extremely accurate in distinguishing classic renal cysts from solid mass lesions or complex cysts.
      (2) **Cystic puncture** is used when ultrasonography cannot provide a diagnosis. The contents are examined, and the presence of blood, fat, or malignant cells indicates the necessity for further evaluation and treatment.
      (3) **CT scan** can help to differentiate cysts, including multilocular cysts, and angiomyolipomas from renal cell tumors.
   c. **Renal arteriography** has long been the standard for the diagnosis of renal cell carcinoma but has been largely replaced by CT.
      (1) Renal tumors are usually quite vascular and have a distorted pattern, including pooling of contrast medium and a tumor "blush" characteristic of neoplasms.
      (2) Vascular encasement, arteriovenous fistulas, and parasitic vasculature from adjacent tissues may also be evident.

5. **Staging.** To determine the appropriate treatment of any neoplasm, the extent or stage of the disease must be determined.
   a. **Staging systems.** The most popular staging system remains that described by Robson. There is also a tumor, node, and metastasis (TNM) classification, which has been used more recently. Both are given in Table 25-3.
   b. **Studies** to assist in the staging of renal tumors include serum liver function tests and chest x-rays and possibly tomography, bone scans, and inferior venacavography. CT scan and ultrasonography have both been valuable in the search for nodal and hepatic metastases and intravascular extension of the tumor. Magnetic resonance imaging (MRI) has been very useful in staging, particularly to demonstrate intracaval tumors, and can be expected to replace contrast radiography of the vena cava.
   c. **Tumor markers** include renin and erythropoietin, although these have not been nearly as valuable nor as extensively studied as the markers for prostatic carcinoma and testicular tumors.

6. **Treatment** must be designed with consideration for the stage of the lesion. Results of treatment of renal cell carcinoma show progressive deterioration with the increasing stage of the disease (Table 25-4).

Table 25-3. Staging of Renal Cell Carcinoma

	Staging System	
Extent of Tumor	**Robson**	**TNM**
Limited within the renal capsule		
Small tumor	A	T1
Large tumor	A	T2
Perinephric fat	B	T3a
Renal vein	C	T3b
Renal vein and infradiaphragmatic		
vena cava	C	T3c
Adjacent organs	D	T4a
Renal vein and supradiaphragmatic		
vena cava		T4b
Lymph nodes (regional)	C	N+
Distant metastases	D	M+

    a. Stage I tumors can be treated with surgical excision of the kidney and tumor by radical nephrectomy.

    b. Stage II tumors can also be treated by radical nephrectomy alone.

    c. Stage III tumors can be treated by radical nephrectomy with surgical excision of the intravascular extension of the tumor.

        (1) When nodal involvement is minimal, complete excision by radical nephrectomy with node dissection may be possible.

        (2) When nodal involvement is extensive, the prognosis is so poor that surgical removal may not be warranted unless the patient has a symptomatic primary tumor.

        (3) Invasion of the renal vein should be treated by excision since such extension does not adversely affect the prognosis.

    d. Stage IV tumors are not excised except for palliative treatment of symptoms. Treatment with progestational agents has not shown a statistically significant benefit. Chemotherapeutic and immunologic agents have also been disappointing.

C. Transitional cell carcinoma of the renal pelvis and ureter

  1. Epidemiology

    a. Transitional cell carcinomas of the renal pelvis and ureter constitute fewer than 5% of urothelial neoplasms in the United States. The remainder are those of the bladder.

    b. The frequency of these lesions appears to be increasing, and in some countries the frequency of transitional cell carcinoma and renal cell carcinoma is nearly equal. Multiple tumors, including bilateral lesions, often occur.

  2. Etiology

    a. Environmental factors, including cigarette smoking and occupational exposure to dyes and rubber products, are associated with an increased risk.

    b. Analgesic nephropathy and Balkan nephropathy (a familial disease prevalent in Yugoslavia) also result in an increased incidence.

  3. Pathology. Transitional cell carcinomas, which represent 90% of renal pelvic tumors, may occur in situ or as papillary (85%) or planar lesions of the neoplastic type. Neoplastic lesions include squamous cell carcinomas (7%), adenocarcinomas, sarcomas, and metastatic lesions.

Table 25-4. Survival of Patients with Renal Cell Carcinoma

Stage	**5 Years (%)**	**10 Years (%)**
I	67	49
II	59	34
III	30	19
IV	7	2

4. Clinical manifestations
   a. Gross hematuria is seen in 70%–95% of patients. **Microscopic hematuria** occurs in an additional 10%.
   b. Other symptoms include flank pain or a palpable mass.

5. Diagnosis
   a. Urinalysis can detect the presence of hematuria. It is necessary to note the urinary pH, since uric acid stones (which can also cause hematuria and appear radiologically as a filling defect) form only in the presence of an acidic urine.
   b. Intravenous urography is usually the initial study and often shows a filling defect.
      (1) A filling defect must then be evaluated further.
         (a) The major distinction to be made is between a urothelial neoplasm and a radiolucent calculus.
         (b) Other diagnoses to be excluded are blood clot and a necrotic papilla.
      (2) In as many as 30% of patients, the involved kidney does not visualize on the urogram, a finding often associated with a high-grade tumor.
   c. Retrograde pyelography offers good radiologic definition of filling defects and is particularly useful in evaluating a nonfunctioning kidney.
   d. Ultrasonography may demonstrate a highly dense echo pattern with an acoustic shadow behind a calculus; tumors show only a mass effect but no shadow.
   e. CT scan can differentiate the very high density of uric acid calculi from tumors, which have essentially the same density as renal parenchyma. Tumors do not increase in density after intravenous administration of contrast medium.
   f. Urine cytology is particularly valuable in diagnosing transitional cell lesions of the ureter and renal pelvis. Voided urine, catheter-collected specimens, or brushed specimens can be used.
   g. Ureteroscopy is an endoscopic technique for the observation and direct biopsy of lesions that cause filling defects. Flexible ureteroscopy has been particularly valuable in the diagnosis of filling defects within the kidney.

6. Treatment of transitional cell carcinomas of the renal pelvis includes **nephroureterectomy** with a cuff of bladder included in the specimen.
   a. More conservative approaches, such as local resection or partial nephrectomy, can be undertaken in a patient with a solitary kidney.
   b. Conservative treatment should be considered for low-grade distal ureteral tumors.
   c. High-grade lesions and those located more proximally in the ureter necessitate nephroureterectomy.

D. Carcinoma of the bladder

1. Epidemiology. Bladder cancer is of major importance throughout the world. The incidence in the United States is approximately 20,000–30,000 new cases with 10,000 deaths a year.

2. Etiology
   a. Many environmental and disease factors have been associated with bladder cancer. These include cigarette smoking, exposure to aniline dyes, and ingestion of artificial sweeteners.
   b. Other risk-increasing agents include phenacetin and benzidine.
   c. Schistosomiasis is associated predominantly with squamous cell carcinoma.

3. Clinical presentation
   a. Although presentation may vary widely, most patients note hematuria among their symptoms. Others are found to have microscopic hematuria alone.
   b. Irritative symptoms with disturbances of urination, pyuria, or a mass have also been presenting features.
   c. The presence or absence of pain is not a distinguishing feature.
   d. A new urinary tract infection with bleeding, particularly in an older patient with a history negative for infections, should be considered suspicious.

4. Diagnosis
   a. Excretory urography is an essential study in any patient with gross hematuria. Although its sensitivity for vesical lesions is poor, filling defects in the bladder are often seen, and lesions of the upper urinary tract can be defined.
   b. Endoscopy with cystoscopy is absolutely essential to evaluate the urethra and bladder mucosa.

     c. Urinary cytology is valuable with high sensitivity for high-grade neoplasms and carcinoma in situ.

  5. Staging. The choice of the appropriate treatment for bladder carcinoma depends upon accurate staging of the disease (Table 25-5).

     a. Endoscopic biopsy and resection of the bladder tumor is the most important step in diagnosis and staging.

       (1) Histologic examination will reveal the **cell type** and the **grade** of the tumor as well as the **depth of invasion**. In general, the extent of infiltration of the primary tumor into the muscular wall of the bladder relates to the extent of regional and distant metastases.

       (2) The **gross appearance** of the mucosa is also important. In the presence of **carcinoma in situ,** the bladder may appear entirely normal or diffusely erythematous and cobble-stoned. Low-grade papillary tumors and high-grade solid-appearing tumors are also characteristic.

     b. Bimanual examination is essential to judge the extent of local disease. Papillary tumors may not be palpable, while a mass is suggestive of an invasive lesion. Any mass extending beyond the bladder must be evaluated further.

     c. Ultrasonograpy has been used to evaluate the extent of local disease. It has had some value in defining the depth of invasion of the primary tumor and in detecting nodal metastases.

     d. CT scan has been most valuable in detecting nodal metastases. It has also been useful in examining the perirectal space for the extent of the primary tumor.

     e. MRI has been used for the evaluation of local and nodal lesions. Its appropriate value remains unknown.

     f. Lymphangiography has not been found to be accurate enough to warrant routine use in bladder cancer patients.

     g. Chest x-rays must be obtained to screen for pulmonary metastases. Pulmonary tomography may increase the sensitivity in detecting pulmonary metastases; CT scan is much less specific and may cause considerable confusion with benign pulmonary lesions when used on a routine basis.

     h. Bone scans are a satisfactory screening technique for bony metastases in patients being considered for major surgical procedures, such as cystectomy. Although bony metastases are uncommon at tumor presentation, they do develop in high-grade invasive lesions and may be the first sign of metastases in these patients.

     i. Cell surface antigens

       (1) There are many antigens on the surface of urothelial cells just as there are on blood cells. These include the ABO (H) blood group antigens, T antigens, and tumor-associated antigens.

       (2) The loss or acquisition of these antigens by tumors has, in some cases, been shown to be related to the biologic behavior of the tumor.

  6. Treatment

     a. Carcinoma in situ consists of mucosa with neoplastic degeneration of the cells but without invasion of the lamina propria.

       (1) Because of the frequent irritative symptoms, the diagnosis is often delayed. Urinary cytologic findings frequently indicate malignancy.

Table 25-5. Staging of Carcinoma of the Bladder

Extent of Tumor	Staging System	
	Jewett-Marshall	**TNM**
Carcinoma in situ	O	TIS
Lamina propria	A	T1
Superficial muscle	B_1	T2
Deep muscle	B_2	T3
Perivesical fat	C	T3
Adjacent organs	D_1	T4
Lymph nodes (regional)	D_2	N1
Lymph nodes (above aortic bifurcation)	D_3	N2
Distant metastases		M

    (2) Because of the possible chronicity of carcinoma in situ and the unpredictability of invasion, **treatment is controversial.**

        (a) Topical chemotherapy has been used as a primary treatment agent with encouraging results.

        (b) If the lesion is widespread and symptoms are prominent or if the tumor extends into the urethra, the prostatic ducts, or the lower ureter, then early cystectomy and urinary diversion may be advisable.

  b. Superficial bladder tumors that have not invaded the muscle can be treated by local **transurethral resection.** Although these tumors seldom progress to invasive lesions, there is a high rate of recurrence or development of new tumors.

    (1) Intravesical chemotherapy has been effective in reducing the recurrence of superficial bladder tumors. Effective agents include thiotepa, ethoglucid (Epodyl), doxorubicin, and mitomycin C.

    (2) Local immunotherapy with bacille Calmette-Guérin (BCG) vaccine has also been effective in reducing recurrences, even in patients who have failed to respond to intravesical chemotherapy.

    (3) Radiotherapy by external beam has been shown to have poor long-term results (a 50% rate of recurrence within 5 years) and considerable complications, such as reduced bladder capacity. Interstitial radiotherapy in one series was more effective, but the true efficacy of this treatment awaits other studies.

    (4) Cystectomy remains a treatment possibility in patients with diffuse superficial lesions who have had a poor response to transurethral resection and intravesical chemotherapy.

  c. Invasive bladder cancer includes any lesion beyond the in situ or intraepithelial stage. Deeply invasive tumors extend more than halfway through the muscle layer or into perivesical fat.

    (1) Intensive local therapy is used in selected patients to eradicate an aggressive tumor, but it is withheld from patients in whom the disease has already metastasized. It is in these patients that accurate staging is particularly valuable.

    (2) Partial cystectomy is used for invasive tumors that have infiltrated too deeply for local resection.

        (a) There must be an adequate margin of normal bladder around the tumor, and selected-site biopsies from the remainder of the bladder should show no evidence of atypia or carcinoma in situ.

        (b) Preoperative radiotherapy and pelvic lymphadenectomy have often been employed as adjuvant therapy.

    (3) Radiotherapy has been an important factor in the treatment of invasive bladder cancer. Fractionated doses totaling 6000–7000 rads to the bladder have been effective in treating some tumors. There remains a significant failure rate; however, the possibility of successful preservation of bladder function without a major surgical procedure maintains radiotherapy as an option in treatment.

    (4) Radical cystectomy remains the primary choice of treatment for deeply infiltrating tumors.

        (a) Radical cystectomy includes removal of the bladder and prostate gland in men and the bladder, urethra, anterior vaginal wall, and usually the uterus in women.

        (b) Although the mortality rate due to this operation has been less than 5% in recent years, the morbidity rate remains at approximately 25%, and patients must endure urinary diversion.

        (c) The role of adjuvant radiotherapy has been controversial. Improved rates of survival have been seen only in patients who have exhibited downstaging of the primary tumor.

E. Testicular tumors

1. Epidemiology

  a. The major testicular tumors in terms of incidence are **seminomas** and **nonseminomatous germ cell tumors** (i.e., embryonal carcinoma with or without seminoma, teratoma, teratocarcinoma with embryonal carcinoma or choriocarcinoma, and pure choriocarcinoma).

  b. Testicular tumors are uncommon, constituting only 2% of all cancers.

  c. Over 50% of testicular tumors are found in men between 20 and 44 years of age.

  d. The frequency of occurrence depends upon the population: The younger groups studied in reports from military institutions have a seminoma rate of 21%–46%, while this rate may increase to 40%–60% in older men.

    e. Neoplasms of the testicle occur less frequently in blacks than in whites.
    f. Cryptorchidism has been reported to increase the incidence of tumors.

2. Clinical presentation. Asymptomatic tumors occur frequently, which emphasizes the need for thorough physical examinations in men, including the genitalia, as well as the need for patient education and training in testicular self-examination.
    a. The commonest presenting complaint is **painless swelling** or enlargement of the testicle. This has been reported in 65%–95% of patients with an additional 10%–15% noting a **painful swelling,** which is frequently confused with epididymitis.
    b. A sense of **testicular heaviness** or dragging has also been reported.
    c. Hydroceles have been associated with 2%–8% of testicular tumors.

3. Diagnosis of a scrotal mass is made by **physical examination,** possibly assisted by ultrasonography and surgical exploration via an inguinal approach.

4. Staging is shown in Table 25-6.
    a. Procedures include chest tomography and CT scan, inferior venacavography, lymphangiography, and abdominal CT.
    b. The **major advance** in the staging of testicular tumors has been the use of **tumor markers.** Serum levels of human chorionic gonadotropin (HCG) and α-fetoprotein have been shown to be elevated in some patients with an existing tumor. The use of these markers has significantly decreased error in staging.

5. Treatment. The treatment of testicular tumors varies with the cell type and with the disease stage.
    a. Seminoma is generally sensitive to irradiation.
        (1) Stage I seminoma. Treatment is fractionated doses totaling 2500–3000 rads to the periaortic and the ipsilateral pelvic and inguinal lymph nodes. Ipsilateral scrotal irradiation and contralateral inguinal nodal irradiation are considered in patients who have had previous scrotal surgery.
        (2) Stage II seminoma that has been detected radiographically or by elevation of β-HCG after orchiectomy is treated with 2500–3000 rads to the periaortic and the ipsilateral pelvic and inguinal lymph nodes.
           (a) Additional doses may be delivered to specific tumor masses.
           (b) Mediastinal irradiation has been routinely applied as well, although its use is being questioned due to the development of effective chemotherapy.
           (c) Retroperitoneal lymphadenectomy may be of value for histologic diagnosis in patients with bulky disease.
           (d) The survival rate for patients with stage I or II seminoma approaches 100%.
        (3) Stage III seminoma has not responded nearly as well to radiotherapy alone and should be treated with combination chemotherapy. A regimen of cisplatin, vinblastine, and bleomycin has been effective. Reduced dosage is necessary after previous radiotherapy.
    b. Nonseminomatous germ cell tumors
        (1) Stage I nonseminomatous testicular tumors can be classified by finding no evidence of tumor spread upon retroperitoneal lymphadenectomy, in addition to a negative metastatic evaluation. Survival has been 100% in these patients.
        (2) Stage II nonseminomatous testicular tumors
           (a) Stage II tumors have been treated by lymphadenectomy.
           (b) Bulky disease benefits from preoperative combination chemotherapy. The role of adjuvant postoperative chemotherapy remains controversial.
           (c) Retroperitoneal node dissection for testicular tumor involves the surgical removal of tissue around the great vessels from the level of the diaphragm, including both renal hilar and ipsilateral perirenal tissue and extending to the common iliac artery contralaterally and to the inguinal ligament ipsilaterally.

Table 25-6. Staging of Testicular Cancer

Extent of Tumor	Stage
Confined to the scrotum	I (or A)
Confined to the retroperitoneum	II (or B)
Beyond the retroperitoneum	III (or C)

(3) Stage III or disseminated testicular tumors
  (a) The discovery of cisplatin and the development of combination chemotherapeutic regimens have markedly increased the response and survival rate of affected patients.
  (b) The response rate has been related to the extent of disease with a 100% response seen among patients with elevated levels of tumor markers as their only indication of dissemination, and a 65% response in patients with advanced pulmonary or abdominal tumors.

F. Prostatic tumors

1. Epidemiology
  a. Prostate cancer, over 95% of which is adenocarcinoma, is uncommon among men under the age of 50 years. The incidence increases rapidly with age, however, and the average patient age at diagnosis is 73 years.
  b. The rates of occurrence and mortality are higher among blacks than whites.

2. Etiology
  a. Genetic and hormonal factors have been implicated.
  b. Exposure to cadmium is also a risk factor.

3. Diagnosis
  a. Prostate cancer is frequently asymptomatic until it reaches an advanced stage.
  b. Low-stage tumors are most often found on routine rectal examination or on prostatectomy for benign indications. Induration or a firm nodule should be considered suspicious for cancer.
  c. The diagnosis of carcinoma can be confirmed by needle biopsy of the suspicious area.

4. Tumor grading.
Various grading systems for prostatic tumors have considered the histologic appearance—both cytologic characteristics and glandular morphology. Survival has been shown to be affected adversely by loss of differentiation.

5. Staging is shown in Table 25-7.
  a. Local tumor extension is staged by **physical examination**. The extent of the tumor mass within the prostatic capsule or its extension beyond the capsule can be determined by **digital rectal examination**.
  b. Although ultrasonography and CT scan may assist in determining local tumor extension, any superiority of these techniques over physical examination is questionable.
  c. The search for metastatic disease should be conducted by **chest x-ray, excretory urography, bone scan,** and **CT scan.**
  d. Acid phosphatase produced by the prostate gland is an extremely valuable **tumor marker**. It is elevated in the serum in 70%–85% of patients with metastatic disease but in fewer than 10%–30% of patients with local disease alone.
  e. Prostate specific antigen is a second useful **tumor marker**. It can be elevated to lower levels with benign prostatic hypertrophy. It is extremely useful to monitor recurrences after treatment of localized carcinoma of the prostate.

6. Treatment
  a. Therapy for prostatic carcinoma is related both to the extent of disease and the status of the patient.
  (1) In approximately 40% of patients, metastases are present at the time of diagnosis.
  (2) In another 40%, the tumor extends beyond the prostatic capsule; in turn, nearly 50% of these patients have clinically undetectable metastases.
  (3) Only in the remaining 20% can cure be obtained by local treatment of the disease.

Table 25-7. Staging of Prostatic Cancer

Extent of Tumor	Stage
Incidental, focal	A_1
Incidental, diffuse	A_2
Prostatic nodule	B_1
Large or multiple nodules, within prostate	B_2
Localized to periprostatic area	C
Distant metastases	D

b. Stage A
   (1) If adenocarcinoma of the prostate gland is localized to a focus involving only a few prostatic chips on transurethral resection of the prostate (stage A_1), survival without recurrence can be expected in over 90% of patients.
   (2) However, if the tumor is diffuse (stage A_2) or of a high grade early on, undetected metastases are likely in approximately 30% of patients.
   (3) Because of this important differentiation between stages A_1 and A_2, some authors have recommended a repeat of transurethral resection in a search for residual tumor.
c. Stage B tumors are the most controversial in terms of treatment. These lesions respond to local ablative therapy, and it has been difficult to determine the most successful treatment. Radical prostatectomy, interstitial radiation with lymph node dissection, and external beam radiation all have their advocates and supporting data.
   (1) The selection of patients for **radical prostatectomy** depends on the patient's status as well as on the tumor. Candidates should be in good medical condition and should have an expected survival of 10–15 years.
      (a) The procedure includes removal of the prostate gland, seminal vesicles, and usually the pelvic lymph nodes.
         (i) Although the operative mortality rate is less than 1%, **morbidity** occurs, with impotence in up to 90% of patients. However, a new modification has lessened this rate by avoiding section of the periprostatic autonomic nerves and 60%–80% of patients maintain patency.
         (ii) Early urinary incontinence occurs in some patients but clears within 6 months in approximately 90% of those affected.
      (b) The survival rate in patients with B_1 lesions has been good. When the tumor has increased from stage B_1 to B_2, the 15-year survival has dropped from 27%–18%.
   (2) Interstitial radiation
      (a) Interstitial radiation by implantation of iodine 125 (^{125}I) seeds has recently been popular for the control of prostatic carcinoma. Lymph node dissection is usually performed as well.
      (b) Long-term survival studies are not yet available, although at 5 years, persistent tumor has been noted in nearly two-thirds of patients initially staged with B or C disease.
   (3) External beam radiation
      (a) Tumoricidal doses of 6500–7000 rads can be delivered in fractionated doses to a locally confined prostatic tumor.
      (b) The 5-year survival rates have been shown to be 75% for stage B and 52% for stage C tumor. Ten-year survival rates decreased to 47% and 28%, respectively.
      (c) Local control, again, is related to the size and grade of the tumor. Histologic evidence of persistent tumor has been seen in significant numbers of patients after any form of radiotherapy, but the biologic significance of these findings remains unclear.
d. Metastatic carcinoma of the prostate gland cannot rely on local ablative therapy alone. Symptomatic urinary obstruction may be treated by resection, but metastases must be treated systemically.
   (1) Castration and **estrogen administration** have long been established as effective therapeutic regimens.
      (a) Orchiectomy rapidly reduces the serum testosterone concentration from normal levels of 500–700 ng/dl to less than 50 ng/dl.
      (b) Estrogen administered in the form of **diethylstilbestrol** suppresses the release of pituitary gonadotropins in a dose-dependent fashion. Doses of 3 mg are necessary. Additionally, the diethylstilbestrol may have a direct effect on the prostate gland.
   (2) Antiandrogen therapy has proved to be useful.
      (a) Androgen synthesis can be obstructed by inhibitors, such as aminoglutethimide, cyproterone, medrogestone, or spironolactone.
      (b) Gonadotropin release can be inhibited by luteinizing hormone-releasing hormone (LH-RH) analogues, such as leuprolide.
      (c) Survival has improved with therapy combining LH-RH analogues with flutamide (an antiandrogen).
   (3) Chemotherapy for the treatment of metastatic carcinoma of the prostate gland has generated considerable interest recently. Some improvement has been demonstrated with single agents, and combination regimens have also been studied.

VII. BENIGN PROSTATIC HYPERTROPHY AND URINARY OBSTRUCTION. Enlargement of the prostate, resulting in urinary obstruction, has long been recognized as a process affecting the aging male. The central glandular portion of the prostate undergoes stromal and epithelial hyperplasia with well-defined nodular growth. The etiology of this hyperplasia remains unknown.

A. Diagnosis relies on the patients' symptoms, the finding of an enlarged prostate gland, and histologic confirmation.

1. The major symptoms, which result from bladder outlet obstruction and, as a group, constitute **prostatism,** include:
   a. Decrease in force of the urinary stream
   b. Hesitancy in initiating the stream
   c. Intermittent stream or dribbling after voiding
   d. Frequency
   e. Nocturia
   f. Hematuria
   g. Calculus formation
   h. Total urinary retention

2. On physical examination, differentiation from carcinoma of the prostate rests to a large extent on the presence or absence of nodules or firm areas within the gland.

B. Treatment may be indicated in patients with severe symptoms, obstruction, or damage extending to the upper urinary tract, and is certainly indicated in those with acute retention.

1. Agents producing α-adrenergic blockade have had some effect in decreasing outlet obstruction and increasing urinary flow rates in patients with benign prostatic hypertrophy.

2. Although hormonal therapy has aroused considerable interest, no regimen has been uniformly beneficial nor outweighed the potential side effects.

3. Balloon dilation has shown some success, particularly in small glands without median lobe enlargement.

4. **Treatment remains surgical** by transurethral resection or open prostatectomy to remove the obstructing intraurethral prostatic tissue.

VIII. NEUROGENIC BLADDER. Damage to the bladder's nerve supply, either motor or sensory, can hinder normal bladder function. Damage may occur from spinal cord trauma, congenital anomalies, or disease states, such as diabetes mellitus or multiple sclerosis.

A. Diagnosis by urodynamic studies

1. **Urinary flow rate.** The normal urinary flow rate is approximately 20–25 ml/sec in men and 25–30 ml/sec in women. Many factors can operate together or independently to alter the flow rate, but obstruction should be considered when a flow rate of less than 15 ml/sec is seen in a patient with a full bladder.

2. **Bladder function** can be evaluated by **cystometry.** The bladder is filled at a known rate with water or carbon dioxide, and the intravesical pressure is recorded and plotted against the volume of fluid introduced. Thus, the contractility of the detrusor muscle and the patient's ability to inhibit this contraction can be monitored.

3. **Urinary sphincter responses** can be studied by measuring the intraluminal pressure of the sphincter and the electrical activity of the muscle via electromyography.

B. Patterns of neurogenic bladder dysfunction

1. Spastic neurogenic bladder can be the outcome of either partial or complete injury of the spinal cord above the sacral level.
   a. There may be spasms with resultant obstruction of the external urinary sphincter, and frequent involuntary contraction of the bladder can be observed.

    b. In affected patients, functional changes result in diminished bladder capacity with urinary incontinence and with increased intravesical pressure that can be transmitted to the kidneys as well.

  2. Uninhibited neurogenic bladder can result from incomplete lesions of the cortex or the pyramidal tracts. Patients experience urinary frequency, urgency, and nocturia. Uninhibited contractions can be noted on the cystometrogram. The patient empties the bladder completely, and there is a sensation of both fullness and emptying of the bladder.

  3. Flaccid or atonic bladder can be caused by injury to the sacral portion of the spinal cord or to the nerves within the cauda equina with resultant loss in the reflex arc to the bladder. Trauma, tumors, and congenital anomalies are the most frequent causes. The patient exhibits a large bladder capacity with low pressures and has no spontaneous detrusor contractions. The most frequent urinary symptom is overflow incontinence.

C. Treatment

  1. Pharmacologic manipulation can be used to affect the bladder directly and reverse the neurologic effect.

    a. Bethanechol has been used for the atonic bladder, often with an α-adrenergic blocking agent, to decrease bladder neck and posterior urethral tone.

    b. Propantheline or oxybutynin have been used for the spastic or uninhibited bladder.

  2. Intermittent catheterization has become the preferred method for mechanical emptying of the bladder. It has major advantages in decreasing the infection and long-term complications that are seen with chronic catheterization.

  3. Bladder stimulators have been used experimentally with encouraging results.

IX. MALE SEXUAL DYSFUNCTION

A. Overview

  1. Male impotence can be defined as the inability to obtain or maintain an erection that is satisfactory for sexual intercourse.

  2. With an increase in public awareness of the options for evaluation and treatment, impotence is no longer accepted as a part of growing old and has been recognized increasingly as a medical problem.

  3. As with many disorders that are manifested by a loss of functional capability, there may be a wide spectrum of sexual disability. Although some patients may have a total loss of erectile ability, others may have intermittent difficulty or problems with maintaining an erection.

B. Diagnosis. Since the therapy for male sexual dysfunction is rather sharply divided between organic and psychological approaches, a search for the major cause of the dysfunction is extremely important.

  1. History. The diagnosis of sexual dysfunction necessarily relies almost entirely on the history given by the patient. Tact and completeness in taking a sexual history are of major importance.

    a. Affected patients are embarrassed by their problem, are often desperate, and are almost apologetic in seeking medical attention.

    b. The history must include the nature of the present problem, its onset and development, contributing psychological and medical factors, the effects of any prior treatment, and the patient's expectations.

    c. History from the patient's sexual partner is valuable in accurately assessing the extent of the dysfunction.

    d. Thorough consideration of **psychological factors** is of paramount importance.

  2. Physical examination. The patient should have a thorough physical examination with particular emphasis on the genitalia and the vascular and neurologic systems.

  3. Laboratory studies

    a. Blood studies should include screening tests for the patient's general health, including a complete blood count and evaluation of the renal, hepatic, and metabolic status.

      b. Hormonal studies should include serum levels of testosterone (total and free), LH, follicle-stimulating hormone (FSH), and prolactin.

      c. Doppler determinations of the penile blood pressure, ultrasonic evaluation of the vessels, or blood flow scans can evaluate blood flow to the penis.

      d. Perineal electromyography will indicate the status of the pudendal nerves.

  4. Monitoring nocturnal penile tumescence (NPT)

      a. Men normally have erections during periods of rapid eye movement (REM) sleep, which has been recognized as a major distinguishing factor between psychogenic and organic erectile failure.

      b. Many techniques have been developed for evaluating these erections, and there is a major advantage of in-hospital evaluation where a laboratory technician can observe and evaluate the quality of each erection.

         (1) NPT can be monitored with **gauges** evaluating the extent and firmness of an erection.

         (2) Stamps or plastic bands graded to break at specific forces also have proven useful.

C. Treatment. A major division in treatment exists between patients with predominantly psychological dysfunction and those with organically based dysfunction. There are, in addition, many patients with both factors who require combination therapy.

  1. Psychological treatment may include sex therapy, individual psychotherapy, marital therapy, and pharmacologic treatment. In a few patients relatively uncommon techniques, such as hypnosis, may be helpful.

  2. Treatment of organic impotence is often directed toward the specific etiology.

      a. Hormonal abnormalities can be corrected in some patients by the replacement of testosterone.

      b. Diabetes-related impotence can occasionally be improved by better control of the diabetes. It is usually based on vascular or neurologic deficits and must be treated accordingly.

      c. Vascular insufficiency usually results from diffuse involvement of the small arteries to the penis. Success with revascularization has been limited mainly to those patients with a single, usually traumatic, lesion. Obstruction of the large pelvic vessels, such as the iliac arteries, can often be treated surgically.

      d. Neurologic disorders have generally not responded to direct treatment.

  3. Penile prostheses

      a. Implantation of a penile prosthesis to provide sufficient rigidity for intercourse has become an increasingly prevalent treatment.

      b. Three general **types** of prostheses are available: a semirigid type, an inflatable type contained within the corpora, and a fully inflatable type, which has the largest number of mechanical failures but provides the most normal-appearing and normal-functioning erection.

  4. Other treatment techniques

      a. Injection of vasodilators directly into the penis has generated considerable interest. This technique has provided satisfactory rigidity for many patients. Short- and long-term complications are not known, and the eventual role of this treatment remains to be determined. Papaverine, phentolamine, and prostaglandin E have been used.

      b. Transrectal stimulation of the nerves to the corpora cavernosa has produced erections in nonhuman primates and has been demonstrated with varying success in human volunteers.

      c. Vacuum-constriction devices have been introduced, which can be placed over the penis, causing penile engorgement with blood that can be contained by means of a rubber band at the base of the penis. Although this technique has been effective in many patients, fear of complications, such as ischemia from prolonged compression at the base of the penis, has concerned some patients.

I. PLASTIC SURGERY as an art and science deals with the reconstruction of body parts altered by trauma, birth defects, or advanced age. It is one of the oldest fields of surgery, having first been described in 700 B.C., in India. In 1818, von Graefe used the term "plastic" in his monograph on nasal reconstruction, and throughout the years since, this term has been associated with surgery that is concerned with form and function.

A. Skin, or the **integumentary system,** is the largest organ in the body.

1. **Three properties** of skin are essential for understanding reconstruction—elasticity, extensibility, and resilience.
   a. **Elasticity** keeps skin in constant tension, owing to underlying collagen fibers. The function of elasticity becomes apparent by its absence in "wrinkle lines" on the face.
   b. **Extensibility** refers to the skin's ability to stretch, which can be seen on abdominal skin during pregnancy.
   c. **Resilience** is noted by the skin's resistance to infection and puncture.

2. **Layers of the skin.** The two principal layers, the dermis and epidermis, have specialized functions.
   a. **The epidermis** is composed of stratified squamous epithelium, which covers the entire body and provides **protection**. Living cells migrate from the innermost level of the epidermis to the surface to form a dead desquamating layer. The migration takes approximately 19 days.
   b. **The dermis,** which serves in a nutritive capacity to the epidermis, is itself composed of two layers.
      (1) The **papillary layer** is composed of fine collagen fibers, ground substance, and capillaries.
      (2) The **reticular layer** is composed of dense collagen, hair follicles, sebaceous glands, sweat glands, and the subdermal plexus.
   c. **The hypodermis, or subcutaneous tissue,** which may contain hair follicles, sweat glands, and nutrient vessels, lies beneath the dermis.

B. Suture materials and wound closure techniques that are available to the surgeon vary, and proper closure requires knowledge of them.

1. **Suture material** can be **classified** according to the body's ability to absorb it.
   a. **Absorbable sutures**
      (1) **Catgut** is made from the small intestine of sheep or cows. It is absorbed by phagocytosis in 2 weeks to 6 months. If it is treated with chromium salts, the rate of resorption is slower.
      (2) **Polyglycolic acid** is a braided polymer of glycolic acid and is stronger than comparably sized catgut. It is absorbed by enzymatic degradation, generally in 2 weeks to 2 months.
      (3) **Polydioxanone** is a monofilament, which is useful for extended wound support. Absorption is by enzymatic degradation and is usually complete by 6 months.
   b. **Nonabsorbable sutures**
      (1) **Organic sutures** include **silk** and **cotton**, which are both braided. They are the most reactive of the nonabsorbable sutures.
      (2) **Synthetic sutures** include **nylon, polypropylene**, and **Dacron**. They evoke minimal tissue reaction.
      (3) **Stainless steel wire** and **clips** are the most inert of the nonabsorbable sutures.

2. **Suture marks** are imprints of the sutures themselves. They result from pressure on the skin during the time that the suture is left in place. They are exacerbated by tension on the wound, edema, large bites of tissue, and infection.

3. A **cosmetically acceptable appearance** is a major goal of all closures.
   a. **Atraumatic handling of tissue** minimizes necrosis and decreases scarring.
   b. **Buried sutures** reduce dead space and decrease tension along skin edges.
   c. **Eversion of the wound edges** results in a level scar with time, while inversion of the edges may result in a concave scar.

4. **Techniques of wound closure** (Figure 26-1)
   a. **Simple interrupted sutures** result in equal full-thickness bites of skin and subcutaneous tissue. As the knot is secured, the underlying subcutaneous tissue helps to draw the skin edges into opposition.
   b. **Vertical mattress sutures** are similar to simple sutures, but an additional bite through the wound edge is used to ensure edge eversion.
   c. **Horizontal mattress sutures** are similar to simple sutures, but an additional bite is taken laterally on the opposite side so that eversion takes place in wounds under tension.
   d. **Subcuticular sutures** are intradermal closures that can be continuous or interrupted; suture material can be absorbable or nonabsorbable. The main advantage is the avoidance of suture marks on the skin.
   e. **Continuous over-and-over sutures** result in a secure closure. They are most commonly used on the scalp, where suture-line marks will be hidden by hair.
   f. **Skin tape** is useful for areas, such as the face, where suture-line scars must be minimized. It is also a useful adjunct for subcuticular closure and for bolstering a wound following early suture removal.

C. **Skin grafts** are segments of epidermis and dermis that have been detached from their native blood supply to be transplanted to another area of the body. A skin graft may be an **autograft**

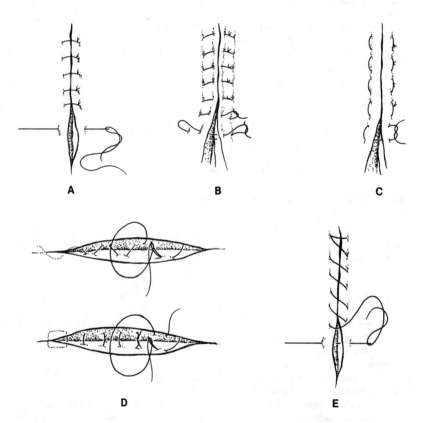

Figure 26-1. Types of wound closures: (A) simple interrupted suture, (B) vertical mattress suture, (C) horizontal mattress suture, (D) subcuticular suture, and (E) continuous over-and-over suture.

(from the same person), an **allograft** (from a genetically dissimilar individual of the same species), or a **xenograft** (from a different species) [see Chapter 24 I A 1].

1. Types. Skin grafts are classified according to thickness.
   a. Split-thickness skin grafts contain the epidermis and a portion of the dermis. They are further subdivided into thin, medium, and thick, based upon the amount of dermis included in the graft (0.010–0.025 inch). The abdomen, buttocks, and thighs are common donor sites.
   (1) Advantages of split-thickness skin grafts include:
      (a) A large supply of donor areas
      (b) Ease of harvesting
      (c) Availability of donor site for reuse in 10–14 days
      (d) Decreased primary contracture
      (e) Coverage of large surface areas
      (f) Ability to be stored for later use
   (2) Disadvantages of split-thickness skin grafts include:
      (a) Cosmetic inferiority to full-thickness skin grafts
      (b) Decreased durability
      (c) Hyperpigmentation
      (d) Increased secondary contracture
   b. Full-thickness skin grafts contain the epidermis and the full thickness of dermis without subcutaneous fat. They are most useful for covering defects on the face or hand that are not amenable to coverage with a skin flap (see I D). A good match of skin color can be obtained from donor sites in the postauricular or supraclavicular areas. Preauricular grafts provide the best color match for the face. The forearm and groin can also serve as donor sites for defects below the clavicle.
   (1) Advantages of full-thickness skin grafts include:
      (a) Cosmetic superiority to split-thickness skin grafts
      (b) Decreased secondary contractures (grafts may be cut as required to fill the defect)
      (c) Increased durability
   (2) Disadvantages of full-thickness skin grafts include:
      (a) Limited donor sites
      (b) Increased primary contracture
   c. Composite grafts are those that are formed of multiple tissues (e.g., a fingertip containing skin, subcutaneous fat, and bone or a segment of ear containing skin and cartilage). These grafts may be effective in young patients or where the distal portion of the graft is less than 1 cm from the blood supply.

2. Grafting procedures
   a. Split-thickness skin grafts are best obtained with specifically designed instruments rather than being taken freehand.
   (1) Methods of obtaining the graft include the following:
      (a) Knives, such as the Humby or Weck, are fitted with an adjustable roller or gauge to determine thickness. The knife is slowly advanced as cutting proceeds in a back-and-forth direction.
      (b) The **drum** (Reese) **dermatome** fixes the epidermis to the drum with glue, which allows the graft to be cut as the drum is rolled back. Grafts cut are of uniform thickness.
      (c) The **electrical dermatome**, such as the Brown or Padgett, has a rapidly oscillating knife and a gauge to adjust depth. Long strips of skin can be removed with this instrument.
   (2) Care of the donor site following the cessation of capillary oozing will aid in re-epithelialization.
      (a) Meshed, nonadherent gauze allows the scab to be incorporated into the dressing. In 2 days, the dressing is dry, and the covering, with the incorporated scab, falls from the wound by 2 weeks.
      (b) Semipermeable membranes trap leukocyte-rich fluid to form an artificial blister, which hastens epithelialization. Patients note diminished pain at the donor site.
   (3) Care of the recipient (grafted) site (see I C 3)
      (a) Hemostasis is necessary to ensure adequate tissue contact.
      (b) When excessive wound drainage or potential infection may be a problem, the graft can be cut and a meshing device can be used to ensure adequate drainage. This technique is also useful for expanding the surface area of a graft. Epithelialization quickly occurs in the meshed interstices following graft "take."

(c) The graft may be fixed to the recipient site by sutures or tapes. External fixation with a "tie-over bolus" dressing (i.e., a large dressing made of gauze or cotton) may be required in areas where immobilization is difficult or where shear forces are expected. The open method, in which the graft is left exposed, may be useful for large surface areas in burn patients, where daily inspection for infection is important.

  b. **Full-thickness skin grafts**
    (1) **Method of obtaining the graft.** The grafts are "harvested" with a freehand technique using a #10 or #15 knife blade. A portion of subcutaneous fat is also harvested, which needs to be excised carefully prior to grafting.
    (2) **Care of the donor site** involves primary skin closure in most instances. Split-thickness skin grafts may be necessary in some cases.
    (3) **Care of the recipient site** is similar to that in split-thickness skin grafts. Tie-over bolus dressings are frequently used.

3. **Survival of skin grafts**
  a. **Vascular recipient beds** are necessary to provide nourishment for the transplant tissues.
    (1) **Imbibition of plasma** supports survival during the first 48 hours. **Fibrin** is laid down, which helps to hold the graft in place.
    (2) **Inosculation** (vascular budding) occurs, and the graft is usually supported by a true circulation by the fourth to seventh day. Generally, a graft begins to turn pink at this time. Lymphatic connections are formed by the fifth day.
  b. **Contact of the skin graft** is essential for inosculation to take place. Factors that can lead to **loss of contact** include:
    (1) **Tension** on the graft
    (2) **Fluid** (blood, serum, or pus) underneath the graft
    (3) **Movement** between the graft and its bed
  c. **Preparation of wounds to be grafted**
    (1) Bone denuded of periosteum, cartilage denuded of perichondrium, and exposed tendon do not support skin grafts; these require a flap procedure.
    (2) **Infected wounds** do not support skin grafts. The critical bacterial concentration appears to be 10^5 organisms per g of tissue, and bacterial counts are useful in determining a wound's suitability for grafting. Mechanical debridement and use of a biologic dressing (i.e., an allograft or a xenograft) help to reduce the bacterial count.

D. **Flaps** are segments of skin and subcutaneous tissues that are moved from one part of the body to another, either retaining or transplanting their vascular supply, which is via a segmental artery through a perforating artery to a cutaneous artery supplying the dermal–subdermal plexus. Because of their intrinsic blood supply, flaps are useful for healing and for covering defects that require padding.

  1. **Types**
    a. **Skin flaps**
      (1) **Random flaps** receive their blood supply from the dermal–subdermal plexus. These flaps lack an anatomically recognized arterial and venous system. Examples include:
        (a) Z-plasty
        (b) V-Y advancement flaps
        (c) Rotation flaps
        (d) Transposition flaps
      (2) **Axial flaps** have a direct cutaneous artery and vein supplying their subdermal plexus. Thus, the blood supply is more reliable than with random flaps, and flaps of greater length may be obtained. Axial flaps may be detached as free flaps and transplanted to other areas of the body, provided that the vessels are large enough. Examples of axial flaps include:
        (a) Forehead flaps
        (b) Groin flaps
        (c) Deltopectoral flaps
    b. **Muscle flaps** provide increased blood supply to an area. Generally, they are used to cover exposed bone and usually are skin grafted. When the overlying skin and subcutaneous tissue are included, they are called **myocutaneous (musculocutaneous) flaps**.
      (1) The blood supply is predictable, and the flaps can be anatomically outlined. The flaps contain muscle with a named artery, which must be identified and preserved.

(2) Muscle flaps have been most useful in reconstruction of the lower extremity and in areas of poor vascularity.

c. Fasciocutaneous flaps involve the transfer of skin, subcutaneous tissue, and the underlying fascia with an anatomically distinct artery. Because there is no mobilization of underlying muscle, there is less functional debilitation. The donor site must be skin grafted, and they are cosmetically inferior to muscle flaps.

d. Free flaps (free tissue transfer) are those in which the native blood supply is completely severed with transplantation of the flap to a separate body area. They can be muscle, myocutaneous, fasciocutaneous, or axial flaps. They can be used to provide function (free neurotized muscle transfer for correction of facial nerve palsy). Revascularization is accomplished by microvascular anastomosis.

2. Uses of flaps include:
    a. Wound closure in areas of poor vascularity (e.g., wounds overlying bare bone, cartilage, nerves, or tendons)
    b. Facial reconstruction (e.g., the nose or lips)
    c. Areas over bone where padding is needed (e.g., the ischial tuberosity in a patient with pressure sores)

3. Vascular patency may be assessed by color, temperature, Doppler flowmetry, fluoroscanning, and laser Doppler.

E. Reconstructive breast surgery. Techniques are available for treating micromastia (small breasts), macromastia (oversized breasts), gynecomastia, and for reconstruction following mastectomy. Because the breast is frequently viewed as a symbol of femininity, there is much emotional overlay in this type of surgery. Careful planning and realistic goals are necessary for patient satisfaction.

1. Micromastia is present when a patient feels she lacks development of one or both breasts.
    a. Treatment is by augmentation with a silicone implant, saline implant, or polyurethane-covered implant. These can be placed either subglandularly (between the breast and pectoralis major muscle) or submuscularly (underneath the pectoralis major muscle).
    b. Complications, although rare, include infections and hematoma formation. A **capsular contracture** may form around the implant, which can lead to asymmetry and discomfort. This may require a subsequent surgical scar release and is commoner when the implant is in the subglandular position.

2. Macromastia is present when the patient feels she has abnormally large breasts. Frequently, macromastia can be debilitating because of neck and back pain. **Ptosis** is present when the nipple has extended below the inframammary fold.
    a. Treatment. A variety of techniques have been described. All involve resecting breast tissue and the inferior breast skin, transposition of the nipple–areolar complex superiorly, and closure of the resultant flap defects. All resected specimens should be examined histologically because occult carcinoma may be present, although rarely.
    b. Complications include hematoma formation, infection, and necrosis.

3. Gynecomastia is enlargement of the male breast. In adolescents, the problem is often transient and regresses spontaneously. It can also occur with various endocrine abnormalities and in association with hepatic disease. Treatment by excision is aimed at restoring normal contour to the breast.

4. Reconstruction of the breast following mastectomy is an alternative to the use of external prosthetic devices. Reconstruction may be performed at the time of mastectomy or delayed for several months; however, the percentage of women who request reconstruction diminishes with increasing time following mastectomy.
    a. If there is adequate soft tissue and the pectoralis major muscle has been preserved, an implant can be used to reconstruct the breast mound. If the quality of the soft tissue is good but limited quantitatively, **tissue expansion** can be used. A tissue expander is a Silastic balloon, which is gradually inflated with saline over months to form a breast mound. It is generally replaced with a permanent prosthesis at a later date.
    b. If the soft tissue is inadequate either quantitatively or qualitatively, vascularized tissue may be transposed. The **latissimus dorsi myocutaneous flap** (with or without a prosthetic implant) and the transverse rectus abdominis myocutaneous (TRAM) are most commonly used.

    c. Totally autogenous breast reconstruction with a **fleur-de-lis latissimus flap** or **TRAM flap** allows the reconstructive surgeon to create a breast mound without an implant. The reconstructed breast feels natural and fluctuates in size with the patient's weight change.

    d. Free flaps are occasionally indicated. The commonest ones are the **free TRAM** and **free gluteus maximus myocutaneous flaps** for breast reconstruction.

    e. Nipple–areola reconstruction is usually done as a second stage. The nipple is reconstructed most commonly with local flaps and a skin graft to reconstruct the areola. If necessary, the nipple–areola complex can be tattooed to increase pigmentation.

    f. Occasionally, a mastopexy or reduction mammoplasty is necessary for the opposite breast to achieve symmetry.

F. Reconstruction of congenital anomalies (see Chapter 29)

    1. Congenital anomalies may result from genetic or environmental factors. In most instances, an initiating environmental factor acts on a genetically predisposed individual. The inheritance risk for most anomalies remains low. The repair and reconstruction of many congenital anomalies do not fall within the scope of plastic surgery; examples include the gastrointestinal anomalies discussed in Chapter 29.

    2. Maxillofacial deformities can be reconstructed by craniofacial surgery.
        a. Soft tissue and bony abnormalities can be reconstructed by a specialized team approach. Examples include:
            (1) Hypertelorism
            (2) Orbital dystopia
            (3) Treacher Collins syndrome
            (4) Facial clefts
            (5) Crouzon's disease
            (6) Apert's syndrome
        b. Cleft lip may be unilateral, bilateral, or incomplete. It is seen in 1 in 1000 births and is commoner in Oriental children and male children. It is less common in blacks. Reconstruction is generally performed at about 3 months of age as determined by the **"rule of tens"**: 10 lb, 10 weeks of age, and 10 g of hemoglobin. Some surgeons prefer to operate in the neonatal period.
        c. Cleft palate may occur as a defect in the primary or secondary palate or both. It occurs in 0.5 in 1000 births.
            (1) Reconstruction is performed before 2 years of age to aid in normal speech development. It commonly involves local flap advancement.
            (2) Secondary bone grafting is indicated prior to eruption of permanent teeth if maxillary discontinuity exists.
            (3) Early attention to nutrition is important as sucking is impaired.

G. Facial trauma frequently accompanies other major trauma. After ensuring adequate ventilation and circulation, attention should be directed initially to areas where trauma is more life-threatening (i.e., the chest and abdomen) [see Chapter 21 I]. Once the patient is stabilized, the facial structures can be systematically examined.

    1. Soft tissue
        a. Lacerations of the face bleed readily because of its rich blood supply. Bleeding is controlled by direct pressure and never by "blind" clamping. Control in the operating room may be necessary.
        b. Lacerations may involve deeper structures, such as the facial nerve and parotid duct.
        c. Most lacerations can be repaired by primary closure, following thorough debridement of all devitalized tissue.

    2. Blunt trauma may result in **contusions** or **associated fractures**.
        a. Many injuries of this type can be initially diagnosed by inspection, noting facial asymmetry, if present.
            (1) Dental malocclusion may signify a mandibular or maxillary fracture.
            (2) Instability of the upper jaw may signify a maxillary or midface fracture.
            (3) Pain on palpation at the nose, depression, or asymmetry may signify a nasal fracture.

(4) Diplopia, malar deformity, enophthalmos, or hypoesthesia of the cheek may signify an orbital blow-out fracture.

    b. Complete radiologic examination is essential. Operative stabilization is usually required.

H. Genitourinary anomalies may interfere with normal urinary function and result in severe psychological problems if not corrected. These congenital anomalies are apparent at birth, and treatment should be initiated at an early age.

    1. Hypospadias is a condition in which the urethral meatus opens on the ventral surface of the penis, scrotum, or perineum.

        a. It occurs in 1 in 300 live male births and is usually associated with downward curvature of the penis caused by fibrous tissue, a condition called **chordee**.

        b. Evaluation of the upper urinary tract is essential as 10% of patients have associated abnormalities.

        c. If present, the chordee is resected, and reconstruction is completed by local skin flap advancement, full-thickness skin grafts to create an urethra, or both.

    2. Epispadias is failure of closure of the dorsal surface of the penis. **Exstrophy of the bladder** occurs when the anterior bladder wall opens on the abdomen. Both represent degrees of the same abnormality.

        a. These are unusual disorders, occurring in 1 in 40,000 births.

        b. Associated upper urinary tract abnormalities are rare.

        c. Treatment is aimed at preserving renal function, which may be accomplished by closure of the bladder defect or excision of the bladder and urinary diversion.

    3. Vaginal agenesis is repaired by vaginal reconstruction, using split-thickness skin grafts. Myocutaneous flaps are used for reconstruction following ablative surgery.

    4. Gender dysphoria is treated surgically by altering sexual appearance to coincide with personality. After careful preoperative evaluation, ablative surgery is performed followed by reconstruction with flaps and skin grafts.

I. Aesthetic surgery is an attempt to improve on nature or to control the body's aging process by surgical means. Changes that occur secondary to aging are the result of decreased elasticity of the skin and loss of subcutaneous fat. Most commonly, procedures are performed on the more noticeable areas of the body (face, neck, abdomen, extremities, and breasts). The expectations of the patient must be realistic; he or she must understand that surgery will alter appearance but not the person.

    1. Rhytidectomy (face-lift) is a procedure that undermines the skin of the face and neck. Excision of redundant pre- and post-auricular skin completes the procedure. Occasionally, the **submuscular aponeurotic system (SMAS)** of the face is plicated at the same operative setting. With this procedure, the skin of the face and neck is tightened giving a more youthful appearance.

    2. Dermabrasion is the physical abrasion of skin. It is most commonly used to treat acne scarring.

    3. Chemical face peel is an induced mild chemical burn to the superficial skin. It is most commonly used to treat fine facial wrinkles.

    4. Blepharoplasty is used to treat **baggy eyelids**. This may be functional in the upper lids as redundant skin may obscure lateral gaze fields. It is accompanied by excision of varying amounts of skin and fat to give a more youthful or "less tired" look to the eyes.

    5. Rhinoplasty is performed to correct congenital or acquired nasal defects. This may be done for aesthetic or functional reasons. The procedure involves a controlled nasal fracture with excision of varying amounts of bone and cartilage.

    6. Abdominoplasty is the excision of excess abdominal fat and skin. In many cases, repair of diastasis recti brought on by pregnancy or prior obesity is performed to tighten the abdominal wall.

    7. Liposuction (suction assisted lipectomy) is a common procedure to treat localized deposits of fat. Subcutaneous fat is aspirated by high-vacuum suction to restore body contour. The patient's fluid status is important as one-third to one-fourth of the aspirated fat is blood. This is not a weight reduction procedure.

8. **Collagen injections and fat autotransplantation** are useful for correcting localized contour irregularities (usually the face). The effect of collagen lasts 3–6 months, necessitating subsequent injections. At this time, fat autotransplantation is somewhat experimental, as the amount of viable harvested fat (by liposuction) cannot be easily assessed clinically.

9. **Breast surgery** is discussed in I E.

II. SKIN LESIONS

A. **Overview.** Many skin tumors can be **diagnosed at an early stage** because of their obvious difference from adjacent skin. They frequently have a **characteristic appearance**, which can aid in planning appropriate therapy.

1. **Examination should be systematic** and based on the gross appearance of the lesion. Inspection can reveal color changes and ulceration. Palpation can reveal fixation to underlying tissues or the involvement of adjacent lymph nodes.

2. **Biopsy** is usually required for accurate diagnosis and can either be **excisional** for smaller lesions or **incisional** for larger ones. In all instances, the biopsy should be carefully planned, as a more radical resection may be necessary. Additionally, cosmetic considerations must be kept in mind.

B. **Benign conditions** are common, and frequently the patient seeks medical attention for cosmetic reasons or from fear of cancer. Only the commoner lesions are discussed in this chapter.

1. **Common warts** (verrucae vulgaris) occur most frequently in the second decade of life and may be transmitted by direct or indirect contact.
   a. **Etiology.** They are caused by a member of the papovavirus family, which invades the stratum spinosum epidermidis, causing papillomatosis.
   b. **Clinical presentation.** The fingers are the commonest location. The lesions have a characteristic rough and elevated surface and can become tender.
   c. **Treatment** involves minimal destruction of normal tissue. In many cases, the warts will resolve spontaneously. Problematic lesions can be treated by:
      (1) Curettage and electrodesiccation
      (2) Freezing with liquid nitrogen
      (3) Chemotherapy with caustic agents

2. **Cysts** are fluid-filled cavities in the subcutaneous tissues; they may resemble solid tumors.
   a. **Epidermal inclusion cysts** develop when epidermal cells are trapped in the subcutaneous tissue. Desquamation leads to the creation of a cavity. Excision is curative.
   b. **Sebaceous cysts** result from blockage of a sweat gland, which causes the accumulation of sebum and the creation of a cyst. Excision is curative and prevents recurrence. If infection is present, the cyst should be incised and drained prior to excision.
   c. **Dermoid cysts** are congenital lesions that may occur later in life. If they occur in the midline (glabellar, nasal), computed tomography (CT) scan is indicated as there may be intracranial communication. Treatment is by excision.
   d. **Ganglia** can occur in areas of weakened retinaculum with outpouching of underlying synovial structures. They occur most commonly on the hands and feet in areas subjected to trauma or inflammation. Excision is curative, but there can be recurrences, which are most probably due to inadequate resection of the ganglion's stalk and base.

3. **Vascular birthmarks** are frequently disturbing to the patient and family because they are cosmetically deforming. They are classified on the basis of their clinical and cellular characteristics.
   a. **Hemangiomas (strawberry marks)** are characterized by increased number of mast cells during the proliferative phase and rapid postnatal growth. These elevated, red, soft, compressible lesions grow rapidly during the first year of life and are most commonly located on the head and neck area and extremities. Spontaneous regression is characteristic. Surgery or steroid therapy is indicated for lesions causing functional impairment (eyes, ears, throat). Rarely platelet consumption occurs. Hemorrhage is uncommon, and usually there is minimal residual scarring.
   b. **Vascular malformations** grow at the same rate as the patient; thus, they may not be obvious at birth. They have a normal number of mast cells and may be subdivided according to the predominant vascular tissue: capillary, venous, lymphatic.

(1) Capillary malformations (capillary hemangioma, port-wine stains) are found on the face, chest, and extremities. They may be associated with Sturge-Weber and Klippel-Trenaunay-Weber syndromes. There is dilatation of the capillaries in the subpapillary, dermal, or subdermal layer. If the tumor is small, excision is curative. Treatment of larger lesions requires careful planning for optimal results. The laser recently has proved to be helpful in treatment.

(2) Venous malformations (cavernous hemangiomas) involve a matrix of mature vessels in the subcutaneous tissues; frequently they involve deeper structures, including muscle. These lesions may sequester platelets. After careful preoperative planning, treatment involves wide excision with attention to the involved structures. Occasionally, direct sclerosant injection may be helpful.

(3) Lymphatic malformations (lymphangioma, cystic hygroma) commonly cause hypertrophy of involved soft tissues. Surgical treatment is excision, and seroma is a common complication.

(4) Arteriovenous malformations frequently remain stable in size and then expand. Treatment is surgical excision.

4. Vascular tumors are frequently benign; they may cause concern because of their prominence.

a. Pyogenic granulomas are papular lesions commonly located on the face, chest, and fingers, which develop rapidly and then stop enlarging after variable periods of growth. The lesions tend to bleed freely. Surgical excision is usually curative.

b. Spider nevi (telangiectasias) occur in all age groups and are commonly located on the face, chest, and extremities. They may arise during pregnancy and in cirrhosis. The lesion consists of a central arteriole with vessels resembling venules radiating from the center. They rarely bleed, and treatment (i.e., laser, electrodesiccation, or cryotherapy) is undertaken primarily for cosmetic reasons.

c. Glomus tumors, which are extremely painful, are located most frequently in the nail beds. Treatment is excision.

5. Lipomas (fat tumors) can be found in any area of the body where fat is normally found, but are commonest on the neck, shoulders, back, and thighs. Malignant transformation is uncommon, and excision is curative.

6. Nerve tumors (see also Chapter 18 IV F 1, 3) are of two varieties.

a. Neurilemomas arise from the Schwann cell sheath, do not cause much pain, and are treated by excision.

b. Neurofibromas involve masses of nerve and fibrous tissue and are related to **von Recklinghausen's disease**. They may undergo malignant degeneration.

7. Seborrheic keratosis is a light- to dark-brown raised papular lesion, which must be differentiated from malignant skin lesions. Treatment is by biopsy followed by curettage and electrodesiccation.

8. Keloids are abnormal accumulations of fibrous tissue, which extend above and beyond an area that was previously traumatized (as opposed to hypertrophic scars that remain within those confines). They occur more commonly in blacks. Treatment is by excision and pressure. Occasionally adjuvant corticosteroid therapy is necessary.

9. Hidradenitis suppurativa may be confused with a tumor, but it is an **infection** of the apocrine sweat glands and subcutaneous tissue most frequently occurring in the axilla or groin. Treatment involves controlling the infection with antibiotics and (if indicated) incision and drainage, followed by excision with either primary closure or a split-thickness skin graft.

C. Premalignant skin lesions are benign lesions with a high likelihood of progressing to invasive squamous cell carcinoma.

1. Actinic keratosis is a rough, scaly epidermal lesion that occurs in areas of the body subjected to chronic sun exposure.

a. It may appear in the third or fourth decade of life, and approximately 10%–20% of the lesions will undergo malignant transformation.

b. If biopsy proves the lesion to be benign, it is treated by excision or cryotherapy. Topical chemotherapy with 5-fluorouracil has been useful in patients with many keratoses.

2. Bowen's disease is intraepidermal squamous cell carcinoma or carcinoma in situ of the skin. It appears as a well-defined, erythematous plaque covered by an adherent scaly yellow crust.

    a. There are no lymphatics in the layer affected, and there is no potential for metastasis.

    b. Bowen's disease occurs mainly in the fourth to sixth decade of life, and arsenical ingestion and viruses have been implicated as etiologic agents. Treatment is similar to that for actinic keratosis.

3. Keratoacanthoma is a locally destructive skin lesion most commonly found on the head, neck, and upper extremities.

    a. Rapid progression of the tumor occurs within a 2–8-week period, followed by spontaneous resolution.

    b. Treatment is excision and biopsy of the lesion; squamous cell carcinoma is found in approximately one-quarter of the lesions biopsied.

D. Nevi (moles)

1. Overview

    a. Nevi are pigmented lesions of the skin that frequently concern the patient because of the fear of malignancy. Because the average white man has 15–20 nevi, total excision is unreasonable.

    b. Clinical diagnosis is of prime importance because **malignant transformation** can occur. In general, however, malignant transformation is rare in children. Also, well-circumscribed lesions and lesions with a uniform color rarely progress to malignancy.

    c. Suspicious looking lesions should be biopsied by excision with a margin of normal skin.

2. Benign pigmented lesions

    a. Junctional nevi are dark, flat, smooth lesions, which range generally from 1–2 cm in diameter. They are occasionally hairy and develop from the basal layer of epidermis. Nevi that are located on the palms and soles are usually junctional. They can develop into malignant melanoma, but this rarely occurs before puberty.

    b. Compound nevi are brown-to-black, well-circumscribed lesions, usually less than 1 cm in diameter. They may be elevated and are frequently hairy, arising from the epidermal–dermal interface and within the dermis. Malignant transformation is rare.

    c. Intradermal nevi are light-colored, well-circumscribed lesions less than 1 cm in diameter. Hairs are usually present, and the cell distribution is in the dermis. Malignant transformation is rare.

    d. Giant pigmented nevi

        (1) These are brown-to-black, hairy lesions with an irregular nodular surface. They frequently involve more than 1 square foot of body surface and arise from the dermis and junctional areas. The lesions are frequently described, in terms of distribution, as "bathing trunk," "vest," "sleeve," or "stocking."

        (2) Malignant degeneration has been estimated at approximately 10%.

        (3) Excision with a margin of normal tissue is indicated, either in stages or with flap reconstruction.

    e. Blue nevi are smooth, hairless lesions measuring less than 1 cm in diameter. They arise in the dermis, and malignant degeneration is rare.

    f. Spitz nevi (**benign juvenile melanomas**) are smooth, round, pink-to-black lesions measuring 1–2 cm in diameter. They have increased cellularity and occur in nests within the upper dermis. Malignant degeneration is rare.

    g. Nevi must be distinguished from **freckles (ephelides)**. These pigmented lesions occur in the basal and upper dermis and have no malignant potential.

3. Treatment

    a. Treatment is indicated for **junctional** and **giant pigmented nevi** because of their malignant potential.

    b. Indications for excision of any pigmented lesion include:

        (1) Changes in color, size, shape, or consistency

        (2) Pain

        (3) Satellite nodules

        (4) Regional adenopathy

    c. Except for large lesions, **excisional biopsy**, with a margin of normal skin, should be performed. Further therapy may be indicated, depending upon the histologic diagnosis and location of the lesion.

d. For large lesions, a full-thickness wedge biopsy, including a small area of normal skin, should be taken.

E. Malignant melanoma (see Chapter 19 X B) is a melanoblastic tumor, which may develop in the skin or eye.

1. **Epidemiology.** The incidence is approximately 13 new cases per 100,000 population a year, representing an increase of 50% in the past decade. The tumor occurs most commonly in the fifth decade of life, and the incidence is approximately equal in men and women.

2. **Etiology. Exposure to sunlight** appears to be an initiating event in the development of melanoma, and fair-skinned whites with frequent direct (overhead) exposure to the sun are most often affected.

3. **Detection** of melanoma is determined by changes in the color, size, or shape of a nevus.
   a. Men are most frequently affected on the back, chest, and upper extremities.
   b. Women are most frequently affected on the back, lower extremities, and upper extremities.

4. **Classification** of melanomas is based on their gross and histologic appearance.
   a. Superficial spreading melanoma accounts for 70% of all melanomas. It can be present on any area of the body but is most frequently found on the back and legs. The median age at diagnosis is the fifth decade. The tumor has irregular borders with a varied color pattern. Cell distribution is in the upper dermis with lateral junctional spread. Generally, the prognosis is good.
   b. Nodular melanoma accounts for 15% of melanomas and occurs most commonly in the sixth decade of life. The tumor is blue-black and may be found on any area of the body. Spread is primarily vertical with rapid dermal invasion, and the prognosis is poor.
   c. Acrolentiginous and mucosal melanomas comprise 10% of all melanomas. They most commonly occur in the fifth decade of life and are distributed on the mucous membranes, palms, and soles. Irregular borders are common, and lesions generally are black but may be amelanotic. Growth occurs slowly in a radial direction; cells are mainly in the upper dermis with occasional deep invasion. The prognosis depends on the depth of invasion and is between that of superficial spreading and nodular melanomas.
   d. Lentigo maligna (melanotic freckle of Hutchinson) is the least common of the melanomas, and it appears most frequently in the seventh decade of life. The lesions are brown-black and contain elevated nodules within a smooth freckle. They occur most frequently on the head, neck, and hand. Growth is slow and in a radial direction, with cells in the upper dermis; vertical extension is infrequent. The prognosis is excellent.

5. **Staging.** Classification of the lesion is imperative for optimal treatment. Histologic evaluation with regard to the depth of invasion as well as the type of tumor is important for determining prognosis. To complete the staging, a thorough history and physical examination are necessary, including a complete blood count, 12-test sequential multiple analysis (SMA-12), urinalysis, and chest x-ray.
   a. Clark's classification assesses the **level of invasion** and has been adopted by the American Joint Committee for Cancer Staging and End Results.
      (1) Level I: The tumor is confined to the epidermis.
      (2) Level II: The tumor invades the papillary dermis.
      (3) Level III: The tumor fills the papillary dermis but does not invade the reticular dermis.
      (4) Level IV: The tumor invades the reticular dermis.
      (5) Level V: The tumor invades the subcutaneous fat.
   b. Breslow method is an additional method that is sometimes used. It involves measuring the depth of invasion precisely in millimeters. However, erroneous estimates of the depth of invasion can occur if ulceration is present.
      (1) Patients with Clark's level I, II, or III lesions and with a depth of invasion that is less than 0.76 mm are at low risk for metastasis.
      (2) Patients with lesions at level IV or V and with a depth of invasion greater than 1.5 mm are at high risk for distant spread.

6. **Treatment** depends on the depth of invasion. Biopsy is by total excision when feasible; otherwise, incisional biopsy is performed. Frozen section is inaccurate in determining the depth of invasion.

a. Excision. There is debate over the previously accepted "5-cm margin."
   (1) For melanoma-in-situ, 0.1–1.0-cm margins are indicated.
   (2) For lesions less than 0.75 mm in thickness, a 1–2-cm margin is generally sufficient.
   (3) For lesions more than 0.75 mm in thickness, 3-cm margins are indicated. The need to excise the underlying fascia is debatable.
b. Resection
   (1) Clinically involved regional lymph nodes with level II, III, IV, or V disease should be resected.
   (2) Prophylactic resection of clinically benign nodes is controversial.
      (a) Some authors recommend prophylactic resection only for patients who are expected to be problems in follow-up, for patients whose tumor overlies a lymph node basin, or for level V disease.
      (b) Other authors have advocated prophylactic resection with invasion greater than 0.75 mm or with Clark's level III, IV, or V disease, feeling that this aids in staging and may enhance survival.
   (3) Postoperative morbidity from lymph node resection needs to be considered when lesions involve the face or lower extremities.
c. Adjuvant therapy is recommended by some authors to prolong the disease-free interval.
   (1) Regional hyperthermic perfusion involves isolating the blood supply of a limb with a pump-oxygenator, enabling high doses of chemotherapy at elevated temperatures (40° C) to be delivered to the limb without the side effects of systemic toxicity. The role of this treatment has yet to be clarified.
   (2) Chemotherapy with dacarbazine (DTIC), carmustine (BCNU), and lomustine (CCNU) has not significantly altered the course of disease.
   (3) Immunotherapy is useful for the control of cutaneous metastases, but visceral metastases have not responded to any significant degree.
   (4) Radiotherapy is strictly palliative and has been used for brain and bone metastases.

7. Prognosis is related to the status of the regional lymph nodes. When disease is confined at the primary site, the 5-year survival rate approaches 80%–90%. If regional lymph nodes are involved, this figure drops to 30%–50%. Patients with distant or visceral metastases are usually dead within 12 months.

F. Other malignant tumors of the skin commonly occur in exposed areas. Generally, they are low-grade and metastasize late. For this reason, they are highly curable.

1. Basal cell carcinoma (see Chapter 19 X A) is the commonest skin tumor seen. It is localized and slow-growing, and it generally occurs in the head and neck. It is found most commonly in individuals of northern European descent.
   a. Etiology. Basal cell carcinoma has also been associated with xeroderma pigmentosum, basal cell nevus syndrome, nevus sebaceous, and unstable burn scars. With the advent of radiation therapy, basal cell carcinomas are being seen with increasing frequency in areas of dermatitis.
   b. Clinical presentation. The lesion has pearly translucent edges, which may become erythematous or pigmented. Frequently, a visible telangiectasia is present. As the lesion grows, it may ulcerate and eventually invade underlying structures. Morphologic types of basal cell cancer include superficial, nodular, pigmented, and morphea-like (sclerosing). Metastatic disease is rare.
   c. Treatment involves complete removal of the tumor to achieve cure. **Biopsy is mandatory** to establish a pathologic diagnosis.
      (1) Curettage and electrodesiccation results in a 95% cure rate, and the technique is acceptable for lesions less than 2 cm in diameter. The disadvantage is the lack of a specimen for determining the adequacy of resection.
      (2) Radiation therapy can be used in areas where tissue preservation is important (e.g., the eyelids). The cure rate is approximately 90%. The disadvantages are that depigmentation and skin atrophy can occur with time.
      (3) Excision with primary closure results in a cure rate approaching 95% and allows inspection of the specimen for adequate margins. If necessary, reconstruction can be performed at the same sitting.
      (4) Mohs' micrographic surgery involves tumor mapping to determine the adequacy of resection. Generally, it is most applicable to recurrent tumors, morphea-like tumors, and those of the nose or perinasal areas. As cure rates approach 99%, immediate reconstruction can achieve excellent aesthetic results.

(5) Cryotherapy is acceptable in certain instances. It has a higher morbidity, and scarring is less predictable than with other techniques.

(6) Topical chemotherapy results in unacceptable cure rates.

d. Recurrent disease requires wide re-excision.

2. Squamous cell carcinoma (see Chapter 19 X A) is second to basal cell carcinoma in occurrence. It may grow rapidly and has the capacity to metastasize via the blood and lymphatic system.

a. Etiology. Exposure to sunlight appears to be a causative factor in that the tumor is commoner on the head and hands. Squamous cell carcinoma may develop from the premalignant lesions already mentioned (see II C) or from old burn scars; it may also occur in people exposed to arsenicals, nitrates, or hydrocarbons.

b. Clinical presentation. The lesion may have satellite nodules or a central area of ulceration that may become encrusted, obscuring deeper invasion. The tumor is common on the lips, in the paranasal folds, and on the axilla. It can be classified as well-differentiated or poorly differentiated squamous cell carcinoma, based upon the histologic examination.

c. Treatment

(1) Treatment is based upon examination of the biopsy specimen.

(a) Excisional biopsy with a cuff of normal tissue is preferred for lesions less than 1 cm in diameter.

(b) Incisional biopsy can be performed for larger lesions or those on the face.

(2) Treatment methods

(a) Electrodesiccation can be used to treat lesions less than 1 cm in diameter. It can also be used in elderly individuals and in patients with a history of repeated tumors.

(b) Excision with primary closure offers the advantage of histologic examination of the specimen. Reconstruction following the excision of large lesions may be required.

(i) Regional lymph node dissection should be performed only if there is clinical evidence of nodal disease.

(ii) Frequently, regional adenopathy may accompany ulcerated lesions. In this case, the lymph nodes should not be excised at the same sitting as the primary tumor, because the nodes will resolve with time if the adenopathy is inflammatory in nature.

(c) Radiation therapy can result in cure with improved cosmetic results in certain instances.

(d) Mohs' surgery (see Chapter 19 X A 3 c) also has been successful in treatment.

3. Sweat gland tumors are rare lesions arising from the eccrine or apocrine glands. They occur in later life and present as a soft tissue mass that has been present for years. Metastases to regional lymph nodes are common, and consideration should be given to regional node dissection at the time of initial excision. The overall 5-year survival rate approaches 40%.

G. Sarcomas of the soft tissue

1. Overview. Sarcomas of the soft tissue constitute only 1% of malignant tumors, and they may occur at any location in the body. Roughly 20 different types have been described, each with a slightly different tendency to metastasize or to invade locally.

a. Clinical presentation. These tumors usually present as an enlarging mass, which is frequently painless. If they occur in deep locations, such as the retroperitoneum, they are often quite large at the time of diagnosis.

b. Diagnosis is made on permanent sections of a representative biopsy. MRI is helpful in determining the extent of the tumor. The biopsy should be planned with the future surgical procedure in mind. Excisional biopsy is indicated for lesions less than 3 cm in diameter; otherwise, incisional biopsy is indicated.

c. Treatment. These tumors are frequently treated inadequately because they have a pseudocapsule, which may lead the surgeon to assume falsely that all of the tumor has been removed. In reality, these tumors extend along tissue planes well beyond their apparent margins.

(1) Wide local excision or amputation is the current accepted treatment. Chemotherapy and postoperative radiotherapy are frequently indicated.

    (2) Limb-sparing surgery is indicated when wide local excision can be accomplished without jeopardizing the function of the extremity (i.e., involvement of major nerves or vessels.)

    (3) Limited surgery with high-dose radiotherapy yields a local recurrence rate similar to that for radical surgery (20%–50%).

  d. The route of metastasis is usually **hematogenous**, and the lungs are the most frequent site of involvement. Lymphatic spread occurs less often and usually late in the course of the disease. Metastatic lesions in the lungs should be resected if the primary tumor is under good control and there is no evidence of other sites of involvement.

2. Major soft tissue sarcomas

  a. Liposarcoma is the commonest of the soft tissue sarcomas in the adult.

    (1) Only 1% arise from preexisting benign lipomas.

    (2) Liposarcomas can occur in any area, including the retroperitoneum.

    (3) They are **treated** by wide excision. The tumors are radiosensitive, and radiotherapy may be helpful in locations where wide excision is not possible.

    (4) Well-differentiated lesions have a 70% 5-year survival rate, while poorly differentiated lesions have only a 20% survival rate at 5 years.

  b. Fibrosarcoma is the second commonest soft tissue sarcoma in the adult.

    (1) These lesions are usually found in an extremity, where they present as a hard, round mass. They are commoner in men than in women and are the commonest sarcoma found in black persons.

    (2) They are radioresistant, and the **treatment** is wide excision. Fibrosarcomas are very prone to local recurrence and must be treated aggressively at the time of presentation.

    (3) Adequately treated fibrosarcomas have a 5-year survival rate of 77%.

  c. Rhabdomyosarcoma arises from skeletal muscle and occurs in both a juvenile and an adult form.

    (1) Embryonal rhabdomyosarcoma usually occurs in children under 15 years of age.

      (a) The head, neck, and genitourinary system are most frequently involved.

      (b) This tumor has recently enjoyed a spectacular increase in the 5-year survival rate. The combination of surgery, radiotherapy, and multidrug chemotherapy now achieves a 70% 5-year survival rate for patients with isolated lesions. If metastases are present, the survival rate is lower but still approaches 40%.

    (2) Pleomorphic rhabdomyosarcoma is the histologic type usually found in adults.

      (a) Wide excision (including amputation, if necessary) is the **treatment** of choice. Chemotherapy is much less effective in this form of the tumor.

      (b) Although lymph node dissections are not done in most cases of sarcoma, they should be done for pleomorphic rhabdomyosarcoma because 25% of patients have regional nodal metastasis.

      (c) The 5-year survival rate is 30%.

  d. Kaposi's sarcoma, which has attracted attention recently in connection with acquired immune deficiency syndrome (AIDS), is a malignant lesion of vascular origin.

    (1) Until recently it was usually seen in the lower extremities of older men. Now, it is often seen in the perianal area in connection with AIDS.

    (2) It usually begins as a single bluish-red macule, and gradually multiple nodules appear and may ulcerate.

    (3) A solitary nodule should be excised, and widespread disease should be treated with radiotherapy. Although there is no cure for systemic Kaposi's sarcoma, patients may live many years.

  e. Lymphangiosarcoma is a peculiar tumor that develops in areas of chronic lymphedema (e.g., in the arm of women with postmastectomy edema, particularly if radiotherapy has also been used). The prognosis is dismal, and there is no effective treatment.

  f. "Benign" sarcomas

    (1) Desmoid tumors are classified as benign fibromatoses that have the capacity to grow to a large size with a high rate of recurrence after excision. They are associated with **Gardner's syndrome**. Usually, they affect the shoulder and trunk and may affect the abdominal wall in parous women.

    (2) Dermatofibrosarcoma protuberans is a slow-growing nodular tumor with a high recurrence rate after excision. Histologically, it exhibits a "cartwheel" pattern of fibroblasts.

    (3) Paraganglioma (chemodectoma, carotid body tumor) presents as a painless mass in the neck overlying the carotid bifurcation. Most tumors are benign. Excision is curative.

27
Neurosurgery
Bikash Bose

I. INTRODUCTION. Neurosurgery involves the surgical management of diseases of the nervous system. In the past two decades, rapid strides have been made in the field with the development of computed tomography (CT scan) for detecting lesions of the brain and spinal cord and with the introduction of operative tools like the operating microscope, the laser, and the ultrasonic aspirator. The **goal of neurosurgical intervention** is to prevent and, if possible, to reverse the loss of neurologic function.

A. Embryology. The entire nervous system is ectodermal in origin.

1. **Neural folds** are thickened ridges on either side of the midline in front of the primitive streak in the embryonic disk. They are formed first.

2. **The neural groove** is the area between the neural folds. With the descent of the primitive streak, there is elongation of both the neural folds and the neural groove.

3. **The neural tube** is formed when the neural folds rise into ridges and finally close around the neural groove. The neural tube closes first in the region of the future hindbrain and then progresses both cranially and caudally.
   a. The **cranial end** of the neural tube forms the future **forebrain (prosencephalon), midbrain (mesencephalon),** and **hindbrain (rhombencephalon).**
   b. The **walls** develop into the **neuronal tissue** and **neuroglia** of the **brain,** and the **cavity** gives rise to the **ventricular system.**
   c. The **caudal end** of the neural tube is modified by the formation of a longitudinal groove called the **sulcus limitans** along the middle portion of each side. This marks the subdivision of the tube into:
      (1) An **alar** (dorsal) **lamina,** which gives rise to the **sensory elements** of the **spinal cord**
      (2) A **basal** (ventral) **lamina,** which gives rise to the **motor elements**

4. **Neural crest.** With the closure of the neural folds, a narrow angular interval is left along the neural tube between it and the primitive body of the ectoderm. Cells at the top of the neural tube at this junction push out into the groove, forming the neural crest.

B. Anatomy. The brain constitutes only 2% of the body weight but requires 18% of the **cardiac output** and 20% of the **oxygen** used by the body. The normal **cerebral blood flow** is about 50 ml/100 g of brain tissue a minute.

1. **Arterial supply to the brain** (see Chapter 7, Figure 7-3) can be divided into an anterior and a posterior circulation.
   a. **The anterior circulation** is derived from the two **internal carotid arteries,** each with its terminal branches, the larger **middle cerebral** and the smaller **anterior cerebral** arteries. These vessels supply mainly the **frontal, temporal,** and **parietal lobes** as well as the **deep gray matter.**
   b. **The posterior circulation** is comprised of two vertebral arteries.
      (1) At the caudal margin of the pons, the vertebral arteries unite to form the **basilar artery.**
      (2) The basilar artery gives off branches supplying the **pons, cerebellum, thalamus,** and (via the **posterior cerebral arteries**) the **occipital lobes.**
   c. **The circle of Willis,** an arterial circle, is formed at the base of the brain between branches of the internal carotid and basilar arteries.
      (1) This arterial circle is fully developed in only about 55% of the population and is of great clinical significance.
      (2) In the event of occlusion of a cerebral vessel (see IX), the blood supply to its territory may be taken over by another vessel via the circle of Willis.

2. **Venous return to the brain** can be divided into two parts.
   a. **Superficial cerebral veins** drain the cortex and subcortical white matter and finally end in the superior sagittal sinus or other basal sinuses (i.e., the transverse, petrosal, or cavernous sinuses).
   b. **Deep cerebral veins** drain the deeper structures (nuclei). The deep veins consist of the paired **internal cerebral** and **basal (Rosenthal) veins**, which finally form the **great vein of Galen** before emptying into the straight sinus.
      (1) All venous blood from the brain returns to the heart via the internal jugular vein.
      (2) Sampling of the jugular bulb blood provides an estimate of cerebral metabolism.

3. **Arterial supply to the spinal cord.** The spinal cord is supplied by the **anterior spinal artery** and the paired **posterior spinal arteries**, reinforced by the **segmental radicular arteries**.
   a. The **anterior spinal artery** gives off the **anterior sulcal artery** in the anterior sulcus, which supplies the anteromedial gray matter.
   b. The **segmental radicular arteries** follow the anterior and posterior roots and join the spinal arteries, forming an arterial circle or **arteria coronae**.
      (1) A large segmental artery at the C5–C6 vertebral level, called the **artery of Lazorthes**, has been described, and a similar artery exists at the thoracolumbar area, termed the **artery of the lumbar enlargement** or the **artery of Adamkiewicz**.
      (2) These segmental arteries are important because their interruption by trauma or surgery can lead to vascular infarction of the spinal cord.

4. **Venous return to the spinal cord** is similar to the arterial supply.
   a. **Anterior longitudinal venous trunks,** consisting of anteromedian and anterolateral veins, drain corresponding areas of the cord. These, in turn, are drained by 6–11 radicular veins draining into the epidural venous plexus.
   b. **Posterior longitudinal venous trunks,** consisting of one posteromedian and paired posterolateral veins, drain the posterior funiculus, the posterior horns, and the white matter in the lateral funiculi. These, in turn, are drained by 5–10 radicular veins into the epidural venous plexus.
   c. **The epidural venous plexus** is located between the vertebral periosteum and the dura mater.
      (1) The plexus consists of two or more anterior and posterior longitudinal veins interconnected at various levels.
      (2) At each intervertebral space, there is an extensive anastomosis with intercostal, thoracic, and abdominal veins.
      (3) None of these venous channels have valves, and, thus, blood from these plexuses may directly enter the systemic circulation and vice versa.

5. **Cerebrospinal fluid**
   a. The cerebrospinal fluid is the third major component within the intracranial compartment, the others being brain tissue and blood.
   b. Normally the total volume of the cerebrospinal fluid is about 150 ml, with 25 ml located in the ventricles. The cerebrospinal fluid is formed at the rate of 0.35 ml/min. About 80% of the cerebrospinal fluid is produced by the choroid plexus, with another 10%–20% formed in the interstitial spaces of the brain.
   c. The **cerebrospinal fluid flows** through the **ventricles** from the lateral to the third and then to the fourth, and **exits** by the **foramina of Magendie** (midline) and **Luschka** (lateral).
      (1) The fluid may then circulate around the spinal cord or pass via the arachnoid villi into the posterior part of the superior sagittal sinus.
      (2) The **arachnoid villi** act as one-way valves, allowing only cerebrospinal fluid to drain into the venous sinus, and they open at a pressure of 5 mm Hg.
      (3) Some of the cerebrospinal fluid is absorbed around the spinal nerve roots.

6. **Functional anatomy of the nervous system.** The following principles form the basis for evaluating and treating neurologic disease.
   a. **Pathophysiologic processes** unique to diseases of the nervous system involve the:
      (1) **Complexity of the functional anatomy** of the nervous system
      (2) **Rigidity of the bony enclosures** of the brain and spinal cord
      (3) **Responses of the nervous system** to injury
   b. **Focal lesions** affect local neurologic function by:
      (1) **Local destruction** of brain tissue
      (2) **Tissue distortion** with functional loss attributable to axonal stretching and consequent damage

(3) Changes in **local blood flow,** causing ischemia or venous congestion

(4) Alterations in the **electrical** or **metabolic activity** of a local area, producing an epileptic focus

  c. Location of the lesion is also important.

    (1) A small focal lesion in the **brain stem** can produce devastating effects.

    (2) A similar lesion in the **frontal (silent) area** may produce no significant neurologic deficit.

C. Pathophysiology

1. Cerebral edema. The brain reacts to different insults by developing edema. Investigators have reported that **acute edema** causes more deterioration in neurologic function than does **chronic edema**—that is, the **rate of formation** of edema is directly proportional to the neurologic deficits.

  a. Types of cerebral edema

    (1) Cytotoxic edema

      (a) Cytotoxic edema is usually seen in the gray matter as a result of a metabolic derangement within the astroglia, leading to an intracellular accumulation of water.

      (b) The blood–brain barrier is preserved.

      (c) This type of edema is common following anoxia and ischemia and in association with Reye's syndrome.

    (2) Vasogenic edema

      (a) Vasogenic edema (also called extracellular white matter edema) results from a breakdown of the blood–brain barrier and the leakage of plasma into the extracellular spaces.

      (b) This is the **commonest type of edema seen clinically,** and it occurs around tumors, abscesses, surgical sites, and areas of ischemia or trauma.

    (3) Interstitial edema. The protein content is low in situations of interstitial edema, which is usually seen in the periventricular region in patients with acute hydrocephalus.

  b. Mechanisms by which edema alters neuronal and axonal function

    (1) Ischemia as a result of increased intracranial pressure and decreased cerebral perfusion pressure

    (2) Decreased oxygen diffusion

    (3) Lipid peroxidation in membranes

2. Intracranial pressure

  a. Types of tissue in the **skull,** which is a rigid box with a volume of approximately 1900 ml

    (1) About 85% is **brain** (5% is extracellular fluid, 45% is glial tissue, and 35% is neuronal tissue).

    (2) About 7% is **blood.**

    (3) About 7% is **cerebrospinal fluid.**

  b. Monro-Kellie hypothesis. Under normal conditions, these three components of the skull (i.e., brain, blood, and cerebrospinal fluid) are in equilibrium, and the intracranial pressure is the sum of the pressure exerted by each one of them.

    (1) To maintain a normal intracranial pressure, a change in one compartment must be followed by **compensatory changes** in the other compartments.

    (2) The **rate of the added volume** is important.

      (a) A slow-growing tumor (e.g., a meningioma) can become quite large before there is any evidence of a change in intracranial pressure or in neurologic function.

      (b) A small but acute mass lesion (e.g., an acute epidural or subdural hematoma) can cause a tremendous increase in intracranial pressure and severe neurologic deficits.

  c. The relationship between intracranial pressure and intracranial volume is described by an exponential curve (Figure 27-1) with an initial flat portion and a later steep portion.

    (1) As the volume of one compartment increases, the volumes of the other compartments must decrease to maintain normal intracranial pressure.

    (2) Beyond a certain point (i.e., beyond the end of the flat portion of the curve), a slight increase in intracranial volume produces a very large increase in intracranial pressure (as evidenced by the steep portion of the curve).

    (3) Equilibrium is maintained mainly by cerebrospinal fluid buffering. With continued volume changes, cerebrospinal fluid buffering becomes exhausted and the elastic

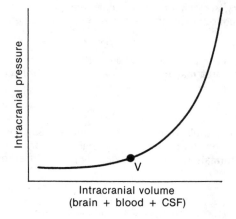

Figure 27-1. The pressure–volume relationship within the intracranial space can be represented by a pressure–volume curve. The intracranial pressure stays within normal limits until a critical volume (V) is reached, above which the pressure rises steeply. *CSF* = cerebrospinal fluid.

properties of the brain substance and the blood vessels play the major buffering role (represented by the steep portion of the pressure–volume curve).

(4) The upper limit of normal intracranial pressure is considered to be 15 mm Hg.

d. Symptoms and signs of increased intracranial pressure (intracranial hypertension) include:
   (1) Headache
   (2) Nausea
   (3) Vomiting
   (4) Clouding of mentation
   (5) Papilledema
   (6) Paralysis of upward gaze (**Parinaud's syndrome**)
   (7) Sixth nerve palsy
   (8) Bulging fontanelles and splitting of sutures (in infants)

3. Herniation. When all compensatory mechanisms have been exhausted and the intracranial pressure continues to rise, the brain "herniates" or shifts towards the low-pressure compartment (the falx and the tentorium divide the interior of the skull into compartments). Various **herniation syndromes** are recognized.

a. Subfalcial herniation is a displacement from one supratentorial compartment to another underneath the falx. It may lead to loss of function in the opposite leg, loss of bladder control, or both.

b. Transtentorial (uncal) herniation
   (1) This is the **commonest type of brain herniation seen clinically** and occurs when the parahippocampal gyrus and uncus of one or both hemispheres is forced down the tentorial notch.
   (2) Uncal herniation may occur as a result of diffuse brain swelling or a supratentorial mass lesion.
   (3) **Neurologic signs** are:
      (a) Progressive deterioration of consciousness
      (b) Ipsilateral pupillary dilatation as a result of third nerve compression
      (c) Contralateral hemiparesis as a result of compression of the cerebral peduncles
   (4) Hemiparesis is ipsilateral in 50% of the cases, while pupillary dilatation is ipsilateral in 80%. Thus, pupillary dilatation is much more reliable in localizing the lesion. In 20% of the cases, the pupillary dilatation occurs on the side opposite to the lesion— a false localizing sign known as the **Kernohan-Woltman notch phenomenon.**

c. Trans–foramen magnum herniation
   (1) The cerebellar tonsils may herniate through the foramen magnum.
   (2) The resultant medullary compression may elicit a Cushing response (i.e., hypertension, bradycardia, and apnea) and may ultimately lead to death.

4. Cerebral blood flow, autoregulation, and cerebral perfusion pressure
   a. Overview
      (1) The **average cerebral blood flow** is normally about **50 ml/100 g of brain tissue a minute,** with the gray matter having a higher flow (i.e., 75 ml/100 g/min) than the white matter (25 ml/100 g/min).

(2) The blood flow is coupled to the local metabolic demands and is highest where the density of synapses is greatest (this is termed **metabolic autoregulation**).

(3) The flow is directly proportional to the **mean arterial pressure** and the radius of the vessel raised to the fourth power (**Poiseuille's law**), and it is inversely proportional to the blood viscosity and the length of the blood vessels. Thus, increasing the caliber of the vessels or decreasing the blood viscosity can increase the flow markedly, and these factors are manipulated in clinical situations to improve cerebral blood flow.

b. Pressure autoregulation describes the observation that normally over a wide range of mean arterial pressure (50–150 mm Hg) the cerebral blood flow remains unchanged at 50 ml/100 g of brain tissue a minute.

(1) This may change focally or globally as a result of head injury, subarachnoid hemorrhage, stroke, or a brain tumor.

(2) If the patient has an intracranial pressure monitor and an arterial line, autoregulation can be tested simply by elevating the systolic blood pressure by 10–15 mm Hg and observing the changes in intracranial pressure.

  (a) If autoregulation is intact, the intracranial pressure should remain unchanged.

  (b) However, if the intracranial pressure passively follows the arterial pressure, it is indicative of impaired autoregulation (vasoparalysis) and is usually a terminal event.

(3) The **cerebral perfusion pressure (CPP)** is equal to the mean arterial pressure (MAP) minus the intracranial pressure (ICP); that is, **CPP = MAP – ICP**. A cerebral perfusion pressure as low as 50 mm Hg can maintain an adequate cerebral blood flow; below 50 mm Hg, the cerebral blood flow decreases steeply. Hence, it is the goal of neurosurgical intervention to **maintain the cerebral perfusion pressure above 50 mm Hg**.

II. EVALUATING THE NEUROSURGICAL PATIENT

A. Personal and family history

1. The patient's history is an important part of the diagnostic armamentarium.

  a. A good history may be the only clue to the diagnosis of either a transient ischemic attack (TIA), which causes no neurologic signs, or a subarachnoid hemorrhage.

  b. It may also help to ascertain the severity of a head injury by identifying periods of anterograde and retrograde amnesia.

  c. It may be necessary to delay taking the history in the event of a life-threatening emergency that requires the physician's immediate attention.

2. The family history helps to rule out congenital lesions, metabolic disorders, neurofibromatosis, Huntington's chorea, and various degenerative central nervous system disorders.

B. Physical examination

1. Vital signs. Simple observation of blood pressure, pulse rate, and respiration can be helpful in localizing a lesion because the vital signs are controlled by central nervous system mechanisms.

2. Hypertension (Cushing response). Cushing first pointed out that compression of the medullary centers by increased intracranial pressure results in hypertension, bradycardia, and short, shallow respirations. The Cushing response is, however, generally considered to be a **terminal response;** when it is noted, irreversible neurologic changes have already taken place.

3. Hypotension in the neurosurgical patient may be produced by interruption of the sympathetic innervation of peripheral vessels, leading to venous pooling. This may be secondary to a hypothalamic, medullary, or spinal cord injury.

4. Patterns of respiration

  a. Lesions in the forebrain can lead to **posthyperventilation apnea**.

  (1) In normal individuals, following a period of hyperventilation, there is a resumption of regular breathing without a delay, although there is a reduction of the tidal volume until normal carbon dioxide partial pressure (P_{CO_2}) is restored.

        (2) Patients with **structural** or **metabolic forebrain damage** do not resume their regular breathing rhythm following hyperventilation, undergoing a period of apnea. Regular respirations are resumed after the Pco_2 returns to the normal level.

    b. Lesions deep in the cerebral hemispheres and involving the **basal ganglia** are associated with **Cheyne-Stokes respiration**.

        (1) Regular periods of hyperpnea alternating with apnea characterize this pattern of breathing.

        (2) The breathing gradually rises in a smooth crescendo and then wanes in a smooth decrescendo.

    c. Lesions in the midbrain can cause **central neurogenic hyperventilation**—deep breathing at a very fast rate, which may lead to severe **alkalosis**.

    d. Lesions in the lower pons can cause **apneustic breathing**—complete cessation of involuntary breathing, leading to respiratory arrest during sleep (**Ondine's curse**).

    e. Medullary lesions can lead to various types of abnormal breathing patterns, which include:

        (1) Cluster breathing (a disorderly sequence of clusters of breaths with irregular pauses in between)

        (2) Ataxic breathing (**Biot's breathing**—periodic breathing in which apneic periods are punctuated by a few irregular deep breaths, lacking the waxing and waning pattern of Cheyne-Stokes respiration)

        (3) Cheyne-Stokes respiration

        (4) Gasping (breathing in which both deep and shallow breaths occur randomly with haphazard intervening pauses and a slow respiratory rate, which may finally lead to apnea)

    f. Kussmaul's respiration, deep rapid breathing similar to central neurogenic hyperventilation, usually occurs as a result of diabetic or uremic acidosis.

5. Hyperthermia. Neurologic disorders can cause severe hyperthermia with body temperatures exceeding 105° F. The commonest **causes** are:

    a. Hyperthyroidism

    b. Heat stroke

    c. Lesions involving the posterior hypothalamus

    d. Status epilepticus

    e. Drug intoxication (e.g., due to isoniazid, amitriptyline, phenothiazines, or carbidopa–levodopa)

    f. Malignant hyperthermia [idiopathic or as a result of a hereditary (autosomal dominant) muscle disease]

    g. Intraventricular hemorrhage

6. Hypothermia. Cold coma may be a result of:

    a. Lesions involving the anterior hypothalamus

    b. Myxedema

    c. Alcohol intoxication

    d. Severe hypoglycemia

    e. Hepatic and renal failure

C. Neurologic evaluation. A detailed neurologic evaluation may not be possible in some emergency situations, such as trauma, in which case it may be necessary to do a **brief examination** to assess the neurologic damage.

1. The level of consciousness should be determined first. Patients may present as:

    a. Alert, awake, and oriented

    b. Lethargic (i.e., sleepy but easily arousable)

    c. Stuporous (i.e., responsive only to noxious stimuli)

    d. Comatose (i.e., not responsive to noxious stimuli)

2. Examination of the pupils. The pupils are examined for their size and reaction to light, and the position and movement of the eyes are noted. A few general rules may be helpful in localizing a lesion:

    a. When a **cortical** lesion is present, the size of the pupil may be 6 mm or larger, and there may be wandering or roving eye movements.

    b. With a lesion in the **basal ganglia**, the pupils may range from 2–3 mm in size and the eyes are deviated downward and inward.

    c. A lesion in the **midbrain** may be associated with pupils that are 4–5 mm in size (midrange), and convergent nystagmus or nystagmus retractorius may be present.

d. A lesion in the **pons** may be associated with pinpoint pupils (1 mm) and with ocular bobbing.

e. When a **medullary** lesion is present, the pupils may be slightly small (2 mm), and there is downbeat nystagmus.

3. Brain stem reflexes, such as the oculocephalic (doll's eye) reflex, and the caloric (oculo-vestibular) responses are checked to rule out irreversible brain stem damage.

4. Motor examination is then performed. In a comatose patient, it may only be possible to assess the response to painful stimuli.

5. Sensory level determination is important in patients with spinal cord lesions (see IV C 1).

6. Deep tendon reflexes and **plantar responses** are checked to distinguish a lower motor neuron lesion from an upper motor neuron lesion.

D. Special diagnostic tests

1. Selective angiography (arteriography). See Figure 27-7 for an example of an angiogram.

    a. This study involves the introduction of a catheter via the transfemoral route (currently the commonest route) into one of the major cerebral vessels (carotids or vertebrals) and the injection of a contrast agent while rapid-sequence x-rays are taken. A definitive picture of the cerebral circulation is obtained.

    b. This is a relatively safe procedure with a morbidity rate that is less than 1%.

2. Myelography

    a. A contrast agent (usually the water-soluble metrizamide) is instilled in the thecal space through a C1–C2 tap or a lumbar puncture.

    b. By the movement of this dye column or its appearance on the x-ray, the nature of the intraspinal lesion can be determined.

3. CT scan has been a major breakthrough in the past decade. The new scanners provide anatomically precise images of the brain and the spinal cord. (See Figures 27-2–27-5 for examples of CT scans.)

4. Magnetic resonance imaging (MRI)

    a. Because MRI looks through bone, it is very helpful in the diagnosis of intraspinal lesions. However, its role is not fully established.

    b. MRI is based on the **principle** that the nuclei of certain elements [e.g., ^{1}H (proton), ^{2}H, ^{13}C, ^{19}F, ^{31}P, and ^{127}I] respond to the application of electromagnetic pulses by absorbing energy and re-emitting it as detectable radio waves.

        (1) These waves can be analyzed by computer and used to obtain morphologic or chemical information about body constituents or to generate detailed anatomic images.

        (2) Several studies have proved the sensitivity of MRI to pathologic changes seen in a broad spectrum of neurologic diseases, especially central nervous system tumors and ischemic lesions.

    c. MRI has rapidly emerged as an **imaging technique** with the potential for providing more diagnostic information in certain situations than any other imaging modality, including CT. The main **advantages of MRI over CT** include:

        (1) Superior contrast between gray and white matter

        (2) Multiplanar or three-dimensional imaging

        (3) Absence of bone artifacts

        (4) High sensitivity to pathologic change

        (5) Absence of any known risks

5. Electromyography

    a. Electromyography involves the recording and study of neuromuscular transmission, such as nerve conduction velocities and the response of muscle to stimulation.

    b. It can help in the evaluation of patients recovering from peripheral nerve injuries and in the diagnosis of entrapment neuropathies.

6. Ultrasonography

    a. This is a very helpful tool in infants as the fontanelle affords easy access to ultrasound imaging.

    b. Currently, ultrasonography is used frequently in the intraoperative diagnosis of lesions located deep within the spinal cord or brain.

III. HEAD INJURIES

A. **Incidence.** Current data show that there are 420,000 new head injuries every year. This number includes hospital admissions only; the overall figures are more impressive. There were 7,560,000 head injuries in the United States in 1976. Of these, 1,255,000 were classified as major head injuries, which included concussion, intracranial hemorrhage, cerebral laceration, cerebral contusion, and crushing of the head.

B. **Classification**

1. Brain injuries following trauma can be classified as:
   a. **Primary**, occurring instantaneously at the time of impact
   b. **Secondary**, resulting from a chain of events triggered by the initial injury. If not controlled, secondary injuries lead to further damage as a result of ischemia, hypoxia, or both.

2. Primary and secondary injuries can be either:
   a. Nonhemorrhagic focal or diffuse **edema**
   b. **Hemorrhages**
      (1) Intra-axial (i.e., intracerebral—within the brain substance)
      (2) Extra-axial [i.e., extracerebral—outside the brain parenchyma (e.g., epidural and subdural hematomas)]

C. **Initial management and assessment**

1. **Immediate care** of a head trauma victim is no different from that of any other injured patient (see Chapter 21 I C 4).
   a. **Priorities**
      (1) **Establishment of adequate ventilation**
      (2) **Control of hemorrhage**
      (3) **Maintenance of peripheral vascular circulation**
   b. **Volume replacement** with colloid or blood products can be used when necessary to reduce the risk that cerebral edema will develop or worsen.
   c. **Stabilization of the neck** with a hard cervical collar (Philadelphia collar) or by sandbags placed on either side of the head is necessary in all patients.
      (1) Fully 10% of patients with severe head injuries have **associated spinal cord injuries**, and consequently all patients with head injuries should be transported as if they had a spinal cord injury.
      (2) Precautions include immobilization of the spine on a hard board and use of a cervical collar until further investigation for spinal cord injury is carried out.
   d. **Blood is drawn** for typing and crossmatching and for other laboratory studies.

2. **Initial examination**
   a. **The type and magnitude of the injuries** can be determined by information gleaned from the initial examination. For example:
      (1) A closed head injury—injury inflicted to the brain without any evidence of scalp laceration
      (2) An injury resulting from a high-speed, nonimpact acceleration–deceleration
      (3) Blunt trauma with or without a scalp laceration or contusion (all scalp lacerations should be checked manually for an underlying skull fracture)
      (4) A penetrating wound from a knife or a bullet (entrance and exit wounds must be sought)
   b. **Location of a fracture** can be determined by certain signs.
      (1) Fractures traversing the base of the skull (**basilar fractures**) often cause ecchymosis behind the ear (**Battle's sign**).
      (2) Anterior basilar fractures often result in periorbital ecchymosis (raccoon's eyes) and subconjunctival hemorrhage.
      (3) Hematotympanum is associated with fractures of the middle fossa.

3. **History.** After the initial management, and if the patient is awake, a quick history should be obtained. The severity of a head injury and the final outcome are directly related to the duration of the unconsciousness, which the history may reveal.

4. **Neurologic evaluation.** A rapid assessment of the patient is performed (see II C).

    a. The Glasgow coma scale (GCS) is now used almost universally in the assessment of the head injury victim. This scale measures three responses:

      (1) Eye opening

        (a) Spontaneous = 4

        (b) In response to command = 3

        (c) In response to pain = 2

        (d) None = 1

      (2) Motor response

        (a) Obeys commands = 6

        (b) Localizes pain = 5

        (c) Withdraws from pain = 4

        (d) Shows flexion (decorticate) response to pain = 3

        (e) Shows extension (decerebrate) response to pain = 2

        (f) None = 1

      (3) Vocal response

        (a) Oriented to person, place, and time = 5

        (b) Confused = 4

        (c) Shows inappropriate speech = 3

        (d) Makes incomprehensible sounds = 2

        (e) None = 1

    b. The GCS score ranges from 3–15.

      (1) The GCS score at 6 hours after trauma is a good predictor of the long-term outcome in head injury (i.e., recovery, disability, vegetative state, or death).

      (2) Adult patients with a 6-hour GCS score below 7 are likely to have a poor outcome; the prognosis is much better in the pediatric population.

    c. Neurologic examinations are repeated periodically; a change of 2 or more in the GCS score is considered significant.

  5. Radiologic studies

    a. CT scans are preferable to skull x-rays in severely injured patients.

      (1) Diagnostic findings

        (a) Hematomas (Figures 27-2 and 27-3) can be easily diagnosed because fresh blood appears hyperdense on a CT scan.

          (i) Epidural hematomas appear as semilunar dense collections with a convexity towards the brain (see Figure 27-2).

          (ii) Acute subdural hematomas have a concavity towards the brain.

        (b) Subarachnoid hemorrhages make subarachnoid spaces appear denser.

        (c) Hemorrhages in the white matter, such as the corpus callosum, internal capsule, and midbrain, suggest a diffuse axonal type of injury (Figure 27-4).

        (d) Cerebral edema (Figure 27-5) can be indicated by the size of the ventricles and basal subarachnoid cisterns.

      (2) If the CT scan is positive, the patient is taken immediately to the operating room for evacuation of hematomas or to the intensive care unit for intracranial pressure monitoring and management of brain swelling.

    b. X-rays

      (1) X-rays of the cervical spine are taken to rule out associated spinal injuries.

      (2) Skull x-rays are used instead of CT scans **to screen for skull fractures** in patients with less severe injuries.

        (a) Intracranial air or clouding of the sinuses suggests a cerebrospinal fluid leak.

        (b) If a fracture line crosses the groove of the middle meningeal vessels, an epidural hematoma should be suspected.

        (c) Basilar skull fractures are very poorly visualized on x-ray and may even be missed on CT scan unless the scan is reviewed carefully. However, clouding of the mastoid air cells or the sphenoid sinus suggests a basilar skull fracture.

D. Management of increased intracranial pressure

  1. Maintenance of an adequate perfusion pressure [see I C 4 b (3)] to **prevent irreversible ischemic injury** to the brain (which is a secondary type of post-traumatic brain injury) is the major goal of treatment of increased intracranial pressure. The patient's cerebral perfusion pressure is maintained above 50 mm Hg by manipulation of the intracranial pressure and the mean arterial pressure.

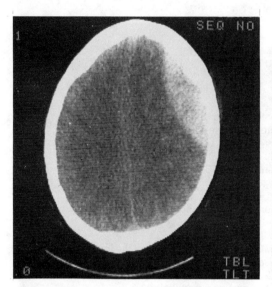

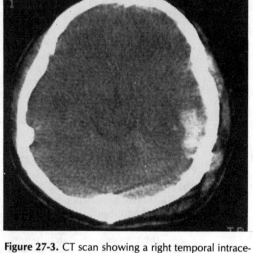

Figure 27-2. CT scan of the head showing a large right frontotemporal epidural hematoma. Acute epidural hematomas have a convexity towards the brain in contradistinction to acute subdural hematomas, which have a concavity towards the brain. Chronic subdural hematomas may resemble acute epidural hematomas but are much less dense.

Figure 27-3. CT scan showing a right temporal intracerebral hematoma following a head injury.

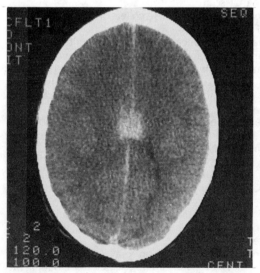

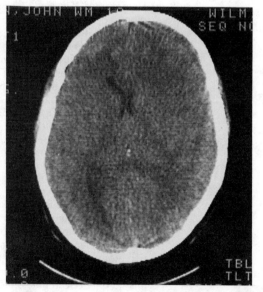

Figure 27-4. CT scan showing evidence of a "bleed" in the corpus callosum. This type of hemorrhage deep in the white matter is seen in diffuse axonal (closed head) injuries.

Figure 27-5. CT scan showing diffuse swelling of the right cerebral hemisphere with effacement of the right lateral ventricle and a midline shift.

2. **Placement of an intracranial pressure monitor** is necessary to control intracranial pressure aggressively.
   a. **Criteria for placement of an intracranial pressure monitor** include one or both of the following:
      (1) A score of 5 or less on the GCS
      (2) Associated systemic complications, such as severe hypotension or hypoxia
   b. **Intracranial pressure measuring devices** (monitors) are of two types:
      (1) **Intraventricular catheter**
         (a) This gives the most accurate measurement and provides the option of removing cerebrospinal fluid to lower the intracranial pressure in an emergency.
         (b) Placement of an intraventricular catheter can be difficult in the presence of diffuse brain swelling with slit-like ventricles.
      (2) **Subarachnoid bolt** (Richmond screw or Philly bolt)
         (a) The subarachnoid bolt is easy to place, gives accurate readings, and is associated with a low infection rate.
         (b) Most head trauma centers use this type of intracranial pressure monitoring device.

3. **Intracranial hypertension** can be managed by a variety of methods. The following therapies can be used in sequence.
   a. **Elevation of the patient's head.** This promotes venous drainage, thereby decreasing intracranial pressure.
   b. **Hyperventilation.** The cerebral vessels respond quickly to a change in the arterial PCO_2. A low PCO_2 causes vasoconstriction, while an elevated PCO_2 causes vasodilatation.
      (1) The PCO_2 is not lowered below 25 mm Hg because the consequent decrease in cerebral blood flow could be counterproductive and also because a problematic respiratory alkalosis develops.
      (2) If the intracranial pressure is not sufficiently lowered by hyperventilation, other therapies have to be used.
   c. **Increasing the serum osmolality** (to around 300 mOsm)
      (1) **Fluid restriction**
         (a) The patient is given only two-thirds of the calculated volume of maintenance fluid (5% dextrose in one-half normal saline solution) to increase the serum osmolality and reduce the transcapillary fluid movement.
         (b) This helps to reduce the cerebral edema, thus lowering intracranial pressure.
      (2) **Hyperosmolar agents**
         (a) The diuretic most commonly used is mannitol, which is administered intravenously in a bolus of 1–1.5 g/kg or by continuous infusion of 0.05–0.15 g/kg/hr. Its effect can be seen in 5–20 minutes. Bolus doses usually are given every 6 hours, and additional doses are given when there is a dangerous rise in intracranial pressure.
            (i) Mannitol is an osmotic diuretic and acts by withdrawing water from the cerebral interstitial spaces if the blood–brain barrier is intact.
            (ii) Repeated use can lead to severe dehydration, hypernatremia, and hyperosmolality. In a patient with hypovolemia, mannitol can cause renal tubular damage.
         (b) **Glycerol** can be administered, either as an intravenous bolus or by continuous infusion, if the patient is refractory to mannitol.
      (3) Serum osmolality and electrolytes have to be measured every 6–8 hours.
   d. **Loop diuretics. Furosemide** is the drug most commonly used and is administered intravenously. The effect of the drug is rapid.
   e. **Corticosteroids**
      (1) Steroids have not been shown to lower the intracranial pressure, but they improve the compliance of the brain (i.e., they shift the pressure–volume curve to the right) and prevent a steep increase in pressure (Figure 27-6).
      (2) Some head injury centers use megadose steroid therapy (i.e., 1 mg/kg of dexamethasone administered intravenously followed by 0.5 mg/kg/day in four divided doses).
   f. **Barbiturates** can be used if all of the previously mentioned efforts fail to lower the intracranial pressure.
      (1) An initial dose of 3 mg/kg of sodium pentobarbital is given intravenously, followed by a maintenance dose of 0.5–3 mg/kg/hr. The effect of the drug occurs within minutes, and an adequate serum level (25–40 mg/L) is maintained. A burst suppression

1 = Normal
2 = Effect of steroids, mannitol,
    and decreasing SAP
3 = Effect of increasing SAP

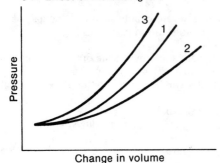

Pressure

Change in volume

Figure 27-6. Changes in pressure–volume curves. *Curve 1* represents a baseline. It has an initial flat portion, which becomes very steep. Steroids, mannitol, and decreasing systemic arterial pressure (*SAP*) improve the cerebral compliance, and the curve moves to the right (*curve 2*). An increase in SAP, on the other hand, causes a stiffening of the brain—that is, a decrease in cerebral compliance (*curve 3*).

pattern on the electroencephalogram suggests that a therapeutic serum level has been reached.

(2) Barbiturates cause myocardial depression, leading to hypotension, and vasopressor agents may be necessary to elevate the mean arterial pressure to maintain an adequate cerebral perfusion pressure.

(3) Although the exact mechanism of action is not known, barbiturates may act by:
   (a) Decreasing cerebral blood flow
   (b) Reducing the metabolic activity of the brain
   (c) Reducing synaptic transmission

g. **Hypothermia** may be used as an adjunct to other therapies. The core temperature of the body is lowered from normal to a temperature that ranges from 89.6°–93.2° F (32°–34° C), which probably decreases the intracranial pressure by reducing cerebral metabolism.

E. **Management of intracranial hemorrhages**

1. **Subarachnoid hemorrhage**, the commonest type of post-traumatic intracranial hemorrhage, usually requires no immediate surgical intervention. However, there is a risk of developing hydrocephalus, and thus, follow-up CT scans are necessary.

2. **Epidural hematomas**
   a. Epidural hemorrhages (those between the skull and dura mater) arise from tears in the middle meningeal artery or vein or in a dural sinus.
   b. The initial impact may result in a temporary loss of consciousness, which is followed by a lucid interval in which the patient is fully awake.
   c. As bleeding continues, a stage is reached when the intracranial pressure rises steeply and there is uncal herniation, causing loss of consciousness, an ipsilateral dilated pupil, and contralateral hemiplegia.
   d. Prompt surgical evacuation makes the difference between a good prognosis and death.

3. **Subdural hematomas**
   a. Subdural hematomas are **classified** according to the **interval of time** between the trauma and the onset of symptoms:
      (1) **Acute** (up to 48 hours)
      (2) **Subacute** (48 hours to 12 days)
      (3) **Chronic** (more than 12 days)
   b. Subdural hematomas arise from tears in the dural sinuses or bridging veins, and they are bilateral in 15% of the cases.
   c. Acute subdural hematomas with a rapid progression of symptoms have a poor prognosis unless they are surgically evacuated.

F. **Management of intracerebral hematomas and cerebral contusions**

1. **Intracerebral hematomas** result from the tearing of small vessels in the white matter and are due to penetrating trauma or acceleration–deceleration injuries.

2. Cerebral contusions. Superficial hemorrhages most commonly occur when the anterior temporal and frontal lobes strike the rough edges of the tentorium (**contrecoup contusion**).
  a. A **coup injury** occurs where the skull strikes the brain underlying the site of impact.
  b. A **contrecoup injury** occurs directly opposite to the impact site.
  c. Thus, if a person is struck on the back of the head, the coup injury would be to the occipital lobe while the frontotemporal tips would sustain the contrecoup injury.

3. Surgical decompression of intracerebral hematomas and cerebral contusions may be necessary when increased intracranial pressure (caused by a mass effect from the accumulated blood and the secondary edema) becomes refractory to medical management.

G. Management of scalp injuries

1. The scalp is made up of **five layers**:
  S —skin
  C —dense subcutaneous tissue
  A —aponeurosis
  L —loose areolar tissue
  P —pericranium

2. The scalp is a **highly vascular** structure, and much blood can be lost from scalp lacerations before they are sutured.
  a. The scalp wound is thoroughly cleansed, debrided, and sutured as soon as possible.
  b. Any laceration greater than 6–8 inches should be closed in the operating room.

H. Management of skull fractures

1. Classification
  a. Linear, stellate, or comminuted describe skull fractures, depending on the complexity of the fracture line.
  b. Depressed fractures are those in which a portion of the vault is displaced inward.
  c. Compound fractures are present if the overlying scalp is lacerated.
  d. Basilar fractures traverse the base of the skull.

2. Operative intervention is necessary to deal mainly with a depressed skull fracture and a compound comminuted skull fracture with underlying cerebral damage.
  a. Depressed skull fractures are usually associated with dural tears and may or may not be accompanied by underlying brain damage. If they are left untreated, scarring may lead to an epileptogenic focus, and, hence, it is necessary to elevate these fractures.
  b. Compound comminuted fractures with damage to the underlying brain are handled by removal of all bony fragments (including those embedded in the brain), thorough debridement, and closure. Failure to remove all bony fragments may lead to the later development of a brain abscess.

I. Management of cerebrospinal fluid leaks

1. Leaks of the cerebrospinal fluid, if mixed with blood, can be **diagnosed** by the **ring (halo) sign**: If drops of cerebrospinal fluid mixed with blood are placed on gauze, a lighter halo forms around a central bloodier area.

2. Most **post-traumatic cerebrospinal fluid fistulas** close spontaneously with **conservative management**, which includes elevating the head to reduce both the intracranial pressure and the cerebrospinal fluid leakage.
  a. In some cases, a drain may have to be placed in the lumbar theca to drain cerebrospinal fluid preferentially through it and allow the fistula to heal.
  b. In extreme cases, operative closure of the leak may be necessary.
  c. The administration of antibiotics in cases of cerebrospinal fluid leaks is controversial, but most surgeons who do use them choose a narrow-spectrum drug, such as nafcillin.

IV. SPINAL CORD INJURIES (see Chapter 28 III B 3 a)

A. Overview

1. Causes. Most spinal cord injuries are caused by automobile accidents, sports injuries, and falls.

    2. Common sites of injury to the vertebral column are the junctions between relatively fixed and mobile segments. These are the:
      a. Lumbosacral junction
      b. Thoracolumbar junction
      c. Cervicothoracic junction

    3. Aims of neurosurgical intervention are:
      a. Preservation of neuronal function
      b. Restoration of bony alignment
      c. Rehabilitation

    4. Associated injuries must be sought. These include:
      a. Hemo- or pneumothorax
      b. Damage to the thoracic aorta
      c. Intra-abdominal or head injuries

B. Initial management

    1. Immobilization of the spine. Great care must be taken to immobilize the spine during transfer of the patient to the hospital from the trauma site.
      a. This can be done by transferring the patient on a firm surface, by use of a hard cervical collar (Philadelphia collar), or both.
      b. It cannot be overemphasized that the **paramedic plays a critical role** in the initial evacuation of patients with spinal cord injuries. Spinal cord injuries can be worsened if proper precautions are not taken during transfer.

    2. Stabilization
      a. The stabilization procedures that are essential for trauma management (see Chapter 21 I C) should be carried out. These are:
        (1) Airway assessment and control
        (2) Establishment of ventilation
        (3) Circulatory support
      b. Patients with **cervical cord injury** may lose their vascular sympathetic tone as a result of the injury and develop **hypotension**. Fluid replacement restores normal blood pressure.
      c. Mannitol, sodium bicarbonate, and methylprednisolone are given intravenously to reduce cord edema and lactic acidosis.

C. Neurologic evaluation

    1. Motor and sensory examinations are performed rapidly to determine the:
      a. Level of the injury. Sensory level determination can be done easily by running a sharp pin lightly across the body to elicit the **triple response of Lewis** (**reflex erythema**—a red line, then a flush, then a wheal), which is diminished or absent below the level of the lesion.
      b. Type of injury (i.e., **complete**, with no function below the level of the injury, or **incomplete**). Important **examples of incomplete injuries** include:
        (1) Central cord injury, which involves the central portion of the cord (the upper extremities are affected more often than the lower extremities)
        (2) Anterior cord injury, which involves the anterior segment of the cord, resulting in muscular weakness, hypoesthesia, and hypalgesia below the level of the lesion
        (3) Brown-Séquard syndrome (hemisection of the cord), which causes contralateral sensory loss and homolateral paralysis

    2. An examination of the sacral segment of the cord (i.e., the bulbocavernosus reflex, the anal twitch, and sacral sensations) must be carried out, because the prognosis is better in patients with preserved sacral reflexes.

D. Radiologic studies. It must be emphasized that in a case of suspected spinal cord injury, the **entire spine must be visualized** with films of good quality before a diagnosis is made.

    1. X-ray studies and CT scans are done to determine the site and extent of bony injury.

    2. Myelography is performed if the bony lesion and the neurologically determined level do not match or if there is a deterioration in the patient's neurologic status.

    3. MRI can delineate intrinsic spinal cord abnormalities, such as cord edema or hemorrhage, better than CT scan or myelography.

E. Treatment

1. **Skeletal traction.** In cases of cervical injuries with fracture dislocations of the spine, skull tongs (such as Gardner-Wells, the most commonly employed) are attached and weights are used to apply traction to the spine. These procedures restore the normal alignment of the vertebral column and relieve the compression of the neural structures.

2. **Surgical intervention**
   a. Previously, patients with spinal cord injuries were managed by immobilization and postural reduction, but there has been a change towards more aggressive surgical management. The **aim** of surgical management is to stabilize the spine and allow early rehabilitation.
   b. **Indications for surgery** may be acute or subacute.
      (1) Immediate surgical intervention is needed in cases of marked neurologic deterioration with myelographic evidence of block.
      (2) Surgery is needed subacutely in patients with incomplete injuries when there is evidence of continued neural compression and the patient, having reached a plateau, fails to show any further neurologic recovery.

F. Long-term complications of spinal cord injuries include:

1. **Pressure sores**, the incidence of which is reduced by the use of a Stryker frame or a rotokinetic (e.g., Rotorest) bed

2. **Flexor spasms**, which can be managed medically with muscle relaxants (e.g., diazepam or baclofen) or in extreme cases by rhizotomy (sectioning the nerve root)

3. **Renal stones, pyelonephritis, and renal failure**

4. **Deep vein thrombosis,** which is the most deadly complication and is diagnosed by:
   a. Maintaining a high index of suspicion
   b. Performing routine impedance plethysmography, iodine 125 (^{125}I)-labeled fibrinogen scanning, and venography, if necessary (see Chapter 8 I B 3)

V. PERIPHERAL NERVE INJURIES (see Chapter 28 III B 3 b)

A. Classification

1. **Neurapraxia** is focal contusion of a nerve, resulting in loss of function. There is continuity of the axons, and the myelin sheaths remain intact.
   a. This type of injury may be due to:
      (1) A direct blow
      (2) Prolonged compression
      (3) Stretching
      (4) A gunshot wound
      (5) A blast injury
   b. Function returns spontaneously in about 6 weeks.

2. **Axonotmesis** is disruption of axons with intact myelin sheaths. The distal axon degenerates. Since the myelin sheaths are in continuity, return of function can be anticipated, because the axon grows back at the rate of 1 mm a day or 1 inch a month.

3. **Neurotmesis** is complete disruption of both the axons and the myelin sheaths. The divided nerves must be approximated for optimal recovery, and there are residual neurologic deficits.

B. Treatment

1. **Indications for immediate surgical repair** are:
   a. Digital nerve injuries
   b. Clean and sharp lacerations

2. **Open injuries of peripheral nerves.** The final extent of the injury is not known for a few weeks.
   a. Nerve repair is, therefore, delayed for 3–4 weeks.
   b. At the time of primary wound repair, the divided ends of the nerves are identified and a suture is tied around the stumps to make identification easier in subsequent repair.

3. **Deep wounds** (e.g., gunshot wounds or deep lacerations). Recovery of function is monitored by serial neurologic examinations and electromyography. Surgical intervention is necessary only when there is lack of optimal recovery.

VI. TUMORS OF THE CENTRAL NERVOUS SYSTEM

A. Incidence

1. Three percent of all cancer deaths are due to brain tumors, which have an incidence of 5/100,000 of the population. The frequency peaks in the sixth decade of life.

2. About 85% of central nervous system tumors are intracranial, while 15% are intraspinal.

3. Fully 25% of central nervous system tumors are metastatic, and 30% of all metastasizing tumors (i.e., lung, breast, skin, gastrointestinal, and urinary tract) have multiple brain metastases.

4. Fifteen percent of all brain tumors occur in children. Among the malignancies of children, central nervous system tumors are second only to leukemia in prevalence.

5. Sixty-five percent of brain tumors in children are infratentorial, and thirty-five percent are supratentorial. This ratio is reversed in adults.

B. Brain tumors

1. **Classification.** Brain tumors can be broadly classified as glial and nonglial, depending upon the cell of origin.
   a. **Glial tumors (gliomas)** constitute 40%–50% of brain tumors.
      (1) They include **astrocytomas** (grades I through IV, depending upon their malignancy), **oligodendrogliomas,** and **ependymomas**.
      (2) Grade IV **astrocytomas (glioblastomas)** that arise in the hemispheres are **the commonest brain tumors** in adults. Low-grade (i.e., grades I and II) midline astrocytomas are the commonest brain tumors in children.
   b. **Nonglial cell tumors**
      (1) This classification is made up of **meningiomas** (arising from arachnoidal cells), **neurilemomas** (arising from nerve sheaths), **medulloblastomas** (of neuroectodermal origin), **pituitary tumors, pineal tumors,** tumors arising from blood vessels, such as **hemangioblastomas** and **endotheliomas,** congenital tumors, such as, **dermoid tumors** and **teratomas,** and **metastatic tumors**.
      (2) Meningiomas account for 15%–20% of brain tumors; neurilemomas account for 10%–15%; and metastatic tumors account for 5%–10%.

2. **Clinical findings**
   a. **Focal neurologic deficits** result from destruction or compression of neuronal tissue either directly by the tumor or indirectly by a decrease in the blood supply.
   b. **Seizures** may occur due to the alteration of neuronal function.
   c. Signs and symptoms of **raised intracranial pressure** may occur, including headache, nausea, vomiting, loss of consciousness, papilledema, and sixth nerve palsy.
   d. A tumor may cause a **mass effect** by one or all of the following mechanisms:
      (1) Growth of the neoplasm
      (2) Edema formation
      (3) Obstruction of cerebrospinal fluid pathways, leading to enlargement of the ventricles and hydrocephalus
   e. **Abnormal endocrine function** may result from a pituitary tumor.

3. **Neurologic evaluation**
   a. A history of progressive neurologic deficits and the neurologic examination give a clue to the diagnosis of brain tumors.
   b. Additional studies may be necessary to pinpoint the lesion. These include:
      (1) Skull x-rays
      (2) CT scans
      (3) Angiography
      (4) MRI

4. **Treatment**
   a. **Medical management** consists of dehydration and administration of large doses of dexamethasone to reduce cerebral edema.

   b. Surgical management. The aim of surgical therapy is cure. However, this is not always possible, and the **main objectives** are:
   (1) To obtain tissue for diagnosis
   (2) To debulk the tumor to reduce its mass effect and make it curable by radiotherapy, chemotherapy, or both
   (3) To prolong survival
   c. Radiation therapy and chemotherapy (intravenous, intra-arterial, or intrathecal) are useful adjuncts in tumor management.

C. Spinal cord tumors

   1. Classification
   a. Extradural tumors
      (1) Extradural tumors are mostly malignant. These grow rapidly and destroy the spinal column.
      (2) Rarely, benign extradural tumors occur, such as meningiomas, neurofibromas, and osteomas.
   b. Intradural-extramedullary tumors. Neurofibromas and meningiomas constitute 90% of these tumors.
   c. Intramedullary tumors are mainly (95%) gliomas. Histologically, they are benign.
      (1) The majority of these tumors are ependymomas (50%) and astrocytomas (45%).
      (2) Ependymomas have a predilection for the conus medullaris and filum terminale.
   d. Metastatic tumors constitute 50% of intraspinal tumors and are commonly from the lungs, breast, lymphoid tissue, prostate gland, kidneys, and thyroid gland.

   2. Clinical presentation
   a. Pain is commonly associated with spinal tumors. **Nocturnal pain** that awakens the patient from sleep, along with a history of progressive weakness, is highly suggestive of an intraspinal neoplasm.
   b. Presenting signs are usually those of **cord compression**:
      (1) Sensory changes below the level of involvement
      (2) Motor weakness
      (3) Bowel and bladder incontinence

   3. Radiologic studies include spinal x-rays, myelography, CT scans, and MRI.

   4. Treatment
   a. Primary tumors
      (1) Medical management includes:
         (a) Intravenous administration of furosemide or mannitol to promote diuresis and reduce cord edema
         (b) Dexamethasone, which also helps in decreasing edema
      (2) Surgical intervention is aimed at:
         (a) Obtaining tissue for diagnosis
         (b) Tumor removal
         (c) Decompression
      (3) The availability of laser surgery and ultrasonic aspirators has made the radical removal of many tumors feasible and safe.
   b. Metastatic lesions
      (1) If they are radiosensitive, metastatic tumors are initially managed with diuretics, dexamethasone, and radiation therapy.
      (2) Surgery is indicated if:
         (a) The tumor is radioresistant
         (b) Radiation therapy fails
         (c) The patient who previously had received a full dose of spinal radiation develops another lesion
      (3) Radiation therapy and chemotherapy are helpful in palliation and in tumor control.

VII. CONGENITAL LESIONS OF THE NERVOUS SYSTEM

   A. Dysraphism. Usually, defective fusion of a raphe is associated with some findings on general physical examination. For example, examination of the back may reveal a tuft of hair, a nevus, a lipoma, abnormal blood vessels, a dimple, or a sinus tract. All of these are highly suggestive of an underlying dysraphic state.

1. Spina bifida
   a. This lesion results from failure of fusion of the vertebral arches.
   b. It may be totally asymptomatic and be found incidentally on spinal x-ray (spina bifida occulta), or it may be symptomatic.
   c. Spina bifida can be associated with other congenital anomalies, such as a dermal sinus, diastematomyelia (splitting of the cord into halves), or neurenteric cysts.

2. Meningocele
   a. This rare lesion is a saclike posterior midline herniation of the dura mater and is usually not associated with any neurologic deficits.
   b. Repair is indicated primarily for cosmetic reasons.

3. Myelomeningocele
   a. Myelomeningocele is herniation of the dura mater and neural elements posteriorly as a result of incomplete closure of the spine.
   b. Neurologic defects are common, and their severity is related to the location of the lesion. Patients with high lesions have a worse prognosis.
   c. Surgical treatment is aimed at closure of the defect.
   d. This lesion may be associated with hydrocephalus secondary to an Arnold-Chiari malformation (i.e., an abnormally low position of the cerebellar tonsils).

B. Hydrocephalus literally means "water head," and the abnormality may be congenital or acquired. It is usually caused by an obstruction of the flow of cerebrospinal fluid.

   1. Etiology. The commonest causes are:
      a. Sequelae of intraventricular hemorrhage in the premature baby
      b. Aqueductal stenosis
      c. Arnold-Chiari malformation
         (1) Type I. The fourth ventricle is above the foramen magnum, but the upper part of the cervical cord is displaced caudally.
         (2) Type II (most commonly seen). There is a downward herniation of the fourth ventricle and the cerebellar tonsils.
         (3) Types III and IV. There is progressive caudal displacement of the cerebellar vermis, pons, and medulla below the foramen magnum.
      d. Dandy-Walker syndrome, in which there is agenesis of the foramina of Luschka and Magendie, resulting in the filling of the posterior fossa with a large cyst and enlargement of the lateral and third ventricles

   2. Clinical findings. Patients may present with bulging fontanelles, scalp vein dilatation, a rapidly increasing head circumference, decreased upward gaze (Parinaud's syndrome), papilledema, lethargy, irritability, nausea, and vomiting.

   3. Treatment. A CT scan is done first to confirm the diagnosis, and then a shunt is placed to divert the ventricular fluid.
      a. A **ventriculoperitoneal shunt** is most commonly used.
      b. In very small infants, the absorptive surface of the peritoneum may be inadequate, warranting the placement of a **ventriculoatrial shunt**.
      c. Cerebrospinal fluid may need to be shunted to the pleural space.

VIII. LESIONS OF THE INTERVERTEBRAL DISKS

   A. Etiology. The intervertebral disks are subjected to everyday wear and tear.

   1. Young adults. Tears in the posterolateral portion of the anulus fibrosus lead to extrusions of the nucleus pulposus, which may result in **nerve root compression**.

   2. Elderly. Desiccation of the disk material results in osteophyte formation, and this leads to **nerve root or spinal cord compression**.

   B. Signs and symptoms of disk herniation are caused by either root compression or cord compression.

   1. In the lumbar area, compression may lead to shooting pains along the distribution of the sciatic nerve. Stretching the nerve root, as is done by straight-leg raising, exacerbates the symptoms.

2. Careful neurologic examination helps in localizing the level of the lesion.

3. Diagnostic tests include:
    a. Plain spinal x-rays
    b. Myelography
    c. Electromyography
    d. CT scan
    e. MRI

C. Treatment

1. Conservative management consists of **bed rest, traction**, and **analgesics** in the acute phase. Once the patient is relieved of the acute pain, **exercise** may help to strengthen the muscles.

2. Indications for surgical therapy include:
    a. Significant motor involvement
    b. Bowel or bladder incontinence
    c. Poor response to conservative therapy
    d. Relapse upon resumption of routine activities following initial pain relief by conservative treatment

IX. CEREBROVASCULAR DISEASE

A. Overview

1. "Stroke" is a term broadly used to describe a category of disorders characterized by a relatively acute onset and an etiology referable to the cerebrovascular system (see Chapter 7 VIII).

2. The main part of a stroke (paralysis or other deficit) is preceded by **warning ischemic attacks** in approximately 80% of cases. Such episodes rarely precede a cerebral embolism or intracerebral hemorrhage but very frequently precede the development of a thrombotic stroke.

B. Subgroups

1. Thrombotic stroke
    a. Overview
        (1) Atheromatous narrowing, thrombotic occlusion, or medial hypertrophy of the arteries supplying the brain results in a cessation of blood flow or a decrease of blood flow below a critical threshold, leading to infarction. It is characterized clinically by a fluctuating course over minutes to days.
        (2) A patient may or may not have warning episodes, that is, **transient ischemic attacks (TIAs)**, prior to a full-blown stroke. An individual suffering from TIAs develops one or more neurologic deficits, which may range from blindness (amaurosis fugax) to hemiplegia and which are sudden in onset and brief in duration, lasting minutes to hours (see Chapter 7 VIII A 3 a)
    b. Lacunar infarction
        (1) The small deep penetrating vessels are occluded as a result of degenerative changes.
        (2) The **sites** that are affected most often are the internal capsule, the thalamus, the pons, and the cerebral white matter.
        (3) Lacunar infarction is manifested as pure motor stroke, pure sensory stroke, dysarthria (slurred speech), "clumsy hand" syndrome, crural paresis and ataxia, ataxia with hemiparesis, or extrapyramidal syndrome.
    c. Carotid circulation thrombosis
        (1) Thrombosis at the **internal carotid artery bifurcation in the neck** commonly results from atherosclerotic degenerative changes, trauma, or fibromuscular dysplasia. Clinical symptoms include amaurosis fugax, headache, and hemispheric dysfunction.
        (2) Internal carotid artery siphon occlusion differs from bifurcation occlusion by the absence of ophthalmic signs and symptoms.
        (3) Anterior cerebral artery occlusion leads to paresis and cortical sensory loss in the contralateral inferior extremity.

(4) Middle cerebral artery occlusion
  (a) The middle cerebral artery is occluded more frequently by emboli than by an in situ stenosis or occlusion.
  (b) Occlusion of the superior trunk of the artery leads to hemiparesis and hemisensory loss, which affect the face and hands more than the legs. Motor aphasia (Broca's aphasia) results if the left hemisphere is involved.
  (c) Occlusion of the inferior trunk of the artery
    (i) Left-sided occlusion leads to Wernicke's aphasia (receptive aphasia) and to right homonymous hemianopia or right superior quadrantanopia.
    (ii) Right-sided occlusion results in constructional dyspraxia, spatial disorientation, and left homonymous hemianopia or left superior quadrantanopia.
d. Vertebrobasilar circulation occlusion (see Chapter 7 VIII B)
  (1) Vertebral artery occlusion leads to lateral medullary infarction with ataxia, decreased pain and temperature sensations, contralateral Horner's syndrome, and hoarseness. It also causes cerebellar infarction, with hemiplegia and dizziness.
  (2) Basilar occlusion results in pontine infarction and is incompatible with life.
  (3) Basilar tip occlusion causes:
    (a) Midbrain and thalamic infarction, leading to pupillary, oculomotor, and motor abnormalities
    (b) Posterior cerebral artery occlusion, resulting in hemianopia, alexia without agraphia (i.e., inability to read without loss of the ability to write), and, occasionally, hemisensory loss and ataxia

2. Embolic stroke. Embolic occlusion of an artery results in infarction.
  a. Etiology
    (1) Eighty percent of the causative emboli are **cardiac in origin.** The cardiac disorders that give rise to emboli are atrial fibrillation, rheumatic heart disease, myocardial infarction, mitral valve prolapse (Barlow's syndrome), and subacute bacterial endocarditis.
    (2) Emboli may also arise from an **atherosclerotic plaque** in the proximal portion of the vessel (these are called artery-to-artery emboli).
  b. Symptoms and signs depend on the vessel that is occluded.

3. Intracerebral hemorrhage
  a. Etiology of intracerebral hemorrhage (bleeding into the brain parenchyma) may be hypertension, arteriovenous malformations, a bleeding diathesis, drug use (anticoagulants, platelet inhibitors), or trauma. The **hemorrhages are located,** in order of frequency, in the putamen (50%), thalamus (20%), pons (10%), cerebellum (10%), and hemispheres (10%). The **onset is usually gradual**.
  b. Signs and symptoms result from:
    (1) Focal destruction, leading to neurologic deficits
    (2) Increased intracranial pressure (see I C 2)
    (3) Herniation (see I C 3)

4. Subarachnoid hemorrhage
  a. Bleeding in the subarachnoid space is usually **secondary to a congenital lesion**, such as a berry aneurysm or an arteriovenous malformation.
  b. The **onset is sudden** with evidence of meningeal irritation (e.g., nuchal rigidity, headache, vomiting, and clouding of consciousness).
  c. Neurologic deficits are related to the location of the aneurysm or arteriovenous malformation.
  d. Vasospasm may develop later on, leading to ischemia and increasing the neurologic deficits.

5. Severe systemic hypotension causes decreased cerebral blood flow, leading to ischemia and infarction in the watershed areas (i.e., the arterial border zones—the areas supplied by the distal ends of two or more arteries).

C. Management of stroke

1. History and neurologic evaluation comprise the initial management of stroke.

2. CT scan is then done.
  a. The CT scan can rule out or suggest:
    (1) Hemispheric infarction

(2) Intraparenchymal hemorrhage
(3) Subarachnoid hemorrhage
(4) Any mass effects
b. The **blood–brain barrier** can be checked by doing a CT scan, following a double-dose injection of contrast medium.
c. If the **CT scan is negative in the face of frequent TIAs**, the patient is given anticoagulant therapy.
   (1) This may be with heparin, dextran, or even, in some centers, simply aspirin and dipyridamole orally.
   (2) Frequent TIAs (**crescendo TIAs**) are managed aggressively with heparin (anticoagulant) and dextran (to decrease blood viscosity) to increase the cerebral blood flow.
d. If there is evidence of **intraparenchymal hemorrhage**, the patient is treated for increased intracranial pressure and cerebral edema (see III D) to reduce the mass effect. **Surgical evacuation** of the hematoma may be necessary if conservative therapy fails.
e. The patient is treated with an **antifibrinolytic agent** such as aminocaproic acid if there is any evidence of **subarachnoid hemorrhage** on the CT scan.

3. Angiogram is obtained as soon as possible to identify the pathology.
   a. According to some investigators, the risks of angiography preclude its use in cases of advanced stroke. However, in most major centers, the risks of angiography have been decreased considerably, so that the benefits far outweigh the risks.
   b. If angiography reveals carotid stenosis or occlusion, middle cerebral artery occlusion, or decreased blood flow in the vertebrobasilar distribution, **surgical therapy** may be necessary to augment the blood supply.
      (1) This may be either a **carotid endarterectomy** (see Chapter 7 VIII F 2) or an extracranial artery to intracranial artery (EC–IC) bypass (Figure 27-7).

A   **B**

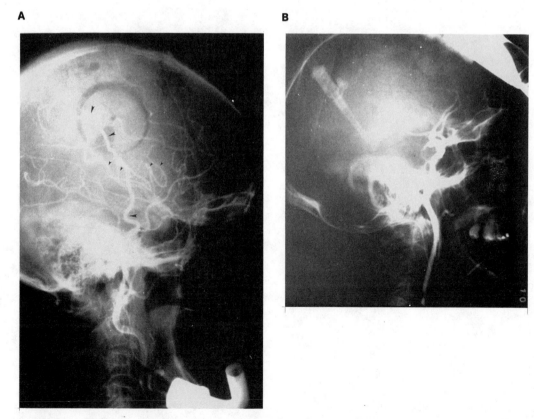

Figure 27-7. (*A*) Cerebral arteriogram showing poor arterial circulation in the territory of the right middle cerebral artery. (*B*) Following a superficial temporal artery to middle cerebral artery (EC–IC) bypass, there is a markedly improved blood supply in the right middle cerebral artery distribution.

(2) A recent international study concluded that EC–IC bypass has no significant benefit over aspirin plus dipyridamole in reducing the risk of stroke. Thus, this procedure is now indicated only when a major cerebral vessel has to be occluded for trapping an aneurysm.

c. Aneurysms and arteriovenous malformations require surgical correction.

X. CENTRAL NERVOUS SYSTEM INFECTIONS

A. **Overview.** Infections of the central nervous system and its coverings are surgically important only if they produce a mass effect, hydrocephalus, or osteomyelitis.

1. **Brain abscesses** and **subdural empyemas** can cause a mass effect.

2. **Osteomyelitis** of the skull and spine can lead to chronic inflammation, abscess, and continued infection of adjacent structures.

B. **Management** of central nervous system infections involves:

1. Identification of the organism

2. Appropriate antibiotic therapy

3. Evacuation of pus

4. Treatment of the source of infection

5. Treatment of the complications of infection, such as mycotic aneurysms, subdural effusions, and hydrocephalus

28
Orthopedic Surgery
Eric L. Hume

I. BONE HEALING

A. Endochondral ossification. By recapitulation of embryologic bone formation, primitive cells of hematogenous origin undergo the following **stages:**

1. **Metaplasia** from initial primitive inflammation

2. **Maturation of cartilage**

3. **Necrosis of cartilage** with **calcification**

4. **Replacement** by woven bone

5. **Remodeling** of the woven bone into mature trabecular and cortical bone

B. Primary bone healing occurs when rigid fixation of a fracture allows cell-to-cell cortical contact.

1. A cutting cone composed of an advancing front of osteoclasts, followed by a vascular bud, and then osteoblastic proliferation, can remodel a fracture gap without the progression of endochondral ossification.

2. This process proceeds more slowly than does endochondral ossification.

C. Failure of bone healing. A **nonunion** is the result of inadequate primary bone healing or endochondral ossification at a fracture site.

1. **Etiologies** include:
   a. Excessive motion at the fracture site
   b. Infection
   c. Severe soft tissue damage with loss of local vascularity
   d. Soft tissue interposition within the fracture gap

2. **Treatment.** Autogenous bone transplantation (bone grafting), surgical fixation, or electrical stimulation of the fracture site are the main management options.

II. INFECTIONS

A. Acute infections

1. **Osteomyelitis**
   a. Clinical presentation. Hematogenous osteomyelitis is not uncommon in childhood.
      (1) In the metaphysis of children's bones, there is a unique capillary venous sinusoid underneath the growth plate. This sinusoid is predisposed by minor trauma to allow organisms from minor bacteremia to initiate an infection.
      (2) The inflammation evoked about this focus devascularizes the surrounding bone and allows the infection to progress.
      (3) The infection can then track to the periosteum and cause a periosteal elevation or, if the metaphysis is intra-articular, as in the hip or shoulder, it can cause a septic arthritis.
   b. Etiology
      (1) Children
         (a) *Staphylococcus aureus* and gram-negative rods predominate as the causative organisms in neonates.

        (b) Osteomyelitis in young children is commonly caused by *Hemophilus* species from ear infections.

        (c) *S. aureus* resumes the role of most likely cause in older children and adolescents.

        (d) A child with a history of minor trauma who does not get better rapidly must be suspected of having osteomyelitis.

    (2) Adults whose immune system is suppressed, drug addicts, and patients with sickle cell anemia are predisposed to osteomyelitis from the hematogenous spread of unusual organisms.

        (a) Patients with immunosuppression and drug addicts are prone to gram-negative infections.

        (b) In sickle cell anemia, the osteomyelitis is most commonly due to *S. aureus*; however, a particularly high incidence of *Salmonella* osteomyelitis has been noted.

        (c) Sexually active patients may have gonococcal septic arthritis.

  c. Diagnosis. A careful physical examination, needle aspiration, a complete blood count, the sedimentation rate, and a bone scan confirm the diagnosis.

  d. Treatment includes appropriate antibiotics and sometimes surgical drainage. Antibiotics for initial treatment are selected to cover the most likely causative organisms.

2. Septic arthritis

  a. Etiology

    (1) Spontaneous joint infections can occur in children or adults, again by the hematogenous spread of the same organisms that cause osteomyelitis in the different age groups.

    (2) Joint disease, as well as immunosuppression, such as occurs in rheumatoid arthritis, can predispose the patient to these joint infections.

  b. Physical examination shows exquisite tenderness, effusion, and pain with minimal motion of the joint.

  c. Diagnosis is confirmed by needle aspiration of the synovial fluid and by finding that the white cell count and sedimentation rate are elevated. Snovial fluid white blood cells are greater than 50,000 with 90% polymorphonuclear neutrophil leukocytes.

  d. Treatment includes decompression of the joint and appropriate intravenous antibiotic therapy.

    (1) Most of the joints of the body except the hip and shoulder can be decompressed satisfactorily by means of needle aspiration.

    (2) The excepted joints, and any joint that does not respond promptly to needle aspiration, should be surgically incised, debrided, and drained promptly.

3. Penetrating wounds that reach a bone or joint can lead to infection. The magnitude of the wound is a major factor related to the severity of the infection.

B. Chronic osteomyelitis

1. Etiology. In today's antibiotic era, chronic osteomyelitis is a different problem from that seen in the past. Most cases are due to postoperative infection after a procedure involving a bone.

2. Clinical presentation

  a. Osteomyelitis involving the **bony cortex** is a particularly frustrating problem. Cortical bone, which has minimal vascularity at best, is even more poorly vascularized as a result of the osteomyelitis. Therefore, white cells, as well as antibiotics, have only limited access to the site of the infection.

  b. The cases that are seen in children may result in limb deformity and growth arrest.

3. Treatment. Attempts to cure chronic osteomyelitis involve removal of foreign material, a thorough debridement of infected bone, good local wound care, and prolonged use of intravenous antibiotics.

  a. Tetracycline bone labeling with a Wood's lamp illumination in the operating room may aid in the debridement of devascularized bone, since well-vascularized bone incorporates the tetracycline, which fluoresces under the Wood's lamp.

  b. Bone defects can be managed with either an open Papineau type of bone graft, in which morselized cancellous bone is packed into an open wound without any soft tissue coverage, or a vascularized bone graft.

  c. The use of muscle flaps and split-thickness skin grafts, employed after the control of infection, completes the treatment.

III. TRAUMA

A. Overview

1. **The extent of an injury** to the musculoskeletal system varies according to the age of the patient, the direction of the causative violence, and the magnitude of the violence.
   a. **The age of the patient** suggests the weak link in the musculoskeletal system.
      (1) In **skeletally immature patients,** the weak link is the growth plate in the ends of the long bones.
      (2) **Young but skeletally mature patients** (16–50 years of age) are more likely to sustain ligamentous injuries because the strength of the mature bone exceeds the strength of the soft tissue supporting the joints.
      (3) In **late middle age, elderly patients** with significant osteoporosis rarely injure the ligaments but instead sustain fractures of the metaphyseal portion of the bone. The metaphysis is usually injured because, as osteoporosis occurs, much of the bone loss is from this metabolically active area.
   b. **The direction of violence** determines which structures are injured. An example is the typical "clipping" injury of the knee with the violence applied to the lateral aspect of the knee, which stretches the soft tissue in the medial side of the knee, causing a medial collateral tear.
      (1) In children or adolescents, a growth plate fracture of the distal femur or proximal tibia is commonest.
      (2) In young adults, ligamentous injuries prevail.
      (3) In older adults, tibial plateau fractures are most likely.
   c. **The magnitude of the violence** is related to its velocity.
      (1) **High-velocity injuries,** as in motor vehicle accidents, tend to cause comminuted complex skeletal injuries. These may be open or compound fractures.
      (2) **Low-velocity injuries,** as occur in sports, are more likely to cause simple, isolated injuries of ligaments, muscles, or bones.

2. **Evaluation of the patient**
   a. **The history** must take into account the above factors.
      (1) A **fall from a height** can frequently lead to calcaneus fracture, hip dislocation, and fracture of the thoracolumbar spine.
      (2) A **motor vehicle accident** in which the patient is thrown forward with knees striking the dashboard frequently causes patellar fracture, femur fracture, and hip fracture or dislocation.
      (3) A **fall on the outstretched upper extremity** will frequently cause fracture of the distal radius, the radial head, or the metaphysis of the humerus at the shoulder.
   b. **Physical examination**
      (1) Musculoskeletal injuries present as bony crepitus at the fracture site, gross limb deformity, or dislocations and local swelling and tenderness at the specific point of injury.
      (2) The integrity of the skin, neural function, and circulatory status must be carefully evaluated when the patient is initially seen and also during the course of treatment. (Specifics are addressed in III B.)

3. **Principles of management**
   a. **Indications for open reduction and fixation**
      (1) **Intra-articular fractures.** The smooth painless function of a joint demands an absolutely smooth contour on the articular surfaces. This is best obtained with direct surgical visualization and internal fixation.
      (2) **Extremity function requiring perfect reduction.** A typical example is a fracture of both bones of the forearm. The shape of the radius and ulna must be anatomic to allow smooth supination and pronation. This is achieved by open reduction and surgical fixation.
      (3) **Unsatisfactory results after closed reduction.** If closed reduction does not give adequate results, open techniques are required.
      (4) **Metastatic tumors** (see IV B)
      (5) **Multiple trauma**
         (a) Patients with multiple-system injuries have a better prognosis if the extremity injuries can be internally fixed or splinted so that the patient can be mobilized at an early date.
         (b) Early mobilization improves pulmonary function and facilitates nursing care and further diagnostic evaluation of the patient.

(6) Injuries in elderly patients
   (a) The elderly patient is able to withstand the complications of prolonged bed rest poorly and does not have the cardiovascular reserves or muscular stamina to allow ambulation after a prolonged period of bed rest.
   (b) Fractures of the weight-bearing bones in the elderly should be surgically fixed, if necessary, to allow early mobilization and ambulation.
 b. Indications for external fixation
   (1) External fixation of fractures is carried out when the soft tissue injuries about the fracture prevent casting or when there is a risk of infection with internal fixation.
   (2) External fixators maintain bone alignment and permit access to the skin for wound care and dressing changes but at the expense of potential infection from the percutaneous pins held with external clamps.
 c. Cast immobilization is the most widely applied and most varied method of fracture care.
   (1) With the increasing awareness of the problems associated with immobilization of the joints, casting techniques have come to include hinges and designs that allow early weight bearing and joint motion.
   (2) These techniques should not be used at the expense of adequate fracture immobilization.

B. Orthopedic emergencies
 1. Open fractures
  a. An open fracture is a surgical emergency because of the:
   (1) Relative susceptibility of bone to infection
   (2) Associated devitalized soft tissue wounds, which may be extensive and which carry a high risk of life-threatening anaerobic infection
  b. Surgical management includes:
   (1) Prophylactic antibiotics, including those effective against gram-positive and anaerobic organisms
   (2) Thorough surgical debridement, ideally within 8 hours after injury
   (3) Inoculation against tetanus, unless this is known to be unnecessary

 2. Vascular injuries. Arterial and venous compromise must be given careful consideration in association with orthopedic trauma. The patient is also at risk for developing **compartment syndromes**. The circulation to the muscles and nerves is compromised by increased tissue pressure.

 3. Neural compromise
  a. Spinal cord injuries (see Chapter 27 IV). Injuries to the spinal column take a very high priority in the initial management of the injured patient.
   (1) Any patient with significant head or face injuries and any patient who is comatose after trauma must be assumed to have a cervical spine fracture.
   (2) Appropriate cross-table lateral x-rays must be obtained. These include x-rays of the cervical spine from the occiput down to and including the first thoracic vertebral body.
   (3) Reduction of any deformity is a surgical priority of the highest order.
  b. Peripheral nerve injuries (see Chapter 27 V)
   (1) Peripheral nerves are frequently injured in association with trauma to the extremities.
   (2) Any such injury must be carefully noted before treatment, both for medicolegal reasons and to indicate the need to restore the anatomic alignment of the extremity to relieve pressure on the peripheral nerve.
   (3) Most peripheral nerve injuries associated with closed injuries to the extremities will recover without nerve exploration. While the nerve is recovering, careful attention must be directed to the muscles and joints to prevent contraction or stretching of the muscles.
   (4) Penetrating wounds have a high incidence of nerve transection and, therefore, should be surgically explored when the patient is stable and an appropriate surgical environment (i.e., a rested staff, magnification, and appropriate instruments) can be obtained.

C. Fractures in children
 1. Overview
  a. Growth plate fractures. The growth plate is weaker than the rest of the long bone in the child.

      (1) A relatively large number of fractures in children disrupt the growth plate with the associated risk of growth problems.

      (2) Patients should be treated with careful, accurate closed reduction of the growth plate, and both patient and parents should be warned about the potential problems.

    b. Buckle fractures

      (1) Because children's bones are relatively flexible in comparison with those of the adult, buckle fractures occur. These fractures are incomplete with more plastic deformation than in adults.

      (2) Buckle fractures can be treated with simple cast protection to prevent further displacement.

    c. Greenstick fractures

      (1) Again, because of the flexibility and plasticity of children's bones, some shaft fractures extend through only one portion or one aspect of the cortex.

      (2) Because of the potential for recurrent angulation despite an initial excellent closed reduction, the remaining cortex of the fractured bone should be disrupted so that the alignment of the bone can be easily obtained.

    d. Oblique and spiral fractures of the long bones; fractures, bruises, burns, or scrapes of various ages; or a suspicious history should alert the physician to the possibility of **child abuse**.

2. Supracondylar fracture of the humerus is associated with a high incidence of injury to the brachial artery and compartment syndromes.

    a. Traction for several weeks may be indicated. However, these fractures may be amenable to closed reduction and casting or percutaneous pinning.

    b. The **neurovascular status** of the extremities should be carefully examined both before and after closed reduction of these injuries. The patient should be admitted to the hospital for these evaluations.

3. Fractures of both forearm bones

    a. In children, these are usually managed with closed reduction and plaster immobilization.

    b. The cast must be carefully molded and the patient observed to ensure that the interosseous space is preserved to maintain forearm supination and pronation after healing.

4. Distal radius fractures

    a. The distal radial metaphysis is a frequent site for buckle fractures.

    b. The distal radial epiphyseal plate is a frequent site for growth plate fractures. The growth plate fracture, if displaced, should have a closed reduction, usually under general anesthesia, with cast immobilization.

5. Femur fractures

    a. In young children aged 2–10 years, femur fractures can most often be managed with closed reduction and plaster spica immobilization.

    b. Usually a small amount of femoral overlap is acceptable.

      (1) The increased vascularity that occurs in response to the injury usually causes overgrowth of the epiphysis on the involved side.

      (2) Without the overlap, the limb is likely to end up longer than the opposite, uninjured extremity.

6. Supracondylar fractures of the femur and fractures of the proximal tibia on physical examination can be easily confused with a ligamentous knee injury.

    a. It is important to remember that skeletally immature individuals almost never have injuries to the ligaments but instead fracture through the growth plates.

    b. When a child's knee is unstable on physical examination, a stress x-ray of the knee should be taken to verify the exact cause and location of the false motion.

7. Tibia fractures

    a. These are frequently open because of the subcutaneous position of the bone. They are also associated with a relatively high incidence of compartment syndromes.

    b. All patients with tibial fractures should be examined for any skin disruption, and the neurovascular status of the leg should be evaluated.

    c. These fractures are well managed in children with plaster immobilization.

D. Fractures in adults

1. Fractures of the spine, hip, the proximal humerus, and the distal radius at the wrist are all quite common in elderly persons with osteoporosis.

   a. In general, the upper extremity fractures can be managed with cast immobilization with an attempt to prevent stiffness, especially at the shoulder.
   b. Because of the weight-bearing function of the hip, open reduction and internal fixation of the fracture or hemiarthroplasty is actually the conservative management, associated with better long-term function and survival of the patient.

2. **Humeral shaft fractures** are associated with a relatively high incidence of radial nerve palsies.
   a. In general, the palsy will recover with immobilization. However, careful attention must be paid to the hand, to prevent stiffness and contractures until the radial nerve recovers.
   b. The fracture may be treated with a sling and humeral cuff with early range-of-motion exercises of the shoulder and elbow and with isometric exercises of the biceps and triceps.

3. **Fractures of both forearm bones**
   a. Because of the precise functional requirements of the forearm, these fractures require open reduction and internal fixation for maximal functional results.
   b. Especially in crushing injuries, the consideration of a compartment syndrome is important.

4. **Finger fractures**
   a. Because of the precise, fine function of the fingers and the problem of stiffness in adults, early range-of-motion exercise of the fingers has a high priority.
   b. Percutaneous pin or plate fixation or early splinting with "buddy" taping are all acceptable methods, assuming that the goal of early motion can be obtained to avoid finger contracture and dysfunction.

5. **Spinal fractures** are associated with high-velocity, high-energy mechanisms of injury. Automobile accidents, motorcycle accidents, and falls from heights are the frequent mechanisms in spinal (and pelvic) fractures.
   a. Treatment of the spinal fracture includes:
      (1) Decompression of the central nervous system as well as peripheral nerves
      (2) Spinal stability for early rehabilitation
   b. Early mobilization is especially important in paraplegics and quadriplegics so that the overwhelming task of rehabilitation can begin promptly.

6. **Femur fractures**
   a. Treatment traditionally has been via traction for 4–6 weeks, until enough healing allows cast immobilization for the duration of the patient's care.
   b. However, improved intramedullary rodding techniques may allow better quadriceps, hip, and knee function with shorter hospital stays.
   c. The decision must be individualized, and the pros and cons of the two options must be carefully explained to the patient.

7. **Tibia fractures** are frequently open and frequently associated with compartment syndromes.
   a. These two associated problems must be anticipated and managed appropriately.
   b. Fractures of the tibia are generally best managed with plaster immobilization and early weight bearing.
   c. The incidence of delayed union or nonunion of tibial fractures is high. In selected instances, plate fixation or intramedullary nail fixation has an important role.

8. **Ankle fractures** are classified according to the degree of instability of the ankle. If ankle fractures are treated successfully, post-traumatic osteoarthritis and delayed ankle instability can be avoided.

E. Dislocations

1. **Shoulder**
   a. Dislocations of the glenohumeral joint are especially common in young adults.
   b. Glenohumeral dislocations frequently recur, especially when management does not include careful immobilization.
   c. These injuries are also associated with axillary nerve palsy.

2. **Hip**
   a. Dislocations of the hip occur in high-velocity injuries, especially automobile accidents.

b. They are associated with fractures of the ipsilateral femur and patella and with contralateral hip fractures or dislocations.

c. They require prompt reduction to lower the risk of a vascular necrosis.

3. Knee

    a. Dislocations of the knee are extreme cases of ligamentous injuries about the knee.

        (1) Ligamentous knee injuries occur more commonly in sports-related activities.

        (2) Total ligamentous disruption and dislocation are associated with violent injuries.

    b. The most important consideration is the common occurrence of injuries to the popliteal artery and vein and to the peroneal nerve. The first step in management of dislocations of the knee is to evaluate the neurovascular status of the lower leg, followed by evaluation of the ligaments and capsule about the knee.

F. Musculotendinous injuries. The musculotendinous unit is most commonly disrupted by overuse but may also be disrupted by forced lengthening of the muscle.

  1. Tear of the rotator cuff

    a. Middle-aged and older patients with intermittent shoulder pain may have an episode of acute pain when the weakened tendon tears.

    b. Most tears are small and may be treated symptomatically.

    c. However, after resolution of the acute symptoms, if the shoulder demonstrates poor muscular function, repair must be undertaken.

  2. Quadriceps disruptions

    a. Middle-aged and older patients, especially those with diabetes mellitus or renal disease, may acutely disrupt the quadriceps mechanism superior to the patella.

    b. Physical examination shows minimal swelling and tenderness.

    c. The patient complains only of weakness in the leg after hearing a "pop" and may be able to raise the leg if the knee is straight. However, the patient is unable to initiate extension against gravity with the knee at 90° of flexion.

    d. Surgical repair is necessary.

  3. Achilles tendon disruptions

    a. The usual patient is middle-aged or older who may have had heel pain. Typically, the patient was trying to bend or to push a heavy object forward, when an audible "pop" was heard.

    b. The patient is usually able to walk, and the symptoms are minimal. Physical examination reveals a palpable defect in the Achilles tendon.

    c. The **Thompson test** may aid in diagnosis. This is performed by squeezing the calf and looking for plantar flexion of the foot. This response is absent with Achilles tendon ruptures.

    d. The treatment is surgical repair or cast immobilization.

  4. Acute muscle ruptures

    a. Any musculotendinous unit may be disrupted by a forced lengthening of the muscle. The disruption usually occurs at the musculotendinous junction but may be within the muscle belly.

    b. These injuries may be very difficult to repair, and the results are variable.

IV. TUMORS

A. Primary bone tumors

  1. Overview

    a. Clinical presentation. The patient with a neoplastic bone lesion presents with pain, swelling, or occasionally, a pathologic fracture induced by minimal trauma. This is true for bony metastases as well as for benign and malignant tumors of bone.

    b. Diagnosis. In addition to differentiating a primary from a metastatic tumor of bone, some metabolic processes, such as hyperparathyroidism and infection, must be carefully considered.

        (1) Physical examination demonstrates the tumor mass, allowing the selection of appropriate x-rays.

        (2) Plain x-rays alone often suggest whether a tumor of bone is benign or malignant.

    (a) **Malignancy** can be expected if the films show:
      (i) A tumor of large size
      (ii) Aggressive destruction of bone
      (iii) Ineffective reaction of the bone to the tumor
      (iv) Extension of the tumor into soft tissue
    (b) **Benign** lesions can be expected if the films show:
      (i) A small, well-circumscribed lytic lesion
      (ii) A thick, sclerotic rim
      (iii) No extension into soft tissue

  (3) **Workup.** If there is any question whatsoever that the tumor is malignant, a careful workup must be performed before biopsy. An incomplete workup or a poorly thought out biopsy is likely to be fatal for the patient or may cost the patient a deforming radical amputation.
    (a) An **appropriate workup** includes **computed tomography (CT scan), magnetic resonance imaging (MRI),** and **technetium-99m (^{99m}Tc) scan** of the involved bone to stage the tumor and delineate its extent and anatomic relationships.
    (b) If **malignancy** is suspected, then **CT scan of the chest** is important to rule out pulmonary metastases. No other metastatic workup is required, since sarcomas metastasize to the lung first.
    (c) **Biopsy** should be performed only after staging has been completed. The biopsy should be carefully planned so that the biopsy incision can be removed with a definitive surgical resection. The biopsy is best planned and performed by the surgeon who will ultimately carry out the definitive surgical procedure. All biopsy incisions should be:
      (i) Longitudinal on the limbs
      (ii) Made through a muscle belly to avoid contaminating intermuscular planes
      (iii) Directed away from neurovascular structures
      (iv) Directed through structures that can be safely and successfully resected to leave a functional limb if radical excision is carried out.

c. Treatment
  (1) **Surgical treatment** continues to be the mainstay of management for both benign and malignant tumors. The **surgical margin,** obviously, varies significantly.
    (a) **Benign tumors** can be adequately treated by intralesional or intracapsular excision of the tumor with or without chemical cautery, electrocautery, or cryotherapy and with or without bone grafting of the defect.
    (b) **Malignant tumors** require at least a 2-cm margin.
    (c) **Metastases.** One or two isolated pulmonary metastases of sarcoma, especially osteosarcoma or chondrosarcoma, should be considered for surgical resection, since the literature shows that this will result in an occasional cure, and certainly a prolonged life span, in these patients.
  (2) **Adjuvant therapy for malignant tumors**
    (a) **Radiation therapy**
      (i) Some tumors, such as Ewing's tumors, are very sensitive to radiotherapy.
      (ii) Some protocols include radiation therapy initially, but in general, radiation therapy is not an important part of the protocol.
    (b) **Chemotherapy,** like radiation therapy, has limited use.
      (i) Ewing's tumors are well known to be very sensitive to various chemotherapeutic regimens.
      (ii) Osteosarcoma appears to be sensitive to some chemotherapeutic agents, and work is under way to delineate the benefits as chemotherapy may allow limb salvage.

2. Types of primary bone tumors
  a. Tumors of bone cell origin
    (1) **Benign osteoid osteoma** is a painful lesion commonly affecting the femur or the tibia.
      (a) **Epidemiology.** It occurs in adolescents with more than 50% of the tumors presenting in patients aged 10–20 years.
      (b) **Histology.** The lesions are benign and are not prone to malignant degeneration. Pathologic examination demonstrates a nidus of disorganized, dense, calcified osteoid tissue, which histologically is benign.
      (c) **Treatment**
        (i) Typically, aspirin offers excellent relief.

(ii) Surgical management is indicated for lesions that are painful. A bone graft may be necessary.

(2) Osteoblastoma is a benign, rare, painful lesion.

    (a) Epidemiology. It occurs most often in the second decade of life.

    (b) Histology. Osteoblastoma appears very similar to osteoid osteoma. One distinguishing feature is its size: An osteoblastoma is defined as a benign bone-forming lesion greater than 2 cm.

    (c) Treatment. Osteoblastomas are cured by surgical excision if symptoms warrant. Bone grafting may be necessary.

(3) Osteosarcoma is a malignant tumor of adolescence.

    (a) Epidemiology. Over 60% of patients with these tumors are aged 10–20 years.

    (b) Clinical presentation

        (i) At least 60% of osteosarcomas occur about the knee at either the distal femur or proximal tibia.

        (ii) Typically, the patient presents with pain and tumefaction.

        (iii) Radiographically, the lesion is typically lytic, but it may be a blastic lesion of the bone. MRI or CT shows that the lesion is ill-defined with soft tissue extension.

    (c) Histology. Histologically, the tumor may be predominantly fibrogenic, chondrogenic, or osteogenic; each of the three types predominates in approximately equal numbers of patients. The **sine qua non** of osteosarcomas is that somewhere within the tumor, bone is being formed by the tumor stroma.

        (i) Although the tumor may look predominantly like a chondrosarcoma or a fibrosarcoma, if bone is being formed by even one small part of the tumor, then by definition the tumor is an osteosarcoma.

        (ii) The distinction is important because the **prognosis** differs significantly for chondrosarcoma and for osteosarcoma: The 5-year survival rate for an osteosarcoma is around 10%–20%. Pulmonary metastases occur early.

    (d) Treatment

        (i) The principal treatment is surgical resection; amputation or limb salvage surgery may be required.

        (ii) Adjuvant chemotherapy seems to have a beneficial effect, and its use is being actively investigated for effects on improving longevity and limb salvage rates.

b. Tumors originating in cartilage

(1) Enchondromas frequently are asymptomatic findings on x-rays, although some present as pathologic fractures.

    (a) Epidemiology. The tumor occurs in patients aged 10–50 and is commonly found in the hand.

    (b) Clinical presentation

        (i) It is typically an intraosseous lytic lesion marked by characteristic "popcorn" calcifications and surrounded by reactive sclerosis.

        (ii) A tumor that appears radiographically to be an enchondroma must be suspected of being a sarcoma if it presents with pain but no pathologic fracture.

    (c) Treatment. When an enchondroma causes a pathologic fracture, curettage and bone grafting are required.

(2) Osteochondromas are benign, easily palpable tumors of bone. They are quite common.

    (a) Clinical presentation

        (i) They grow during adolescence, as does any cartilage portion of bone. If pain or growth occurs after skeletal maturity, malignant degeneration must be suspected and excisional biopsy is warranted.

        (ii) Osteochondromas may be symptomatic because of their prominence or because of a resultant fracture or neurovascular compression.

    (b) Treatment. If symptoms warrant it, osteochondromas can be excised, including the soft tissue covering and cartilage. Bone grafting is generally not necessary.

(3) Chondroblastomas are less common cartilage tumors that almost always occur within the epiphysis of long bones.

    (a) Epidemiology. Over 70% of these tumors occur during the second decade of life. They are very rare if the growth plates have closed.

    (b) Clinical presentation. They are benign lesions, but a very small percentage undergo malignant degeneration.

    (c) Treatment. They frequently require excision and bone grafting.

(4) Chondromyxoid fibromas are relatively rare tumors.
    (a) Epidemiology. They usually occur in the first and second decades of life.
    (b) Clinical presentation. The tumor is a relatively large, well-defined lytic lesion with a sclerotic rim, found in the metaphysis juxtaposed to the growth plate. It may present with pathologic fracture.
    (c) Treatment. Curettage and bone grafting may be required for treatment.
(5) Chondrosarcoma is a primary malignant tumor of adulthood that sometimes develops in preexisting benign cartilage lesions.
    (a) Epidemiology. It occurs with an essentially constant incidence in patients of all ages from 10–70 years.
    (b) Clinical presentation
        (i) Typically, the tumor presents with pain and tumefaction.
        (ii) X-rays may show a lytic lesion with or without stippled calcification.
        (iii) The tumor is locally recurrent, rather than showing early pulmonary metastases as does osteosarcoma.
    (c) Treatment is surgical with the goal of obtaining a 2-cm margin of tumor-free tissue.

c. Other primary tumors
    (1) Giant-cell tumors occur in the epiphyseal–metaphyseal region of long bones, especially about the knee in the femur and tibia. The lesions are benign but are problematic because of their propensity to recur locally.
        (a) Epidemiology. Giant-cell tumors occur in young adults with the peak occurrence in patients between the ages of 20 and 30. The patient almost always is skeletally mature.
        (b) Clinical presentation. The lesion usually extends to the subchondral plate of the joint. It is a lytic lesion, fairly well circumscribed with some ballooning of the cortex.
        (c) Histology. The lesion is characterized histologically by the giant cells found in a benign stroma. The giant cell nuclei and the stroma nuclei are identical in appearance.
        (d) Treatment. Curettage is often accompanied by cryotherapy, phenol chemocautery, or electrocautery. The lesion may be packed with polymethylmethacrylate bone cement, or bone grafting may be done. Recurrence usually requires wide resection of the involved bone.
    (2) Unicameral bone cysts are lytic lesions of bone that occur in older children in the metaphyseal region that extends to the growth plate. The proximal end of the humerus is the commonest site.
        (a) Clinical presentation. Typically, the patient presents with a pathologic fracture, and ultimately the cyst may resolve in response to this trauma.
        (b) Treatment. Unicameral bone cysts may be managed with intralesional steroid injections administered under radiographic control. Multiple injections may be required, which presents a problem in growing children.
    (3) Ewing's sarcoma is a disease of childhood and adolescence. It occurs evenly among individuals under the age of 20 years.
        (a) Clinical presentation
            (i) Typically, the patient presents with significant tumefaction and pain in the involved area.
            (ii) The history, physical examination, and x-ray findings mimic those of osteomyelitis.
            (iii) Radiologically, the lesion is seen to be a lytic bone lesion with some periosteal reaction.
        (b) Histology. Histologically, this is a tumor of small round cells, which may form pseudorosettes reminiscent of neuroblastoma.
        (c) Treatment. The relative roles of chemotherapy, radiation therapy, and surgical therapy are being evaluated.
            (i) These tumors are sensitive to both chemotherapy and radiotherapy, and together these modalities have a significant cure rate.
            (ii) However, new information suggests that patients are at risk of forming osteosarcoma in the radiated bone during early adulthood.
    (4) Fibrosarcoma is a tumor that occurs in adulthood, between the ages of 20 and 70.
        (a) Clinical presentation
            (i) It is predominantly a lytic lesion, occurring in the femur and tibia about the knee.

        (ii) It presents with pain and an x-ray appearance of a purely lytic lesion of bone.

     (b) Histology. Histologic examination shows sheets of spindle cells in a herring-bone pattern and with various amounts of atypism.

     (c) Treatment is wide surgical excision.

   (5) Multiple myeloma

     (a) Epidemiology. Whether this lesion is a primary tumor of bone or of bone marrow is argued. Whatever its classification, it is a common tumor that occurs in patients aged 30 years and older with a peak in incidence at 50–60 years.

     (b) Clinical presentation

       (i) Multiple myeloma is characterized by overproduction of monoclonal immunoglobulins or immunoglobulin subchains (Bence Jones protein).

       (ii) The initial presentation is often a pathologic fracture, frequently of the spine or long bones.

       (iii) The diagnosis should be suspected when lytic lesions are found in a patient with anemia, an elevated sedimentation rate, and elevated serum calcium levels.

     (c) Diagnosis

       (i) The diagnosis can be made by serum or urine electrophoresis or immunophoresis in 95% of cases, but 5% of myeloma patients are nonsecretors of M protein (immunoglobulins or Bence Jones protein).

       (ii) Biopsy of the bone marrow to identify secreting and nonsecreting tumors shows plasma cells replacing the marrow. The percentage of bone marrow replacement offers some prognostic information.

     (d) Treatment is by a combination of chemotherapy and radiation therapy with surgical fixation of pathologic fractures to improve the quality of life.

B. Metastatic disease. Tumors metastatic to the skeletal system are far commoner than primary musculoskeletal tumors. Primary tumors that metastasize to bone include carcinomas of the breast, lung, prostate, thyroid, and kidney, or, indeed, almost any type of tumor.

   1. Diagnosis

     a. Most bony metastatic disease presents with pain in the involved bone. Metastatic bone disease may be the initial presentation of a malignancy.

     b. Radiographs show most bone lesions to be lytic. With some breast tumors and most prostatic tumors, the bone has a blastic appearance.

     c. Bone scans are helpful when a single symptomatic lytic lesion is found on initial x-rays.

       (1) If the bone scan shows multiple lesions, the likelihood of metastatic disease is high.

       (2) Bone scanning may also demonstrate a lesion that is more surgically accessible for biopsy.

   2. Treatment

     a. The likelihood of pathologic fracture is relatively high, and **prophylactic fixation** of long bones with metastatic lesions should be considered in the following situations:

       (1) If the lesion involves more than half of the circumference of the long bone

       (2) If the length of the lesion in the long bone is greater than the diameter of the bone

     b. Treatment of most metastatic lesions in bones is radiation therapy. If the pain does not respond to irradiation, a pathologic fracture has probably occurred or is about to occur, and it should then be fixed. Pathologic fractures in general should be fixed internally, using a combination of metal implants plus methylmethacrylate bone cement to manage bone loss.

V. ARTHRITIS

  A. Classification

    1. Degenerative joint disease includes:

     a. Osteoarthritis with Heberden's nodes and symmetric hip, knee, and spine involvement

     b. Post-traumatic arthritis of the isolated joint

    2. Rheumatoid arthritis and its variants include the autoimmune group of inflammatory diseases in which the hyaline articular cartilage is attacked by a local invasive pannus.

    3. Crystal deposition diseases include **gout** and **calcium pyrophosphate deposition disease**. These usually present as an isolated hot, inflamed joint.

4. Infectious arthritis (see II A 2) also presents as an isolated hot, inflamed joint.
   a. This is the one form of arthritis that requires immediate emergency care.
   b. Diagnosis can be made by aspirating the joint fluid and examining it microscopically and by cell count, sugar determinations, and culture.

B. Nonoperative management

   1. Nonsteroidal anti-inflammatory drugs (NSAIDs)
      a. These are especially important in rheumatoid arthritis, which requires a long-term maintenance regimen.
      b. The crystalline and degenerative joint diseases require NSAIDs during acute flare-ups but do not respond to long-term management with these drugs.

   2. Gold and remittive agents, as the second level of drugs, have an important place in the rheumatoid arthritis armamentarium. They are indicated when the patient has not been successful with the NSAIDs.

   3. Corticosteroids
      a. These provide the third level of care for rheumatoid arthritis when NSAIDs fail to quiet the inflammation. They can be used:
         (1) Systemically if multiple joint involvement or generalized disease is the problem
         (2) Locally by instillation into a single joint that has been identified as the most bothersome.
      b. Degenerative joint disease and rheumatoid arthritis occasionally benefit from instillation of corticosteroid into the joint.

   4. Immunosuppressants are a last level of drugs for uncontrolled rheumatoid arthritis.

   5. Exercise has an important place in all forms of arthritis after the acute joint inflammation has been controlled. The exercise is designed to maintain a full range of joint motion as well as to maintain muscle strength by exercising the joint through a limited, painless arc of motion.

C. Operative management

   1. Types of surgical procedures
      a. Arthroplasty, or **total joint replacement,** is the newest addition to the surgical management of joint disease.
         (1) It can be used for joints destroyed by any of the arthritides; however, postinfectious arthritis is a relative contraindication to arthroplasty because of the increased risk of infection around the implant.
         (2) Arthroplasty is indicated for the relief of pain predominantly in patients who are usually older and less active.
         (3) At the present state of the art, the "life expectancy" for a hip or knee arthroplasty implant is about 15 years, depending on the functional requirements and weight of the patient.
      b. Arthrodesis
         (1) In this procedure, the joint surfaces are excised and the extremity is immobilized so that the joint heals in a fixed position.
         (2) Arthrodesis is indicated for the relief of pain, especially in young individuals.
            (a) The results of arthrodesis are very durable and long-lasting.
            (b) Any patient who is young or has a high functional demand should be considered for arthrodesis rather than arthroplasty.
      c. Osteotomy
         (1) Cutting a bone and realigning a joint may alter the mechanics enough to give significant, although incomplete, relief of pain.
         (2) To be successful, the procedure must not completely destroy a joint but must leave some remaining articular surface.
         (3) Osteotomy is designed to transfer weight-bearing onto this relatively normal articular surface.

   2. Specific examples
      a. Hip
         (1) Total hip arthroplasty was the first successful replacement and is by far the commonest hip procedure done today.
         (2) Hip arthrodesis is a very successful means of providing a functional joint for young individuals with only local disease.

    (3) **Osteotomies about the hip** are becoming more popular again and have a place, albeit limited, in the surgical management of the hip.
  b. **Knee**
    (1) **Arthroplasties** have become more durable and more widely accepted.
    (2) **Coventry osteotomy,** in which the weight-bearing axis of the body is transferred to the usually more normal lateral condyle of the knee, is still the standard of care for early degenerative disease in active or middle-aged patients.
    (3) **Arthrodesis** is a reliable procedure for the unstable, painful knee in young individuals.
  c. **Foot and ankle.** In general, **arthrodesis** of the midfoot joints is indicated for painful involvement of the subtalar or midfoot joints. Ankle arthrodesis is also the standard of care, although ankle **arthroplasty** has a place for certain conditions in patients with extremely limited functional requirements, especially severe rheumatoid arthritis.
  d. **Shoulder.** The shoulder is not a weight-bearing joint, and degenerative disease of this joint is less common. However, total shoulder **arthroplasties** are beginning to show promise in the treatment of degenerative disease and rheumatoid arthritis.
  e. **Elbow. Arthroplasty** with prosthetic components is still a procedure with limited indications. Elbow **arthrodesis** affords good pain relief, as does excisional arthroplasty without the addition of prosthetic components.
  f. **Wrist and hand. Arthroplasty** with Silastic implants often allows functional, painless motion of wrist and hand joints, especially in patients with rheumatoid arthritis. Patients with severe wrist involvement, especially from post-traumatic degenerative disease, are well managed by **arthrodesis** of the involved joint.

VI. PEDIATRIC ORTHOPEDICS

  A. **Congenital dislocation of the hip** is commonest in female neonates, especially if the child is firstborn and was in the breech presentation. The condition is bilateral in 10% of the patients.

  1. **Diagnosis** can be made within the first 2 weeks after birth, once relaxin is gone from the child's circulation.
    a. **Physical examination**
      (1) The examiner can feel a click on reduction of the dislocated hip **(Ortolani's sign).**
      (2) The examiner is able to dislocate the hip with the hip flexed to 90° **(Barlow's test).**
      (3) Other physical findings, especially if the dislocation is unilateral, include asymmetry of the gluteal fold and asymmetric leg lengths, demonstrated by the height of the knee when the hips are flexed to 90°.
    b. **X-rays** confirm the diagnosis.

  2. **Treatment.** A hip that is still dislocatable after 2 weeks of age should be treated.
    a. Initial management is with a Pavlik harness.
    b. Double and triple diapering probably has no significant effect on the dislocation.

  B. **Scoliosis**

  1. **Etiology**
    a. The commonest form of scoliosis in the United States is the **idiopathic scoliosis** that occurs in adolescent females, beginning at the age of about 11 or 12 and progressing until growth is completed.
    b. Scoliosis can also be the result of neuromuscular paralysis, painful lesions, radiation, thoracic surgery, and congenital anomalies.

  2. **Clinical presentation**
    a. Scoliosis most commonly occurs as a right thoracic curve, but thoracolumbar, lumbar, and double curves can occur.
    b. Thoracic curves are most noticeable because of the associated chest rotation and deformity, creating a rib hump.
    c. If the scoliosis is severe, exceeding about 60°, significant cardiopulmonary complications can occur.

  3. **Treatment**
    a. **Braces.** The **Milwaukee** and **Boston braces** are relatively recent additions to the management of scoliosis. They may eliminate the need for surgery in many patients.

        (1) The brace is not expected to correct a curve that is already established when the diagnosis is made but is meant to prevent the scoliosis from advancing into a cardio-pulmonary or serious cosmetic problem.

        (2) Typically, patients are placed into braces:

           (a) If the curve measures about 20° in a patient with significant growth still remaining

           (b) If the scoliosis, even with a smaller angle, is clearly progressing during a period of observation

    b. Surgery

        (1) A variety of surgical techniques are available, but the one most commonly performed is **Harrington rod fixation** with bone graft fusion of the spine over the area of the curve.

        (2) Significant, although never complete, correction is obtained, and the long-term results are maintained by the bone graft's healing and fusing the spine in the corrected position.

C. Foot deformities constitute a large part of pediatric orthopedic practice.

  1. Etiology

    a. Idiopathic foot deformities are quite common and include **metatarsus adductus, talipes equinovalgus (clubfoot),** and **planovalgus**.

    b. A careful neurologic evaluation must be done to make sure that the foot deformity is not due to a **neuromuscular disorder**. Poliomyelitis, cerebral palsy, myelomeningocele, diastematomyelia, and Charcot-Marie-Tooth muscular atrophy can all present with foot deformities.

    c. Congenital dislocated hips must be ruled out whenever a child presents with a foot deformity.

  2. Flatfoot seldom represents a significant problem and does not need treatment unless it causes symptoms or unless the neurologic examination is abnormal.

  3. Clubfoot requires early treatment.

    a. Repeated manipulation and casting will correct the deformity in some cases.

    b. However, if the foot is relatively resistant to manipulation and casting, surgery is needed.

        (1) In recent years, surgical soft tissue releases before age 1 year have shown a better prognosis than manipulation and casting.

        (2) Recurrence of the clubfoot despite correction remains a problem until the cartilaginous anlage of the child's foot has become the fixed osseous bone of the adolescent.

  4. Neuromuscular foot disorders

    a. Treatment of the "neuromuscular foot" includes initial correction to a plantigrade neutral foot, either by manipulation of the very immature foot or by osteotomy and fusion of the more mature adolescent foot.

    b. Once the foot alignment is corrected, then muscle transfers are carried out to prevent deformity. Tendons are transferred to replace the function of a paralyzed foot or to weaken the function of a spastic foot.

29
Pediatric Surgery

Charles W. Wagner

I. INTRODUCTION. Pediatric surgery has evolved as a subspecialty for several reasons. First, infants and children differ from adults physiologically as well as anatomically. For example, their nutritional needs and fluid and electrolyte management are not the same as for adults. Thus, specialized knowledge is required for the care of pediatric surgical patients. Second, infants and children also differ to some extent in the types of disorders that require surgical management. For example, in infants, congenital malformations require prompt correction, and specialized knowledge is needed. The full discussion of specialized pediatric considerations is far too extensive to be covered in this book; therefore, only certain topics have been touched on. For more complete information, the reader is referred to standard textbooks on pediatric surgery.

II. CONGENITAL HERNIAS (see Chapter 2 V)

A. Inguinal hernia. Repair of an inguinal hernia remains the commonest general surgical procedure in the child. The defect is due to nonfusion of the processus vaginalis, not to a breakdown of the floor of the inguinal canal.

1. Incidence
  a. Inguinal hernia occurs in 1%–3% of all children.
     (1) The hernia is on the right about 60% of the time, on the left about 30% of the time, and bilateral between 10% and 15% of the time.
     (2) The male:female ratio is 6:1.
  b. In premature infants, the incidence is one and one-half to two times greater.
  c. There is an increased incidence of hernias in patients with hydrocephalus who are treated by ventriculoperitoneal shunts.

2. Clinical presentation
  a. The age at diagnosis is in infancy with about 35% of patients presenting before the age of 6 months.
  b. The classic history and clinical presentation is that of a mass or bulge in the groin, scrotum, or labia, usually occurring at times of abdominal pain. The mass usually disappears after the straining or crying has been resolved, but it is for the most part easily reducible.
  c. If no mass is present, one may feel the thickened spermatic cord, which represents the nondistended hernia sac. This has been described as the **"silk glove" sign**.
  d. If no hernia is identified but the patient's history is both classic and reliable, then most surgeons feel that surgery is indicated.

3. Incarceration
  a. In boys, the risk associated with a hernia is the chance of incarceration of the intestine.
     (1) Intestinal ischemia and obstruction can occur.
     (2) With time, the entrapped bowel becomes edematous enough to compress the spermatic vessels and cause testicular ischemia with resultant damage or necrosis.
  b. In girls, the intestine does not usually incarcerate into the hernia, but the ovary may. While ischemia of the ovary may result, this is not usually the case.
  c. Treatment includes reduction of the incarcerated hernia, hydration of the patient, and herniorrhaphy.
     (1) These steps should all be done within 48–72 hours.

      (2) Reduction is performed with or without sedation by gentle, continuous pressure on the incarcerated intestine.

      (3) Almost all hernias in children will reduce. However, the chance of reducing necrotic intestine is very low.

   4. Herniorrhaphy. A hernia should be repaired soon after it is diagnosed unless there is a major medical reason not to use general anesthesia. In most children, the repair can be done as outpatient surgery without hospitalization.

     a. Herniorrhaphy in the child consists of identifying the sac, dissecting the spermatic structures free, and ligating the sac high at the internal ring of the inguinal canal. Very rarely is there a need for a floor repair.

     b. Complications of the procedure include damage to the vas deferens, vascular injury to the testes, recurrence of the hernia, and iatrogenic cryptorchidism.

      (1) Recurrence can be associated with both Hunter's syndrome and Elhers-Danlos syndrome.

      (2) Iatrogenic cryptorchidism occurs when the testicle has been mobilized from the scrotum but not properly replaced. Unlike regular cryptorchidism, in which the testes may later descend, the testes will remain in the abnormally high position with iatrogenic cryptorchidism.

B. Diaphragmatic hernias are communications through the diaphragm that allow abdominal contents to migrate into the thoracic cavity.

   1. Incidence. The incidence of this defect is 1 in 4000 live births.

   2. Etiology. Two underlying anatomic defects are common; both result from the failure of the surrounding tissues to fuse in utero.

     a. Foramen of Bochdalek is a posterolateral diaphragmatic defect.

      (1) This hernia (Figure 29-1) is the commonest congenital hernia.

      (2) It occurs most often in the left hemidiaphragm. It is bilateral in fewer than 10% of infants.

     b. Foramen of Morgagni is an anterior diaphragmatic defect. It is much less common and generally results in less severe problems.

   3. Diagnosis of herniation of abdominal contents into the thorax is based primarily on impaired ventilatory capacity. The earlier that respiratory distress is noted in the infant, especially if it occurs during the first 24 hours, the more severe the impairment and the worse the prognosis.

     a. Physical examination reveals the following:

      (1) Tachypnea, dyspnea, use of accessory muscles for ventilation, cyanosis, and nasal flaring

      (2) Decreased or absent breath sounds on the affected side

      (3) Heart sounds that are shifted away from the affected side

      (4) Bowel sounds in the affected hemithorax

      (5) Scaphoid abdomen due to the migration of abdominal contents into the chest

     b. Chest x-ray has signs typical of herniation, such as:

      (1) A loculated gas pattern in the affected hemithorax

      (2) A mediastinal shift away from the hernia

      (3) Atelectasis of the unaffected lung

      (4) The presence of the nasogastric tube in the affected hemithorax after passage of the tube through the nose or mouth

   4. Preoperative management

     a. Gastrointestinal decompression should be performed via nasogastric or orogastric tube.

     b. A pneumothorax in the unaffected hemithorax should be sought and, if present, treated with a chest tube.

     c. Attempts to correct the respiratory insufficiency preoperatively will be futile until the herniated contents are returned to the abdomen.

   5. Operative management is based on the following principles:

     a. Surgical reduction of the herniated contents back into the abdomen (through an abdominal incision); this can immediately relieve the distress

     b. Repair of the hernia defect

     c. Exploratory laparotomy to diagnose associated congenital anomalies; intestinal malrotation is often associated with this hernia

     d. Insertion of a chest tube into the affected hemithorax

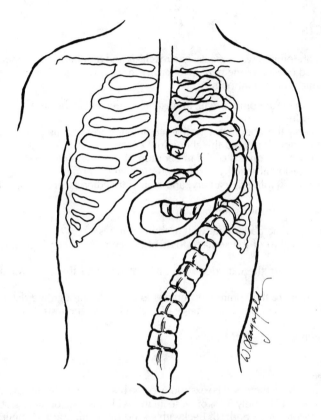

Figure 29-1. Bochdalek hernia.

    e. Careful monitoring of the infant's acid–base balance and respiratory function
    f. Creation of a gastrostomy for decompression of the gastrointestinal tract

6. Postoperative management is aimed primarily at maintaining adequate ventilation and perfusion, and includes the following:
    a. Respiratory support on a ventilator as needed with monitoring of arterial blood gases
    b. Treatment of atelectasis of either lung and the prevention of retained secretions
    c. Use of chest tube suction on the affected side to stabilize the mediastinum in the midline
    d. Observation for contralateral pneumothorax and rapid treatment if it occurs
    e. Adequate gastrointestinal compression
        (1) The abdomen is small and may not be able to hold all of the contents after reduction.
        (2) The loss of the "right of domain" of the abdominal contents will greatly distend the abdomen and raise intra-abdominal pressures.
        (3) Abdominal distention will significantly impair both thoracic excursion and venous return from the lower body.
    f. Extracorporeal membrane oxygenation (ECMO) to support the patient with severe respiratory insufficiency after surgical repair

7. Prognosis for the infant with a diaphragmatic hernia is a function of the hernia's preoperative severity and the time of its presentation.
    a. The immediate mortality rate is 50% or more.
    b. The resolution of respiratory insufficiency in the postoperative period depends on the maturity of the contralateral lung.
        (1) The ipsilateral lung is almost always hypoplastic when a diaphragmatic hernia is present and, therefore, does not aid in respiratory function during the immediate postoperative period.
        (2) If the infant survives, the lung will eventually develop.

    c. No permanent respiratory difficulties have been noted in later life once the acute pulmonary insufficiency has resolved.

III. ABDOMINAL WALL DEFECTS

A. Types. There are two types of abdominal wall defects: **gastroschisis** and **omphalocele**. Although the abdominal contents are located outside of the peritoneal cavity in each type, the similarities, both developmental and therapeutic, end at that point.

  1. Gastroschisis is an opening in the abdominal wall, immediately adjacent to the umbilicus, which is located in the normal position.

    a. During fetal development, the abdominal wall is completely formed, but the peritoneal cavity does not enlarge enough to hold the abdominal contents.

    b. The protruding viscera, which consists of the midportion of the small intestine, the spleen, stomach, colon, and occasionally the liver, has no protective covering.

    c. The intestine is edematous, semirigid, leathery, and matted together as a result of chemical peritonitis.

    d. Associated anomalies and syndromes are rare.

  2. Omphalocele is an opening in the abdominal wall at the umbilicus.

    a. It is due to incomplete closure of the somatic folds of the anterior abdominal wall in the fetus.

    b. Unless ruptured, a sac covers the extruded visceral contents, and there are no signs of chemical peritonitis.

    c. The liver and small bowel are the commonest organs to protrude through the defect.

    d. The omphalocele may be a part of the **pentalogy of Cantrell,** which consists of:

      (1) Omphalocele

      (2) Diaphragmatic hernia

      (3) Cleft sternum

      (4) Absent pericardium

      (5) Intracardiac defects

    e. If the caudal folds are involved, there will be exstrophy of the bladder or exstrophy of a cloaca.

    f. Associated anomalies. Approximately 50% of these infants will have one or more associated anomalies, including trisomies 13 and 18, Beckwith's syndrome, and cardiac, neurologic, and genitourinary malformations.

B. Diagnosis of either gastroschisis or omphalocele is obvious. Further studies may be required on an infant with omphalocele to define any associated problems. The associated anomalies may dictate the management approach in these patients.

C. Preoperative management is similar in both disorders.

  1. Gastrointestinal decompression, intravenous fluids, and antibiotics are instituted.

  2. Albumin should be given for the hypoproteinemia associated with both of these disorders.

  3. Protection of the abdominal contents is imperative, especially because the escape of moisture and heat is considerable in these patients.

    a. In the unruptured omphalocele, this is done by wrapping antibiotic-soaked gauze around the sac to prevent it from drying out.

    b. A gastroschisis or a ruptured omphalocele is protected with moist antibiotic-soaked gauze under a plastic covering (Saran wrap, an intestinal bag, or a plastic tracheostomy bag).

  4. When the patient with gastroschisis has a small defect and a swollen intestine, kinking of the vascular supply may occur at the edge of the defect. This vascular compromise may be prevented by placing the infant on its side.

  5. The outcome of gastroschisis is related to the condition of the intestines at the time of surgery.

D. Operative management differs somewhat for the two disorders. However, the goal in both conditions is to cover the abdominal viscera either with prosthetic material or with the abdominal wall itself.

1. **Gastroschisis.** Primary closure involves decompressing the gastrointestinal tract and stretching the abdominal wall over the defect.
   a. If the closure is excessively tight, the blood supply to the intestine, abdominal wall, or lower extremities will be compromised. To avoid this complication, it is better to cover the exposed organs temporarily with prosthetic materials.
      (1) Currently, Silastic sheeting is used because it is nonreactive and allows the gradual reduction of the viscera into the abdominal cavity.
      (2) **Staged repair** requires daily reduction under sterile conditions. Reduction should be completed within 10 days to minimize the risk of infection.
   b. A gastrostomy is placed for decompression in either method of treatment.

2. **Omphalocele.** The choice of procedures includes primary closure, staged repair, or, for an unruptured omphalocele, nonoperative management. The important factor is the size of the defect.
   a. The greater the size of the defect, the less the peritoneal cavity has enlarged with adequate musculature of the abdominal wall, and with a large defect, primary closure may involve too much tension.
      (1) An alternative method of treatment is to cover the defect with skin flaps, leaving the resultant ventral hernia to be repaired at a later date.
      (2) A Silastic sheeting can be used to stage the repair; by keeping tension on the prosthetic sac, the Silastic sheet will stretch the abdominal wall enough to accommodate the herniated viscera.
      (3) As with a staged repair of gastroschisis, closure must be accomplished within 10 days.
   b. **Nonoperative management** offers an alternative in patients with associated anomalies.
      (1) The sac is coated with tincture of merbromin (Mercurochrome).
      (2) An eschar will form with subsequent coverage by granulation tissue.
      (3) Repair of the resultant ventral hernia can be done at a later date.
      (4) The risks associated with this method are rupture of the sac, requiring subsequent repair in an infected area; sepsis; undiagnosed intestinal atresia; mercury poisoning; and a prolonged hospitalization.
   c. As with gastroschisis, a gastrostomy is placed for decompression.

E. Postoperative management

1. With primary closure, respiration may be inhibited if the reduced abdominal contents compress the diaphragm. Patients may require muscular paralysis and mechanical ventilation until the abdomen stretches enough to accommodate the viscera.

2. Venous return may be compromised due to compression of the inferior vena cava.
   a. For vascular access, upper extremity veins should be used.
   b. The legs may show signs of venous obstruction and resultant edema.

3. With staged repair, the patient needs to be observed after each daily reduction for both respiratory compromise and decreased venous return due to increased abdominal pressure.

4. With both primary and staged repairs, patients will require hyperalimentation because intestinal motility and absorption are slow to return.

5. After repair of an unruptured omphalocele, intestinal function is not as delayed as in gastroschisis; however, hyperalimentation may still be needed.

F. Prognosis

1. **Gastroschisis,** while more difficult to manage initially, has very few long-term problems.
   a. Intestinal strictures may occur at the site of evisceration and will require resection at a later date.
   b. The mortality rate, formerly around 30%, has improved greatly with the use of hyperalimentation and is now less than 10%. Mortality is related to sepsis and the viability of the gastrointestinal tract at the time of surgery.
   c. With resection for intestinal gangrene, short bowel syndrome may develop.

2. **Omphalocele.** The outcome for omphalocele is related to the size and location of the defect and to the presence of associated anomalies. The overall mortality rate ranges from 20%–60%.

IV. ESOPHAGEAL ATRESIA AND TRACHEOESOPHAGEAL MALFORMATIONS occur once in every 3000 live births. They encompass a spectrum of lesions that can vary greatly in their time of presentation and in their treatment. There is a high incidence of associated maldevelopments in other organ systems that may complicate the treatment of these patients.

A. **Types of lesions** (Figure 29-2)

1. **Esophageal atresia** (proximal pouch) **with a distal tracheoesophageal fistula** is the commonest type; it occurs in 86% of the cases.

2. **Pure esophageal atresia** (proximal and distal blind pouches) without fistula occurs in 7% of cases.

3. **Tracheoesophageal fistula without atresia** (H fistula) occurs in 5% of cases.

4. **A proximal and a distal tracheoesophageal fistula is combined with a proximal atresia** (the uncommonest type) in 2% of cases.

B. **Associated anomalies.** In approximately 40% of these patients, other malformations are present in one or more organ systems.

1. **An endocardial cushion defect** affects the heart, the commonest single involved organ.

2. **The VATER complex,** a well-recognized anomaly complex, involves vertebral and anal defects, tracheoesophageal fistula, and radial limb dysplasia or renal abnormalities.
   a. The complex may be fully or partially demonstrated; that is, one or any combination of lesions may occur.
   b. If it seems to be partial, the complete complex must be ruled out.

C. **Diagnosis** of esophageal atresia and tracheoesophageal fistula is usually made soon after birth, when the affected infant exhibits some form of respiratory distress.

1. **Physical examination**
   a. **Aspiration of material from the upper pouch** will cause some symptoms.
      (1) The infant may appear to be salivating excessively and may show continuous drooling.
      (2) The aspiration may also cause coughing spasms, intermittent choking, or cyanosis that develops when the infant is feeding.
   b. **Continuous aspiration of gastric secretions** occurs if a fistula is present. This aspiration is more severe and more harmful than that from the upper pouch.
   c. Tachypnea and signs of pneumonia may develop.
   d. A scaphoid abdomen due to the unused gastrointestinal tract accompanies a pure atresia.

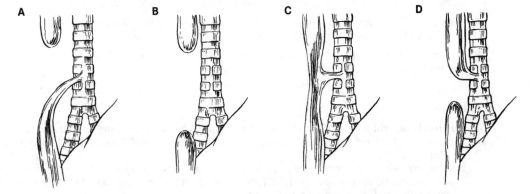

Figure 29-2. Esophageal atresia. (*A*) Esophageal atresia with distal tracheoesophageal fistula, (*B*) proximal and distal blind pouches without fistula, (*C*) H fistula, and (*D*) esophageal atresia with proximal tracheoesophageal fistula. (Adapted from Altman RP, et al: Pediatric surgery. In *Principles of Surgery*, 5th ed. Edited by Schwartz SI, et al. New York, McGraw-Hill, 1989, pp 1637–1678.)

     e. Attempts to pass a tube through the nose into the stomach will fail, since the tube will stop in the blind pouch of the esophagus, confirming the suspicion of esophageal atresia.

  2. X-rays of both the chest and the abdomen are important, both in diagnosis and in preparation for treatment.

     a. The chest film will show the blind upper pouch with the failure of passage by the gastric tube.

     b. A gas-free abdomen is characteristic of a pure atresia.

     c. Hyperventilation, atelectasis, or pneumonia must be evaluated so that the proper surgical approach (i.e., immediate versus delayed repair) can be chosen.

     d. Identification of the aortic arch is also necessary for proper surgical management.

     e. The length of the esophageal defect can be measured on a lateral film.

D. Preoperative management. Several steps are taken once the diagnosis is made.

  1. Decompression of the proximal pouch by means of a sump tube with constant suction (Replogle tube) is required.

  2. An upright position is maintained, using a "chalasia chair."

  3. Gastrostomy is performed if delayed repair is chosen.

     a. This prevents further gastric aspiration.

     b. It also provides a route for preoperative feedings if surgery is delayed for an extended period.

  4. Stretching the proximal pouch daily in pure atresia will shorten the defect in preparation for eventual repair.

E. Operative management. Primary repair at the time of presentation can be done if the defect is less than 2 cm and there are no signs of pneumonitis. **Delayed repair** may be needed if the defect is greater than 2 cm or extends the length of 2½ vertebral bodies. At the time of surgery, the approach is the same for either immediate or delayed repair.

  1. Broad-spectrum antibiotic therapy is begun.

  2. If not previously done, a gastrostomy may be performed, although this measure is controversial.

  3. An extrapleural dissection through the hemithorax opposite the aortic arch is currently favored to prevent the complication of an empyema from occurring as the result of an anastomotic leak.

  4. The tracheoesophageal fistula is repaired.

  5. A primary esophagostomy is performed.

     a. Care is taken during dissection of the distal esophagus, as the blood supply is tenuous.

     b. An adequate length of esophagus is necessary to create a tension-free anastomosis and is obtained by dissecting the proximal pouch. The use of myotomies may aid in gaining length for closure.

  6. A drain is placed in the extrapleural space.

F. Postoperative management is directed at potential pulmonary and esophageal problems.

  1. The infant is extubated as soon as possible to protect the tracheal repair.

  2. Vigorous pulmonary toilet is necessary to clear up any previous pneumonia and to prevent the need for reintubation.

     a. Reintubation may disrupt either the esophageal repair or the tracheal repair, or both.

     b. There is also a degree of tracheal malacia, which compromises pulmonary function.

     c. Chest percussion is mandatory to prevent early postoperative problems.

  3. The infant is kept in a chalasia chair because esophageal functions at first will not be adequate to control secretions.

  4. Esophagotracheal suction is done carefully and with a specifically defined length of tubing. Disruptions of the esophagus can occur during placement of a suction catheter through the anastomotic line.

  5. The esophagus is evaluated at 7 days by means of a barium swallow.

     a. If no leak is present, oral feedings are started and, if tolerated, the extrapleural drain is removed.

    b. Prior to this, the gastrostomy, if present, may be used for constant feedings.

  6. Surgical follow-up is critically important. There are well-recognized problems that can develop, which can have a drastic effect on the outcome in these patients.

    a. Esophageal dysmotility and its concomitant problems are major concerns.

      (1) The patient may develop a **dilated proximal pouch** with resultant aspiration or tracheal compression.

      (2) The patient may also have severe **gastroesophageal reflux** and aspiration.

        (a) Anastomotic stricture, once thought to be solely related to ischemia at the suture line, is now considered to be a consequence of esophagitis from gastroesophageal reflux.

        (b) If gastroesophageal reflux can be implicated in postoperative problems, an **"antireflux" procedure,** usually a Nissen fundoplication, is recommended.

    b. Recurrent fistulas were formerly considered to be a relatively common potential problem, but in recent studies they have been rare.

  7. Prognosis is related to the size of the patient, the condition of the lungs, and the presence or absence of associated anomalies. Patients have been grouped into three categories:

    a. Group A—100% survival: Patients weigh over 2500 g, have no associated anomalies, and no signs of pneumonitis.

    b. Group B—80% survival: Patients either:

      (1) Weigh 1800–2500 g

      (2) Weigh over 2500 g but have mild pneumonitis

      (3) Have one or more associated anomalies that are not life-threatening

    c. Group C—43% survival: Patients either:

      (1) Weigh less than 1800 g

      (2) Have severe pneumonitis

      (3) Have a life-threatening anomaly

V. MALROTATION OF THE INTESTINE is the abnormal placement and fixation of the midgut into the peritoneal cavity (Figure 29-3). The involved portion of the gut includes all of the small intestine from the ampulla of Vater to the proximal two-thirds of the transverse colon. Malrotation can occur independently or can be associated with other malformations, such as diaphragmatic hernia, omphalocele, and gastroschisis.

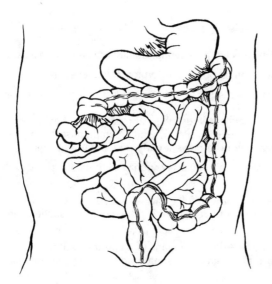

Figure 29-3. Malrotation and volvulus of the midgut.

A. Overview

1. **Normal in utero development.** The midgut develops extra-abdominally. It then migrates intraperitoneally, where it undergoes a 270° rotation. The results are as follows:
   a. The cecum ends up in the right lower quadrant.
   b. The right colon becomes fixed in the right paracolic gutter.
   c. The duodenum becomes fixed in the retroperitoneal location with the superior mesenteric artery passing over the duodenum.

2. **Displacements caused by malrotation**
   a. The cecum is not in the right lower quadrant, and the duodenum does not pass posteriorly to the superior mesenteric artery.
   b. Instead of the base of the small bowel being fixed from the ligament of Treitz to the cecum in the right lower quadrant, the whole midgut is anchored on the superior mesenteric artery.
   c. Various stages of fixation of the cecum can be seen, but it usually is fixed to the right upper quadrant with the fibrinous bands (Ladd's bands) that extend across the second portion of the duodenum.

3. **Sequelae to malrotation.** Two serious problems may accompany this lesion, which must, therefore, be handled expeditiously.
   a. **Intestinal obstruction** can result from adhesive bands across the second portion of the duodenum fixing to the right upper quadrant.
   b. A **midgut volvulus,** which is more serious than intestinal obstruction, can also occur.
      (1) This develops when the intestine twists on its vascular pedicle (the superior mesenteric artery) and causes ischemia as well as obstruction of the entire midgut.
      (2) The result can be catastrophic with gangrene of the entire small bowel.

B. Clinical presentation

1. Bilious vomiting is the usual presenting symptom.

2. Passage of a bloody stool is a late occurrence and implies ischemia with necrosis of the bowel mucosa, bowel wall, or both.

3. The infant may appear normal with hemodynamic stability or may be dehydrated and in shock.

C. Early diagnosis of malrotation is crucial to prevent the development of a volvulus with resulting intestinal gangrene. Therefore, when malrotation in an infant is suspected and cannot be ruled out, all efforts are made to confirm the diagnosis rapidly.

1. **X-rays** are very useful in making the diagnosis.
   a. The plain film may demonstrate the **"double-bubble"** sign, produced by intestinal gas confined to the stomach and duodenum with no gas in the residual, unused gastrointestinal tract. In a newborn infant with bilious vomiting, this is an indication for surgery.
   b. The upper gastrointestinal (GI) series may demonstrate an abnormally located ligament of Treitz, the presence of the duodenum to the left of midline, duodenal obstruction, or a "beaked" end in the barium column at the point of the intestinal twist.

2. Prompt **surgical exploration** is imperative if the diagnosis of malrotation is suspected but cannot be ruled out because approximately 50% of infants with obstructive malrotation will have a volvulus.

D. Operative management. Surgical procedures for malrotation vary with the presence or absence of volvulus and the status of the intestine.

1. **Simple malrotation** is treated by the **Ladd procedure**.
   a. This consists of releasing the adhesive bands and mobilizing the duodenum.
   b. The cecum is placed in the left upper quadrant and the duodenum in the right lateral abdomen so that both organs will be in positions that should prevent intestinal obstruction or ischemia.
   c. An appendectomy is performed, and the remaining abdominal contents are examined for other anomalies, such as a duodenal web.

2. **Malrotation with volvulus** requires several **preliminary steps**.
   a. The first step is counterclockwise detorsion of the midgut volvulus.
   b. The bowel is then examined for viability and for areas of necrosis.

(1) If small areas of gangrene are present, resection is performed, followed by the Ladd procedure.
(2) If large amounts of the midgut appear necrotic, long lengths of bowel are not resected. Instead, the bowel is untwisted and the abdomen is closed and then re-explored 24 hours later. This second look allows marginally viable tissue to recover, hopefully minimizing the amount of bowel to be resected.

E. Prognosis

1. The recurrence of a **midgut volvulus** following surgical exploration and a Ladd procedure occurs in as many as 10% of cases, usually in the immediate postoperative period.

2. The long-term sequelae are minimal after repair of **simple malrotation**. However, when **extensive intestinal resection** is required, the result depends strongly on the amount of intestine remaining. Extreme resections result in severe malabsorption and even in death.

VI. INTESTINAL ATRESIA

A. Duodenal atresia and stenosis occur because the second portion of the duodenum fails to recanalize in the early embryonic stages. The lesion may be complex, partial, or in the form of a web (which is identified by an upper GI study).

1. **Associated anomalies**
   a. **Trisomy 21** occurs in 30% of infants with duodenal malformations.
   b. **Cardiac lesions** and various elements of the **VATER** complex are present in many infants.
   c. **Annular pancreas** may be present with the pancreas forming a ring around the duodenum. This anomaly is now thought to result from the malformation, rather than being a cause of duodenal stenosis.

2. **Diagnosis** is usually made from two simple findings.
   a. Bilious vomiting that occurs soon after birth in a nondistended infant suggests a high obstruction.
   b. Abdominal x-rays show the classic **double-bubble sign,** which is air in the stomach and a proximally dilated duodenum.
      (1) This suggests duodenal obstruction but can also be seen with malrotation.
      (2) While duodenal atresia or stenosis in itself is not life-threatening, malrotation is (see V).
         (a) If delay in treatment is being considered in the patient with a double-bubble x-ray, a barium contrast study to rule out malrotation is necessary.
         (b) This may be a barium enema to localize the cecum or an upper gastrointestinal study to see the duodenal sweep.

3. **Preoperative management**
   a. Gastric decompression and fluid resuscitation are performed as needed.
   b. Broad-spectrum antibiotic therapy is begun.
   c. Since these lesions have a high association with other more critical anomalies, stabilization and evaluation of these lesions may be done prior to surgery. However, this can only be done if malrotation is ruled out as the cause of duodenal obstruction.

4. **Operative management** has as its goal the reestablishment of a patent gastrointestinal tract.
   a. The site of obstruction is identified.
   b. Usually a duodenoduodenostomy can be performed. If not, a duodenojejunostomy is a good alternative. Gastrojejunostomy is contraindicated.
   c. If a **web** is present, the duodenum is opened at the site of obstruction, the web is excised, and the duodenum is closed. Care must be taken to identify the ampulla of Vater, for it is also located on the mesenteric side of the web.
   d. If an **annular pancreas** is present, care is taken not to damage this structure.
      (1) In no circumstance is the pancreas divided.
      (2) The annular pancreas is not the obstructing lesion (the duodenal stenosis is), and the mortality rate is extremely high among patients in whom division of the annular pancreas is performed.
      (3) The annular pancreas can usually be bypassed by a duodenoduodenostomy.

      e. Because 15% of the patients have other gastrointestinal atresias, a thorough search is undertaken to ensure the patency of the entire gastrointestinal tract.

      f. A gastrostomy is performed for gastrointestinal decompression.

  5. Postoperative management is simple but requires patience.

      a. Gastrointestinal decompression is important to protect the suture line and prevent possible aspiration.

      b. The return of gastrointestinal function is slow not only because of gastric and duodenal dysfunction but also because the distal intestine is small due to disuse.

      c. Nutritional support by hyperalimentation may be needed.

  6. Prognosis. Long-term results of surgery are good. Mortality in these patients is related to prematurity of the infant and to associated anomalies.

B. Jejunal, ileal, and colonic atresias are caused by in utero vascular accidents that result in ischemia of a segment of bowel with consequent stenosis or atresia. The **ileum** is most commonly affected; the **jejunum** and **colon** less often. The severity of the lesion is related to the size of the vascular arcade that was affected in utero.

  1. Associated anomalies. Since these are not embryonic maldevelopments, associated anomalies are much less common than with duodenal atresia. However, approximately 10% of patients have **cystic fibrosis**.

  2. Clinical presentation. The diagnosis is suspected when an infant develops bilious vomiting after 24 hours of life.

      a. The degree of abdominal distention will vary with the level of the obstruction.

      b. The passage of meconium does not rule out an atresia, since the gastrointestinal tract was intact before the vascular accident.

      c. All patients with small bowel or colonic atresia should have an early evaluation for cystic fibrosis.

  3. Diagnosis

      a. Abdominal x-rays show various degrees of obstruction, depending on the level of the atresia or stenosis.

         (1) The picture can be confused with meconium ileus.

         (2) In atresia, air–fluid levels are present, whereas with a meconium ileus there is only distended bowel, without fluid levels, and a soap-bubble appearance.

      b. Contrast studies are helpful in both diagnosis and management.

         (1) A barium enema will reveal colonic lesions and perhaps low ileal lesions.

         (2) Hirschsprung's disease, meconium ileus, and other congenital disorders may also be ruled out, making diagnosis of the atresia more certain.

  4. Preoperative management includes gastrointestinal decompression and fluid replacement. Broad-spectrum antibiotics are begun.

  5. Operative management. Surgery is performed to re-establish intestinal continuity.

      a. The current **procedure of choice** is an end-to-end intestinal anastomosis.

         (1) This may be difficult because of the marked size disparity of the bowel, with the proximal bowel dilated and the distal, unused bowel small in size.

         (2) Because of this, tapering of the proximal bowel may aid in the repair.

      b. The distended bowel has been found to have varying degrees of impaired motility. Thus, gastrointestinal function may be extremely slow to return.

      c. A gastrostomy is placed to allow decompression, prevent aspiration, and protect the suture line.

      d. A thorough abdominal examination for **multiple atresias** is performed. Their overall occurrence rate is 6%, but the frequency is high with ileal atresia and very low with colonic atresia.

      e. In a patient with **both an atresia and meconium ileus,** the distal intestine may contain inspissated small bowel secretions. In this case, the site of inspissation should be irrigated with a 4% acetylcysteine (Mucomyst) solution to relieve any potential obstruction before the atresia is repaired.

  6. Postoperative management involves decompression and patience.

      a. Hyperalimentation may be needed until the gastrointestinal tract begins to function.

      b. Malabsorption, if present, may prolong recovery time.

7. **Prognosis.** Since associated anomalies are few, survival is a function of the prematurity of the infant. Current results show a survival rate of nearly 100%.

C. **"Apple-peel" atresia,** a severe form of small bowel atresia, is known by this name because of its appearance.

1. This occurs when there is a large vascular accident to one or more of the mesenteric arcades in utero.

2. There is loss of intestinal length and atresia of the remaining distal intestine.

3. In these patients, return of gastrointestinal function is very prolonged, and malabsorption is common.

VII. IMPERFORATE ANUS (Figure 29-4). Abnormal termination of the anorectum has a clinical spectrum that ranges from a fistulous opening in the perineal area or a colourethral fistula to a completely blind ending of the rectum. The incidence of these malformations ranges from 1 in 1500 to 1 in 5000 live births. The male:female ratio is 2:1.

A. **Types.** While there are many proposed classifications for imperforate anus, the simplest division is on the basis of sex and the relationship to the levator ani.

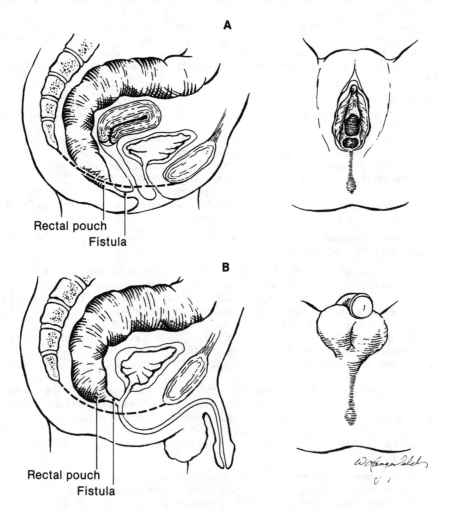

Rectal pouch
Fistula

Rectal pouch
Fistula

Figure 29-4. Imperforate anus in the female (A) and in the male (B).

1. **Infralevator (low) type.** The rectum passes through the puborectalis sling. This type is commoner in girls.

2. **Supralevator (high) type.** The rectum does not pass through the puborectalis sling. This type is commoner in boys.

B. **Associated anomalies** are common in patients with imperforate anus.

1. **The genitourinary tract** is the most commonly involved organ system.
   a. Malformations include renal agenesis, renal dysplasia, hypospadias, epispadias, and bladder exstrophy.
   b. These findings have been reported in up to 40% of patients with imperforate anus.

2. **Other organ systems** involved are:
   a. **Gastrointestinal tract** (in 15%), most often as a tracheoesophageal fistula
   b. **Heart** (in 7%)
   c. **Skeletal system** (in 6%)
      (1) Defects include hemivertebrae, sacral agenesis, and spina bifida.
      (2) While sacral agenesis may not physically affect the patient, it may have some implications for the successful function of the surgically created anus.

C. **Diagnosis** of imperforate anus appears easy; however, determining the extent of the **lesion** is critical for appropriate management.

1. **Physical examination.** The first step is a thorough examination of the perineum and, in girls, the vaginal vault.
   a. A fistula in the perineal area may be found.
   b. The patient may have a fistulous tract, which opens:
      (1) In girls, to the apex of the vagina
      (2) In boys, to the posterior urethra
   c. In boys, meconium in the urine should be sought. This occurs only if there is a fistula between the rectal pouch and the urinary tract.
   d. **Problems in patients with fistulas**
      (1) They may develop symptomatic **urinary tract infections**.
      (2) They may also develop a **hyperchloremic acidosis** due to reabsorption of chloride by the colonic mucosa.
         (a) This is characterized by lethargy, tachypnea, and elevation of the serum chloride and the blood urea nitrogen.
         (b) While the condition may resolve with time, treatment with bicarbonate may be required, and, if the condition is severe or not correctable, division of the rectal pouch–urinary tract fistula may be necessary before the time of the definitive procedure.

2. **X-rays.** If no external fistula is identified, it must be determined if the rectum has traversed the puborectalis sling. Using a cross-table lateral x-ray of the pelvis, one may identify the extent of the rectum by visualizing the end of the infracolonic air.
   a. A line drawn from the posterior portion of the symphysis pubis to the tip of the coccyx (the **pubococcygeal line**) aids in differentiating the infralevator from the supralevator type.
   b. Air visible in the bladder suggests a posterior urethral fistula, which implies a supralevator type.
   c. If the distance from the tip of the colonic air column to the anal dimple is greater than 2 cm, the lesion is supralevator in type. Ultrasound examination may be more accurate in defining the distance.

D. **Operative management**

1. **Infralevator type.** If an **external fistula** is identified, there are several alternatives in the initial management.
   a. If the fistula can be dilated, it may function satisfactorily until the patient is older, at which time the opening can be relocated to the correct site (**Pott's anal transfer**).
   b. If the mucosa is close to the opening, the fistula may be enlarged by a procedure known as a **Denis Brown cutback**.
   c. These procedures are commoner in girls because the infralevator type of imperforate anus occurs more often in girls.

2. Supralevator type. The treatment for the supralevator type of imperforate anus is initially the formation of a colostomy, followed by formation of a neorectum and anus at about 1 year of age.

E. Postoperative management will depend on the type of imperforate anus. Basically, the **goal of treatment** in these patients is to have a socially accepted, continent child. These children require patience during toilet training; they usually are trained between 3 and 5 years of age.

1. Infralevator types will require constant dilations until the stool obtains bulk.

2. Supralevator types will require colostomy care until the definitive procedure can be performed. With the formation of a new anus, the patient may require dilations to prevent strictures.

F. Prognosis

1. The mortality rate among patients with imperforate anus is directly related to the associated anomalies.

2. Functional morbidity is directly related to:
a. Inappropriate management
b. Associated neurologic dysfunction due either to spina bifida or to sacral agenesis

VIII. HIRSCHSPRUNG'S DISEASE

A. Overview

1. Hirschsprung's disease is caused by the congenital absence of parasympathetic ganglia cells in the wall of the gastrointestinal tract.
a. As a result, the affected portions of the bowel are unable to relax and allow effective peristalsis to occur.
b. Hirschsprung's disease always involves the rectum and extends proximally with no skip areas. Any other part of the gastrointestinal tract, or even the entire tract, may also be involved.

2. There is a male predominance of 4 to 1 except when the entire colon is involved. In that situation, the frequency ratio is reversed with females predominating.

3. Some 30% of patients with Hirschsprung's disease have a relative afflicted with the disease.

B. Clinical presentation. Hirschsprung's disease may go **undiagnosed** for years following birth. It should be **suspected** in any patient with a chronic unexplained illness who has an abnormal bowel pattern dating back to early infancy.

1. Newborns with Hirschsprung's disease present with a history of nonpassage of meconium.
a. Meconium is usually passed within 24 hours after birth in term infants and within 48 hours in premature infants.
b. Distention and bilious vomiting are common.
c. Physical examination in the newborn reveals a distended abdomen.
   (1) Occasionally, loops of stool-filled bowel may be palpated.
   (2) Rectal examination shows the ampulla or rectal vault to be empty and the sphincter tone to be increased. Classically, on removal of the examining finger, there is an explosion of watery stool.

2. Infants and older children have a history of obstipation and constipation as well as a failure to thrive.
a. Bouts of diarrhea, vomiting, and abdominal distention may herald the development of enterocolitis.
b. Enterocolitis is sometimes associated with Hirschsprung's disease. If untreated, it has a high mortality rate.

C. Diagnosis is confirmed by x-ray and tissue studies.

1. Abdominal x-rays reveal air–fluid levels and a distended bowel. Often no air is seen in the rectum.

2. Barium enema shows spasm and a narrowed lumen in the affected bowel.
a. A **transition zone** is present, showing a dilated proximal gut and a narrowed distal gut.
   (1) This represents the most distal area in which ganglia cells are present.
   (2) In most patients, this zone will be in the rectosigmoid segment of the colon.

    b. In total colonic Hirschsprung's disease or with a longer segment involving the small bowel, the findings may not be as clear, and the transition zone may not be identified.

  3. **Follow-up x-ray** is obtained in 24 hours when the barium enema is inconclusive in a newborn with suspected Hirschsprung's disease. The appearance of residual barium in the bowel is very suggestive of Hirschsprung's disease.

  4. **Tissue confirmation**

    a. **Biopsy specimens** are examined for the presence of Auerbach's plexus in the muscular layer. The specimen can be obtained by either of two procedures, both of which require bowel preparation and general anesthesia.

      (1) Seromuscular biopsy of the bowel wall at laparotomy

      (2) Full-thickness transrectal biopsy

    b. **Suction biopsy technique** has been developed recently.

      (1) With this procedure, the biopsy specimen is examined for Meissner's plexus in the submucosal layer.

      (2) The procedure can be performed at the bedside with little risk to the patient.

      (3) While the procedure is simple, it produces small specimens and requires an experienced pathologist for a correct interpretation.

D. Preoperative management. Once the diagnosis is made, the patient is prepared for surgery.

  1. If enterocolitis is present preoperatively, the patient will require parenteral antibiotics and gastric decompression. In addition, rectal decompression and irrigations with saline or an antibiotic solution are performed.

  2. The usual surgical approach is to perform a colostomy in an area of intestine that has ganglia cells. Failure to perform this will result in a patient who will be functionally obstructed.

  3. Once the gastrointestinal tract is patent, the child can be fed orally.

E. Operative management. Definitive corrective surgery is usually done at the age of at least 1 year or at a weight of 20 lbs or more.

  1. **Goals of surgery.** While there are different operative procedures for the definitive repair, all have two goals in common:

    a. Removal of most or all of the involved intestine

    b. Re-establishment of a functional, continent anus

  2. **Procedures.** The three operations most commonly performed are the Swensen, Duhamel, and Soave procedures.

    a. **Swensen procedure** is the standard operation, but it is difficult to perform and today is not done by most pediatric surgeons.

      (1) The involved colon is excised to within 1 cm of the anal mucocutaneous margin.

      (2) The bowel is then sutured to the cuff of distal anorectal segment, thus establishing gastrointestinal continuity.

    b. **Duhamel procedure**

      (1) The involved colon is excised to the level of the peritoneal reflection within the abdomen.

      (2) The proximal normal bowel is tunneled between the sacrum and rectum and is then anastomosed end-to-side to the low anorectum.

    c. **Soave procedure**

      (1) In this operation, the involved colon is also excised to the level of the peritoneal reflection.

      (2) The mucosa is removed in the remaining rectum.

      (3) The proximal normal bowel is pulled through the stripped anorectal segment and sutured to the anorectal junction.

  3. **Sequelae.** Enterocolitis may occur, albeit rarely, following these operations. Because the mortality rate is as high as 60%, early diagnosis and treatment are critical.

F. Prognosis for infants properly treated for Hirschsprung's disease is excellent.

  1. Anal dilation may be intermittently necessary if constipation occurs secondary to the retained aganglionic internal anal sphincter.

  2. Problems of incontinence and fecal soiling occasionally occur.

IX. AGNOGENIC DISORDERS OF INFANCY

A. Pyloric stenosis. In this condition, there is hypertrophy of the muscular layer of the pylorus, which causes gastric outlet obstruction. The hallmark symptom is nonbilious projectile vomiting.

1. **The etiology** of the condition is unknown. However, there are consistent elements that imply a hereditary, genetic basis.
   a. It is a male-predominant disease; the male:female ratio is 4:1.
   b. The offspring of a woman with pyloric stenosis have a 10-fold greater than normal chance of developing pyloric stenosis.
   c. The condition is commoner in whites than in blacks.

2. **Clinical presentation.** Pyloric stenosis occurs early in life, usually between the ages of 2 weeks and 2 months.
   a. The history is one of nonvomiting at birth, a gradual onset of vomiting, and final progression to nonbilious projectile vomiting.
   b. The vomiting may lead to dehydration.
   c. A hypochloremic, hypokalemic metabolic alkalosis may be present; this varies with the degree of dehydration.
   d. Jaundice is present in 10% of the infants. It is felt to be due to a deficiency of glucuronyl transferase and resolves after surgical treatment of the pyloric stenosis.

3. **Diagnosis**
   a. **Physical examination** can often provide the diagnosis.
      (1) Palpation of a midepigastric mass in the right upper quadrant of an infant with projectile vomiting is the sine qua non of pyloric stenosis. However, finding the mass may require experience, persistence, and patience.
      (2) Complete evacuation of the stomach by nasogastric tube may aid in finding the mass.
   b. **Upper GI series** may be helpful in diagnosis. The findings include:
      (1) Gastric retention of 3–4 hours
      (2) Elongation and narrowing of the antrum
      (3) A "string" sign or "railroad track" sign (one or two thin barium tracts, respectively, through the pylorus)
      (4) A mass effect on the antrum
      (5) Nonprogression of a peristaltic wave through the pylorus to the duodenum
   c. **Ultrasonography** has become a quick and accurate method of diagnosis.
      (1) The length of the pylorus is measured, and if greater than 15 mm, pyloric stenosis is suspected.
      (2) The width of the muscular wall is measured, and if greater than 4 mm, pyloric stenosis is suspected.

4. **Preoperative management**
   a. Correction of the alkalosis and volume deficits is necessary.
      (1) This is done by fluid replacement and potassium supplementation.
      (2) Adequate hydration is determined by voiding patterns (the normal infant voids four to five times a day).
      (3) Alkalosis correction is measured by the serum bicarbonate, which should be less than 28 mEq/dl, or serum chloride, which should be greater than 92 mEq/dl before surgery is considered.
   b. Gastric decompression may also be instituted to protect against aspiration.

5. **Operative management.** The surgical procedure is pyloromyotomy. This involves incision of the serosa over the pylorus and division of the hypertrophic muscle of the antrum but not the duodenum. The stomach is not entered.

6. **Postoperative management**
   a. The patient may be started on feedings of glucose and water or an electrolyte infant formula (e.g., Pedialyte) 4–6 hours after surgery.
   b. Vomiting will occur in 50%–80% of the patients due to gastric atony or acute gastritis.
      (1) This is usually self-limited.
      (2) Occasionally, the patient will benefit from gastric lavage with half-strength bicarbonate solution.
   c. Feedings are advanced on a prescribed schedule with full feedings usually being reached by 24 hours after surgery. The patient may be discharged at this point.

   d. Complications
     (1) Duodenal perforation is the major complication.
       (a) Its danger is not so much its occurrence as overlooking the problem at the time of surgery.
       (b) The perforation is handled by simple repair, nasogastric decompression for 24–48 hours, and antibiotics.
       (c) If it is recognized and handled appropriately, the major difficulty is an extended hospital stay.
       (d) If it is missed, the morbidity is severe, and the incidence of mortality is significant.
     (2) Apnea may also occur in the early postoperative period.
       (a) The patient should, therefore, have an apnea monitor in place for the first 24 hours postoperatively.
       (b) Postoperative apnea is associated with a serum carbon dioxide level greater than 28 ml/dl.

  7. Prognosis. Once treated, pyloric stenosis does not recur, and long-term studies indicate no sequelae, such as ulcer disease, food intolerance, or hiatal hernia. There are also no problems with growth and development.

B. Biliary atresia is a disease that affects the development of the biliary duct system both intra- and extrahepatically. It occurs once in every 25,000 births.

  1. The etiology of the disease is unknown. Many possible causes have been implicated but not confirmed, including viral infections, hereditary factors, neonatal hepatitis, and malformation of the extrahepatic ductal system. Biliary atresia appears to develop after birth. While isolated fetal cases have been described in Japan, none has been reported in the United States.

  2. Types. Classically, biliary atresia is divided into correctable and noncorrectable types. However, the current feeling is that biliary atresia represents a progressive spectrum of disease and that these divisions have little bearing on the eventual outcome.
   a. Correctable biliary atresia occurs in 20% of the cases.
     (1) There is a **normal common bile duct** that becomes atretic at some distal point.
     (2) It is called "correctable" because the duct can be anastomosed to a jejunal conduit.
   b. Noncorrectable biliary atresia. There is **no macroscopic biliary system** in the portal triad. Until the Kasai operation, there was no successful procedure to establish bile drainage of the liver.

  3. Clinical presentation. Clinically, the child presents from 4 weeks to 4 months of age as a healthy but jaundiced infant with few other complaints. Some patients have associated light stools.
   a. Laboratory studies will show a conjugated hyperbilirubinemia.
   b. Liver function studies may or may not be abnormal, depending on the degree of liver damage from the cholestasis.

  4. Diagnosis. The most important rule of thumb is that **persistent jaundice** beyond the first month of life must be evaluated. This may not affect the outcome in patients with medical causes of conjugated hyperbilirubinemia (for whom no effective therapy may exist). However, the prognosis of surgery for biliary atresia is related to the age at diagnosis.
   a. The workup is designed to differentiate true anatomic obstruction of the biliary tree from other causes of hyperbilirubinemia.
     (1) TORCH (**t**oxoplasmosis, **o**thers, **r**ubella, **c**ytomegalovirus, and **h**erpes simplex virus) titers are checked for possible infection.
     (2) Serum electrophoretic patterns are examined for α_1-antitrypsin deficiency.
     (3) Ultrasonography is performed to examine for dilation of the biliary ducts and for the presence or absence of a gallbladder.
     (4) Nuclear scans employing technetium-99m (^{99m}Tc)-labeled iminodiacetic acid derivatives (PIPIDA, HIDA, DECIDA) look for biliary excretion into the gastrointestinal tract.
     (5) Percutaneous liver biopsy is very helpful in experienced hands. If it shows bile duct proliferation in the face of hepatocellular necrosis, one should suspect biliary atresia.
   b. If biliary atresia cannot be ruled out by these methods, the child should undergo **diagnostic laparotomy**.
     (1) If **intraoperative cholangiography** demonstrates a normal patent biliary system, a **wedge biopsy** of the liver is taken and the surgical procedure is ended.

(2) If patency cannot be demonstrated, the porta hepatis is explored in an effort to find the atretic duct.

(3) If an extrahepatic duct can be found, a Roux-en-Y loop of jejunum is anastomosed to it. This is the so-called **correctable biliary atresia**.

(4) If the common duct cannot be found, the dissection is then carried to the hilus of the porta hepatis and a **Kasai procedure** (hepatoportal enterostomy) is performed. This involves anastomosing a loop of jejunum to the liver hilus, incorporating the area where the common bile duct should be.

   c. In some centers, primary liver transplantation has been used with good success. The limiting factor remains the availability of donor organs.

5. Prognosis
   a. Two factors influence the outcome of the Kasai operation:
     (1) **Age** of the patient at surgery
       (a) The best results are obtained in patients 8–12 weeks old.
       (b) To date, there have been no long-term survivors among patients who were repaired when more than 20 weeks old. This is due to the irreversible liver damage that results from the cholestasis.
     (2) **Microscopic stage** of the biliary tree examined from the hilar dissection specimen
       (a) Patients with ductules greater than 120 μ in diameter have a good prognosis.
       (b) Patients with ductules smaller than 70 μ have a very poor prognosis.
       (c) A "gray zone" occurs when the ductules are between 70 and 120 μ. While bile drainage may occur, resolution of the jaundice and reversibility of the liver disease may or may not occur.
   b. Currently, about 60% of the patients with biliary atresia undergo a **surgical repair**.
     (1) However, only a little more than one-half of these patients have a resolution of jaundice and a return to normal liver function.
     (2) One-third of all patients with biliary atresia who undergo surgery will be successfully treated by current surgical techniques. (These are United States results.)
   c. Until recently, if initial surgery failed to reverse the liver changes, no alternative was available. However, now **liver transplantation** allows one-half of the patients with failed hepatoportal enterostomies to be treated more successfully.

C. Necrotizing enterocolitis is an ischemic disorder of the intestine in the newborn.

1. Etiology. While the etiology and underlying mechanism of the disease are unknown, many causes have been implicated, including bacterial infection, hypoxia, umbilical artery catheterization, aortic thrombosis, and hyperosmolar feedings.

2. Clinical presentation
   a. The **basic defect** is an ischemic or hypoxic insult, which causes intestinal mucosal sloughing. This may lead to bacterial invasion with subsequent intestinal gangrene and perforation.
   b. The patients are usually born prematurely or have a low birth weight (75% weigh less than 2000 g at birth). The disease usually occurs within the first 2 weeks of life.
   c. **The first signs** are usually formula intolerance and abdominal distention. These may be associated with the passage of either heme-positive or grossly bloody stools.
   d. **Associated perinatal problems** include premature rupture of the membranes, prolonged labor, amnionitis, umbilical artery catheterization, respiratory distress, apneic episodes, cyanosis, or delivery-room resuscitation.

3. Diagnosis
   a. **Laboratory findings** include leukopenia, thrombocytopenia, a low hematocrit, low serum sodium levels, metabolic acidosis, and coagulation defects.
   b. **Abdominal x-rays** are used to aid in diagnosis and to follow the patient's clinical course. Initial findings include distended, edematous intestines, intramural air (pneumatosis), portal vein gas, an isolated persistent distended loop of bowel, or free intraperitoneal air, suggesting intestinal perforation.

4. Medical management. The primary management remains medical. This includes gastrointestinal decompression with a large oral or nasogastric tube, parenteral antibiotics, fluids, and nutritional support.

5. **Operative management.** Although the disease is primarily a medical disorder, approximately 25% of all infants who develop necrotizing enterocolitis require surgery for its complications (perforation, gangrene, or intestinal stricture).
   a. **Absolute indication** for surgery in the acute stage is **intestinal perforation**.
      (1) This can usually be documented by the abdominal x-ray.
         (a) A cross-table lateral or left lateral decubitus position is used.
         (b) Films are obtained every 4–6 hours or as clinically indicated.
      (2) If perforation occurs, it is **treated** by resection of the involved intestine.
         (a) The gastrointestinal tract is diverted with either a jejunostomy or an ileostomy and colostomy.
         (b) A gastrostomy is performed to allow gastric decompression and nutritional support.
      (3) Primary reanastomosis of the normal bowel is done only in patients with limited disease or an isolated perforation.
      (4) In the severely ill patient with perforation, a major resective procedure may not be tolerated. In this situation, placement of peritoneal drains (using local anesthesia) may be acceptable treatment.
   b. **Relative indications** for surgery include:
      (1) Increasing signs of peritonitis (erythema or edema of the abdominal wall)
      (2) Failure of the patient to stabilize after 12 hours of optimal medical treatment (the patient shows persistent acidosis, apnea, or hypothermia)
      (3) A persistent distended loop of bowel seen on serial x-rays
      (4) Palpation of an abdominal mass
      (5) A **stricture** with subsequent intestinal obstruction
         (a) This problem usually occurs 3–6 weeks after the acute episode.
         (b) Strictures are treated by resection and primary anastomosis once the patient is nutritionally prepared for surgery.

6. **Postoperative management** includes continued medical management of the primary disease as well as routine postsurgical care.
   a. The infant is treated with antibiotics, gastrointestinal decompression, and hyperalimentation.
   b. Progression of the disease may occur, requiring further surgery for additional perforations.
   c. Oral feedings are not started until 10–14 days after resolution of the acute disease. Dietary adjustments may be necessary until the mucosa has regenerated and undergone functional maturation.
   d. The enterostomy can be closed during the initial hospitalization or at a later date.
   e. **Management of the stoma** can be difficult.
      (1) Local problems include prolapse, degeneration of the surrounding skin, or mucosal irritation.
      (2) Physiologic problems include fluid losses, electrolyte abnormalities, and intolerance of the diet.
      (3) Early recognition and treatment of these difficulties are necessary to prevent further complications.

7. **Prognosis**
   a. The mortality rate is 20% among patients who require only medical management for necrotizing enterocolitis.
   b. The mortality rate among patients requiring surgery is 50%, reflecting the greater severity of the disease in this group.
   c. **Long-term morbidity** is relatively low after recovery from necrotizing enterocolitis.
      (1) It is principally related to concomitant problems, such as intraventricular cerebral hemorrhage, chronic pulmonary insufficiency, or associated cardiac problems.
      (2) A patient who has had an extensive bowel resection may develop a short bowel syndrome (see Chapter 12 II E) requiring a change of diet or nutritional support.

X. SOLID TUMORS. The two commonest solid tumors of childhood are Wilms' tumor and neuroblastoma. While **other tumors** occur (rhabdomyosarcoma, Ewing's tumor, osteogenic sarcoma, and various brain tumors), neuroblastoma and Wilms' tumor illustrate the multidisciplinary approach that is currently used in the management of childhood tumors. They also illustrate an outstanding example of successful management (Wilms' tumor) and the need for continued research to improve current poor results (neuroblastoma).

A. Wilms' tumor. Wilms' tumor can involve either the entire kidney or a part of it. Bilateral involvement occurs in 3%–10% of the cases.

1. **Etiology.** Mesodermal, mesonephric, and metanephric origins have been proposed for this tumor.

2. **Incidence.** It has been estimated that there are 500 new cases of Wilms' tumor per year in the United States.

3. **Clinical presentation**
   a. An asymptomatic flank mass is usually discovered by the parents or on routine physical examination. It is smooth, lobulated, and commonly mobile.
   b. Other complaints or findings include abdominal pain, hematuria, and anorexia.
   c. Hypertension occurs in about 10% of the patients.
   d. The age at presentation is between 1 and 4 years; most patients are between 1 and 3 years old.
   e. The tumor rarely crosses the midline but may appear to do so because of its size.

4. **Associated anomalies**
   a. Wilms' tumor has been associated with congenital anomalies, such as aniridia, hemihypertrophy, Beckwith's syndrome, sexual ambiguity, cryptorchidism, urinary tract anomalies, and abnormal karyotypes.
   b. **Congenital mesoblastic nephroma** is a distinct renal tumor of infancy related to Wilms' tumor.
      (1) To date about 70 cases have been reported.
      (2) The tumor usually presents soon after birth as an abdominal mass.
      (3) Nephrectomy alone is the current therapy and is curative.

5. **Diagnosis**
   a. **Intravenous pyelography** may reveal findings that range from compression of the collecting system to complete nonfunction of the kidney. Calcifications are seen in 10% of the patients.
   b. **Chest x-ray** will reveal lung metastasis, the commonest site.
   c. **Venogram** may be indicated to identify tumor extension into the vena cava.
   d. **Computed tomography (CT scan)** may both identify the tumor and lung metastasis.
   e. **Ultrasonography** with Doppler can both identify the location of the mass and the presence or absence of tumor in the inferior vena cava.

6. **Staging** of Wilms' tumor is as follows.
   a. **Stage I:** The tumor is limited to the kidney and can be resected with the capsule intact.
   b. **Stage II:** The tumor extends beyond the kidney; when resected, the capsule is found to be involved.
   c. **Stage III:** There is residual nonhematogenous tumor in the abdomen; the capsule is ruptured; implants are not completely resected.
   d. **Stage IV:** There is hematogenous metastasis to the liver, lungs, bone, or brain.
   e. **Stage V:** Bilateral involvement is present.

7. **Management** of Wilms' tumor involves a **multidisciplinary approach**.
   a. **Surgery** is the mainstay of treatment.
      (1) The timing of surgery depends on the stage of the tumor (i.e., stage IV or V)
      (2) The operation includes:
         (a) An exploratory laparotomy
         (b) Examination of the opposite kidney
         (c) Resection of the tumor
         (d) Periaortic node dissection or sampling
      (3) Because of the relatively good prognosis, even with extensive disease, resection of other organs in an effort to remove the tumor is acceptable.
   b. **Chemotherapy** currently involves the use of dactinomycin (actinomycin D) and vincristine.
      (1) These are given after surgery in patients with stage II or III Wilms' tumor and in some patients with stage I tumor.
      (2) They are given preoperatively in stage IV and V disease.
      (3) Adriamycin is added to the chemotherapy regimen for patients with advanced disease.
   c. **Radiotherapy** is used to treat extensive disease (stage III–V). There are many **complications** after high-dose radiotherapy, including secondary cancers in children; interference with growth and development of bones, joints, and muscles; radiation pneumonitis, radiation enteritis; and cardiotoxicity.

8. **Prognosis.** Survival appears to be related to the histology of the tumor. This is reported as favorable and unfavorable and will now dictate treatment protocols. Current 2-year survival rates are as follows:
   a. **Stage I:** 90%
   b. **Stage II:** 80%–85%
   c. **Stage III:** 70%–75%
   d. **Stage IV:** 60%–65%
   e. **Stage V:** 50%

B. **Neuroblastoma** is a neoplasm of adrenal and neural crest origin.

1. **Incidence.** It occurs in 1 of every 10,000 live births and is the commonest extracranial solid tumor of childhood. It occurs in the early age-group with 50%–60% presenting by age 2 years.

2. **Types.** There are several **major variants** of neuroblastoma.
   a. **Classic neuroblastoma** is a highly undifferentiated, immature malignant tumor that is un-encapsulated and diffusely infiltrates the surrounding tissue.
   b. **Ganglioneuroma** is a benign, well-encapsulated tumor containing fully differentiated mature ganglia cells.
   c. **Ganglioneuroblastoma** is an intermediate or transitional form consisting of both primitive undifferentiated neuroblasts and mature differentiated ganglia cells. It can occur with or without encapsulation.

3. **Etiology.** While they may occur anywhere along the sympathetic chain, the majority (65%) of these tumors arise from adrenal or nonadrenal retroperitoneal sites.

4. **Clinical presentation**
   a. Most patients **present** with a complaint of an abdominal mass.
   b. Neurologic symptoms may occur, resulting from compression of nerve trunks or from extension of the tumor into the extradural space (**"dumb-bell" tumor**).
   c. Horner's syndrome has been reported.
   d. Other symptoms include acute cerebellar ataxia and **opsoclonus** (sustained, irregular, multidirectional spontaneous conjugate eye movements).
   e. **Metastatic spread** can involve the liver, lungs, skin, bone marrow, and bone.
      (1) Skin lesions are firm, nontender, and bluish; biopsy will provide the diagnosis.
      (2) The orbit is a common site of bony metastasis with consequent periorbital ecchymosis and proptosis.

5. **Diagnosis** of the tumor may be obtained by various laboratory means.
   a. **Bone marrow** aspiration may reveal typical neuroblastoma cells.
   b. **Urinalysis.** The tumor may synthesize various catecholamines.
      (1) The excretion products include vanillylmandelic acid (VMA) and homovanillic acid.
      (2) These can be checked in both spot urine samples and in 24-hour urine collections.
   c. **Radiologic studies**
      (1) Skeletal surveys or bone scans may show metastatic lesions.
      (2) Chest x-rays will confirm or rule out pulmonary metastasis.
      (3) The mainstay of radiologic testing for adrenal neuroblastoma is **intravenous pyelography**. This will show a suprarenal mass compressing the kidney and causing the collecting system to take on a "drooping lily" appearance.
      (4) Calcifications are seen much more often on abdominal x-rays in neuroblastoma than in Wilms' tumor.
      (5) Sonography may be of aid in identifying the mass.
      (6) A CT scan may not only aid in localizing the primary tumor but also may be a sensitive test for identifying hepatic metastasis.
   d. Liver function is documented and routine blood studies are done. Anemia will be present in about 40%–60% of the patients at the time of diagnosis.

6. **Staging** for neuroblastoma is as follows:
   a. **Stage I:** The tumor is confined to the organ or structure of origin and is completely excised.
   b. **Stage II:** The tumor extends beyond the organ or structure of origin but does not cross the midline.
   c. **Stage III:** The tumor extends across the midline.
   d. **Stage IV:** Remote disease is present and involves the skeleton, organs, soft tissue, or a distant lymph node group.

e. **Stage IV-S:** The tumor is stage I or II; remote disease is present but is confined to one or more of the following sites: liver, skin, or bone marrow.

7. **Medical/surgical management.** A rational approach to the treatment of neuroblastoma requires a combined approach employing the surgeon, radiation oncologist, chemotherapist, and pediatrician.

   a. **Surgery.** While complete surgical removal is desirable, most patients (60%) present with metastatic disease. Neuroblastoma is unlike Wilms' tumor, in which aggressive surgery in the face of advanced disease is associated with good results.

   b. **Radiation** is used as an adjuvant for resected or partially resected primary tumors and as palliative therapy for symptomatic metastases.

   c. **Chemotherapy** includes the use of cyclophosphamide, vincristine, adriamycin, and dacarbazine (DTIC). The exact therapeutic protocol has not been developed, and other agents are currently under investigation.

   d. **Autologous bone marrow transplant** with tumor cell purge is now being used for advanced stages or recurrent disease. Initial reports are encouraging with survival rates markedly better than reported with standard therapy.

8. **Prognosis.** Neuroblastoma remains as one of the few childhood tumors that has not responded dramatically to modern antitumor therapy. A child diagnosed today has the same dismal prognosis as a child diagnosed over 20 years ago.

   a. **Factors that influence survival**

      (1) **Age.** The younger the child at diagnosis, the better the outlook; this is independent of staging.

      (2) **Stage.** The more advanced the disease, the worse the prognosis; however, stage IV-S has a relatively good prognosis (60% survival).

      (3) **Location.** Abdominal neuroblastoma has a worse outlook than extra-abdominal neuroblastoma.

      (4) **Site of metastasis.** Patients presenting with bony lesions have a mortality rate near 100%.

      (5) **Presentation.** Patients presenting with opsoclonus have a higher survival rate than those presenting without it.

   b. **Overall survival rates** are as follows:

      (1) **Stage I:** 64%

      (2) **Stage II:** 54%

      (3) **Stage III:** 28%

      (4) **Stage IV:** 5%

      (5) **Stage IV-S:** 61%

Part VII Special Subjects

STUDY QUESTIONS

Directions: Each question below contains four or five suggested answers. Choose the **one best** response to each question.

1. Which of the following statements is true concerning soft tissue injuries in the trauma patient?

(A) Palpable pulses rule out arterial injury
(B) Fasciotomies are frequently required in conjunction with vascular repair
(C) Stab wounds or missile tracts near major vessels can be closed if there is no sign of major arterial or venous hemorrhage
(D) Exposed nerves can be left open as granulation tissue will readily cover them
(E) Attached bones should be removed to speed healing

2. All of the following statements regarding electrical burns are true EXCEPT

(A) they are usually deeper and more severe than indicated by the surface appearance
(B) blood vessels, nerves, and bone have the lowest resistance to electrical current
(C) muscle necrosis may be markedly underestimated
(D) all patients with high-voltage electrical injury need continuous cardiac monitoring
(E) mannitol may be used to maintain high-level urine output, especially with myoglobinuria

3. Which of the following statements concerning hypersplenism is true?

(A) Primary hypersplenism is commoner in men than in women
(B) Primary hypersplenism does not respond to splenectomy
(C) Splenic vein thrombosis can cause secondary hypersplenism and bleeding from esophageal or gastric varices
(D) Portal hypertension usually causes severe secondary hypersplenism
(E) Spontaneous thromboembolic events are common in the early postoperative period after splenectomy for primary hypersplenism

4. Which of the following statements concerning Hodgkin's disease is true?

(A) The prognosis for affected individuals remains poor
(B) Stage II classification indicates involvement of the nodal regions on both sides of the diaphragm
(C) The spleen is not usually removed during staging laparotomy
(D) Staging laparotomy reveals unsuspected abdominal disease in 25% of stage I or II patients
(E) Staging laparotomy is useful in patients with stage IV disease

5. Trauma can cause rupture of the spleen or it can occur spontaneously. True statements regarding a ruptured spleen include

(A) the area around small capsular tears should be resected
(B) when massive splenic injury is accompanied by other intra-abdominal injuries, there should be an attempt to salvage the spleen
(C) the spleen can be removed with impunity since it has little known immunologic function
(D) delayed rupture of a subcapsular splenic hematoma usually occurs within 2 weeks of the injury
(E) none of the above

6. Postsplenectomy sepsis is best characterized by

(A) occurrence within 2 years of splenectomy
(B) a 10% incidence following splenectomy for traumatic injury
(C) the greatest risk of development in elderly patients
(D) a sudden and catastrophic onset of symptoms

7. Which of the following presenting symptoms of breast cancer is commonest?

(A) Isolated axillary enlargement
(B) Nipple discharge
(C) Breast mass
(D) Mammographic findings of microcalcifications
(E) Nipple changes and desquamation

8. All of the following statements regarding nipple discharge are true EXCEPT

(A) intraductal papilloma is the commonest cause of serosanguineous nipple discharge
(B) up to 10% of all pathologic nipple discharges are due to a malignant process
(C) if a mass is present in association with the discharge, it should be followed nonoperatively
(D) patients with nipple discharge should be evaluated with mammography and cytology of the discharged fluid
(E) when no mass is present but the quadrant of the discharge can be localized, a quadrantectomy is indicated

9. Which of the following donor types is likely to offer the greatest chance for renal graft survival?

(A) One-haplotype match, living related donor
(B) Two-haplotype match, living related donor
(C) Cadaver allograft donor
(D) Isograft donor
(E) Xenograft donor

10. Which of the following conditions in a potential cadaver donor would make the kidneys unacceptable for transplantation?

(A) Deep coma
(B) Colon cancer 3 years previously
(C) Serum creatinine level of 1.5 mg/dl (normal: 1.4 mg/dl)
(D) Gunshot wound to the head
(E) Endotracheal intubation

11. Likely causes of anuria following renal transplantation include all of the following EXCEPT

(A) acute tubular necrosis
(B) accelerated acute rejection
(C) ureteral obstruction
(D) azathioprine toxicity
(E) renal artery thrombosis

12. True statements regarding liver transplantation include all of the following EXCEPT

(A) patients with end-stage liver disease who have a low likelihood of surviving 1–2 years are candidates
(B) donors are matched with recipients based on blood and HLA type
(C) donor livers are preserved in University of Wisconsin solution
(D) leakage of the biliary duct in a transplant recipient may be due to hepatic artery thrombosis
(E) survival is approximately 70% at 1 year

13. A 24-year-old woman was admitted to the hospital complaining of dysuria and urinary frequency. She was found to have a temperature of 101° F, pyuria, and bacteriuria. Her chest was clear and her abdomen normal on physical examination. Tenderness was noted at the costovertebral angle. This patient should be treated with

(A) antibiotics for 1 day
(B) antibiotics for 1 week
(C) antispasmodics
(D) fluids and observation
(E) bethanechol

14. What organism most frequently causes a renal infection?

(A) *Staphylococcus aureus*
(B) *Staphylococcus epidermidis*
(C) *Escherichia coli*
(D) *Proteus mirabilis*
(E) *Pseudomonas aeruginosa*

15. All of the following factors adversely affect the survival of patients with renal cell carcinoma EXCEPT

(A) invasion of the perinephric fat
(B) invasion into the liver
(C) nodal metastases
(D) invasion into the renal vein
(E) a solitary pulmonary metastasis

16. Prostate specific antigen has been found to be most useful to

(A) differentiate between prostatitis and prostatodynia
(B) screen for carcinoma of the prostate
(C) select patients with stage A_2 carcinoma of the prostate
(D) follow patients for recurrence after treatment of localized carcinoma of the prostate
(E) predict survival of patients before treatment of carcinoma of the prostate

17. A test that has been most effective in distinguishing between organic and psychogenic impotence is

(A) determination of serum testosterone level
(B) perineal electromyography
(C) Doppler determination of penile blood pressure
(D) nocturnal penile tumescence monitoring
(E) intracavernosal injection of prostaglandin E_1

18. The best suture material for a simple interrupted closure is

(A) silk
(B) catgut
(C) polyglycolic acid
(D) polypropylene
(E) none of the above

19. Factors that impair wound healing include all of the following EXCEPT

(A) excessive use of cautery
(B) excessive tension
(C) lack of hemostasis
(D) drains
(E) inversion of wound edges

20. All of the following methods are useful for wound coverage EXCEPT

(A) split-thickness skin graft
(B) full-thickness skin graft
(C) muscle or myocutaneous flap
(D) free flap
(E) fat autotransplantation

21. Which of the following statements concerning breast reconstruction is true?

(A) The percentage of women who request reconstruction diminishes over time following mastectomy
(B) Reconstruction should never be performed at the time of mastectomy
(C) Silastic implants are usually placed immediately beneath the skin to reconstruct breast fullness
(D) Although breast fullness can be accomplished, the nipple–areolar complex can not be reconstructed
(E) Reduction mammoplasty is seldom necessary for the opposite breast to achieve symmetry

22. In patients with malignant melanoma, prognosis is most dependent on

(A) lymph node status
(B) depth of invasion
(C) histologic grading of the tumor
(D) classification of the melanoma
(E) anatomic location on the body

23. The diagnosis of Parinaud's syndrome could be based on all of the following findings EXCEPT

(A) papilledema
(B) hydrocephalus, visible on CT scan
(C) a mass lesion involving the right cerebral hemisphere
(D) a mass lesion in the posterior part of the third ventricle
(E) upward gaze palsy

24. All of the following measures are likely to be helpful in the management of cerebral edema EXCEPT

(A) restricting fluids to two-thirds of maintenance
(B) administering osmotic agents (e.g., mannitol and glycerol)
(C) monitoring intracranial pressure
(D) maintaining PCO_2 in the 40–45 mm Hg range
(E) administering barbiturates

25. A 24-year-old man sustained a crush injury to his right shoulder. On examination, a 3-inch laceration is found, extending into the axilla and with no apparent involvement of the underlying muscles. Neurologic examination of the right upper extremity shows deltoids to be 2^+ and triceps to be 2^+. No other muscle contractions are seen. The proper management of this patient should include all of the following measures EXCEPT

(A) evaluation of the vascular supply to the limb
(B) immediate exploration of the brachial plexus
(C) thorough debridement of the wound and primary closure
(D) tetanus prophylaxis
(E) periodic neurologic examinations of the limb

Questions 26 and 27

A 36-year-old male motorcycle rider came in with complaints of a pain radiating down his right lower extremity. Initial examination shows a positive straight-leg raising test at 30° on the right side. There is a decreased pinprick sensation in the right L5–S1 dermatome, and the right ankle reflex is depressed.

26. Initial management would consist of all of the following EXCEPT

(A) plain x-rays of the lumbosacral spine
(B) analgesics or anti-inflammatory medicine
(C) bed rest
(D) pelvic traction, heat, and ultrasound treatment to the lower back
(E) emergency myelogram

27. The patient did not respond to 4 weeks of conservative treatment, and his symptoms worsened. A CT scan of the lumbosacral spine showed a large herniated disc at L4–L5 lateralized to the left. Further management would consist of

(A) conservative treatment for another 4 weeks
(B) a left sided L4–L5 discectomy
(C) nerve blocks
(D) referral to a pain clinic
(E) myelogram or MRI

(end of group question)

Questions 28 and 29

A 40-year-old white woman is brought to the emergency room after being found unresponsive following a sudden onset of severe headaches at work. She had been in good health until then. In the emergency room, her blood pressure is 180/100, and her respirations are irregular and of Cheyne-Stokes type. She is agitated and does not follow commands but moves all of her extremities spontaneously.

28. Initial management of this patient would consist of all of the following EXCEPT

(A) 6 L oxygen by nasal cannula
(B) rapid awake intubation and hyperventilation
(C) starting an intravenous line with lactated Ringer's solution
(D) CT scan of the head
(E) lower the systolic blood pressure to around 120–130 mm Hg

29. The most likely diagnosis is

(A) subarachnoid hemorrhage due to a ruptured cerebral aneurysm or arteriovenous malformation
(B) hypoglycemic coma
(C) conversion reaction
(D) myxedema
(E) addisonian crisis

(end of group question)

30. All of the following are causes of fracture nonunion EXCEPT

(A) calcium deficiency
(B) excessive fracture motion
(C) soft tissue damage
(D) infection
(E) excessive immobilization

31. Management of chronic osteomyelitis would include all of the following techniques EXCEPT

(A) use of antibiotics
(B) debridement
(C) bone graft (Papineau)
(D) plaster cast immobilization
(E) use of muscle flaps

32. All of the following are indications for open fracture reduction and internal fixation EXCEPT

(A) open fracture
(B) functional requirements
(C) unsatisfactory closed reduction
(D) multiple trauma
(E) intra-articular fracture

33. Which of the following situations requires true emergency care?

(A) Closed tendon rupture
(B) Comminuted fracture of the femur
(C) "Boxer's" fracture of the hand
(D) Open fracture of the ankle
(E) Subperiosteal hematoma of the tibia

34. The most dangerous aspect of compound fractures is

(A) bleeding
(B) skin loss
(C) anaerobic infection
(D) bone loss
(E) muscle loss

35. Which of the following statements about hip dislocations is true?

(A) They require urgent reduction
(B) They have a high recurrence rate
(C) They occur with minor trauma
(D) They rarely are associated with other injuries
(E) They usually are dislocated anteriorly

36. The commonest causative factor in tendon ruptures is

(A) overuse
(B) severe trauma
(C) a stab wound
(D) a fall from a height
(E) a congenital defect

37. Treatment of an incarcerated congenital inguinal hernia involves

(A) immediate operation to prevent the reduction of necrotic intestine

(B) evaluation of the child's state of hydration, after reduction of the hernia

(C) observation after reduction of the hernia until the child is old enough to undergo surgery

(D) observation after reduction until the processus vaginalis has clearly fused

(E) surgery of the small intestine in both male and female patients

38. Characteristics of gastroschisis include all of the following EXCEPT

(A) multiple congenital anomalies in most cases

(B) abdominal wall defect lateral to the umbilicus

(C) no protective covering over the protruding viscera

(D) edematous bowel and hypoproteinemia

(E) delayed gastrointestinal function requiring total parenteral nutrition

39. Malrotation of the gut is characterized by all of the following statements EXCEPT

(A) two potential problems are intestinal obstruction at the duodenum and midgut volvulus that produces obstruction and ischemia of the small intestine

(B) malrotation is a diagnosis of exclusion and is considered only after other causes of obstruction are ruled out

(C) bilious vomiting is a common presenting symptom

(D) the "double-bubble" sign is often seen on x-rays of the abdomen

(E) the long-term outlook is very good in patients treated for simple malrotation without volvulus

40. All of the following statements about necrotizing enterocolitis are true EXCEPT

(A) approximately 25% of patients require surgery

(B) it occurs most commonly in term newborns

(C) the intestinal mucosa sloughs due to hypoxia and ischemia

(D) abdominal x-rays aid greatly in diagnosis and management

(E) supportive management is currently the treatment of choice

Directions: Each question below contains four suggested answers of which **one or more** is correct. Choose the answer

A   if **1, 2, and 3** are correct
B   if **1 and 3** are correct
C   if **2 and 4** are correct
D   if **4** is correct
E   if **1, 2, 3, and 4** are correct

41. Trauma is the leading cause of death among people under 35 years of age. Of trauma victims, it can be said that

(1) over one-half of deaths result from motor vehicle accidents
(2) some 10%–15% have serious multisystem injuries
(3) patient management requires adherence to an established order of priority
(4) prophylactic antibiotics and tetanus prophylaxis should be administered routinely

42. Certain steps are essential during the early management of trauma victims, including

(1) airway assessment and control
(2) cardiac resuscitation
(3) insertion of venous access lines
(4) suturing of all facial lacerations

43. When a trauma patient is in profound shock, management involves

(1) subclavian lines and saphenous vein cutdowns
(2) crystalloid solutions, followed by packed red blood cells if the hematocrit is less than 25%
(3) uncrossmatched type-specific blood cells
(4) initial use of type O-negative blood, if available, if there is no time for blood typing

44. A patient with multiple injuries is brought to the hospital. Which of the following management procedures is appropriate in the emergency room to control the hemorrhage?

(1) Applying pressure on the wounds with gauze pads
(2) Hemostats used proximally and distally to control arterial-type bleeding in the base of deep puncture wounds
(3) Pneumatic splints and medical antishock trousers to tamponade bleeding and increase peripheral resistance
(4) Suturing closed actively bleeding missile tracts or stab wound sites

45. A young man is brought to the emergency room with multiple injuries following an automobile accident. Management of his thoracic injuries would involve

(1) upright chest x-rays obtained as soon as possible
(2) monitoring the electrocardiogram and central venous pressure for evidence of cardiac contusion or tamponade
(3) contrast studies of the esophagus to look for perforation
(4) thoracotomy if bleeding from a chest tube exceeds 100 ml/hr

46. True statements concerning peritoneal lavage of the trauma patient with abdominal injuries include

(1) it is useful for unconscious patients
(2) the open technique is safest and most reliable
(3) the lavage is positive if gross blood or fecal matter are found in the lavage aspirate
(4) the patient's bladder need not be empty prior to lavage

47. The surgical treatment of abdominal injuries involves

(1) a generous midline incision
(2) obtaining hemostasis as a first priority
(3) mobilization and palpation of the pancreas and duodenum if a central upper abdominal retroperitoneal hematoma is present
(4) exploration of lower abdominal and pelvic retroperitoneal hematomas

48. Correct statements regarding burn wound care include which of the following?

(1) Cold compresses may be applied to relieve the pain of 25% second-degree burns
(2) Topical antibiotics are usually recommended for deep second- and third-degree burns
(3) Systemic antibiotics are usually indicated immediately for third-degree burns
(4) Escharotomy may be urgently required and performed prior to transfer to a burn center

49. Functions of the spleen include

(1) removal of abnormal red blood cells
(2) storage of over one-half of the body's platelets
(3) production of opsonins and immunoglobulin M (IgM)
(4) production of new red blood cells under normal physiologic conditions

50. Absolute indications for splenectomy include

(1) primary splenic tumors
(2) splenic abscess
(3) hereditary spherocytosis
(4) autoimmune hemolytic anemia

51. Idiopathic thrombocytopenic purpura is characterized by

(1) an acute form found in children
(2) a female:male ratio of 3:1
(3) a chronic form found in adults
(4) decreased peripheral platelets and bone marrow megakaryocytes

52. Factors that may increase the risk of developing cancer of the breast include

(1) chronic cystic mastitis with atypia
(2) previous contralateral breast cancer
(3) breast cancer in a maternal grandmother
(4) breast cancer in a paternal grandmother

53. True statements concerning hormone receptors in breast cancer include

(1) elevated hormone receptors indicate a better prognosis
(2) as hormone receptor status may change over time, treatment should depend on the most recent determination of receptor status
(3) therapy with male hormones is useful in treating premenopausal patients
(4) if a patient does not respond to one form of hormonal therapy, a different hormone should be tried

54. Contraindications to renal transplantation in a potential recipient include

(1) positive tuberculin test, but no other evidence of active tuberculosis
(2) an unhealed duodenal ulcer
(3) polycystic kidneys
(4) the presence of antiglomerular basement membrane antibody in the blood

55. True statements concerning transplant rejection include

(1) acute rejection involves lymphocytic infiltration of the kidney
(2) hyperacute rejection involves preformed antibodies against the new kidney
(3) chronic rejection involves vascular intimal thickening and scarring
(4) accelerated acute rejection usually involves a second-set, or anamnestic, response

56. Immunosuppressive drug therapy can be complicated by

(1) cushingoid facies
(2) cytomegalovirus infection
(3) hypertension
(4) central nervous system tumors

57. Long-term complications of renal transplantation include

(1) skin cancers
(2) coronary artery disease
(3) lymphoma
(4) hyperlipidemia

58. A 40-year-old woman with a history of recurrent urinary tract infections was found on urinary culture to have *Proteus mirabilis* in a concentration of 10^5 organisms/ml. An abdominal radiogram showed a branched calculus in the right kidney. Excretory urography demonstrated bilateral function and showed that the calculus essentially filled the entire collecting system on that side. There is moderate blunting of the calyces. The ureter was patent. This patient should be treated with

(1) shock wave lithotripsy
(2) administration of antibiotics
(3) percutaneous nephrostomy
(4) nephrectomy

59. A 35-year-old woman has passed two urinary calculi and required ureteroscopic removal of a large distal ureteral stone. In a search of a metabolic basis for her stone disease, which of the following studies should be included?

(1) A 24-hour urine collection for citrate
(2) Serum protein electrophoresis
(3) Serum calcium and 24-hour urine collection for calcium
(4) Serum oxalate

SUMMARY OF DIRECTIONS

A	B	C	D	E
1,2,3 only	1,3 only	2,4 only	4 only	All are correct

---

60. A 10-year-old boy was injured while riding a bicycle, which struck the edge of a curb. Which of the following observations suggest that the patient has a significant urethral injury?

(1) A small amount of blood located at the urethral meatus
(2) A perineal ecchymosis
(3) Inability to void to give a urine sample
(4) A palpable lower abdominal mass

61. A 53-year-old man was seen in a urologist's office with a history of a single episode of gross, painless hematuria. The physical examination revealed nothing, and the urinalysis was normal, demonstrating only an occasional white blood cell. His initial evaluation should include

(1) excretory urography
(2) cystourethroscopy
(3) urinary cytology
(4) ultrasonography

62. Evaluation of a patient with erectile failure should include determination of

(1) urinary esterase
(2) serum testosterone levels
(3) serum chorionic gonadotropin levels
(4) penile blood pressure

63. The survival of a skin graft requires

(1) an adequate vascular bed for the graft
(2) good contact of the skin graft with the recipient bed
(3) absence of gross infection in the recipient bed
(4) careful removal of periosteum from bone prior to grafting

64. Common warts (verrucae vulgaris) have which of the following characteristics?

(1) They occur most frequently in the third decade of life
(2) They are caused by papovaviruses
(3) Most will not resolve spontaneously and require treatment such as desiccation
(4) The fingers are the commonest location

65. True statements concerning lipomas include which of the following?

(1) They can be found in any location of the body where fat is usually found
(2) Malignant transformation is common
(3) Simple excision is curative
(4) They can be caused by trauma to areas of fatty tissue

66. Indications for excision of a pigmented nevus include

(1) a sudden change in color, size, or shape
(2) development of pain in the lesion
(3) the appearance of satellite lesions in the area of a previously existing nevus
(4) unexplained regional adenopathy

67. Joint arthroplasty, or total joint replacement, is a recent addition to the operative management of joint diseases. True statements about this useful new procedure include which of the following?

(1) It is limited to rheumatoid arthritis
(2) It is a permanent repair
(3) It is indicated for young, active patients
(4) It is used to relieve pain

68. Management of a diaphragmatic hernia should include

(1) preoperative placement of nasal or gastric tube and chest x-ray
(2) preoperative placement of a chest tube on the ipsilateral side to re-expand the compressed lung
(3) the use of extracorporeal membrane oxygenation in the presence of postoperative respiratory insufficiency
(4) preoperative respiratory support with mask ventilation to prevent a contralateral pneumothorax

69. A neonatal tracheoesophageal fistula has which of the following characteristics?

(1) Associated congenital defects are common, with the heart the most commonly involved organ

(2) Failure to pass a nasogastric tube into the stomach is very suggestive of a tracheoesophageal fistula

(3) The length between the blind pouch and the fistula is important in determining the time of surgery

(4) Gastroesophageal reflux is uncommon and has no bearing on the development of esophageal stricture

70. A 4-week-old white boy whose mother has been breast-feeding him is noted to be jaundiced. The history reveals an increased intolerance to feeding, nonbilious vomiting, and weight loss. There is no relevant family history, as this is the first-born child. What can be said about the management of this case?

(1) The vomiting and jaundice call for an immediate workup to identify or exclude biliary atresia

(2) Palpation of the abdomen in this patient would reveal a mass

(3) The infant needs to be changed to a formula, since feeding intolerance accompanied by jaundice has been related to breast milk

(4) Both physical examination and serum electrolytes in this infant would reveal findings of pyloric stenosis

Directions: The groups of questions below consist of lettered choices followed by several numbered items. For each numbered item select the **one** lettered choice with which it is **most** closely associated. Each lettered choice may be used once, more than once, or not at all.

Questions 71–75

Match each of the findings on physical examination with the appropriate clinical stage.

(A) T1N0
(B) T1N1
(C) T2N2
(D) T3N0
(E) None of the above

71. 1.0-cm tumor with mobile ipsilateral axillary adenopathy

72. 2.5-cm tumor with fixed ipsilateral axillary nodes

73. 5.5-cm tumor with no axillary adenopathy

74. 1.5-cm tumor with fixed ipsilateral axillary nodes

75. 1.0-cm tumor with no axillary adenopathy

Questions 76 and 77

For each condition associated with breast cancer, select the therapy that is most appropriate.

(A) Modified radical mastectomy
(B) Adjuvant chemotherapy
(C) Primary radiation therapy
(D) Oophorectomy
(E) Close observation

76. Noninvasive lobular carcinoma in situ

77. Myelosuppression

ANSWERS AND EXPLANATIONS

1. The answer is B. [*Chapter 21 I C 5 d (3) (d)*] Palpable pulses do not rule out arterial injury as intimal tears can be present with intact pulses distally. Fasciotomies will almost always be required for vascular injuries, particularly if any length of time has passed before repair. The reason is that postoperative swelling will be extensive and will lead to necrosis of muscle in closed fascial spaces. Stab wounds or missile tracts near major vascular structures require arteriography to rule out injury to the structures. This should be done whether or not obvious bleeding is seen. Exposed nerves must be covered with normal muscle or fat following repair. Attached bones should generally be left in situ to speed healing.

2. The answer is B. [*Chapter 21 II E 6*] Electrical burns are usually deeper and more severe than indicated by the surface appearance, and muscle involvement may be markedly underestimated by attention to surface wounds alone. All patients with electrical burns need continuous cardiac monitoring as myocardial infarction is a well-described postinjury. Because electrical energy is converted to heat as it traverses the body along the path of least resistance, such as the blood vessels and nerves, muscles closest to bone, which has high resistance and, thus, generates the most heat, incur the most damage. Oliguria is common in patients with electrical burns and can be managed with mannitol. The administration of mannitol is mandatory in the presence of myoglobinuria.

3. The answer is C. [*Chapter 22 II A 1, 3, B 1, 2*] Primary hypersplenism is a diagnosis of exclusion and is commoner in women than in men. It can be cured by splenectomy. Portal hypertension is a common cause of secondary hypersplenism, but it is usually mild and not clinically significant. Splenic vein thrombosis usually is a result of pancreatitis. It can lead to splenic congestion and resultant secondary hypersplenism. Varices in the distal esophagus and stomach develop from pressure transmitted via the short gastric veins between the spleen and the stomach. Bleeding may be severe. Splenectomy is curative and will stop both the bleeding and the hematologic complications. Although the platelet counts may rise following splenectomy, spontaneous thromboembolism is uncommon.

4. The answer is D. [*Chapter 22 IV I 2 c, 3 b (1)*] Hodgkin's disease is now treatable, and patients have a good chance of cure or long-term survival. Proper staging is essential. A classification of stage II Hodgkin's disease indicates two or more involved nodal areas on the same side of the diaphragm. The spleen should be removed during laparotomy; if it is not, it may need to be radiated, a procedure that may damage the left kidney and left lung, which are both in the field of radiation. Histologic examination may reveal involvement of the spleen and change the staging of the disease. Patients with stage IV disease are not candidates for staging since their treatment will not be changed by the procedure.

5. The answer is D. [*Chapter 22 V A 4, C 1, 3*] In virtually all isolated splenic injuries, an attempt should be made to salvage the spleen; however, when other severe intra-abdominal injuries are involved, splenectomy is indicated. Small capsular tears will stop bleeding with pressure and topical application of hemostatic agents and do not require resection. Delayed rupture usually is the result of a subcapsular splenic hematoma that ruptures within 2 weeks 75% of the time. The spleen is important as a source of opsonins and immunoglobulins, and postsplenectomy sepsis is now a well-recognized entity.

6. The answer is A. [*Chapter 22 VI D 1 a–c*] Postsplenectomy sepsis usually begins as a mild influenza-like syndrome. Progression to death, after shock develops, is usually rapid. Young patients, especially those who are less than 4 years old, are at greatest risk. Postsplenectomy sepsis following trauma is rare (occurring in 0.5%–0.8% of cases), but it still has a higher occurrence than in the general population. A polyvalent pneumococcal vaccine should be given to all splenectomized patients; however, it will only protect against 80% of pathogenic pneumococci.

7. The answer is C. [*Chapter 23 III B 1*] Although axillary node enlargement, nipple discharge as well as nipple changes and desquamation, and microcalcifications may be signs of breast cancer, an isolated breast mass is the commonest mode of presentation, occurring in 85%–90% of patients. For this reason, routine physical examination as a means of surveillance in high-risk patients and the teaching of breast self-examination are the most important aspects of the management of this condition.

8. The answer is C. [*Chapter 23 III B 1 b (4)*] Most nipple discharges are benign (physiologic), presenting as serosanguineous discharge from an intraductal papilloma; however, 10% of pathologic nipple discharges are due to carcinomas. If there is an associated mass, it should be biopsied. Quadrantectomy is indicated if the abnormal duct can be identified.

9. The answer is B. [*Chapter 24 I A 1, 2, E 2 b*] The genotypes of a related donor and recipient are more compatible than those of an unrelated donor and recipient. In a two-haplotype match all antigens are matched; in a one-haplotype match, only 50% of the antigens are matched.

10. The answer is B. [*Chapter 24 I A 2 b (1)*] A history of cancer in a potential donor is an absolute contraindication to organ donation. The only exception to this would be a preexisting primary central nervous system tumor restricted to the cranial vault. The minimally elevated creatinine level is not a contraindication to organ donation.

11. The answer is D. [*Chapter 24 I C 2 a, c, D 1 d, F 1 b (1), (2)*] Azathioprine toxicity is not associated with anuria; rather, it usually causes leukopenia. Acute tubular necrosis generally resolves in 7–14 days, resulting in normal renal function. Accelerated acute rejection is treated with high-dose prednisone but with a poor success rate. When anuria is present, a high index of suspicion is necessary to diagnose ureteral obstruction or renal artery thrombosis early enough to salvage the kidney.

12. The answer is B. [*Chapter 24 II A 1, B 5, 6, D 3, G*] Unlike kidneys, no attempt is made to match livers based on HLA type or crossmatch. The size of the organ donor should be matched to within 10%–20% of the recipient. Generally, blood group matching is used. Exceptions to this do occur if a recipient is extremely unstable and an organ of a different blood type becomes available.

13. The answer is B. [*Chapter 25 I C; II B 4*] The signs and symptoms of the patient described in the question suggest a renal infection. Simple pyelonephritis responds well to antibiotic therapy but requires more than 1 day of therapy to prevent recurrences. Single-day therapy is adequate for bladder infections. Antispasmodics may minimize some of the symptoms of frequency, but bethanechol could be expected to increase such symptoms.

14. The answer is C. [*Chapter 25 II B 2, D 2, E 2*] *Escherichia coli* is responsible for over 90% of all renal infections, both initial and recurrent. The presence of other organisms should raise the suspicion of prior antibiotic therapy or complicating factors, such as anatomic abnormalities.

15. The answer is D. [*Chapter 25 VI B 5, 6 c (3); Table 25-3*] Renal vein involvement by renal cell carcinoma does not adversely affect the prognosis. Such a tumor should be excised surgically. Invasion of the perinephric fat, invasion into the liver, nodal metastases, and pulmonary metastasis worsen the prognosis and may determine changes in the therapeutic approach.

16. The answer is D. [*Chapter 25 VI F 5 e*] Prostate specific antigen is specific for the prostate but not for carcinoma of the prostate. It may be elevated in inflammatory conditions and benign prostatic enlargement. It is not directly related to stage or prognosis of carcinoma of the prostate but may be useful to monitor recurrences after treatment of localized prostatic carcinoma.

17. The answer is D. [*Chapter 25 IX B 4*] Measurement of serum testosterone levels, perineal electromyography, and penile blood pressure are nonspecific and are not uniformly causally related to erectile failure. The intracavernosal injection of prostaglandin E_1 can result in erection in patients without an erectile deficit and in those with both psychogenic and organic causes of erectile failure. Nocturnal penile tumescence monitoring is the most effective study that distinguishes between physical and psychogenic causes for impotence.

18. The answer is D. [*Chapter 26 I B 1 b (2)*] Catgut and polyglycolic acid are both absorbable suture materials and are, therefore, prone to degradation and tissue reaction. Silk is reactive and could cause irritation. Polypropylene is unbraided, relatively inert, and exerts minimal tissue reaction.

19. The answer is D. [*Chapter 26 I B 2, 3 a, c*] Cautery, tension, and bleeding can result in tissue necrosis secondary to compromised blood supply. Inversion of the wound edge causes lack of dermal apposition (facilitates wound healing). Drains, by themselves, do not directly effect wound healing.

20. The answer is E. [*Chapter 26 I C 1 a, b, D 1 b, d*] Split-thickness grafts, full-thickness grafts, muscle flaps, and free flaps are all useful for providing soft tissue coverage. Split-thickness skin grafts are mainly used for coverage of burn wounds or where secondary contracture is desired. Full-thickness skin grafts offer excellent cosmesis, especially on the face. Muscle and free flaps can augment wound blood supply and diminish chances of infection. Fat autotransplantation is not a method of wound coverage. It is used for soft tissue augmentation.

21. The answer is A. [*Chapter 26 I E 4*] The percentage of women requesting reconstruction diminishes as the time since mastectomy increases. Reconstruction may be performed at the time of mastectomy if plastic surgeons skilled in this technique are available. The Silastic implants are placed beneath the pectoralis muscle and not beneath the skin. The nipple–areolar complex can be reconstructed, usually with tissue taken from the opposite breast or from the labia. It is frequently necessary to do a reduction mammoplasty on the opposite breast to achieve symmetry. Women can now be offered satisfactory breast reconstruction following mastectomy, and postmastectomy reconstruction represents one of the major areas of advancement in plastic surgery in recent times.

22. The answer is A. [*Chapter 26 II E 7*] The status of the regional lymph nodes is the best predictor of survival rates for malignant melanoma. However, the depth of invasion, the histologic grading of the tumor, the classification of the melanoma, and the anatomic location on the body all play a role in the prognosis.

23. The answer is C. [*Chapter 27 I C 2 d (6)*] Parinaud's syndrome consists of upward gaze paralysis, usually resulting from pressure in the pretectal area. A pineal tumor could cause obstructive hydrocephalus, leading to Parinaud's syndrome, and would be seen on the CT scan as a lesion in the posterior part of the third ventricle. A tumor involving a cerebral hemisphere would be unlikely to produce Parinaud's syndrome.

24. The answer is D. [*Chapter 27 III D*] In patients who develop severe brain edema, fluids must be restricted and osmotic agents may be necessary to keep the serum osmolality in the 300–320 mOsm range. The use of intracranial pressure monitoring helps in following the course of the edema and in determining the time for therapeutic intervention. The cerebral microvasculature is most responsive to changes in the arterial P_{CO_2}. Hyperventilation (hypocapnia) reduces the cerebral blood volume and, thus, decreases the intracranial pressure, almost instantaneously. In severe cases, P_{CO_2} has to be kept in the 20–25 mm Hg range to control intracranial hypertension. Barbiturates can rapidly reduce the intracranial pressure, although their role in improving the eventual outcome is debatable.

25. The answer is B. [*Chapter 27 V; Chapter 28 III B 3 b*] The patient obviously has a brachial plexus injury. In this case, the peripheral pulses should be evaluated, and if they are present, exploration of the brachial plexus would not be done. If there is any vascular injury that requires operative repair, it would be reasonable to inspect the brachial plexus at the time that the repair is made. In general, crush injuries of peripheral nerves do not require acute intervention.

26 and 27. The answers are: 26-E, 27-E. [*Chapter 27 VI B 1 a (1)*] The patient described in the question developed acute lumbar radiculopathy. The commonest cause would be a lumbar sprain or a herniated disc. Initial management would consist of x-rays of the lumbosacral spine, bed rest, pelvic traction, heat, ultrasound treatments, anti-inflammatory medication, muscle relaxants, and anlagesics. After 4 weeks of conservative treatment, CT scan showed a herniated disc at L4–L5 lateralized to the left. However, the symptomatic side is the right side; thus, the CT scan findings do not explain the clinical findings. A myelogram or an MRI would be necessary as a further workup. Indeed, the patient was found to have a tumor on myelography. Subsequent surgery confirmed an ependymoma.

28 and 29. The answers are: 28-A, 29-A. [*Chapter 27 III D; IX B 4, C*] The patient described in the question most likely has a subarachnoid hemorrhage. Intubation has to be done very carefully, taking precautions not to raise the intracranial pressure as this could precipitate a fatal rebleed. The patient can be sedated with barbiturates and lidocaine intravenously to reduce cough reflex and intracranial pressure. Also, muscle relaxants are used prior to intubation. Five percent dextrose in water can worsen cerebral edema and, thus, is contraindicated. The blood pressure is controlled very strictly and kept at normotensive levels to reduce the risk of rebleeding from an aneurysm.

30. The answer is A. [*Chapter 28 I C*] A failure of bone healing or endochondral ossification defines a nonunion. Causes include excessive motion at a fracture site, soft tissue damage, and infection. Tibia fractures classically need early weight-bearing to stimulate healing. Calcium deficiency is not known to cause nonunions.

31. The answer is D. [*Chapter 28 II B 3 a–c*] Chronic osteomyelitis can be difficult to cure. Therapeutic principles include removal of all foreign material, thorough debridement of infected, devascularized bone, correction of bone defects with a bone graft, good local wound care, and prolonged use of intravenous antibiotics. Muscle flaps and split-thickness grafts are employed after the infection is controlled. The affected region is not immobilized in a plaster cast; this would reduce blood circulation to a site that is already poorly vascularized and, therefore, would hinder, not promote, control of the infection.

32. The answer is A. [*Chapter 28 III A 3 a, b, B 1*] An open fracture is a surgical emergency because of the risks of infection. Surgical management includes thorough debridement, use of appropriate prophylactic antibiotics, and, if needed, tetanus inoculation. Functional requirements—for example, the need for an absolutely smooth contour within a joint—may call for open reduction and surgical fixation of a fracture, as may unsatisfactory results after closed reduction of a less complicated type of fracture. Internal fixation is valuable when early mobilization is especially important, as in patients with multiple injuries and in elderly patients.

33. The answer is D. [*Chapter 28 III B*] Open fractures constitute surgical emergencies not only because bone is relatively susceptible to infections, but more importantly because the devitalized soft tissue, which inevitably accompanies open fractures, is a likely target for a life-threatening anaerobic infection. Other orthopedic emergencies include vascular compromise, spinal cord injuries, and peripheral nerve injuries.

34. The answer is C. [*Chapter 28 III B 1 a*] Anaerobic infection is the most dangerous complication of open fracture. Bleeding can be controlled by pressure dressings. Devitalized soft tissue and bone, which is debrided to lessen the risk of infection, can be reconstructed later.

35. The answer is A. [*Chapter 28 III E 2 c*] Hip dislocations occur in high-velocity injuries and are frequently associated with other fractures, such as fractures of the femur and patella. They require prompt reduction as avascular necrosis is associated with a prolonged time before reduction.

36. The answer is A. [*Chapter 28 III F*] Disruptions of the musculotendinous unit are most commonly associated with overuse. The typical patient is middle-aged or older, who often gives a history of unusual, strenuous exertion. Torn or ruptured tendons require surgical repair.

37. The answer is B. [*Chapter 29 II A 3 c*] A congenital inguinal hernia is due to nonfusion of the processus vaginalis, which is highly unlikely to fuse after birth. The treatment of an incarcerated hernia is reduction, hydration of the patient, and herniorrhaphy. Essentially, all incarcerated hernias can be reduced without the fear of reducing a necrotic intestine. The hernia in a girl contains ovary, not intestine, and, therefore, after reduction it can be treated in a less urgent fashion.

38. The answer is A. [*Chapter 29 III A 1, C 2*] Gastroschisis is an abdominal wall defect located laterally to the umbilicus. Because there is no umbilical covering, the viscera is exposed to amnionic fluid, causing edema of the organs and loss of protein from the fetus. Because of this, the gastrointestinal tract is slow to function and the newborn requires total parenteral nutrition. There are few associated anomalies with gastroschisis.

39. The answer is B. [*Chapter 29 V A 3, B 1, C 1, D, E*] Simple duodenal obstruction is the commoner of the two potential problems of malrotation, but volvulus with ischemia of the midgut is the more critical since delay in treatment may cause complete loss of the midgut. If a diagnosis of malrotation is entertained, the infant must quickly be evaluated, and if malrotation cannot be excluded rapidly, then an immediate surgical exploration is carried out. Bilious vomiting is an early and common symptom and dictates a surgical evaluation. Simple malrotation, once treated, has no long-term sequelae associated with it, and the outlook is excellent.

40. The answer is B. [*Chapter 29 IX C 2–5*] Approximately 25% of infants with necrotizing enterocolitis require surgery usually for perforation or stricture of the intestine. The basic problem is an ischemic or hypoxic insult that damages the intestinal mucosa in premature newborns. Abdominal x-rays both show the findings of necrotizing enterocolitis as well as illustrate free air from perforations. Management includes correcting the ischemia or hypoxia and supporting the patient with total parenteral nutrition.

41. The answer is E (all). [*Chapter 21 I A*] Trauma is the leading cause of death among people under 35 years of age. More than one-half of deaths in this group result from motor vehicle accidents. Multisystem injuries occur in 10%–15% of trauma victims. Mortality can be reduced by efficient handling of the injured patients; this begins with skilled emergency medical technicians; rapid transport of patients to trauma centers, and trauma centers that are staffed by professional personnel trained in delivering rapid care to seriously injured patients. Prophylactic antibiotics and tetanus prophylaxis should be administered routinely to all patients suffering severe traumatic injuries.

42. The answer is A (1, 2, 3). [*Chapter 21 I C 2, 3*] The initial assessment of the critically injured patient determines the ultimate outcome. The patient should be examined for chest wall motion and cyanosis. If ventilation is unsatisfactory, corrective measures must be taken quickly. Early intubation is important and should be carried out without neck extension, since the status of the cervical spine often is not known. Ventilation can then be performed. Cardiac resuscitation may be required if the patient is asystolic or severely hypovolemic. Venous access lines should be placed rapidly, and the two most effective means for doing so are subclavian puncture and saphenous vein cut-down. Lacerations of the face can cause bleeding; however, these are not high-priority injuries during the initial evaluation of the critically injured patient.

43. The answer is E (all). [*Chapter 21 I C 3 c, d*] The subclavian vein is useful for percutaneous placement of large bore venous catheters. In addition, the saphenous vein can be quickly isolated at the ankle and is similarly useful. It is important to remember that the saphenous vein will be flaccid and empty in a hypovolemic patient and may resemble a tendon during the cut-down. This vein can almost always be cannulated and will provide a conduit for the rapid administration of fluid. Crystalloid solutions should be started as soon as the patient reaches the emergency room when shock is present. If the hematocrit is low, packed cells are indicated, and usually these can be obtained within a matter of minutes. If the patient is in profound shock and there is no time even for blood-typing, O-negative blood can be used. If the patient initially responds to the saline infusion, uncrossmatched type-specific blood is preferred, particularly if the patient has no history of prior transfusion.

44. The answer is B (1, 3). [*Chapter 21 I C 3 f*] When a patient presents with hemorrhage in the emergency room, the application of direct pressure on bleeding wounds with manually held gauze pads is usually effective and safe. No attempt should be made to clamp blindly arterial bleeders in the emergency room. Compression of the wound should be carried out until the patient can be moved to the operating room, where definitive repair of these injuries can be accomplished. Pneumatic splints and antishock trousers are useful in tamponading bleeding and increasing peripheral vascular resistance. One advantage of these devices is that they increase peripheral vascular resistance without the pharmacologic effects of pressor agents. Stab wounds and missile tracts should never be sutured in the emergency room but should be packed until definitive repair of the underlying injury can be accomplished in the operating room.

45. The answer is E (all). [*Chapter 21 I C 5 a*] Upright films of the chest should be obtained as soon as possible after a patient with chest injuries arrives in the emergency room. A significant finding would be pneumothorax, fluid in the chest cavity, or evidence of widening of the mediastinum. Penetrating injuries that traverse the mediastinum are an indication for contrast studies of the esophagus and arteriography of the great vessels to rule out injury to these vital structures. If significant fluid or pneumothorax is present, a chest tube should be inserted. If there is a continuing massive air leak and the lung fails to re-expand, a ruptured or lacerated bronchus should be suspected. Bleeding through a chest tube at a rate greater than 100 ml/hr is an indication for thoracotomy for control of the bleeding.

46. The answer is A (1, 2, 3). [*Chapter 21 I C 5 b (2)*] Peritoneal lavage is used when the need for abdominal exploration is unclear. It is especially useful if the patient is unconscious or neurologically impaired as that patient will not be able to give information regarding abdominal pain. With the open technique, a small incision is made below the umbilicus, and the perineum is visualized directly, so that the catheter is placed under direct vision. Upon placement of this catheter, if more than 10 units of gross blood are aspirated, the tap is considered positive, and exploratory laparotomy is performed. If aspiration is negative, 1 L of saline is infused and then aspirated. If there are more than 100,000 red cells/ml, more than 5000 white blood cells/ml, evidence of bile, particulate matter, or bacteria in the effluent, the lavage is considered positive. It is essential to empty the patient's bladder and stomach prior to doing the lavage, as a distended bladder or stomach may be inadvertently entered.

47. The answer is A (1, 2, 3). [*Chapter 21 I C 5 b (4)*] A midline incision should be made for all abdominal explorations. Hemostasis should be controlled by clamping obvious bleeders and packing areas where the bleeding site is not immediately obvious. At this time, the anesthesiologist can catch up with volume loss, and the patient can be stabilized before a systematic exploration is undertaken. Retroperitoneal hematomas in the pelvis should not be explored unless they show evidence of arterial pulsation or rapid expansion. In the upper abdomen, these retroperitoneal hematomas must be explored since they are frequently associated with injuries of the duodenum, pancreas, and bile ducts.

48. The answer is C (2, 4). [*Chapter 21 II D 1–5, E 3*] Cold compresses may be applied to relieve the pain of partial-thickness burns if the burns cover less than 10% of the body surface area. If the burns cover a larger area, cold compresses will cause an unacceptable lowering of the body temperature. Topical antibiotics are usually recommended for deep second-degree and third-degree burns. Systemic antibiotics are usually not indicated. Although escharectomy is best performed at a burn center, it may be urgently required in circumferential extremity wounds, causing distal circulation impairment, and in circumferential trunk or neck wounds, causing respiratory impairment.

49. The answer is B (1, 3). [*Chapter 22 I B 1 b, 2 a, b*] Primarily, the spleen functions as a blood filter that removes senescent or abnormal red blood cells and cellular debris and as a producer of opsonins and antibodies, particularly immunoglobulin M (IgM). Approximately one-third of the body's platelets are stored in the spleen. Under normal circumstances, red blood cells are not produced by the spleen.

50. The answer is A (1, 2, 3). [*Chapter 22 III A–C; IV C*] Primary splenic tumors, splenic abscess, and hereditary spherocytosis are absolute indications for splenectomy. Idiopathic autoimmune hemolytic anemia occurs most often in women over 50 years of age. Antibodies against red blood cells are found, and the direct Coombs' test is positive. The disease may be self-limited and mild. If it persists, it should be treated with steroids; splenectomy is considered if steroids are ineffective or contraindicated.

51. The answer is A (1, 2, 3). [*Chapter 22 IV D 1–3*] Idiopathic thrombocytopenic purpura is characterized by a decreased platelet count with increased megakaryocytes in the bone marrow. The acute form, which occurs in children under the age of 16, resolves spontaneously in 80% of cases. The condition occurs three times as often in women as in men. Splenectomy produces a sustained remission in 70% of patients who do not respond to or who relapse after steroid therapy.

52. The answer is A (1, 2, 3). [*Chapter 23 III A 2*] Family history and antecedent contralateral breast cancer are the most significant risk factors for developing breast cancer. As far as is known presently, however, only maternal family history is significant; paternal family history of female breast cancer does not carry an increased risk of developing the disease. A patient with chronic cystic mastitis has a slightly increased risk.

53. The answer is A (1, 2, 3). [*Chapter 23 III F 4, G 3 a (2), H 2 a, b*] The estrogen receptor status is a predictor of responsiveness to hormonal therapy, and estrogen-positive tumors often have a better prognosis than estrogen-negative tumors, all other things being equal. Patients who do not respond to one form of hormonal therapy generally will not respond to another form. Male hormones are useful in treating both premenopausal and postmenopausal patients.

54. The answer is C (2, 4). [*Chapter 24 I B 2 a, 4 b, 5, 7 c, F 3 b*] Unhealed duodenal ulcers may become worse with bleeding or perforation, if steroids are given after renal transplantation. Circulating anti-glomerular basement membrane antibodies will attack the new kidney as well as the original kidneys, resulting in rapid destruction of the graft. Therefore, both duodenal ulcer disease and autoimmune diseases characterized by glomerular basement membrane antibodies should be inactive before proceeding with transplantation.

55. The answer is E (all). [*Chapter 24 I F 1 b (1)–(4)*] There are four types of renal transplant rejection, classified according to the time of rejection in relation to the operation and the type of immune response involved. Hyperacute rejection results from preformed antibody and complement deposition on vascular endothelium followed by activation of the coagulation system; it occurs in the operating room. Accelerated acute rejection occurs within 1 week following transplantation and probably is a second-set, or anamnestic, response involving both cellular and humoral elements. Acute rejection usually occurs within 3 months following the operation and is characterized by T-lymphocyte–mediated infiltration of vascular and interstitial renal elements. Chronic rejection occurs over a period of months to years and involves both cellular and humoral destructive events. Chronic rejection is associated with vascular intimal thickening and tubular atrophy.

56. The answer is E (all). [*Chapter 24 I F 2 b, 4 a (1), (4), d*] Infections are the most dangerous sequelae of transplantation and subsequent immunosuppression. Central nervous system tumors are 300 times commoner than in control populations. Other long-term complications include malignancy, aseptic necrosis of the hip or knee as a result of steroid therapy, and cataracts. Cyclosporine A has been reported to cause hypertension, especially in children.

57. The answer is E (all). [*Chapter 24 I F 4*] Malignancy is more likely to occur following transplantation because of the immunosuppressive therapy administered. The incidence of primary cancers is 100 times greater than in controls. Vascular complications, including hypertension, hyperlipidemia, coronary artery disease, and cerebral vascular disease, are common after both dialysis and transplantation.

58. The answer is A (1, 2, 3). [*Chapter 25 I C; IV D 2 b, 4 c*] Percutaneous debulking and shock wave lithotripsy of any remaining fragments has been very effective in treating branched calculi. This is a typical infectious stone with *Proteus mirabilis* in the urine, and antibiotics should be administered prior to, during, and after treatment. Nephrectomy should be considered only if there is markedly decreased function.

59. The answer is B (1, 3). [*Chapter 25 IV E 1 a, c*] Citrate functions as an inhibitor of stone formation. Urinary levels of citrate may be diminished in several stone-forming conditions, and it can be replaced by oral administration of potassium citrate. Determination of serum calcium is essential in a search for hyperparathyroidism, while the urinary output is important for a diagnosis of hypercalciuric conditions.

60. The answer is E (all). [*Chapter 25 V B 1 a–e, 2*] The findings listed in the question (i.e., blood in the urethral meatus, perineal ecchymosis, inability to void, and a palpable lower abdominal mass) are among the classic indications of a urethral injury. Although any one of these findings is suggestive of a urethral injury, together they are not necessarily diagnostic. A urethrogram is the most useful diagnostic study and should be performed before attempts at catheterization or repair of the injury.

61. The answer is A (1, 2, 3). [*Chapter 25 VI C 4 a, 5 a, b, d, f, g*] Gross painless hematuria suggests a urologic malignancy. Evaluation should include studies of the entire urinary tract. An excretory urogram is more sensitive for calculi and urothelial tumors throughout the upper urinary tract than is ultrasonography, which can be used in the evaluation of renal masses. Cystoscopy gives direct inspection of the urethra and bladder and is sensitive for epithelial neoplasms. Urinary cytology is a noninvasive, sensitive test for urothelial malignancies.

62. The answer is C (2, 4). [*Chapter 25 IX B 3 a–d*] The evaluation of the patient with erectile failure should include serum testosterone and penile blood pressure determinations. Measuring serum levels of testosterone, follicle-stimulating and luteinizing hormones, and prolactin may indicate hormonal abnormalities, which can be treated appropriately. Penile blood pressure determinations may indicate inadequate penile blood flow. When this is related to obstruction of major pelvic vessels, revascularization procedures can be used. Because revascularization of small vessels has not been particularly successful, treatment by implantation of a prosthesis may be indicated.

63. The answer is A (1, 2, 3). [*Chapter 26 I C 3 a–c*] A well-vascularized recipient bed is essential to provide nourishment for the transplanted graft. The graft is initially supported by plasma imbibition and within several days will become vascularized through a process of vascular budding. Contact between the graft and the vascular bed is essential, and any infected wound will not support a skin graft. Bone denuded of periosteum will not support a skin graft, nor will cartilage denuded of perichondrium.

64. The answer is C (2, 4). [*Chapter 26 II B 1*] Common warts occur most frequently in the second decade of life and may be transmitted by direct or indirect contact. They are caused by a member of the papovavirus family. The fingers are the commonest location, and the lesions have a characteristic rough, elevated surface and can become tender. Many of these warts resolve spontaneously, and only problematic lesions should be treated. This is usually accomplished by electrodesiccation or by chemotherapy with caustic topical agents.

65. The answer is B (1, 3). [*Chapter 26 II B 5*] Lipomas, which are tumors composed of fat cells, can be found in any area of the body where fat is usually found. They are most commonly found on the neck, shoulders, back, and thighs. Malignant transformation is extremely uncommon, and simple excision is curative.

66. The answer is E (all). [*Chapter 26 II D 3 b*] Malignant melanoma can arise from preexisting nevi, particularly those that have a junctional component. Sudden changes in color, size, and shape as well as pain, satellite lesions, and unexplained regional adenopathy all warrant immediate excision and pathologic examination of the nevus.

67. The answer is D (4). [*Chapter 28 V C 1 a, b*] Joint arthroplasty, which is indicated for the relief of pain, can be used to repair a joint destroyed by any of the arthritides except, perhaps, postinfectious arthritis. It is used predominantly in patients over the age of 65, in part at least, because the repair is not permanent. The "life expectancy" of an arthroplasty implant is about 15 years at present. By contrast, the results of arthrodesis are long-lasting. In this procedure, the joint surfaces are fused so that the joint heals in a fixed position. Because the results are more durable, arthrodesis rather than arthroplasty is the preferred procedure for young, active patients.

68. The answer is B (1, 3). [*Chapter 29 II B 4, 6*] A newborn with a diaphragmatic hernia presents with respiratory failure of varying intensity. The herniated abdomen contents compress the contralateral or functional lung as the gastrointestinal tract becomes filled with air. Management to prevent this includes gastric tube decompression and the avoidance of mask ventilation. Chest x-ray confirms the diagnosis and the location of the defect. The involved lung is small due to decompression by the abdominal contents and cannot be expanded by a chest tube either pre- or postoperatively. Extracorporeal membrane oxygenation has shown improved survival in the patients with prolonged respiratory failure after repair.

69. The answer is A (1, 2, 3). [*Chapter 29 IV B 1, C 1 e, E, F 6 a (2)*] In tracheoesophageal fistula, there is a high incidence of associated defects. Affected organs include the heart (most commonly involved), the kidneys, and bone. Other gastrointestinal anomalies are also common. The hallmark of tracheo-esophageal fistula is a blind proximal pouch that will not allow passage of a nasogastric tube. A gap of greater than 2 cm (2½ vertebral bodies) may require delayed repair. Gastroesophageal reflux is now felt to be the primary reason for postoperative stricture formation in the patient with tracheoesophageal fistula.

70. The answer is C (2, 4). [*Chapter 29 IX A 1–4*] The infant described in the question has a typical history of pyloric stenosis. Jaundice occurs in about 10% of these infants, and it resolves after pyloromyotomy. The diagnosis is usually made by palpation of a mobile midepigastric mass. Correction of dehydration and correction of serum potassium and serum carbon dioxide deficits are necessary before surgery.

71–75. The answers are: 71-B, 72-C, 73-D, 74-E, 75-A. [*Chapter 23 III E*] Clinical stage is determined by tumor size, palpable adenopathy, and symptoms of distant disease. Tumors less than 2 cm in diameter are indicated by T1, tumors 2–5 cm, by T2, and tumors over 5 cm, by T3. Mobile ipsilateral adenopathy (nodal involvement) is indicated by N1, while fixed adenopathy is indicated by N2.

76 and 77. The answers are: 76-E, 77-B. [*Chapter 23 III F 1 a (2), G 1 b, 2 a, 3 a (1) (b)*] The choice of surgical procedure for the treatment of breast cancer is based on the clinical staging, on the pathologic cell type and its invasive characteristics, and on factors relating to the operative risk of the patient. Modified radical mastectomy, the current standard surgical procedure for the treatment of breast cancer, removes a generous amount of skin, the entire breast, the pectoralis minor muscle, and the axillary contents inferior to the axillary vein. This procedure is very effective in preventing local recurrence of disease but has the disadvantage of causing an obvious deformity.

Noninvasive lobular carcinoma is an in situ carcinoma that has a 15%–20% chance of developing into frank adenocarcinoma within 20 years. The opposite breast is involved by adenocarcinoma as often as the breast containing the noninvasive lobular carcinoma. Either prophylactic bilateral mastectomy or close long-term observation is appropriate therapy.

Adjuvant therapy is treatment designed to eradicate occult distant metastasis or local residual tumor in patients with positive axillary nodal involvement. Chemotherapy is the commonest form of adjuvant therapy, resulting in improvement in both the disease-free interval and the overall survival of premeno-pausal women. Side effects, however, include myelosuppression, which requires monitoring of bone marrow function, and immunosuppression, particularly against infection. Oophorectomy as adjuvant therapy has been shown to have no effect on long-term survival rates, although it perhaps prolongs the disease-free interval prior to recurrence.

Comprehensive
Exam

Introduction

One of the least attractive aspects of pursuing an education is the necessity of being examined on what has been learned. Instructors do not like to prepare tests, and students do not like to take them.

However, students are required to take many examinations during their learning careers, and little if any time is spent acquainting them with the positive aspects of tests and with systematic and successful methods for approaching them. Students perceive tests as punitive and sometimes feel that they are merely opportunities for the instructor to discover what the student has forgotten or has never learned. Students need to view tests as opportunities to display their knowledge and to use them as tools for developing prescriptions for further study and learning.

A brief history and discussion of the National Board of Medical Examiners (NBME) examinations [now the United States Medical Licensing Examination (USMLE)] are presented here along with ideas concerning psychological preparation for the examinations. Also presented are general considerations and test-taking tips as well as how practice exams can be used as educational tools. (The literature provided by the various examination boards contains detailed information concerning the construction and scoring of specific exams.) Before the various NBME exams were developed, each state attempted to license physicians through its own procedures. Differences between the quality and testing procedures of the various state examinations resulted in the refusal of some states to recognize the licensure of physicians licensed in other states. This made it difficult for physicians to move freely from one state to another and produced an uneven quality of medical care in the United States.

To remedy this situation, the various state medical boards decided they would be better served if an outside agency prepared standard exams to be given in all states, allowing each state to meet its own needs and have a common standard by which to judge the educational preparation of individuals applying for licensure.

One misconception concerning these outside agencies is that they are licensing authorities. This is not the case; they are examination boards only. The individual states retain the power to grant and revoke licenses. The examination boards are charged with designing and scoring valid and reliable tests. They are primarily concerned with providing the states with feedback on how examinees have performed and with making suggestions about the interpretation and usefulness of scores. The states use this information as partial fulfillment of qualifications upon which they grant licenses.

Students should remember that these exams are administered nationwide and, although the general medical information is similar, educational methodologies and faculty areas of expertise differ from institution to institution. It is unrealistic to expect that students will know all the

---

The author of this introduction, Michael J. O'Donnell, holds the positions of Assistant Professor of Psychiatry and Director of Biomedical Communications at the University of New Mexico School of Medicine, Albuquerque, New Mexico.

material presented in the exams; they may face questions on the exams in areas that were only superficially covered in their classes. The testing authorities recognize this situation, and their scoring procedures take it into account.

The Exams

The first exam was given in 1916. It was a combination of written, oral, and laboratory tests, and it was administered over a 5-day period. Admission to the exam required proof of completion of medical education and 1 year of internship.

In 1922, the examination was changed to a new format and was divided into three parts. Part I, a 3-day essay exam, was given in the basic sciences after 2 years of medical school. Part II, a 2-day exam, was administered shortly before or after graduation, and Part III was taken at the end of the first postgraduate year. To pass both Part I and Part II, a score equalling 75% of the total points available was required.

In 1954, after a 3-year extensive study, the NBME adopted the multiple-choice format. To pass, a statistically computed score of 75 was required, which allowed comparison of test results from year to year. In 1971, this method was changed to one that held the mean constant at a computed score of 500, with a predetermined deviation from the mean to ascertain a passing or failing score. The 1971 changes permitted more sophisticated analysis of test results and allowed schools to compare among individual students within their respective institutions as well as among students nationwide. Feedback to students regarding performance included the reporting of pass or failure along with scores in each of the areas tested.

During the 1980s, the ever-changing field of medicine made it necessary for the NBME to examine once again its evaluation strategies. It was found necessary to develop questions in multidisciplinary areas such as gerontology, health promotion, immunology, and cell and molecular biology. In addition, it was decided that questions should test higher cognitive levels and reasoning skills.

To meet the new goals, many changes have been made in both the form and content of the examination. These changes include reduction in the number of questions to approximately 800 in Step 1 and Step 2 of the USMLE to allow students more time on each question, with total testing time reduced on Step 1 from 13 to 12 hours and on Step 2 from 12.5 to 12 hours. The basic science disciplines are no longer allotted the same number of questions, which permits flexible weighing of the exam areas. Reporting of scores to schools include total scores for individuals and group mean scores for separate discipline areas. Only pass/fail designations and total scores are reported to examinees. There is no longer a provision for the reporting of individual subscores to either the examinees or medical schools. Finally, the question format used in the new exams is predominately multiple-choice, best answer.

The New Format

New questions, designed specifically for Step 1 are constructed in an effort to test the student's grasp of the sciences basic to medicine in an integrated fashion. The questions are designed to be interdisciplinary. Many of these items are presented as vignettes, or case studies, followed by a series of multiple-choice, best-answer questions.

The scoring of this exam is altered. Whereas, in the past, the exams were scored on a normal curve, the new exam has a predetermined standard, which must be met in order to pass. The exam no longer concentrates on the trivial; therefore, it has been concluded that there is a common base of information that all medical students should know in order to pass. It is anticipated that a major shift in the pass/fail rate for the nation is unlikely. In the past, the average student could only expect to feel comfortable with half the test and eventually would complete approximately 67% of the questions correctly, to achieve a mean score of 500. Although with the standard setting method it is likely that the mean score will change and become higher, it is unlikely that the pass/fail rates will differ significantly from those in the past. During the first testing in 1991, there was not differential weighing of the questions. However, in the future, the NBME will be researching methods of weighing questions based on both the time it takes to answer questions vis à vis their difficulty and the perceived importance of the information. In addition, the NBME is attempting to design a method of delivering feedback to the student that will have considerable importance in discovering weaknesses and pinpointing areas for further study in the event that a retake is necessary.

Since many of the proposed changes will be implemented for the first time in June 1991, specific information regarding actual standards, question emphasis, pass/fail rates, and so forth were unavailable at the time of publication. The publisher will update this section as information becomes available as we attempt to follow the evolution and changes that occur in the area of physician evaluation.

Materials Needed for Test Preparation

In preparation for a test, many students collect far too much study material only to find that they simply do not have the time to go through all of it. They are defeated before they begin because either they leave areas unstudied, or they race through the material so quickly that they cannot benefit from the activity.

It is generally more efficient for the student to use materials already at hand; that is, class notes, one good outline to cover or strengthen areas not locally stressed and for quick review of the whole topic, and one good text as a reference for looking up complex material needing further explanation.

Also, many students attempt to memorize far too much information, rather than learning and understanding less material and then relying on that learned information to determine the answers to questions at the time of the examination. Relying too heavily on memorized material causes anxiety, and the more anxious students become during a test, the less learned knowledge they are likely to use.

Positive Attitude

A positive attitude and a realistic approach are essential to successful test taking. If concentration is placed on the negative aspects of tests or on the potential for failure, anxiety increases and performance decreases. A negative attitude generally develops if the student concentrates on "I must pass" rather than on "I can pass." "What if I fail?" becomes the major factor motivating the student to **run from failure rather than toward success**. This results from placing too much emphasis on scores rather than understanding that scores have only slight relevance to future professional performance.

The score received is only one aspect of test performance. Test performance also indicates the student's ability to use information during evaluation procedures and reveals how this ability might be used in the future. For example, when a patient enters the physician's office with a problem, the physician begins by asking questions, searching for clues, and seeking diagnostic information. Hypotheses are then developed, which will include several potential causes for the problem. Weighing the probabilities, the physician will begin to discard those hypotheses with the least likelihood of being correct. Good differential diagnosis involves the ability to deal with uncertainty, to reduce potential causes to the smallest number, and to use all learned information in arriving at a conclusion.

This same thought process can and should be used in testing situations. It might be termed **paper-and-pencil differential diagnosis**. In each question with five alternatives, of which one is correct, there are four alternatives that are incorrect. If deductive reasoning is used, as in solving a clinical problem, the choices can be viewed as having possibilities of being correct. The elimination of wrong choices increases the odds that a student will be able to recognize the correct choice. Even if the correct choice does not become evident, the probability of guessing correctly increases. Just as differential diagnosis in a clinical setting can result in a correct diagnosis, eliminating incorrect choices on a test can result in choosing the correct answer.

Answering questions based on what is incorrect is difficult for many students since they have had nearly 20 years experience taking tests with the implied assertion that knowledge can be displayed only by knowing what is correct. It must be remembered, however, that students can display knowledge by knowing something is wrong, just as they can display it by knowing something is right. **Students should begin to think in the present as they expect themselves to think in the future.**

Paper-and-Pencil Differential Diagnosis

The technique used to arrive at the answer to the following question is an example of the paper-and-pencil differential diagnosis approach.

> A recently diagnosed case of hypothyroidism in a 45-year-old man may result in which of the following conditions?

(A) Thyrotoxicosis
(B) Cretinism
(C) Myxedema
(D) Graves' disease
(E) Hashimoto's thyroiditis

It is presumed that all of the choices presented in the question are plausible and partially correct. If the student begins by breaking the question into parts and trying to discover what the question is attempting to measure, it will be possible to answer the question correctly by using more than memorized charts concerning thyroid problems.

- The question may be testing if the student knows the difference between "hypo" and "hyper" conditions.
- The answer choices may include thyroid problems that are not "hypothyroid" problems.
- It is possible that one or more of the choices are "hypo" but are not "thyroid" problems, that they are some other endocrine problems.
- "Recently diagnosed in a 45-year-old man" indicates that the correct answer is not a congenital childhood problem.
- "May result in" as opposed to "resulting from" suggests that the choices might include a problem that **causes** hypothyroidism rather than **results from** hypothyroidism, as stated.

By applying this kind of reasoning, the student can see that choice **A,** thyroid toxicosis, which is a disorder resulting from an overactive thyroid gland ("hyper") must be eliminated. Another piece of knowledge, that is, Graves' disease is thyroid toxicosis, eliminates choice **D**. Choice **B,** cretinism, is indeed hypothyroidism, but it is a childhood disorder. Therefore, **B** is eliminated. Choice **E** is an inflammation of the thyroid gland—here the clue is the suffix "itis." The reasoning is that thyroiditis, being an inflammation, may **cause** a thyroid problem, perhaps even a hypothyroid problem, but there is no reason for the reverse to be true. Myxedema, choice **C,** is the only choice left and the obvious correct answer.

Preparing for Board Examinations

1. **Study for yourself.** Although some of the material may seem irrelevant, the more you learn now, the less you will have to learn later. Also, do not let the fear of the test rob you of an important part of your education. If you study to learn, the task is less distasteful than studying solely to pass a test.

2. **Review all areas.** You should not be selective by studying perceived weak areas and ignoring perceived strong areas. This is probably the last time you will have the time and the motivation to review **all** of the basic sciences.

3. **Attempt to understand, not just memorize, the material.** Ask yourself: To whom does the material apply? When does it apply? Where does it apply? How does it apply? Understanding the connections among these points allows for longer retention and aids in those situations when guessing strategies may be needed.

4. **Try to anticipate questions that might appear on the test.** Ask yourself how you might construct a question on a specific topic.

5. **Give yourself a couple days of rest before the test.** Studying up to the last moment will increase your anxiety and cause potential confusion.

Taking Board Examinations

1. In the case of the USMLE, be sure to **pace yourself** to use time optimally. Each booklet is designed to take 2 hours. You should use all your allotted time; if you finish too early, you probably did so by moving too quickly through the test.

2. **Read each question and all the alternatives carefully** before you begin to make decisions. Remember the questions contain clues, as do the answer choices. As a physician, you would not make a clinical decision without a complete examination of all the data; the same holds true for answering test questions.

3. **Read the directions for each question set carefully.** You would be amazed at how many students make mistakes in tests simply because they have not paid close attention to the directions.

4. It is not advisable to leave blanks with the intention of coming back to answer the questions later. Because of the way Board examinations are constructed, you probably will not pick up any new information that will help you when you come back, and the chances of getting numerically off on your answer sheet are greater than your chances of benefiting by skipping around. If you feel that you must come back to a question, mark the best choice and place a note in the margin. Generally speaking, it is best not to change answers once you have made a decision, unless you have learned new information. Your intuitive reaction and first response are correct more often than changes made out of frustration or anxiety. **Never turn in an answer sheet with blanks.** Scores are based on the number that you get correct; you are not penalized for incorrect choices.

5. **Do not try to answer the questions on a stimulus–response basis.** It generally will not work. Use all of your learned knowledge.

6. **Do not let anxiety destroy your confidence.** If you have prepared conscientiously, you know enough to pass. Use all that you have learned.

7. **Do not try to determine how well you are doing as you proceed.** You will not be able to make an objective assessment, and your anxiety will increase.

8. **Do not expect a feeling of mastery** or anything close to what you are accustomed. Remember, this is a nationally administered exam, not a mastery test.

9. **Do not become frustrated or angry** about what appear to be bad or difficult questions. You simply do not know the answers; you cannot know everything.

Specific Test-Taking Strategies

Read the entire question carefully, regardless of format. Test questions have multiple parts. Concentrate on picking out the pertinent key words that might help you begin to problem solve.

Words such as "always," "all," "never," "mostly," "primarily," and so forth play significant roles. In all types of questions, distractors with terms such as "always" or "never" most often are incorrect. Adjectives and adverbs can completely change the meaning of questions—pay close attention to them. Also, medical prefixes and suffixes (e.g., "hypo-," "hyper-," "-ectomy," "-itis") are sometimes at the root of the question. The knowledge and application of everyday English grammar often is the key to dissecting questions.

Multiple-Choice Questions

Read the question and the choices carefully to become familiar with the data as given. Remember, in multiple-choice questions there is one correct answer and there are four distractors, or incorrect answers. (Distractors are plausible and possibly correct or they would not be called distractors.) They are generally correct for part of the question but not for the entire question. Dissecting the question into parts aids in discerning these distractors.

If the correct answer is not immediately evident, begin eliminating the distractors. (Many students feel that they must always start at option A and make a decision before they move to B, thus forcing decisions they are not ready to make.) Your first decisions should be made on those choices you feel the most confident about.

Compare the choices to each part of the question. **To be wrong,** a choice needs to be incorrect for only part of the question. **To be correct,** it must be **totally** correct. If you believe a choice is partially incorrect, tentatively eliminate that choice. Make notes next to the choices regarding tentative decisions. One method is to place a minus sign next to the choices you are certain are incorrect and a plus sign next to those that potentially are correct. Finally, place a zero next to any choice you do not understand or need to come back to for further inspection. Do not feel that you must make final decisions until you have examined all choices carefully.

When you have eliminated as many choices as you can, decide which of those that are left has the highest probability of being correct. Remember to use paper-and-pencil differential diagnosis. Above all, be honest with yourself. If you do not know the answer, eliminate as many choices as possible and choose reasonably.

Vignette-Based Questions

Vignette-based questions are nothing more than normal multiple-choice questions that use the same case, or grouped information, for setting the problem. The NBME has been researching question types that would test the student's grasp of the integrated medical basic sciences in a more cognitively complex fashion than can be accomplished with traditional testing formats. These questions allow the testing of information that is more medically relevant than memorized terminology.

It is important to realize that several questions, although grouped together and referring to one situation or vignette, are independent questions; that is, they are able to stand alone. Your inability to answer one question in a group should have no bearing on your ability to answer subsequent questions.

These are multiple-choice questions, and just as is done with the single best answer questions, you should use the paper-and-pencil differential diagnosis, as was described earlier.

Single Best Answer—Matching Sets

Single best answer—matching sets consist of a list of words or statements followed by several numbered items or statements. Be sure to pay attention to whether the choices can be used more than once, only once, or not at all. Consider each choice individually and carefully. Begin with those with which you are the most familiar. It is important always to break the statements and words into parts, as with all other question formats. **If a choice is only partially correct, then it is incorrect.**

Guessing

Nothing takes the place of a firm knowledge base, but with little information to work with, even after playing paper-and-pencil differential diagnosis, you may find it necessary to guess the correct answer. A few simple rules can help increase your guessing accuracy. Always guess consistently if you have no idea what is correct; that is, after eliminating all that you can, make the choice that agrees with your intuition or choose the option closest to the top of the list that has not been eliminated as a potential answer.

When guessing at questions that present with choices in numerical form, you will often find the choices listed in an ascending or descending order. It is generally not wise to guess the first or last alternative, since these are usually extreme values and are most likely incorrect.

Using the Challenge Exam to Learn

All too often, students do not take full advantage of practice exams. There is a tendency to complete the exam, score it, look up the correct answers to those questions missed, and then forget the entire thing.

In fact, great educational benefits can be derived if students would spend more time using practice tests as learning tools. As mentioned earlier, incorrect choices in test questions are plausible and partially correct or they would not fulfill their purpose as distractors. This means that it is just as beneficial to look up the incorrect choices as the correct choices to discover specifically why they are incorrect. In this way, it is possible to learn better test-taking skills as the subtlety of question construction is uncovered.

Additionally, it is advisable to go back and attempt to restructure each question to see if all the choices can be made correct by modifying the question. By doing this, four times as much will be learned. By all means, look up the right answer and explanation. Then, focus on each of the other choices and ask yourself under what conditions they might be correct? For example, the entire thrust of the sample question concerning hypothyroidism could be altered by changing the first few words to read:

> "Hyperthyroidism recently discovered in . . . ."
> "Hypothyroidism prenatally occurring in . . . ."
> "Hypothyroidism resulting from . . . ."

This question can be used to learn and understand thyroid problems in general, not only to memorize answers to specific questions.

In the practice exams that follow, every effort has been made to simulate the types of questions and the degree of question difficulty in the USMLE Step 1. While taking these exams, the student should attempt to create the testing conditions that might be experienced during actual testing situations.

Summary

Ideally, examinations are designed to determine how much information students have learned and how that information is used in the successful completion of the examination. Students will be successful if these suggestions are followed:
- Develop a positive attitude and maintain that attitude.
- Be realistic in determining the amount of material you attempt to master and in the score you hope to obtain.

- Read the directions for each type of question and the questions themselves closely and follow the directions carefully.
- Guess intelligently and consistently when guessing strategies must be used.
- Bring the paper-and-pencil differential diagnosis approach to each question in the examination.
- Use the test as an opportunity to display your knowledge and as a tool for developing prescriptions for further study and learning.

The USMLE is not easy. It may be almost impossible for those who have unrealistic expectations or for those who allow misinformation concerning the exam to produce anxiety out of proportion to the task at hand. It is manageable if it is approached with a positive attitude and with consistent use of all the information that has been learned.

Michael J. O'Donnell

QUESTIONS

Directions: Each question below contains five suggested answers. Choose the **one best** response to each question.

1. In a patient who presents with Cushing's syndrome with elevated plasma cortisol and low plasma adrenocorticotropic hormone levels, the most likely cause of the syndrome is

(A) a basophilic adenoma of the pituitary gland
(B) an oat cell carcinoma of the lung
(C) bilateral adrenal cortical hyperplasia
(D) an adrenal cortical adenoma
(E) a malignant islet cell tumor of the pancreas

2. An elderly patient with a crush injury to the knee is most likely to sustain

(A) tibial plateau fracture
(B) growth plate fracture of the femur
(C) anterior cruciate tear
(D) meniscus tear
(E) posterior cruciate tear

3. Correct statements concerning postoperative drainage tubes include all of the following EXCEPT

(A) an underwater-seal drain is necessary when draining the pleural space
(B) sump drains can be used as continuous irrigation catheters because they allow collected material to drain continuously into a reservoir at a lower level
(C) rigid drains may erode through the wall of a hollow viscus or blood vessel, resulting in a gastrointestinal fistula or local hemorrhage
(D) a T tube is used to drain bile following common duct exploration until spasm of the sphincter of Oddi resolves
(E) open drains increase the risk of bacterial wound infection

4. A patient is found to have a soft, breathy voice 24 hours after undergoing general anesthesia with endotracheal intubation. Which of the following statements about this patient's condition is true?

(A) Laryngeal surgery may be necessary soon
(B) Speech therapy is indicated
(C) Complete voice rest should be instituted
(D) This patient probably has contact ulcers
(E) No treatment is necessary

5. A 3-month-old child has a soft, irregular, compressible, enlarging, posterior neck mass. This most likely represents a

(A) thyroglossal cyst
(B) teratoma
(C) abscess
(D) cystic hygroma
(E) paraganglioma

6. A patient with chronic pancreatitis has moderate pain that does not require narcotics. Acceptable methods of treatment would include which of the following?

(A) Puestow procedure
(B) Ninety-five percent pancreatectomy
(C) Distal pancreatectomy with intestinal drainage of the pancreatic duct
(D) Medical management alone
(E) Duval procedure

Questions 7 and 8

A 25-year-old man was involved in a motor vehicle accident. Paramedics who rescued him stated that it appeared as if he had been thrown from the car. He was found unresponsive. In the emergency room, his blood pressure is 60/40, heart rate is 120, and respirations are diaphragmatic. Both lower extremities are fractured.

7. The initial management of this patient would consist of all of the following EXCEPT

(A) endotracheal intubation
(B) volume replacement with Ringer's lactate solution
(C) peritoneal lavage
(D) cervical, thoracic, and lumbar spine x-rays
(E) x-rays of the chest and lower extremities

8. After the initial resuscitation, the patient's blood pressure is 100/60. Peritoneal tap is negative, and cervical spine x-ray shows 5-mm subluxation of C5 on C6. Further management would consist of all of the following EXCEPT

(A) mannitol 50 g
(B) volume replacement to raise the blood pressure
(C) application of a soft collar and transfer to a rotokinetic bed
(D) CT scan of the head
(E) CT of the cervical spine (C5–C6)
(end of group question)

9. A physician is called to the operating room to evaluate a patient with a large open fracture of the distal third of the tibia. The reconstructive options would include all of the following EXCEPT

(A) cross-leg flap
(B) fasciocutaneous flap
(C) free flap (microvascular flap)
(D) muscle flap
(E) skin graft

10. Achalasia of the esophagus is suspected on the basis of an x-ray film showing

(A) multiple strictures of the esophagus
(B) diffuse dilatation of the esophagus
(C) "corkscrew" appearance of the esophagus
(D) a diverticulum in the cricopharyngeal muscle
(E) reflux of barium into the esophagus

11. All of the following patients are at increased risk of developing deep venous thrombosis or pulmonary embolism EXCEPT

(A) an obese woman who needs a gastric bypass
(B) a woman with a history of congestive heart failure who needs an appendectomy
(C) a 32-year-old woman who is scheduled for a left colectomy for carcinoma
(D) a 25-year-old man who is scheduled for inguinal herniorrhaphy
(E) a 36-year-old man who had experienced spinal cord injury

12. A 5-year-old patient has a midline neck mass, which moves with swallowing and is located just below the hyoid. The mass is most likely to be a

(A) branchial cleft cyst
(B) cystic hygroma
(C) teratoma
(D) thyroglossal duct cyst
(E) laryngeal papilloma

13. A patient who has undergone a radical mastectomy with inadequate soft tissue coverage desires breast reconstruction. The technique least likely to be successful is

(A) silicone implant alone
(B) silicone implant with latissimus dorsi myocutaneous flap
(C) transverse rectus abdominis myocutaneous flap
(D) silicone implant with transverse rectus abdominis myocutaneous flap
(E) free flap

Questions 14–16

A 55-year-old man presents with a 1-week history of vomiting. An obstruction series shows a markedly dilated stomach.

14. Appropriate initial evaluation and treatment should include all of the following EXCEPT

(A) insertion of an intravenous catheter
(B) insertion of a nasogastric tube
(C) administration of metaclopramide to increase the rate of gastric emptying
(D) administration of intravenous H_2-blockers
(E) insertion of a Foley catheter

15. Which of the following sequelae is most likely seen with this problem?

(A) Hypertension
(B) Electrolyte disorders
(C) Fever
(D) Liver function abnormalities
(E) Hyperglycemia

16. Which of the following statements concerning the treatment of this patient is true?

(A) He will most likely require surgery
(B) Medical therapy will most likely be successful
(C) There is a high risk of recurrence after appropriate treatment
(D) Treatment can often be done on an outpatient basis
(E) There are many treatment alternatives
(end of group question)

17. Wilms' tumor has been associated with all of the following conditions EXCEPT

(A) aniridia
(B) hemihypertrophy
(C) hypertension
(D) bilateral polycystic kidneys
(E) Beckwith's syndrome

18. Patients requiring surgery should be treated by blood transfusions to maintain a hemoglobin level (1 lb) of 10 g/dl in all of the following situations EXCEPT

(A) Hb of 8 g/dl in a patient with coronary artery disease
(B) Hb of 8 g/dl in a patient with a ruptured spleen
(C) Hb of 7 g/dl in a patient on parenteral nutrition for a small bowel fistula
(D) Hb of 7 g/dl in a patient with chronic renal failure
(E) Hb of 8 g/dl in a patient with a history of congestive heart failure

19. A patient who previously was treated with a parietal cell vagotomy for an intractable duodenal ulcer presents 6 months later with a recurrence. Workup confirms the Zollinger-Ellison syndrome, and localization studies suggest a gastrinoma in the area of the tail of the pancreas. Management should entail

(A) H_2-receptor antagonists
(B) total gastrectomy
(C) subtotal gastrectomy and completion of the vagotomy
(D) exploration and resection, if feasible, of the gastrinoma
(E) gastrin-receptor blockers

20. Tension pneumothorax may cause all of the following problems EXCEPT

(A) hypoxia
(B) acidosis
(C) decreased venous return to the heart
(D) decreased cardiac output
(E) dullness to percussion on the side of the pneumothorax

21. All of the following immunologic criteria are routinely examined prior to transplantation from a cadaver donor EXCEPT

(A) HLA-A and -B locus typing
(B) crossmatch compatibility
(C) mixed lymphocyte reaction
(D) ABO blood group compatibility
(E) HLA-DR locus typing

22. A 21-year-old man who was involved in an automobile accident is brought to the emergency room. On admission, his blood pressure is 80/60, respirations are purely diaphragmatic, and he has a right-sided Horner's syndrome. Cervical spine x-rays show a C4 on C5 fracture dislocation but C7 cannot be visualized. Which of the following statements about management of this patient is correct?

(A) Repeat cervical spine films are not necessary as there is very little likelihood of fracture at another level
(B) Vasopressor agents have to be administered immediately to raise the blood pressure
(C) Attention must be given to maintaining an adequate airway
(D) Administration of mannitol is unnecessary
(E) The nature of the cervical injury is a contraindication to the use of traction as part of therapy

23. Which of the following statements regarding the anatomy of the esophagus is true?

(A) The gastroesophageal junction is 40 cm from the incisors and the entire esophagus is approximately 24 cm in length
(B) It is made up of mostly striated muscle
(C) It is innervated by the phrenic nerve
(D) The lower esophageal sphincter is a separate and distinct muscle band
(E) The muscle fibers of the left crus of the diaphragm form most of the esophageal hiatus

Questions 24–26

A 26-year-old woman presents with a 6-month history of bloody diarrhea, weight loss, and crampy abdominal pain. You are concerned about the possibility of inflammatory bowel disease.

24. An appropriate first step toward the diagnosis would be

(A) upper gastrointestinal endoscopy
(B) small bowel mucosal biopsy
(C) mesenteric angiography
(D) barium enema
(E) abdominal CT scan

25. Workup reveals an inflammatory process within the colon with skip areas. The rectum is spared. The most likely diagnosis is

(A) ischemic colitis
(B) ulcerative colitis
(C) amebic dysentery
(D) Crohn's disease
(E) toxic megacolon

26. Initial treatment should include

(A) surgical resection of the involved bowel
(B) steroids and sulfasalazine
(C) hyperalimentation
(D) nasogastric suction, intravenous fluids, and bowel rest
(E) oral antibiotics

(end of group question)

27. A 69-year-old woman with known aortic stenosis is admitted to the hospital in congestive heart failure. Cardiac catheterization reveals a gradient across the aortic valve of 32 mm Hg. (A year ago, the gradient was 50 mm Hg.) Wedge pressure is 26 mm Hg. Cardiac index is 1.8 L/m$_2$. Which of the following statements about this case is true?

(A) The gradient was measured incorrectly
(B) Aortic valve replacement should be carried out urgently
(C) The degree of stenosis has decreased
(D) Rapid profound diuresis should be induced
(E) Administration of nitrates would be indicated

28. The commonest cause of secondary hypersplenism is

(A) splenic vein thrombosis
(B) lymphoma
(C) portal hypertension
(D) sarcoidosis
(E) Felty's syndrome

29. A 14-year-old girl presents to the physician with a history of slowly progressive swelling in her right lower extremity, which began 4 months ago. Initially, this involved the dorsum of her foot and now has progressed to involve the calf and distal portion of the thigh. Which of the following statements is true regarding this patient?

(A) The patient should have an immediate lymphangiogram to establish the diagnosis
(B) The patient should be warned that she may develop ulceration and hyperpigmentation of the skin of her lower extremity
(C) This patient would benefit from groin exploration with lymphaticovenous anastomosis
(D) It is rare that patients with this problem can be successfully treated nonoperatively
(E) The patient should be warned that she will require meticulous foot care to prevent recurrent infectious episodes

30. Liposuction is best characterized by which of the following statements?

(A) It is useful as a weight reduction technique
(B) It is useful in removing localized fatty deposits in the hip area
(C) It is generally performed under topical anesthesia on an outpatient basis
(D) It is used to treat baggy eyelids
(E) None of the above

31. A 25-year-old man is admitted with a history of sudden onset of severe midepigastric abdominal pain. Upright chest x-ray reveals free intraperitoneal air. Correct therapy for this patient is

(A) upper endoscopy
(B) barium swallow
(C) Gastrografin swallow
(D) observation
(E) laparotomy

32. Operative treament of reflux esophagitis includes all of the following EXCEPT

(A) Nissen fundoplication
(B) Heller procedure
(C) Belsey Mark IV operation
(D) Hill repair
(E) esophageal resection if strictures are present

33. Medical treatment for reflux esophagitis includes all of the following EXCEPT

(A) weight loss
(B) H$_2$-receptor antagonists
(C) antacids
(D) calcium channel blockers
(E) abstinence from smoking and alcohol use

Questions 34–37

A 59-year-old patient undergoes a craniotomy for a benign meningioma. On the tenth postoperative day, he is noted to have a swollen left calf and thigh.

34. The least accurate method to diagnose the etiology of the swollen leg is

(A) physical examination
(B) left leg venogram
(C) ^{125}I fibrinogen scan
(D) impedance plethysmography
(E) duplex ultrasonography

35. If deep venous thrombosis is documented, initial treatment should include

(A) subcutaneous heparin therapy
(B) intravenous heparin therapy
(C) thrombolytic therapy with urokinase
(D) aspirin therapy
(E) warfarin treatment

36. While on anticoagulants at a therapeutic level for deep venous thrombosis of the left leg, the patient begins to bleed from a stress ulcer in the stomach. The best treatment option is to

(A) continue anticoagulants at a lower dose and administer blood
(B) switch to another form of anticoagulation
(C) stop anticoagulants and observe
(D) stop systemic anticoagulants and administer a thrombolytic agent directly into the femoral venous system
(E) stop anticoagulants and interrupt the inferior vena cava

37. After recovery from the acute illness, the patient returns in 6 months, complaining of persistent leg swelling. Optimal long-term management as initial treatment is

(A) chronic diuretic therapy
(B) venous thrombectomy
(C) venous bypass using an autologous vein
(D) venous bypass using a prosthetic graft
(E) support hose

(end of group question)

38. A patient has had a persistent area of pneumonitis in the right lung for 2 months. What is the next step in the workup?

(A) Continuous observation with monthly chest x-rays
(B) Workup with multiple fungal skin tests and begin antifungal therapy
(C) Addition of broad-spectrum antibiotics
(D) Repetition of sputum cultures and accordant treatment
(E) Bronchoscopy with biopsy brushings and washings

39. Correct statements concerning acute suppurative parotitis, an inflammatory disorder of the parotid gland, include all of the following EXCEPT

(A) it is usually found in debilitated, dehydrated patients with poor oral hygiene
(B) it is usually caused by *Staphylococcus aureus*
(C) it presents as a painless swelling of the gland
(D) it is usually treated by hydration, antibiotics, and measures to promote salivation
(E) it may require surgical drainage if conservative measures fail

40. An absolute predictor of success in below-knee amputation includes which of the following?

(A) A pulsatile pulse volume recording in the calf
(B) A transcutaneous PO_2 greater than 40 mm Hg at the site of the amputation
(C) Sensation in the dorsal aspect of the foot
(D) Absence of gangrene above the ankle
(E) None of the above

41. A 3-year-old boy is brought to the emergency room after drinking an unknown amount of Liquid Plummer. Following resuscitation and antibiotic administration, the child should

(A) have an X-ray of his chest to look for free fluid
(B) undergo endoscopy
(C) be observed and placed at bed rest
(D) be taken directly to the operating room
(E) have his gastric contents alkalinized

42. A 14-year-old boy was in a motor vehicle accident and is brought to the emergency room. On admission, his blood pressure is 80/40, heart rate is 120, and his respirations are very irregular. The patient is unresponsive. He has a 5-cm laceration in the right temporal area. The right pupil is 6 mm and nonreactive, while the left pupil is 4 mm and reactive. Initial management would consist of all of the following EXCEPT

(A) intubation and hyperventilation
(B) immediate surgery
(C) mannitol
(D) CT scan of the head
(E) peritoneal lavage, chest x-ray, and cervical spine x-rays

43. All of the following complications of renal transplantation are likely to threaten the patient's life EXCEPT

(A) active peptic ulcer disease
(B) acute diverticulitis
(C) pulmonary aspergillosis
(D) glomerulonephritis
(E) angina pectoris

44. The most effective way to prevent infection in a dirty traumatic wound is to

(A) administer tetanus toxoid
(B) administer intravenous antibiotics
(C) apply a skin graft
(D) repeat surgical debridement
(E) administer topical antibiotics

45. An obese 60-year-old man complains of cramping pain in his right calf, which occurs after walking three blocks. The pain occurs predictably and is promptly relieved by rest. The patient admits to a history of hypertension and smoking one pack of cigarettes a day. Physical examination reveals absent popliteal and pedal pulses in the involved lower extremity. Initial treatment of this patient would be

(A) admission to the hospital and arteriography, followed by balloon dilatation of the superficial femoral artery

(B) admission to the hospital and arteriography followed by femoral–popliteal bypass

(C) initiation of medical treatment with pentoxifylline

(D) initiation of aspirin therapy

(E) initiation of nonoperative therapy, including weight loss, exercise, control of hypertension, and cessation of smoking

46. Which of the following statements is true regarding the energy stores of the human body?

(A) Body stores of carbohydrate as glucose and glycogen are adequate to provide the body's energy needs for 7 days of starvation

(B) Protein contains the highest amount of energy for each gram of any tissue

(C) During the earliest phase of starvation, protein provides a ready source of caloric needs

(D) Fat comprises less than 10% of healthy adult men

(E) Fat contains 9 kcal/g of stored energy

47. Indications for surgery in a newborn infant with either active or resolved necrotizing enterocolitis include all of the following EXCEPT

(A) free intraperitoneal air

(B) portal vein gas

(C) ileal stricture documented on barium studies

(D) a persistent loop of distended bowel on abdominal films associated with a palpable abdominal mass

(E) erythema of the abdominal wall with persistent acidosis after optimal medical treatment

48. A patient who has had a previous appendectomy presents in the emergency room with a history of abdominal pain, cramps, vomiting, and anorexia. A mechanical small bowel obstruction is seen on abdominal x-ray. He has no fever, his white blood count is normal, and he has no acidosis or hypotension, although his serum potassium level is 2.8 mEq/L. Which of the following is the best treatment?

(A) Immediate surgery for lysis of adhesions

(B) Correction of hypokalemia over 3–6 hours, followed by surgery

(C) Correction of hypokalemia over 24 hours, followed by surgery

(D) Observation for signs of complications due to intestinal obstruction

(E) Insertion of a gastrointestinal tube into the small bowel

49. A patient presents with a small, fast-growing lesion on the upper extremity, which has been present for the past 2 weeks. This most likely represents

(A) squamous cell cancer

(B) keratoacanthoma

(C) basal cell cancer

(D) junctional nevus

(E) seborrheic keratosis

50. The commonest complication following splenectomy is

(A) subphrenic abscess

(B) atelectasis

(C) hemorrhage

(D) necrosis of the gastric wall

(E) deep venous thrombosis

51. A 56-year-old man with gallstones has stable angina well controlled with nitrates. If he undergoes elective cholecystectomy, which of the following statements is true?

(A) He has no increased risk for cardiac complications as compared to patients without angina

(B) He has a 14% incidence of perioperative myocardial infarction after major surgery

(C) He should have cardiac catheterization prior to elective surgery

(D) He should routinely have bacterial endocarditis prophylaxis

(E) He would have a lower morbidity with spinal anesthesia rather than general anesthesia

52. A 43-year-old woman with no previous history of breast disease presents with a 2-cm mass in the upper inner right breast. An aspiration is performed. Biopsy should be performed if

(A) the fluid is greenish-black
(B) the cytology on the fluid reveals no suspicious cells
(C) the fluid is yellow, and there is a small residual mass
(D) the mass recurs in 1 year
(E) a mass appears in the upper outer quadrant in 2 months

Questions 53–55

A 32-year-old male executive with longstanding Crohn's disease presents with complete small bowel obstruction. At laparotomy, there is scarring of the distal ileum and cecum, causing obstruction. There is a 10-cm segment of mid–small bowel with moderate, nonobstructive Crohn's disease.

53. Which of the following operative procedures should be performed at this time?

(A) Radical resection of the involved segment of mid–small bowel, all of the ileum, the cecum, and the right colon
(B) Resection of the distal ileum and right colon with the involved mesentery and lymph nodes
(C) Bypass of the obstructing segment with a side-to-side anastomosis between the ileum and right colon and no resection
(D) Stricturoplasty of the obstruction plus resection of the short involved segment of mid–small bowel
(E) Resection of the distal ileum and cecum

54. Postoperatively, the patient requires an indwelling bladder catheter for 5 days to treat urinary retention. He does well until the tenth postoperative day, at which point he develops a fever of 103° F, right lower quadrant pain, and an ileus. The midline wound is not inflamed. The most likely development is

(A) blind loop syndrome
(B) pyelonephritis
(C) recurrent Crohn's disease
(D) intra-abdominal abscess
(E) pseudomembranous enterocolitis

55. After successful surgery and discharge from the hospital, which of the following statements is now true?

(A) If the diseased bowel was removed, prednisone and metronidazole can best prevent recurrence
(B) The chance of cure is greater than 60%
(C) The recurrence rate is greater than 50% over the next 5–10 years
(D) If the terminal ileum was removed, the risk of recurrence is less
(E) If the terminal ileum was removed, the patient will require long-term therapy with oral iron to prevent anemia

(end of group question)

56. Metastases to regional lymph nodes are common with all of the following cancers EXCEPT

(A) basal cell carcinoma
(B) squamous cell carcinoma
(C) sweat gland tumors
(D) acrolentiginous melanoma
(E) pleomorphic rhabdosarcoma

57. A patient with normal renal function has a serum sodium concentration of 120 mEq/L and does not appear to be dehydrated. This patient most likely has

(A) a total body sodium deficit
(B) dilutional hyponatremia
(C) a contracted blood volume
(D) diabetes insipidus
(E) Cushing's disease

58. Which of the following factors is most helpful in differentiating ectopic Cushing's syndrome from Cushing's syndrome of pituitary origin?

(A) Absence of diurnal variation in cortisol secretion
(B) Results of a low-dose dexamethasone suppression test
(C) Determination of urinary free cortisol
(D) Determination of plasma adrenocorticotropic hormone (ACTH) levels
(E) Differential ACTH levels in jugular versus peripheral venous blood samples

59. In a 60-year-old patient with jaundice of 2 weeks' duration and with no history of abdominal pain, a markedly distended gallbladder seen on ultrasound is most likely secondary to which of the following diagnoses?

(A) Common duct obstruction from a stone
(B) Common duct obstruction from pancreatitis
(C) Common duct obstruction from a carcinoma of the head of the pancreas
(D) Acute cholecystitis
(E) Alcoholic hepatitis

Questions 60 and 61

60. Estimates of the extent of burns in an adult patient with first-degree burns on the face and neck, second-degree burns on the anterior chest and abdomen and ventral left, and third-degree circumferential burns on the left thigh and leg are

(A) 23%
(B) 41%
(C) 45%
(D) 50%
(E) none of the above

61. Estimate of initial fluid requirements, using the Parkland formula, in an 80-kg patient with the above burn estimate is

(A) approximately 11,000 ml Ringer's lactate to be infused at 455 ml/hr for the first 24 hours
(B) approximately 11,000 ml Ringer's lactate to be infused at 690 ml/hr for 8 hours and followed by a rate of 345 ml/hr for 16 hours
(C) approximately 5000 ml colloid and 6000 ml crystalloid to be infused at 690 ml/hr for 8 hours and followed by a rate of 345 ml/hr for 16 hours
(D) approximately 14,400 ml Ringer's lactate to be infused at 900 ml/hr for 8 hours and then 450 ml/hr for 16 hours
(E) none of the above

(end of group question)

62. Ligation of the superior thyroid artery above the superior pole of the thyroid gland may result in

(A) injury to the recurrent nerve
(B) injury to the vagus nerve
(C) devascularization of the inferior parathyroid gland
(D) injury to the hypoglossal nerve
(E) injury to the external branch of the superior laryngeal nerve

63. Which of the following statements about inguinal hernias in infants is true?

(A) They are bilateral in 60% of cases
(B) They can cause bowel obstruction or testicular injury
(C) They are no commoner in premature infants than in term infants
(D) They require repair of the muscular floor of the canal
(E) If incarcerated, they should not be reduced

64. A 56-year-old woman with an endotracheal tube in place is being mechanically ventilated at a tidal volume of 800 ml, respiratory rate of 12/minute, a fraction of inspired oxygen of 50%, and 10 cm H_2O of positive end–expiratory pressure, suddenly develops tachycardia with multiple premature contractions, hypotension, and hypoxia. The most likely cause is

(A) retained tracheobronchial secretion
(B) pulmonary embolus
(C) cardiac arrhythmia
(D) pneumothorax
(E) myocardial infarction

65. A 67-year-old man presented initially after a single episode of gross painless hematuria. An excretory urogram demonstrated a 1.5 mm round filling defect in the right lower renal infundibulum. The best study to obtain next is

(A) urinary cytology
(B) cystoscopy
(C) ultrasonography
(D) retrograde pyelography
(E) ureteroscopy

66. An elderly woman is admitted with weakness, anemia, weight loss, and a palpable abdominal mass. She has a colon carcinoma. The most likely anatomic site is the

(A) rectum
(B) sigmoid colon
(C) left colon
(D) transverse colon
(E) cecum

67. The commonest cause of intestinal obstruction in adults is

(A) carcinoma of the colon
(B) carcinoma of the small bowel
(C) adhesive bands
(D) incarcerated inguinal hernia
(E) diverticulitis

68. Which of the following would be the most appropriate measure in the management of a patient with a spontaneous complete collapse of a lung for the first time?

(A) Observation with daily chest x-rays
(B) Aspiration of air with a needle, followed by observation
(C) Thoracotomy to biopsy the site of pneumothorax
(D) Chest tube drainage of the pleural space
(E) Thoracotomy and pleural abrasion to prevent recurrence

69. There are three basic phases in wound healing that ultimately lead to the return of tissue strength. All of the following statements about these phases are true EXCEPT

(A) there is no increase in wound strength during the lag phase
(B) capillaries migrate into the wound during the proliferative phase
(C) an uncomplicated wound has good resistance to infection from surface contamination in the earliest phase
(D) wounds attain breaking strength equivalent to normal tissue during the maturation phase
(E) neutrophils and macrophages are the predominant cell types during the early phases

70. A 50-year-old patient has a 3-cm villous-appearing tumor at 6 cm within the rectum. Biopsy shows that it is a villous adenoma. The most acceptable next step in management is to

(A) observe the lesion for signs of malignancy
(B) reassure the patient that these are not premalignant lesions
(C) fulgurate the lesion
(D) locally irradiate the lesion
(E) surgically excise the lesion

71. A small boy who is brought to the emergency room by his parents is found to have a spiral fracture of the femur with a variety of ecchymoses. What is the most likely cause of the injuries?

(A) Automobile hit-and-run accident
(B) Fall from a tree
(C) Child abuse
(D) Fall from a bicycle
(E) Hockey-stick injury

72. The degree of left-to-right shunting across a large atrial septal defect is dependent upon the

(A) force of the left atrial contraction
(B) pressure gradient between the left and right atrium
(C) enlargement of the right atrium
(D) difference in the right and left ventricular compliance during ventricular diastole
(E) velocity of the electrical conduction in the right ventricle

73. A 27-year-old man presents for repair of an easily reducible right inguinal hernia. On physical examination, the patient has scleral icterus, a tender liver measuring 18 cm by palpation, and noticeable asterixis. Preoperative management of this patient should include

(A) initial vaccination for hepatitis B virus
(B) general anesthesia for herniorrhaphy to reduce patient agitation
(C) preoperative transfusion with fresh frozen plasma to counteract coagulopathy
(D) futher medical evaluation before the hernia is repaired
(E) prophylaxis for alcohol withdrawal

74. A patient presents with hypertension, hypokalemia, polyuria, and muscle weakness. After being placed on a salt-loading diet, the plasma potassium falls lower, and there is a marked kaliuresis. The aldosterone levels are high, and the plasma renin levels are below normal. Which of the following studies should be performed next?

(A) Idocholesterol scan
(B) CT scan of the adrenal glands
(C) Selective arteriography
(D) Selective adrenal venous sampling
(E) Ultrasound of the retroperitoneum

75. A patient with persistent cavitary atypical tuberculosis has been treated for 3 months with isoniazid, rifampin, and streptomycin. His sputum remains positive, and he has experienced two episodes of mild hemoptysis. Appropriate treatment now would be

(A) to continue present therapy
(B) to add ethambutal to current drug regimen
(C) thoracoplasty
(D) cavernostomy
(E) resection

76. The carcinoid syndrome can be diagnosed by finding which of the following metabolites in the urine?

(A) 5-Hydroxytryptamine
(B) Serotonin
(C) Metanephrine
(D) 5-Hydroxyindoleacetic acid
(E) Vanillylmandelic acid

77. The lower esophagus of a patient is inadvertently perforated during esophagoscopy. A barium swallow done immediately after perforation demonstrates that a small amount of barium is leaking into the left pleural space. What is the most acceptable method of treatment?

(A) Observation alone
(B) Observation plus antibiotics
(C) Insertion of a left chest tube
(D) Prolonged esophageal intubation
(E) Drainage and surgical repair of the injury

78. All of the following statements concerning angiography are true EXCEPT

(A) angiographic dye is hypertonic and may cause renal failure
(B) arterial digital subtraction angiograms give superior images when compared to intravenous digital subtraction angiograms
(C) hand claudication is a complication of brachial artery angiography
(D) limb ischemia after angiography is most likely due to vasospasm
(E) retroperitoneal hematomas may occur following translumbar aortography

79. A patient who has been admitted to the hospital for an elective surgical procedure has a recent history of heavy aspirin use. The safest course of action in this case is to

(A) proceed with the surgery, paying particular attention to meticulous hemostasis
(B) proceed with the surgery, after ensuring that properly crossmatched platelets are available should excess bleeding occur
(C) proceed with the surgery after transfusion of 8 units of platelets immediately prior to the incision
(D) delay the surgery for 7 days, instructing the patient to avoid all aspirin and aspirin-containing products
(E) delay the surgery only if it involves additional anticoagulation, such as open heart surgery

80. Clinical pictures of Hirschsprung's disease include all of the following EXCEPT

(A) a term infant with nonpassage of meconium stool at 48 hours of life
(B) a 2-month-old boy with failure to thrive and foul-smelling diarrhea
(C) a barium enema that illustrates a normal colon in a 6-month-old girl with constipation
(D) x-rays in a newborn that show a distended abdomen with a ground-glass appearance
(E) a higher incidence in boys with a more complex form in girls

81. Most patients with primary hyperparathyroidism have as their underlying pathology

(A) four-gland hyperplasia
(B) single-gland adenoma
(C) parathyroid carcinoma
(D) multiple adenomas
(E) asymmetric hyperplasia

82. A 45-year-old woman who has had a hysterectomy presents to the emergency room with abdominal pain and vomiting. A mechanical small bowel obstruction is seen on the abdominal x-ray. The most likely cause for this obstruction is

(A) carcinoma of the colon
(B) small bowel cancer
(C) adhesions
(D) incarcerated inguinal hernia
(E) diverticulitis

83. A 50-year-old chronic alcoholic with known cirrhosis is noted to have a mass in the right lobe of his liver and an elevated α-fetoprotein level. What is the most likely diagnosis?

(A) Hepatocellular adenoma
(B) Hepatocellular carcinoma
(C) Metastatic carcinoma of the colon
(D) Regenerating nodule of cirrhosis
(E) Focal nodular hyperplasia

84. Which of the following statements concerning breast cancer is true?

(A) By the age of 70, 20% of all women in the United States will have contracted carcinoma of the breast
(B) The incidence of carcinoma of the breast is somewhat increased in the sun belt
(C) High socioeconomic status is associated with a low risk of developing breast cancer
(D) The age-adjusted mortality rate and incidence of breast cancer have shown no appreciable change since the 1930s
(E) Parity has no effect on the risk of developing breast cancer

85. A 60-year-old woman who received radiation therapy for cancer of the cervix 20 years previously undergoes a laparotomy and lysis of adhesions for a distal small bowel obstruction. Ten days later, she developed an enterocutaneous fistula through the wound. Which of the following conditions is likely to prevent spontaneous closure of this fistula?

(A) Right lower lobe pneumonia
(B) A history of small bowel obstruction
(C) A history of radiation therapy
(D) Advanced age of the patient
(E) Duodenal ulcer

86. True statements concerning the anatomy of the parotid gland include all of the following EXCEPT

(A) it is the largest of the salivary glands
(B) the fascia of the gland is quite tight
(C) the facial nerve and its branches run through the gland
(D) the gland has two true anatomic lobes separated by the facial nerve
(E) drainage of saliva is via Stensen's duct

87. Which of the following characteristics would favor the diagnosis of a benign lesion in a patient with a solitary pulmonary nodule?

(A) A diameter greater than 5 cm
(B) Cavitation
(C) A peripheral location
(D) Heavy, concentric calcification within the lesion
(E) Calcium flecks within the lesion

88. A 15-year-old girl has recurrent abdominal cramping and melena. Physical examination reveals increased pigmentation on her lips and buccal mucosa. Her sister has a similar history and similar physical findings. What is the most likely diagnosis?

(A) Pseudopolyposis
(B) Familial polyposis
(C) Villous adenoma
(D) Juvenile polyposis
(E) Peutz-Jeghers syndrome

89. Diagnosis and treatment for an infant with hypertrophic pyloric stenosis include all of the following EXCEPT

(A) rehydration with oral electrolyte formula in an attempt to prepare the child for surgery
(B) correction of the electrolytes with intravenous therapy
(C) placement of a nasogastric tube for gastric decompression
(D) confirm the diagnosis with an abdominal ultrasound, if the examination is inconclusive for pyloric stenosis
(E) check serum electrolytes to ensure that the alkalosis is corrected prior to surgery

Questions 90 and 91

A 54-year-old woman has a 2-year history of hypertension with occasional attacks of palpitations, sweating, and headaches. Physical examination and baseline serum electrolytes are normal.

90. The next step in the workup of this woman should be

(A) serum aldosterone and renin levels
(B) serum cortisol level
(C) 24-hour urine for metanephrine, vanillylmandelic acid, and catecholamines
(D) 24-hour urine for 17-hydroxycorticosteroids
(E) salt-loading followed by serial measurements of potassium in the serum and urine

91. After obtaining the results of the screening test, the abnormality should be anatomically localized with

(A) selective adrenal arteriography
(B) selective venous sampling of the inferior vena cava
(C) CT of the abdomen
(D) radionuclide scan
(E) laparotomy

(end of group question)

92. Hoarseness following radiation therapy for a left superior sulcus lung carcinoma is usually secondary to

(A) vocal cord paralysis due to radiation injury
(B) radiation scarring of the larynx
(C) tumor involvement of the left recurrent laryngeal nerve
(D) continued cigarette smoking
(E) central nervous system metastasis

93. A patient whose job involves worldwide travel presents with a complaint of right upper quadrant pain. Examination reveals hepatomegaly and eosinophilia. The most likely diagnosis is

(A) hepatocellular carcinoma
(B) hepatitis B
(C) echinococcal cyst
(D) choledochal cyst
(E) *Candida albicans* abscess of the liver

94. A 7-year-old child presents with an infected draining sinus in the midline of the neck over the thyroid cartilage. After appropriate drainage and antibiotics, the infection resolves, and ultrasound of the neck reveals a cystic structure separated from the thyroid gland. Appropriate treatment would be excision of the cyst and

(A) the thyroid isthmus
(B) the thyroid cartilage
(C) the medial portion of the cricoid cartilage
(D) the medial portion of the hyoid bone
(E) none of the above

95. The correct management protocol for a patient who receives a penetrating injury to the arm includes all of the following EXCEPT

(A) if active immunization occurred more than 5 years previously, a toxoid booster is recommended
(B) if the wound is clean and the patient has never been immunized, it is safe to give tetanus toxoid in three separate doses
(C) penicillin provides good prophylaxis against *Clostridia tetani* infections
(D) if the wound is dirty and the patient has never been immunized, passive immunization with human tetanus immune globulin is recommended
(E) adequate debridement of devitalized tissue is essential

96. After a thorough diagnostic workup, a patient is found to have Zollinger-Ellison syndrome. Which of the following statements can be made about this syndrome?

(A) It is a postoperative complication of ulcer surgery that leads to postprandial vomiting
(B) It is also known as "cast syndrome" and is due to duodenal obstruction by the superior mesenteric artery
(C) It is an obstruction of the gastric outlet caused by a pyloric ulcer
(D) It is a form of severe duodenal ulcer disease caused by a gastrin-secreting pancreatic tumor
(E) It is seen in psychotic persons who repeatedly ingest foreign objects

97. A 45-year-old man reported the acute onset of severe right flank pain. He denied any voiding symptoms or hematuria. A urinalysis showed 5–10 red blood cells/high-power field. The most appropriate diagnostic study is

(A) CT scan
(B) retrograde ureteropyelogram
(C) excretory urogram
(D) ultrasonography
(E) MRI

98. A patient undergoes cervical exploration for primary hyperparathyroidism. At surgery, one grossly enlarged gland and three normal-sized glands are found. The enlarged gland is removed, and frozen section shows a hypercellular parathyroid. One of the normal glands is biopsied, and frozen section shows normal parathyroid. The next morning, the patient's calcium level is 7.5 mg/dl, down from a preoperative level of 11.3. The patient feels well and is asymptomatic. Treatment should include

(A) intravenous calcium
(B) oral calcium and vitamin D
(C) oral calcium alone
(D) intravenous phosphorus
(E) none of the above

99. Which of the following lesions in a patient with renovascular hypertension would be most responsive to percutaneous balloon dilatation?

(A) A midrenal artery lesion caused by a fibromuscular dysplasia
(B) An atherosclerotic lesion at the orifice of the renal artery
(C) Multiple atherosclerotic lesions in the hilar branches of the renal artery
(D) Multiple fibromuscular dysplastic lesions in the hilar renal arteries
(E) None of the above

100. A 45-year-old man is seen in the emergency room after vomiting bright red blood. He has no previous symptoms. He drinks one alcoholic beverage a day. The most reliable method for locating the lesion responsible for the bleeding is

(A) upper GI series
(B) exploratory laparotomy
(C) upper endoscopy
(D) arteriography
(E) radionuclide scanning

101. Surgery is not considered an appropriate initial form of therapy for which of the following lesions?

(A) Amebic abscess
(B) Echinococcal cyst
(C) Multiple large hepatic bacterial abscesses
(D) Choledochal cyst
(E) Hepatocellular carcinoma

102. A 60-year-old man with cancer of the stomach has a subtotal gastrectomy with removal of lymph nodes along the greater and lesser curvature and along the celiac access, splenectomy, and removal of the greater omentum, all removed as a single specimen. Which of the following best describes the procedure that was performed?

(A) Wide local excision
(B) Radical local resection
(C) Super radical resection
(D) Debulking procedure
(E) Radical en block resection

103. Which of the following statements concerning patients with dialysis-dependent chronic renal failure is true?

(A) They should be transfused to a hemoglobin of 10 g/dl prior to surgery
(B) They should not be dialyzed for 48 hours prior to surgery
(C) They require Foley catheterization to monitor urine output accurately
(D) They may develop intractable hyperkalemia after administration of succinylcholine
(E) They may develop coagulopathy resistant to cryoprecipitate

104. The initial management of stable angina pectoris should include all of the following EXCEPT

(A) coronary angiography
(B) medical therapy with nitrates, β-blockers, and antihypertensive medications
(C) a low-fat diet
(D) coronary artery bypass
(E) graded exercise program

105. The bacterial organism most likely to cause hematogenous osteomyelitis in a 3-year-old child is

(A) *Escherichia coli*
(B) *Hemophilus influenzae*
(C) *Staphylococcus aureus*
(D) *Neisseria gonorrhoeae*
(E) *Pseudomonas aeruginosa*

106. Massive bleeding from the lower gastrointestinal tract is occurring in a 55-year-old, otherwise healthy man. Initial management, after continued bleeding equivalent to 1 unit of blood, would be

(A) emergency laparotomy and total colectomy with ileoproctostomy
(B) emergency laparotomy and colostomy with operative endoscopy
(C) arteriography to identify the bleeding site after anoscopy and sigmoidoscopy have ruled out a distal site
(D) infusion of vitamin K and fresh frozen plasma
(E) colonic irrigation with iced saline solution

107. A physician considering a preoperative regimen for elective colon surgery should know that

(A) perioperative intravenous antibiotics effective against aerobes and anaerobes obviate the need for a mechanical bowel preparation
(B) an effective mechanical bowel preparation reduces the concentration of bacteria per gram of stool and is adequate preparation alone for surgery
(C) oral antibiotics, if indicated, should be started at least 1 week prior to surgery
(D) the level of aerobes in the stool is about 1/1000 of that of anaerobes
(E) oral antibiotics must be absorbed to be effective as part of a bowel preparation regimen

108. A diabetic patient in a hyperosmolar, non-ketotic state has a blood glucose level of 850 mg/dl and a serum sodium of 130 mg/dl. His sodium level corrected for the hyperglycemia is

(A) 130
(B) 134
(C) 138
(D) 142
(E) 146

109. Indications for resection of a lung abscess include all of the following EXCEPT

(A) obstructive carcinoma
(B) rupture into the pleural space
(C) massive hemoptysis
(D) failure to respond to prolonged antibiotic therapy
(E) history of foreign body aspiration

Questions 110–112

A young man presents to the emergency room with the acute onset of severe abdominal pain. His blood pressure is 70 systolic. His abdomen is rigid.

110. Appropriate initial measures would include all of the following EXCEPT

(A) obtaining a complete blood count
(B) inserting an intravenous catheter
(C) obtaining a detailed history, including a family and travel history
(D) inserting a Foley catheter
(E) obtaining blood specimen for type and cross

111. The test most likely to yield a diagnosis would be

(A) a white blood count
(B) a sedimentation rate
(C) an abdominal flat plate
(D) an obstruction series
(E) a barium enema

112. The choice of operation for this patient would depend least on

(A) medical condition of the patient
(B) duration of symptoms
(C) degree of peritoneal soiling
(D) previous symptoms of epigastric pain
(E) patient's body habitus
(end of group question)

113. An elevated parathyroid hormone level with a low serum calcium value would be compatible with the diagnosis of

(A) primary hyperparathyroidism
(B) secondary hyperparathyroidism
(C) tertiary hyperparathyroidism
(D) hypoparathyroidism
(E) none of the above

114. Which of the following patients with a femoral fracture is best treated with an intramedullary rod?

(A) A 6-year-old bicycle rider
(B) An adult who has been in an automobile accident
(C) An adult with an infected nonunion
(D) A 2-year-old child abuse victim
(E) A neonate with birth trauma

115. A 60-year-old postmenopausal woman presents with a 2.5-cm mass in the lower inner right breast. The excisional biopsy reveals an invasive ductal carcinoma. All of the following studies should be obtained as part of this woman's evaluation EXCEPT

(A) bone scan
(B) contralateral mammogram
(C) liver function studies
(D) chest radiograph
(E) CT scan of the head

116. A 40-year-old woman presents with bowel obstruction. At surgery, the cause is found to be an ileal carcinoid tumor that is 2.5 cm in diameter. Which of the following statements concerning this woman's condition is true?

(A) If liver metastases are present, no bowel resection should be done due to the poor prognosis
(B) Carcinoid tumors frequently arise in the heterotopic gastric mucosa of a Meckel's diverticulum
(C) An appendectomy should be performed
(D) Inspection of the entire small bowel in search of other carcinoids is necessary
(E) If liver metastases are present, the patient may develop the carcinoma syndrome

117. What anatomic landmark distinguishes an indirect hernia from a direct hernia?

(A) Femoral vein
(B) Inferior epigastric vessels
(C) Spermatic cord
(D) Transversalis fascia
(E) Processus vaginalis

118. A 25-year-old woman with Grave's disease has failed to achieve remission despite appropriate doses of propylthiouracil for 1 year. Appropriate therapy at this point would be

(A) propylthiouracil for another year
(B) methimazole for 1 year
(C) subtotal thyroidectomy
(D) ^{131}I therapy
(E) propylthiouracil plus propranolol for 1 year

119. A patient was referred by his family physician because of a mass in his leg. All of the following radiologic studies are part of the initial workup of this patient EXCEPT

(A) plain radiography
(B) CT of the mass and area
(C) CT of the chest
(D) a scan of the liver and spleen
(E) a bone scan

120. All of the following conditions are associated with esophageal carcinoma EXCEPT

(A) Barrett's esophagus
(B) hiatal hernia
(C) chronic reflux esophagitis
(D) excessive smoking and alcohol
(E) achalasia

121. A biliary tract tumor, such as a Klatskin tumor, occurring at the hepatic duct confluence is most accurately diagnosed with which of the following tests?

(A) An upper GI series
(B) Intravenous cholangiography
(C) Percutaneous transhepatic cholangiography
(D) Hepatic scintiscanning
(E) Liver biopsy

122. A 50-year-old man has a right upper lobe cavitary lesion that is 4 cm in diameter and of unknown age. Which one of the following tests is most likely to establish the diagnosis?

(A) Bronchography
(B) Computed tomography
(C) Bronchoscopy with biopsy brushings and washings
(D) Percutaneous needle aspiration of the cavity contents
(E) An immunologic skin test

123. Which of the following antithyroid agents blocks the peripheral conversion of T_4 to T_3?

(A) Radioiodine
(B) Propranolol
(C) Propylthiouracil
(D) Methimazole
(E) Iodine

124. After hospitalization for a parasternal knife wound, a young man is monitored. All of the following may be anticipated EXCEPT

(A) distended neck veins
(B) hypotension
(C) pulsus paradoxus
(D) increased heart sounds
(E) pleural effusion

125. A 60-year-old woman undergoes a left radical nephrectomy for a hypernephroma. During the procedure, 1 L of blood is lost, and no blood is given as replacement. The patient is taken to the recovery room, still intubated and asleep. A postoperative hemoglobin is 6.5, and transfusion with the first of 2 units of packed red blood cells is begun. Fifteen minutes later, the nurse notes diffuse bleeding from the sites of intravenous catheters, from the incision, and through the drain that was left in the operative bed. The patient's urine, which was clear, is now pink-tinged. Which of the following statements about this patient's condition is true?

(A) The patient is having an allergic reaction to the transfused blood
(B) Diphenhydramine should be administered immediately
(C) The patient is having a febrile reaction to the transfused blood due to antigens on white cells or platelets, which contaminate packed red blood cell transfusions
(D) The patient should be treated immediately with epinephrine and steroids
(E) The patient should receive fluids and mannitol

126. All of the following statements concerning fibrocystic disease of the breast without atypia are true EXCEPT

(A) painful bilateral cystic masses change during the menstrual cycle
(B) excisional biopsy may be indicated
(C) the chance of developing cancer is enhanced five to seven times
(D) usual onset is the third or fourth decade of life
(E) needle aspiration may be helpful in diagnosis

127. In a patient with hemorrhage from a suspected diverticulum in the colon, what is the minimal rate of hemorrhage that can usually be visualized by selective mesenteric angiography?

(A) 0.1 ml/min
(B) 0.5 ml/min
(C) 5 ml/min
(D) 15 ml/min
(E) 50 ml/min

128. Correct statements concerning prophylactic antibiotics and surgery include which of the following?

(A) They should be administered for 24 hours before and at least 48 hours after surgery
(B) They are useful when there is a risk of infection at the operative wound site
(C) Broad-spectrum antibiotics are the treatment of choice
(D) They are beneficial when used to sterilize infected protheses
(E) None of the above

129. A 63-year-old smoker complains of dyspnea, wheezing, and nonproductive cough. Chest x-ray appears normal, but CT scan reveals an intraluminal mass located in the distal trachea. The most likely diagnosis is

(A) adenoid cystic carcinoma
(B) carcinoid tumor
(C) squamous cell carcinoma
(D) mucoepidermoid carcinoma
(E) squamous papilloma

130. During a pre-employment physical examination, a 50-year-old man is found to have an asymptomatic thyroid nodule. The nodule is well circumscribed and freely moveable. There is no associated cervical lymphadenopathy and no family history of thyroid malignancy. Which of the following studies will best determine the nature of the thyroid enlargement?

(A) ^{99m}Tc thyroid scan
(B) ^{131}I thyroid scan
(C) Thyroid ultrasonography
(D) Fine-needle aspiration of the thyroid
(E) Serum thyrocalcitonin assay

131. All of the following are Haagensen's criteria for inoperability of breast carcinoma EXCEPT

(A) nipple inversion with eczematoid changes
(B) peau d'orange
(C) supraclavicular adenopathy
(D) arm edema
(E) a parasternal tumor

132. The arterial replacement prosthesis of choice for a femoropopliteal bypass graft in a young man is

(A) a Dacron tube graft
(B) an umbilical vein allograft
(C) an autogenous arterial graft
(D) an autogenous saphenous vein graft
(E) an arterial allograft

133. A woman has undergone a cholecystectomy and common duct exploration. Two stones were removed, and a T tube was placed in the common duct. On the seventh postoperative day, her serum bilirubin level remains elevated, and she has an episode of crampy pain that radiates to her back. What is the next step in the management of this patient?

(A) Begin therapy with drugs to "dissolve" gallstones
(B) Remove the T tube
(C) Clamp off the T tube
(D) Return the patient to the operating room
(E) Perform T-tube cholangiography

134. A patient with total occlusion of the right superficial femoral artery would most likely present with symptoms in which of the following locations?

(A) Hip and buttock
(B) Thigh
(C) Calf
(C) Foot
(E) None of the above

135. A 45-year-old executive is seen because of vomiting bright red blood. There are no previous symptoms. The man admits to drinking one alcoholic drink a week and has no other significant history. In the hospital, he bleeds 5 units of blood prior to endoscopy. The most likely diagnosis is

(A) gastritis
(B) duodenal ulcer
(C) esophagitis
(D) Mallory-Weiss tear
(E) esophageal varices

Directions: The groups of questions below consist of lettered choices followed by several numbered items. For each numbered item select the **one** lettered choice with which it is **most** closely associated. Each lettered choice may be used once, more than once, or not at all.

Questions 136–140

For each statement listed below, select the diagnosis that is most likely to be associated with it.

(A) Acute tubular necrosis
(B) Hyperacute rejection
(C) Accelerated acute rejection
(D) Acute rejection
(E) Chronic rejection

136. No crossmatch compatibility

137. Usually temporary, lasting 1–10 days and related to the harvest and preservation of the kidney

138. Effectively treated with high-doses of prednisone, antilymphocyte globulin, or orthoclone

139. Second-set immune response that occurs within the first week of transplantation

140. Slow decline in renal function over months or years that results from humoral and cellular events

Questions 141–145

For each condition listed below, select the treatment that would be most appropriate.

(A) Cryoprecipitate
(B) Factor VIII concentrate
(C) Fresh frozen plasma
(D) Albumin
(E) Fresh whole blood

141. Volume expansion

142. Acute hemorrhage

143. von Willebrand's disease

144. Replacement of clotting factors

145. Fibrinogen deficiency

Questions 146–150

Match the following.

(A) Squamous cell carcinoma of the larynx
(B) Papillary carcinoma
(C) Hodgkin's lymphoma
(D) Atypical mycobacteria
(E) Infected congenital cyst

146. Slow-growing, painless neck mass, fever, malaise, and weight loss

147. Slow-growing, painless neck mass, cough, and hoarseness

148. Slow-growing, painless neck mass with a history of childhood irradiation

149. Slow-growing, painless neck mass with fixation to overlying skin and a draining ulcer

150. Fast-growing, painful, red, warm neck mass, fever, and chills

Questions 151–155

For each urologic neoplasm listed below, select the diagnostic study that is appropriate for that neoplasm.

(A) Acid phosphatase
(B) Arteriography
(C) Human chorionic gonadotropin
(D) Cystoscopy
(E) Retrograde pyelography

151. Testicular tumor

152. Prostatic carcinoma

153. Renal cell carcinoma

154. Transitional cell carcinoma of the renal pelvis

155. Carcinoma of the bladder

Questions 156–160

Match the following.

(A) Hyperplastic polyp
(B) Villous adenoma
(C) Hamartomatous polyp
(D) Tubular adenoma
(E) Inflammatory polyp

156. Referred to as a pseudopolyp

157. Commonest polyp of the adult colon

158. Juvenile polyp

159. Highest malignant potential

160. Associated with familial polyposis

Questions 161–165

The following table lists the oxygen saturation of each cardiac chamber as measured at cardiac catheterization (RA = right atrium; RV = right ventricle; LA = left atrium; LV = left ventricle; PA = pulmonary artery; and AO = aorta). Match each set of parameters with the condition with which it is most likely to be associated.

Oxygen Saturation (in %)

	RA	RV	LA	LV	PA	AO
(A)	65	85	95	95	85	95
(B)	65	65	95	95	85	95
(C)	85	85	95	95	85	95
(D)	50	50	95	85	50	70
(E)	40	40	98	98	98	40

161. Tetralogy of Fallot

162. Atrial septal defect

163. Transposition of the great arteries

164. Ventricular septal defect

165. Patent ductus arteriosus

Questions 166–170

For each multiple endocrine adenomatosis (MEA) syndrome or pancreatic tumor, select the clinical feature that is most characteristic of it.

(A) Elevated serum calcium level
(B) Elevated serum thyrocalcitonin level
(C) Severe watery diarrhea
(D) Abdominal pain secondary to peptic ulceration
(E) Distorted body habitus

166. MEA type I (Wermer's syndrome)

167. MEA type II (Sipple's syndrome)

168. MEA type III (mucosal neuroma syndrome)

169. Pancreatic gastrinoma (Zollinger-Ellison syndrome)

170. Pancreatic cholera

Questions 171–175

For each characteristic below, select the disorder with which it is most likely to be associated.

(A) Gastric ulcer
(B) Duodenal ulcer
(C) Stress ulceration
(D) Chronic gastritis
(E) Prepyloric ulcer

171. Brought on by ischemia

172. Carries increased risk of cancer

173. Causes gastric outlet obstruction

174. Associated with blood group O

175. Associated with parietal cell antibodies

Questions 176–180

For each pathologic entity listed below, select the most appropriate therapy.

(A) Thymectomy
(B) Treatment with anticholinesterases
(C) Thymectomy with radiation therapy
(D) Radiation therapy and chemotherapy
(E) Partial thymectomy

176. Benign thymoma

177. Malignant thymoma

178. Ocular myasthenia gravis with a grossly normal thymus gland

179. Generalized myasthenia gravis with a grossly normal thymus gland

180. Generalized myasthenia gravis with a benign thymoma

ANSWERS AND EXPLANATIONS

1. The answer is D. [*Chapter 16 II E 3, 4*] All of the conditions listed in the question except for adrenal cortical adenoma cause Cushing's syndrome by producing increased levels of adrenocorticotropic hormone (ACTH). Basophilic adenomas of the pituitary cause bilateral adrenal cortical hyperplasia as a result of increased ACTH production. Adrenal cortical hyperplasia does not occur de novo but results from excessive stimulation of the adrenals by ACTH from an extra-adrenal source, whether it be pituitary or nonpituitary in origin. Both oat cell carcinoma of the lung and malignant islet cell tumors of the pancreas are sources of ectopic ACTH production and result in increased plasma levels of ACTH. While adrenal cortical adenomas can also cause Cushing's syndrome, they autonomously produce increased amounts of cortisol without being dependent on ACTH production; they actually suppress endogenous ACTH production.

2. The answer is A. [*Chapter 28 III A 1 b (3)*] The extent of an injury to the musculoskeletal system varies according to the age of the patient, direction of the causative violence, and magnitude of the violence. The age of this patient suggests the weak link in the musculoskeletal system. In elderly patients, ligament injury is rare, and fracture of the metaphyseal portion of the bone is more likely. Growth plate fractures are more likely in children, and soft tissue injuries are commonest in young adults.

3. The answer is B. [*Chapter 2 I A 1 a (2), b, c, 4 d, 5 c (1)*] Various types of tubes are used in surgery to permit drainage that is either abnormal, such as pus, or is a normal body fluid that cannot be handled normally by the body. An underwater-seal drain, a type of closed drain, is useful for draining the pleural space because it prevents air and fluid from reentering the body. A T tube is used to drain bile following common duct exploration until spasm of the sphincter of Oddi resolves. Rigid drains may erode through the wall of a blood vessel or a hollow viscus, a complication that may be minimized by using soft drains or removing drains early. Open drains allow free movement of bacteria because they are not sealed at either end and as a result, carry a high risk of deep wound infection. Sump drains are double-lumen catheters that allow air or irrigation fluid to enter through one lumen while suction is applied to the other lumen. Gravity drains allow collected material to drain into a reservoir at a lower level.

4. The answer is A. [*Chapter 18 IV J 6*] The situation described in the question is typical in cases of an arytenoid dislocation. This lesion is commonly caused by endotracheal intubation or traumatic extubation. It requires early, accurate diagnosis and prompt reduction to prevent joint fixation. Until an accurate diagnosis is made, no specific vocal treatment should be attempted. Complete voice rest should be avoided as this would reduce any residual motion in the cricoarytenoid joint. Speech therapy is not indicated in a patient with a dislocated arytenoid until reduction is attempted. Contact ulcers also result from traumatic or prolonged intubation. However, the presenting symptoms are usually pain and cough and do not involve significant change in the vocal quality.

5. The answer is D. [*Chapter 18 III E 2*] Cystic hygroma and teratoma are the only lesions listed in the question that would be clinically significant at 3 months of age. The description of an irregular, compressible mass is specific for cystic hygroma. They can undergo progressive enlargement, compressing the airway and brachial plexus. Treatment is surgical.

6. The answer is D. [*Chapter 15 II D 4, 5*] Surgical management of chronic pancreatitis should be reserved for the patient who has intractable pain despite intensive efforts at medical management, because the surgical procedure may be difficult, may carry significant risk, and may not resolve the pain.

7. The answer is A. [*Chapter 27 IV B 2*] While managing a patient with multiple trauma, the possibility of head and spinal cord injury must be considered. Since the patient described in the question was found unresponsive and also had diaphragmatic breathing, concomitant head and spinal cord injury are possible. In such a situation, endotracheal intubation is contraindicated and nasotracheal intubation or intubation with a flexible bronchoscope is preferred. Colloids, blood products, and balanced salt solution, such as Ringer's lactate, are preferred for volume replacement, as plain 5% dextrose and water can worsen cerebral edema.

8. The answer is C. [*Chapter 27 IV B, E*] Patients with a high cervical spinal cord injury are usually hypotensive as a result of the disruption of the sympathetic nervous system. Volume replacement usually restores the blood pressure to normal. Since the cervical spine x-rays confirmed a significant injury at the C5–C6 level, skeletal traction using Gardner-Wells tongs is used to realign the spine and remove compression of the spinal cord. A soft collar does not immobilize the spine. A CT scan of the spine is indicated to evaluate the extent of the spinal injury. A CT scan of the brain should also be done to rule out any intracranial pathology. Mannitol is an osmotic agent and is used in spinal injuries to reduce the cord edema.

9. The answer is E. [*Chapter 26 I C 3 c, D 2*] In large open fractures (grade III), vascularized tissue is necessary to provide optimum soft tissue to permit bone healing. In distal lower extremity injuries, free flaps are usually the best choice. Muscle flaps, fasciocutaneous flaps, and cross-leg flaps have their role in selected cases. A skin graft will not reliably "take" on an open fracture devoid of periosteum.

10. The answer is B. [*Chapter 10 II B 3 a*] In achalasia, the normal peristalsis in the body of the esophagus is absent, resulting in diffuse esophageal dilatation that can be seen on x-ray films. A corkscrew appearance is characteristic of esophageal spasm, and reflux of barium indicates inadequate functioning of the lower esophageal sphincter. A diverticulum visible in the area of the cricopharyngeal muscle is a Zenker's or pharyngoesophageal diverticulum, caused by dysfunction in the upper esophageal sphincter.

11. The answer is D. [*Chapter 8 II B 3–6*] Patients who are undergoing uncomplicated surgery (e.g., inguinal herniorrhaphy) and who are otherwise young and healthy are not at risk for developing pulmonary embolism. Obesity, a history of congestive heart failure, spinal cord injury, and carcinoma do place the surgical patient at increased risk for pulmonary embolism and deep venous thrombosis.

12. The answer is D. [*Chapter 18 III B 3*] A midline neck mass that is mobile with swallowing is indicative of a thyroglossal duct cyst. These are infrahyoid in 65% of the cases, suprahyoid in about 20%, and at the hyoid in 15%. In half of the cases, they present by age 10. Branchial cleft cysts can occur anywhere between the external auditory canal and the clavicle. Cystic hygromas are found in the neck, most commonly in the posterior triangle, and are usually noted soon after birth. Teratomas are generally unilateral and cause tracheal compression or deviation. They are most commonly noted at birth. Laryngeal papillomas in children are usually multiple and may involve the airway from the epiglottis to the bronchi.

13. The answer is A. [*Chapter 26 I C 3, E 4*] Following radical mastectomy, a skin graft is used to reconstruct the chest wall defect. Any technique in breast reconstruction will require vascularized soft tissue coverage. An implant may or may not be necessary. A skin graft alone will not provide adequate soft tissue coverage for the implant.

14. The answer is C. [*Chapter 11 II C 3*] Because the stomach is so dilated, decompression is necessary with a nasogastric tube. This patient would likely need rehydration, and a Foley catheter is used to monitor the urine output in response to hydration. H_2-blockers may be of some benefit, but giving metaclopramide, which stimulates gastric motility, is contraindicated until it is proven, usually by an upper gastrointestinal series, that no mechanical obstruction to gastric emptying exists.

15. The answer is B. [*Chapter 11 II C 3 a*] Prolonged vomiting causes excessive losses of hydrochloric acid from the stomach, leading to a metabolic alkalosis. This also is often associated with hypokalemia.

16. The answer is A. [*Chapter 11 II C 3 c*] Patients with gastric outlet obstruction from ulcer disease usually do not respond to medical therapy and require surgery. Vagotomy with antrectomy or drainage is done with good relief of the problem.

17. The answer is D. [*Chapter 29 X A 3 c, 4*] Wilms' tumor has been associated with a number of congenital anomalies, including aniridia, hemihypertrophy, Beckwith's syndrome, sexual ambiguity, cryptorchidism, and other genitourinary defects. Hypertension is seen in about 10% of the patients with this common childhood tumor of the kidney. Wilms' tumor is not associated with polycystic kidneys.

18. The answer is D. [*Chapter 3 I C 3 a; IV B 3 a (1)*] Most physicians accept a hemoglobin level of 10 g/dl of blood prior to major surgery. Thus, preoperative blood replacement is recommended when excessive blood loss is anticipated, when the patient has significant coronary artery disease or a history of congestive heart failure, after a preoperative hemorrhage, in hypoxia, and in the presence of sepsis or malnutrition. However, the patient with chronic renal failure and no other complications tolerates a hemoglobin level of 7–8 g/dl well for most surgical procedures.

19. The answer is D. [*Chapter 17 II C 5*] The first goal of treatment for patients with Zollinger-Ellison syndrome should be removal of the causative tumor, since about 60% of these tumors are malignant; however, it is possible to localize these tumors in only 20% of cases. If the primary tumor cannot be controlled or is metastatic, then H_2-receptor blockers are used to control the end-organ response to the hypergastrinemia. Total gastrectomy is also effective in controlling the end-organ (stomach) response and should be employed in patients who fail or are unable to tolerate medical (H_2-receptor antagonist) treatment. Although under investigation, gastrin-receptor antagonists are not clinically available. Subtotal gastrectomy does not control the primary tumor and is inadequate in preventing recurrent ulceration in Zollinger-Ellison syndrome patients.

20. The answer is E. [*Chapter 4 II A 2 b*] A tension pneumothorax results in collapse of the lung with decreased breath sounds and tympany on the ipsilateral side. This distorts the mediastinum, resulting in decreased venous return and decreased cardiac output with resultant hypoxia and acidosis.

21. The answer is C. [*Chapter 24 I A 3 a–c*] Although the mixed lymphocyte reaction may be used to predict success in kidney transplantation from a cadaver donor, the test is not usually performed because it requires 5–7 days. Cadaver kidneys must be transplanted within 1–2 days following removal.

22. The answer is C. [*Chapter 27 IV A–E*] In cases of suspected cervical spine trauma, the importance of visualizing all cervical vertebrae cannot be overemphasized. When there is difficulty in visualizing the C7 vertebra, using special views (e.g., Swimmer's) or simply pulling the arms down and taking a lateral film may be beneficial. High cervical cord injuries result in a sympathectomy and, thus, may give rise to a Horner's syndrome and systemic hypotension as a result of peripheral vasodilatation. In these cases, adequate blood pressure is restored by volume replacement rather than by the use of vasopressor agents. Hematomas can develop in front of the vertebral bodies, jeopardizing the airways. Therefore, attention must be given to maintaining adequate airways. It has been postulated that cord edema develops following the initial injury, which further embarrasses the microcirculation and aggravates the injury. Thus, osmotic agents, such as mannitol, are administered to decrease the cord edema and reduce the extent of injury. Fracture dislocations of the cervical spine are treated by traction, applied by means of skull tongs and weights.

23. The answer is A. [*Chapter 10 I A 1 a–c, C, D 3*] The gastroesophageal junction is 40 cm from the incisors, and the entire esophagus is approximately 24 cm in length. The esophagus passes through the right crus of the diaphragm. It is composed of both striated and smooth muscle cells and is innervated principally by the vagus nerve. The lower esophageal sphincter represents a region of increased resting pressure in the esophagus but does not consist of distinct muscle fibers.

24. The answer is D. [*Chapter 13 X B 5 c*] Of the diagnostic options listed, the barium enema would have the highest yield for the least risk in the diagnosis of inflammatory bowel disease.

25. The answer is D. [*Chapter 13 X A 1 b*] Ulcerative colitis represents a continuous disease beginning in the rectum. Skip areas are characteristic of Crohn's disease and are not seen in ulcerative colitis.

26. The answer is B. [*Chapter 13 X A 2 a (1), (2)*] The patient described in the question is best managed by an initial course of steroids and sulfasalazine. If she does not respond, bowel rest and nutritional support would need to be considered.

27. The answer is B. [*Chapter 6 I B 1 b, d (4), e (1)*] The 69-year-old woman described in the question has left ventricular failure for untreated aortic stenosis. Cardiac failure has led to a decreased cardiac output, causing the gradient to be less. The noncompliant hypertrophied ventricle is preload dependent; therefore, brisk diuresis or nitrate administration could lead to systemic hypotension, coronary ischemia, and death. The only solution is to relieve the mechanical obstruction to left ventricular outflow.

28. The answer is C. [*Chapter 22 II B 1*] Secondary hypersplenism is caused by an identifiable underlying disease. The commonest mechanism of action is portal hypertension, which can lead to passive splenic congestion. The hypersplenism associated with portal hypertension is usually mild and clinically insignificant; thus, isolated splenectomy is not indicated.

29. The answer is E. [*Chapter 8 III A 1 a (2), 2, 3*] The patient described in the question presents with a classic history of primary lymphedema. Since this occurred in her teens, it would be classified as lymphedema praecox. This diagnosis is made by history and physical examination; lymphangiography is seldom required. Unlike swelling in the lower extremities secondary to postphlebitic syndrome, patients with lymphedema rarely develop ulceration or skin discoloration. Treatment for lymphedema consists of elevation and chronic compression with an elastic stocking. Intermittent compression devices are occasionally useful. This patient would not be a candidate for lymphaticovenous anastomosis, which is an operation designed for decompression obliteration of the proximal lymphatics in the groin or pelvis. Patients with lymphedema are prone to develop recurrent infections. *Streptococcus* is the most likely etiologic agent. When infection occurs, it must be treated early and aggressively, usually with penicillin, and if recurrent episodes continue, prophylactic penicillin may be indicated.

30. The answer is B. [*Chapter 26 I I 7*] Liposuction (suction assisted lipectomy) is a safe outpatient procedure usually performed under general or regional anesthesia. It is not a method for weight reduction, and it is not considered safe to treat baggy eyelids. Liposuction is most useful for removing localized deposits of fat to improve body contour.

31. The answer is E. [*Chapter 9 I F 1 c (1)*] Free air within the peritoneal cavity signals perforation of a hollow viscus. It is present in about 80% of gastroduodenal perforations. Because free peritoneal air is rarely secondary to other causes, additional studies would not be necessary in this patient prior to laparotomy.

32. The answer is B. [*Chapter 10 II B 4 b, D 4 b (2); III B 1, 3*] Reflux esophagitis occurs because of incompetence of the lower esophageal sphincter. The Nissen fundoplication, Belsey Mark IV operation, and the Hill repair are all used to increase the competency of the lower esophageal sphincter and to treat gastroesophageal reflux. The consequence of chronic gastroesophageal reflux is stricturing of the esophagus. In those cases of severe stricturing, esophageal resection may be required. The Heller procedure is a long myotomy of the esophagus and is used to treat diffuse esophageal spasm or achalasia.

33. The answer is D. [*Chapter 10 II C 4 b, D 4 a*] Gastroesophageal reflux can be treated medically in most patients. Weight loss, antacids, H_2-receptor antagonists, and abstinence from smoking and alcohol are all recommended for patients suffering from gastroesophageal reflux. Calcium channel blockers, which have a tendency to relax smooth muscle, may be detrimental in patients with gastroesophageal reflux.

34. The answer is A. [*Chapter 8 I B 3 c (1)–(4)*] Physical examination is the least likely method to diagnose the cause of acute leg swelling. Currently, such a patient would undergo duplex ultrasonography or venography to confirm the presumed diagnosis of deep venous thrombosis. Impedance plethysmography will detect increased resistance to venous flow but does not identify the cause. [125]I fibrinogen scanning will identify ongoing thrombosis, but the scan takes 24 hours to complete and is, thus, not useful in acute situations.

35. The answer is B. [*Chapter 8 I B 3 d (1)*] Subcutaneous heparin therapy in its current form is not acceptable treatment for deep venous thrombosis. Thrombolytic therapy would be contraindicated in a patient with a recent craniotomy as it would increase the risk of hemorrhage. Aspirin therapy has no role in the treatment of deep venous thrombosis. Warfarin can be used once the patient is discharged but not as the initial treatment. Transition from intravenous heparin to warfarin therapy should occur on the 4th or 5th postheparin day.

36. The answer is E. [*Chapter 8 I B 3 d (1)–(3)*] Hemorrhage is a significant complication in the presence of anticoagulation; thus, anticoagulants should be discontinued in a patient who has a bleeding ulcer. Observation would be dangerous in a patient with deep venous thrombosis due to the risk of life-threatening pulmonary emboli. Thrombolytic agents are contraindicated in this patient, and injection of thrombolytic agents into the area of a femoral venous thrombus is not standard therapy.

37. The answer is E. [*Chapter 8 I B 3 e (1)*] Support hose is the mainstay of treatment for patients with chronic postphlebitic syndrome. Thrombectomies have been unsuccessful, and the efficacy of venous bypass has yet to be established. There is interest in transplanting venous valves and segments of a vein to replace short-segment thromboses, but this is still experimental at present. Prosthetic grafts have no role in venous reconstruction. Chronic diuretic therapy may be useful for short-term therapy but is certainly not optimal long-term management for this problem.

38. The answer is E. [*Chapter 4 I B 2 b (1)*] Persistent pneumonitis should be aggressively investigated as an indicator of an occult carcinoma impinging upon a bronchial segment. Bronchoscopy and further workup should be performed. If the question remains unresolved, then lung biopsy or resection should be carried out.

39. The answer is C. [*Chapter 20 V A*] Acute suppurative parotitis is usually a staphylococcal infection that develops in debilitated patients who are dehydrated and who cannot maintain good oral hygiene. Elderly, debilitated postoperative patients are particularly at risk. Medical management consists of hydration, use of antibiotics, and measures to promote salivation. If these measures fail, surgical drainage is mandatory. The gland is usually very painful due to stretching of the fascia enclosing the gland.

40. The answer is E. [*Chapter 7 IV C 2 e (2)*] An absolute method for predicting amputation healing is currently not available. Both a pulsatile pulse volume recording in the calf and a transcutaneous PO_2 greater than 40 mm Hg are useful in indicating probable healing but do not guarantee success. Sensation in the foot and absence of gangrene above the ankle likewise have no absolute predictive value. Approximately 80% of patients will heal a below-knee amputation in the absence of obvious ischemia of the midcalf.

41. The answer is B. [*Chapter 10 III A 1, 2*] Ingestion of a caustic material causes burns in the mouth, pharynx, and esophagus. As part of the initial evaluation and treatment, these patients should undergo prompt endoscopy. Once the area of initial damage has been visualized, the endoscopy should be halted, and the patient should be treated, depending on the clinical condition. The patient should undergo repeat endoscopy in 2 weeks to evaluate the full extent of the caustic burn.

42. The answer is B. [*Chapter 27 III D 1–3*] Although the patient described in the question seems to have an intracranial mass lesion, other severe intrathoracic or intra-abdominal injuries, which could be life-threatening, must be ruled out. Thus, administering mannitol and hyperventilation would give a few extra minutes for chest x-ray, cervical spine x-ray, and peritoneal tap. If necessary, a combined trauma team could then simultaneously handle the brain, thoracic, and abdominal injuries.

43. The answer is D. [*Chapter 24 I B 2, 5, 7 c, d, F 3, 4 a*] Although the recurrent development of glomerulonephritis may destroy the transplanted kidney, it is not directly life-threatening. An acute or chronic infection, whether bacterial, viral, or fungal, and myocardial infarction are the commonest causes of death in transplant recipients.

44. The answer is D. [*Chapter 1 III D 6 c (1) (b), (2)*] The most effective way to prevent infection in a dirty traumatic wound is debridement with irrigation. Any person with a penetrating injury must receive tetanus prophylaxis if previous immunization cannot be documented; however, adequate debridement of devitalized tissue is also essential. Although prophylactic antibiotics can reduce the incidence of wound infections, they are probably of little benefit for grossly contaminated wounds. Topical antibiotics are used most appropriately for burns of the skin. Skin grafts are used to cover large open wounds that are covered by healthy granulation tissue.

45. The answer is E. [*Chapter 7 I A 2, B 1 a–c*] The patient described in the question has a typical history and physical examination of a patient with superficial femoral artery occlusion. He has a relatively minor degree of claudication. Initial treatment should include control of risk factors, including normalizing the patient's blood pressure, cessation of smoking, and weight loss. The patient should be instructed to begin an exercise program to improve collateral circulation in the involved extremity. Many patients respond well to this form of therapy.

46. The answer is E. [*Chapter 1 II A 1, B 1*] Fat, because it is hydrophobic and, hence, is not hydrated like protein and carbohydrates, is the most energy-dense reservoir. The body contains less than 300 g of carbohydrate, which provides less than 1000 kcal of energy and which is exhausted after less than 24 hours of starvation. Protein stores, which contain 4 kcal/g, are not easily accessible as an energy source except after prolonged starvation. The body's protein is present in muscle, circulating proteins, intracellular enzymes, and structural proteins. All of these are important for maintaining body integrity and are conserved early in starvation. Healthy adult men generally have 20%–25% of their body weight stored as fat.

47. The answer is B. [*Chapter 29 IX C 5*] The absolute indications for surgery in an infant with necrotizing enterocolitis include intestinal perforation as demonstrated by free intraperitoneal air and a stricture requiring resection to relieve the bowel obstruction. Perforation occurs in active necrotizing enterocolitis and may require formal laparotomy or placement of an intraperitoneal drain. A persistent loop of distended bowel associated with the mass usually indicates perforation with possible abscess formation. In most cases, this will not resolve except with surgery. Erythema of the abdominal wall with persistent acidosis indicates complete necrosis of some part of the intestine and requires exploration for correction of the problem. Portal vein gas has been found to be an early finding associated with the disease. By itself, it now has no surgical implications.

48. The answer is B. [*Chapter 9 I H 6*] As long as the patient has no evidence of a strangulating process, which usually causes acidosis, leukocytosis, and hypotension, it is safe to postpone exploration for several hours while fluids and electrolytes are corrected. It is potentially dangerous to begin general anesthesia in the presence of hypokalemia, and it is certainly unwarranted to observe the patient for complications because the commonest complications of intestinal obstruction would be perforation of the bowel followed by sepsis. Most surgeons do not initially treat small bowel obstruction with a long intestinal tube.

49. The answer is B. [*Chapter 26 II C 3*] Keratoacanthomas are benign lesions with a rapid growth phase. Frequently, this alarms patients, which prompts the initial consultation. The lesions should be excised and biopsied. The other lesions mentioned are relatively slow-growing.

50. The answer is B. [*Chapter 22 VI A*] Atelectasis is the commonest complication following splenectomy. This may be seen readily on chest x-ray in the investigation of postoperative fever. Hemorrhage is rare following splenectomy if meticulous surgical technique is followed. Subphrenic abscess occurs in 5%–8% of patients and should be considered as a cause of late postoperative fever. Injury to adjacent structures is rare but occasionally occurs when ligating the short gastric vessels. Thrombocytosis is common after splenectomy but actual thrombotic complications occur in fewer than 5% of patients.

51. The answer is A. [*Chapter 3 II B 3*] Patients with chronic stable angina have no increased risk for cardiac complications as compared to patients without angina. However, patients who are well maintained on an antianginal regimen before surgery must be maintained on effective antianginal therapy in the perioperative period as well.

52. The answer is C. [*Chapter 23 III B 1 a, b*] Aspiration of any palpable breast mass should be performed as part of the initial evaluation. Aspiration is considered successful and biopsy is not required as long as the mass disappears completely, the fluid is not bloody, the cytology is not suspicious, and the mass does not recur within 2 months. If these criteria are not met, then biopsy is warranted.

53. The answer is E. [*Chapter 12 II B 5*] When surgery is necessary to treat complications of Crohn's disease, the operations done are "conservative" as defined by the length of the resection. Thus, when an obstructive lesion is present, only a short length of bowel needs to be resected. Therefore, to remove the described obstruction, the distal ileum and cecum should be removed. Radical resections are not necessary, do not reduce the risk of recurrence, and may ultimately contribute to short bowel syndrome if several resections are needed over long periods of time. Additionally, resection of mesentery and lymph nodes, as for a cancer operation, are not necessary. Bypass procedures without resection are reserved for only the worst cases. A stricturoplasty is occasionally appropriate for short symptomatic strictures in the small bowel only.

54. The answer is D. [*Chapter 2 II B 3; Chapter 12 II B 5*] The second postoperative week is the usual time for the development of complications, such as abdominal wound dehiscence, intestinal anastomotic breakdown, superficial wound infection, and intraperitoneal abscess. Blind loop syndrome is rare, and while it does cause pain and diarrhea, it does not cause fever and ileus. Pyelonephritis usually causes flank pain. Crohn's disease does not recur immediately and does not cause the signs described in the question unless complications have occurred. Pseudomembranous enterocolitis causes tenderness over the transverse colon and occasionally over the descending colon, with diarrhea.

55. The answer is C. [*Chapter 12 I B 2 f, g; II B 4–6*] The prognosis of Crohn's disease, which requires surgery, is not good as 50% of patients will require additional surgical procedures within 5 years of the first operation. Thus, the chance of cure is less than 50%. Medical therapy, including anti-inflammatory and antibiotic drugs, has not proven effective at preventing disease recurrence. Removal of the terminal ileum has no effect on disease recurrence or iron absorption; however, the absorption of vitamin B_{12} will be significantly impaired.

56. The answer is A. [*Chapter 26 II F 1 b*] Basal cell carcinoma metastasizes infrequently. Squamous cell carcinoma can metastasize to the regional lymph nodes, and sweat gland tumors, melanomas, and pleomorphic rhabdomyosarcomas are known for their metastatic potential.

57. The answer is B. [*Chapter 1 I C 2 e*] If a patient with hyponatremia (i.e., a deficiency of salt in the blood) does not show signs of dehydration, then it is likely that he or she is overhydrated, resulting in dilutional hyponatremia, which is not a true sodium deficit. The blood volume would be overexpanded, and the total body sodium would be normal. Diabetes insipidus produces hypernatremia and dehydration. Cushing's disease can cause overhydration due to salt retention, but this is much less likely.

58. The answer is E. [*Chapter 16 II E 3, 4 b*] Both ectopic and pituitary Cushing's syndrome result in a loss of diurnal variation in plasma cortisol levels. Although adrenocorticotropic hormone (ACTH) may be high with ectopic Cushing's syndrome, both high and normal values are found in the pituitary type. Although high-dose dexamethasone usually suppresses urinary secretion of 17-hydroxycorticosteroids in pituitary Cushing's syndrome but not in ectopic Cushing's syndrome, a low-dose suppression (2 g/day) will not help to differentiate the two types. However, jugular ACTH levels, particularly petrosal venous samples, are higher in patients with pituitary Cushing's syndrome but not in ectopic Cushing's syndrome.

59. The answer is C. [*Chapter 15 III A 2 c (1) (a)*] Painless jaundice in the presence of a distended gallbladder is most likely secondary to a carcinoma of the head of the pancreas. Occasionally, a common duct stone will not cause pain, but this is unusual. A patient with distal common bile duct obstruction usually has a history of repeated bouts of pancreatitis. Acute cholecystitis is associated with pain. Alcoholic hepatitis usually does not cause a distended gallbladder, and the patient will have an associated history of alcohol abuse.

60 and 61. The answers are: 60-C, 61-B. [*Chapter 21 II A 1, 2, C 2; Figure 21-1*] The management of the burned patient depends on the depth, extent, and location of the burned area. The extent of burns is determined by the "rule of nines," where the body surface area (BSA) is divided into anatomic areas, each of which is 9% (or a multiple thereof) of the total BSA. Thus, first-degree burns on the face and neck (9%), second-degree burns on the anterior chest (18%), and third-degree burns on the left thigh (18%) equal 45% of the BSA.

Major burns (20% or more of the BSA) require fluid resuscitation. Fluid resuscitation should begin with lactated Ringer's solution, and the volume to be given is calculated for adults as follows:

% BSA burned x kg of body weight x 2–4 ml of electrolyte solution

62. The answer is E. [*Chapter 16 I B 2 a–c*] The external branch of the superior laryngeal nerve is intimately intertwined with the branches of the superior thyroid artery, necessitating ligation of the branches of the artery where they join the superior pole of the gland. Ligation at a more proximal level may result in injury to the superior laryngeal nerve. The recurrent laryngeal and vagus nerves are well removed from injury during dissection in this area. Although 10% of superior parathyroid glands derive their blood supply from the superior thyroid artery and may be devascularized during mobilization of the superior pole of the gland, the inferior parathyroids are always supplied by the inferior thyroid artery and are not at risk of injury during dissection in this area. The hypoglossal nerve crosses the internal carotid artery at a much higher level and is not at risk at all during thyroid operations.

63. The answer is B. [*Chapter 29 II A 1 a, 3 a, c, 4 a*] Inguinal hernias occur in 1%–3% of all children. They are commoner on the right (60%), and 10%–15% are bilateral. The complications include intestinal obstruction and testicular injury due to incarceration. For the most part, an incarcerated hernia is treated by reduction and repair within 24–48 hours. Because the inguinal hernia in a child is congenital due to nonfusion of the processus vaginalis, floor repair is not necessary in most cases.

64. The answer is D. [*Chapter 4 II A 2*] The sudden onset of tachycardia and hypotension indicate an acute physiologic alteration. Primary arrhythmia would be unlikely to cause such findings. Retained secretions or myocardial infarction usually have a progressively worsening presentation. Although pulmonary embolus could well explain the situation described in the question, when a patient is being mechanically ventilated, pneumothorax must be considered first and rapidly treated.

65. The answer is C. [*Chapter 25 VI B 4 b (1), C 5 c, D 4 b, c*] Ultrasonography is a noninvasive study, which can delineate between radiolucent calculi and soft tissue lesions. Cytology is less sensitive for low-grade transitional cell carcinoma, and therefore, negative cytology is not definitive. Cystoscopy should be performed to evaluate the bladder, but in this clinical setting, the filling defect should be evaluated first. Retrograde pyelography and ureteroscopy may be needed to define the lesion, but the simple noninvasive study of ultrasonography should be performed first.

66. The answer is E. [*Chapter 13 VIII A 5 a, b*] Cecal lesions are likely to be silent until they become very large. They cause heme-positive stools from a slow, chronic blood loss. The resultant anemia is so insidious in its onset that it often does not cause symptoms until late in the course.

67. The answer is C. [*Chapter 9 II A 2 a*] Obstructing adhesive bands following abdominal surgery are the commonest cause of intestinal obstruction. Although inguinal hernias were the commonest cause in the early 1900s, the policy of repairing hernias electively has greatly reduced this problem. Colonic tumors are the third commonest cause. Acute diverticulitis can, on occasion, cause complete obstruction, but it more commonly produces incomplete obstruction.

68. The answer is D. [*Chapter 5 II A 4*] Simple insertion of a chest tube will cure most patients with a spontaneous pneumothorax. Observation or aspiration is usually not successful and thoracotomy with pleural abrasion is reserved for recurrent cases or cases with a persistent air leak or incomplete lung expansion.

69. The answer is D. [*Chapter 1 III A 2 a, B 1–3*] The lag phase of wound healing occurs during the first several days. Neutrophils predominate for the first 48 hours, after which the macrophages become active. There is no increase in wound strength at this time; however, an uncomplicated wound has good resistance to infection from surface contamination in this phase. The proliferative phase is characterized by the migration of fibroblasts and capillaries into the wound, although neutrophils and macrophages continue to be abundant. The maturation phase of wound healing occurs when the cellular activity in the wound diminishes. Wounds rarely attain the same breaking strength that was present in the tissue prior to injury. Some wounds reach 80% of the original strength, but this may require years.

70. The answer is E. [*Chapter 13 VII B 4 b, D*] Villous adenoma carries about a 35% risk of developing into an adenocarcinoma, and as many as one-third of all specimens are already invaded. Often a biopsy of only one location will not reveal cancer. Because a carcinoma may be present, the adenoma should be excised in its entirety. Local excision is acceptable if no invasion is present. Most authorities would recommend excision over fulgeration to allow adequate pathologic examination of the specimen.

71. The answer is C. [*Chapter 28 III C 1 d*] The spiral fracture of a long bone, combined with the variety of bruises, should lead one to suspect a case of child abuse. Other suspicious lesions include unusual oblique fractures, fractures of various ages in different extremities, and burns or scrapes in various locations and of various ages. Inconsistencies between the type of lesion seen and the history of how it occurred can also be a clue. Abuse of a child is now reportable by law in all states.

72. The answer is D. [*Chapter 6 II D 2*] The presence of a large atrial septal defect causes pressure equalization in both atria. Since atrial flow (emptying) occurs during ventricular diastole, the flow across the atrial septal defect is dependent on the relative compliances of the left and right ventricles. Since the right ventricle is more compliant and, therefore, distensible, flow will be left to right across the atrial septal defect. The greater the differential in compliance, the greater the magnitude of the shunt.

73. The answer is D. [*Chapter 3 V A 2*] Clearly the patient described in the question presents with stigmata of significant liver disease and should have further evaluation prior to elective surgery. Hepatitis serology, liver function tests, coagulation parameters, and a careful history, including a history of alcohol and substance abuse, should be taken.

74. The answer is B. [*Chapter 16 II F 5 a–c*] The patient has a presumed diagnosis of Conn's syndrome, primary hyperaldosteronism, the commonest cause of which is a solitary adrenal adenoma. Ultrasound is not helpful in localizing these adenomas. Arteriography is invasive, and the diagnosis can usually be made more easily with a CT scan or MRI in about 80% of the patients. Selective venous sampling and iodocholesterol scans can be used when the CT or MRI fail to demonstrate the lesion.

75. The answer is E. [*Chapter 5 III C 2*] Atypical pulmonary tuberculosis frequently exhibits a high degree of drug resistance; thus, failure to respond over a 3-month period indicates the need for additional treatment. Persistent cavitary disease, positive sputum, and hemoptysis are indications for resection. Experience has also shown that changing drug therapy or adding minor drugs does not influence the course of the disease. Cavernostomy and thoracoplasty are older methods that are rarely, if ever, employed today.

76. The answer is D. [*Chapter 12 II A 2 c (3) (b)*] The carcinoid syndrome is caused by the release of serotonin and other vasoactive substances produced by the tumor. Serotonin, or 5-hydroxytryptamine, is broken down in the liver and lungs into 5-hydroxyindoleacetic acid (5-HIAA), which is excreted in the urine. An abnormally high level of 5-HIAA in the urine is diagnostic of the carcinoid syndrome.

Metanephrine and vanillylmandelic acid are breakdown products of catecholamines, and elevated urine levels are diagnostic of catecholamine-secreting tumors (e.g., pheochromocytoma).

77. The answer is E. [*Chapter 10 V C 1, 2*] Recognized perforation of the esophagus is most safely treated by thoracotomy and repair of the injury with wide drainage. Failure to carry out these measures may result in a life-threatening infection.

78. The answer is D. [*Chapter 7 I C 2 a–f*] Invasive tests for the assessment of peripheral vascular disease include digital subtraction angiography and conventional arterial angiography. Arterial digital subtraction angiography gives superior images as compared to digital intravenous subtraction angiography and can be repeated due to the small amount of contrast needed for each image. Conventional arterial angiography demonstrates the vascular anatomy by the selective injection of contrast medium intra-arterially. Acute renal failure may result from the nephrotoxicity of the dye. Brachial artery catheterization is frequently performed for cardiac catheterization or for angiography when the lower extremity vessels are unsuitable; however, hand claudication may result. Translumbar aortography is performed by catheterizing the suprarenal aorta posteriorly via a long needle. This study is used when neither the femoral nor the brachial arteries are suitable; however, retroperitoneal hematomas may complicate this procedure. Although ischemia after angiography may be caused by vasospasm, this is a rare occurrence; the occlusion is more often the result of technical problems, such as simple thrombosis at the needle insertion site, thrombi formed on the angiogram catheter, or release of an atherosclerotic plaque during catheter manipulation.

79. The answer is D. [*Chapter 1 IV A 2 b (3), B 1 c, C 1 a (1)*] In a truly elective situation, patients should stop aspirin use at least 1 week prior to surgery. The platelet deficit caused by aspirin lasts for the full life of the platelets—that is, about 7 days. After this time, if aspirin is avoided, the platelets will be normal. Although disorders of platelet function are treated by transfusions of normal platelets preoperatively if the surgery is urgent, the cost and the potential complications from their use are not justified in an elective case.

80. The answer is D. [*Chapter 29 VIII A 2, B 1, 2, C 2*] Hirschsprung's disease may present in either newborns or older infants. A term newborn should pass meconium at 24 hours. The older child usually presents with constipation and failure to thrive but may present with overflow diarrhea or diarrhea of Hirschsprung's enterocolitis. While there is a male predominance, females usually have the long-segment disease (total colonic). Because of this, the barium enema may show a nondistended colon, which may be interpreted as normal. Newborns with abdominal distention due to Hirschsprung's show air–fluid levels on x-ray not the ground-glass appearance that is seen in meconium ileus.

81. The answer is B. [*Chapter 16 III C 1 b (1)–(4)*] Approximately 90% of cases of primary hyperparathyroidism are caused by single-gland adenomas. Between 8%–10% of cases are due to four-gland hyperplasia, and 1% or less are caused by parathyroid carcinoma or multiple adenomas.

82. The answer is C. [*Chapter 9 II A 3 a*] Obstructing adhesive bands following abdominal surgery are the commonest cause of intestinal obstruction. They may be diffuse or solitary. Management consists of surgical lysis of the obstructing bands.

83. The answer is B. [*Chapter 14 I D 1 b (2), d (1)*] Alpha-fetoprotein is a protein secreted by embryonal hepatocytes and is present at levels of 400 ng/ml in up to 85% of patients with hepatocellular carcinoma. It has a high sensitivity as a diagnostic "marker" in hepatocellular carcinoma, as it is not often present in other disorders with the exception of hepatoblastoma, a tumor of children.

84. The answer is D. [*Chapter 23 III A 1, 2*] The incidence of carcinoma of the breast is decreased in the sun belt and increased in the north central states. Approximately 10% of women will have breast cancer by the age of 70. High socioeconomic status and nulliparity are associated with an increased risk for developing a breast cancer. The fact that age-adjusted mortality has not changed since 1930 indicates that therapy has not improved significantly since that time.

85. The answer is C. [*Chapter 2 IV B 5*] Fistulas between the gastrointestinal tract and the skin can undergo spontaneous closure when the patient is provided with adequate nutrition, fluids, and electrolytes. There are five problems that prevent spontaneous closure: (1) obstruction of the bowel distal to the fistula (in this patient, the problem has been fixed); (2) foreign body at the fistula; (3) badly damaged bowel at the fistula (e.g., radiation injury or Crohn's disease); (4) cancer at the fistula; and (5) epithelialization of the fistula tract.

86. The answer is D. [*Chapter 20 I A 1–3, B*] The parotid is the largest salivary gland. The tight fascia is the reason for the severe pain that occurs if the gland swells acutely. The gland probably does not have two true lobes, although this concept is useful in planning resections of the parotid gland. The facial nerve runs through the gland, and preservation of the nerve is essential in surgery for benign conditions of the parotid gland. Drainage of saliva is via Stensen's duct.

87. The answer is D. [*Chapter 5 IV B 5 a*] Calcification within a solitary pulmonary lesion, especially if it is in a concentric or popcorn-like pattern, favors a benign diagnosis. No growth shown on chest x-rays taken over 1–2 years also suggests a benign lesion. A diameter greater than 1–2 cm suggests a malignant lesion. All solitary pulmonary lesions are peripheral, and so this location would not help to distinguish a benign from a malignant lesion. Cavitation occurs with both carcinoma and infection. Small flecks of calcium within the lesion suggests malignancy.

88. The answer is E. [*Chapter 13 VII E 3 a (2), (3)*] The history of the patient described in the question is typical of Peutz-Jeghers syndrome. The association of recurrent bouts of colicky pain with pigmented spots on the lips and oral mucosa is striking. A sibling with similar symptoms is a clue to the hereditary nature of the disorder.

89. The answer is A. [*Chapter 29 IX A 2, 3*] The diagnosis of hypertrophic pyloric stenosis can usually be made by physical examination and palpation of an abdominal mass. However, if the history is suspicious and a mass cannot be demonstrated, ultrasound is an accurate and quick means of confirming the diagnosis. The child usually presents with various stages of dehydration and alkalosis. Both need to be corrected prior to surgery. Placement of a nasogastric tube will aid in the comfort of the patient, relieve the gastric distention as well as improve the postoperative feeding schedule. Once the diagnosis of pyloric stenosis has been made, any attempt at oral rehydration will be hazardous as well as unsuccessful.

90 and 91. The answers are: 90-C, 91-C. [*Chapter 16 II G 3–5*] The patient presented in the question has clinical signs (hypertension) and symptoms (attacks of palpitations, sweating, and headaches) of a pheochromocytoma. A normal physical examination would make Cushing's syndrome less likely. Patients with Conn's syndrome usually have abnormalities in serum electrolytes, particularly hypokalemia. Twenty-four–hour urine for metanephrines, vanillylmandelic acid, and catecholamines will reveal abnormalities in 95% of patients with pheochromocytomas and should be ordered next to confirm the suspected diagnosis biochemically. Measurements of serum aldosterone and renin and salt loading with subsequent measurements of urine and serum potassium would be indicated if Conn's syndrome was suspected. Serum cortisol and urine for 17-hydroxycorticosteroids would be indicated if Cushing's syndrome was suspected.

Once a pheochromocytoma is diagnosed biochemically, CT scan will localize the tumor anatomically in about 95% of the cases. The other tests can be ordered if CT does not reveal any abnormality. Laparotomy should be performed after anatomic localization studies are performed.

92. The answer is C. [*Chapter 4 I B 2 a*] Tumor involvement of the left recurrent laryngeal nerve within the thorax is the usual cause of hoarseness in superior sulcus lung carcinoma. Therefore, when hoarseness develops after radiation therapy, it indicates failure of therapy to control the tumor.

93. The answer is C. [*Chapter 14 I F 4 a, b (3)*] An echinococcal parasitic infestation of the liver causes a cyst to form within the parenchyma. Diagnostic serologic tests are now available. The major risk of this infestation is either spontaneous rupture with resultant shock or leakage at the time of surgery with the formation of new cysts.

94. The answer is D. [*Chapter 16 I C 5 c*] Thyroglossal duct cysts present as midline neck masses between the hyoid bone and the thyroid isthmus. Excision is recommended to prevent recurrent infection. They are always connected to the base of the tongue and traverse the middle of the hyoid bone. Thus, curative resection involves the central portion of the hyoid bone and the tract all the way to the base of the tongue. The thyroid gland, thyroid cartilage, and cricoid cartilage are usually not involved.

95. The answer is C. [*Chapter 2 II A 5*] Any person with a penetrating injury must receive tetanus prophylaxis if previous immunization was not recent or cannot be documented. A previously immunized person should be given a booster dose if none has been given within the past 5 years. A patient with a clean injury who has never been immunized may be given tetanus toxoid in three separate doses. A patient with a dirty wound who has never been immunized should be given passive immunization with human tetanus immune globulin. Adequate debridement of devitalized tissue and removal of all foreign matter is also essential. The efficacy of antibiotics for prophylaxis of tetanus-prone wounds is unproven. Although *Clostridia* are very susceptible to penicillin, the nature of a tetanus-prone wound prevents delivery of antibiotic to the wound, and hence, antibiotic prophylaxis is not helpful.

96. The answer is D. [*Chapter 11 II B 2 d; Chapter 17 II C*] The Zollinger-Ellison syndrome causes a virulent form of duodenal ulcer disease. The syndrome is due to the oversecretion of gastrin by a gastrinoma, a tumor of the non-beta islet cells of the pancreas. Because the cells of origin are part of the amine precursor uptake and decarboxylation (APUD) system, gastrinomas and other types of tumors arising from cells of this system are known as apudomas. In the Zollinger-Ellison syndrome, the excess gastrin production causes an overproduction of gastric acid, which leads to the severe ulcer symptoms.

97. The answer is C. [*Chapter 25 IV C 2 b*] An excretory urogram can demonstrate a calculus if it is radiopaque and can indicate the site of obstruction. Ultrasonography may indicate hydronephrosis but may not demonstrate a ureteral calculus. A CT scan can give much of the same information as an excretory urogram, but it is more expensive and can miss a calculus, depending on the width of the tomographic cuts. A retrograde ureterogram is invasive and should be avoided if a less invasive study will suffice.

98. The answer is E. [*Chapter 16 III C 1 h (1)*] Postoperative hypocalcemia usually occurs after successful treatment for primary hyperparathyroidism. In the absence of significant bone disease, this is usually temporary. If the patient is asymptomatic, no treatment is required.

99. The answer is A. [*Chapter 7 VII D 1*] Fibromuscular dysplasia frequently causes lesions in the midportion of the renal artery. Many physicians feel that transcutaneous dilatation of these lesions is the most acceptable first choice for management of these lesions. Patients with osteal atherosclerotic lesions do not fair well with balloon dilatation. Aortorenal bypass is the acceptable procedure in this situation. Patients with multiple lesions caused by atherosclerosis or fibromuscular dysplasia in the renal hilar vessels are best repaired operatively.

100. The answer is C. [*Chapter 9 III E 1*] Upper endoscopy is the most reliable method for locating precisely the site of upper gastrointestinal bleeding. Endoscopy can be used in most situations except when bleeding is massive. If bleeding is so rapid that exsanguination is imminent, laparotomy is indicated.

101. The answer is A. [*Chapter 14 I F 3 c*] Amebic abscesses respond to parenteral antibiotics, particularly metronidazole. Bacterial abscesses require adequate drainage. Echinococcal cysts require adequate evacuation and sterilization. Choledochal cysts and hepatocellular carcinomas should be resected when feasible.

102. The answer is E. [*Chapter 1 VI H 1 c*] An appropriate operation to attempt to cure a gastric cancer removes all or most of the stomach with the lymph node draining areas. This includes the lymph nodes along the lesser curvature and the celiac plexus superiorly and along the greater curvature and the splenic hilum inferiorly. To remove the lymph nodes from the splenic hilum requires a splenectomy. Additionally, as the omentum's blood supply is derived primarily from the stomach and since it may be a source of metastatic spread, it is removed during this operation. This operation is a radical resection with en block excision of the lymphatic drainage. Wide local resections do not include the lymphatic drainage. The same is also true for radical local resections. Super radical resections are much larger procedures, which include adjacent viscera. A debulking procedure is a palliative procedure, which attempts to remove gross disease only, knowing that microscopic disease is left behind.

103. The answer is D. [*Chapter 3 IV B 2 a, 3 b (1), (3), (5)*] Patients with chronic renal failure can tolerate a hemoglobin level of 7–8 g/dl for most surgical procedures. Routine dialysis should be undertaken 24 hours prior to elective surgery to minimize the effects of intravenous heparin (given with dialysis), to allow the patient to stabilize post-treatment, and to treat the signs or symptoms of uremia or coagulopathy. Bleeding tendencies may also be treated with cryoprecipitated plasma. The use of neuromuscular-blocking agents may precipitate severe hyperkalemia, which must be treated immediately. Bladder catheterization is unnecessary in chronic renal failure patients.

104. The answer is D. [*Chapter 6 I E 4, 5*] Initially, angina pectoris is managed with medical therapy. Nitrates, β-blockers, and antihypertensive medicines are frequently effective in ameliorating the symptoms. In addition, the patient is encouraged to modify his or her life-style to eliminate all risk factors. Cardiac catheterization and coronary angiography provide the most accurate means of determining the extent of coronary artery disease. Surgical treatment is indicated if the angina is intractable or unstable. In selected lesions, such as left main coronary artery obstruction or three-vessel coronary artery disease, surgery is the preferred treatment.

105. The answer is B. [*Chapter 28 II A 1 b (1) (b)*] Hematogenous osteomyelitis is not uncommon in childhood. *Staphylococcus aureus* and gram-negative rods predominate as the causative organisms in neonates. Young children commonly have ear infections with *Hemophilus influenzae,* which may cause osteomyelitis. *S. aureus* is again the most likely cause of osteomyelitis in older children and adolescents. *S. aureus* and *Salmonella* may be the causative agents of this disease in adults.

106. The answer is C. [*Chapter 9 IV B, C*] Arteriography is most often used as the initial evaluation step for continued bleeding after anorectal bleeding sources have been eliminated by endoscopy. Arteriography allows identification of diverticular bleeding as well as an angiodysplastic lesion of the right colon. Barium enema may also be used in the initial management. Surgery is generally not indicated until 4–6 units of blood have been shed. Coagulation products are of no use unless the patient has abnormal clotting studies. Saline lavage of the colon is not a routine procedure.

107. The answer is D. [*Chapter 2 II F 1 c*] In normal human stool, there are 10^8–10^9 aerobes per gram of stool and 10^{11} anaerobes per gram of stool. An effective preparation of the colon must include the removal of gross feces (mechanical preparation) plus the use of oral, nonabsorbable antibiotics to lower bacterial concentrations of the remaining colonic contents. While intravenous antibiotics may provide additional help in lowering the incidence of both wound and intraperitoneal infections, this is controversial. Oral antibiotics used to decrease the numbers of intraluminal bacteria are usually nonabsorbable.

108. The answer is D. [*Chapter 3 VI F 2 a*] Serum sodium levels must be corrected for elevated glucose levels by a factor of 1.7 mg/100 mg over normal glucose.

109. The answer is B. [*Chapter 5 III A 2 c*] Rupture of a lung abscess into the pleural space produces empyema thoracis, which is *initially* treated by tube thoracostomy and continued antibiotic therapy. If this is inadequate, open drainage (decortication with or without resection) may be necessary. The remaining choices are all indications for resectional therapy.

110. The answer is C. [*Chapter 11 II C 1 a*] The patient described in the question is in shock. He needs to be resuscitated with intravenous fluids. Once his condition has stabilized, a secondary assessment, including a more detailed history, may be obtained.

111. The answer is D. [*Chapter 11 II C 1 a*] The white blood count and sedimentation rate are nonspecific tests. In a patient with peritonitis and a possible ruptured viscus, a barium study is ill-advised. An abdominal flat plate will not demonstrate free air from the perforation. An upright chest x-ray, part of an obstruction series, is necessary for this.

112. The answer is E. [*Chapter 11 II C 1 b*] Consideration involved in choosing the best operation for a patient with a perforated duodenal ulcer include the medical stability of the patient, previous history of peptic ulcer disease, and the amount of peritoneal contamination from the perforation. The patient's size is usually not a consideration.

113. The answer is B. [*Chapter 16 III C 1 d (1) (b) (ii); Figure 16-2*] In secondary hyperparathyroidism, the secretion of parathyroid hormone (PTH) increases the response to chronic hypocalcemia. Both calcium and PTH levels are elevated in primary and tertiary hyperparathyroidism. In hypoparathyroidism, calcium and PTH levels are below normal.

114. The answer is B. [*Chapter 28 III A 3 a (5), D 6 b, c*] Acute intramedullary rodding of closed femoral fracture in multiple trauma has become a standard of care to improve mobilization and decrease complications of trauma, such as pulmonary complications, bed sores, joint immobility, and urinary tract infections. Open growth plates in children preclude intramedullary rodding for routine fracture care. Infection is a contraindication to intramedullary rodding.

115. The answer is E. [*Chapter 23 III D 2*] The preoperative evaluation determines if there is evidence of disease beyond the breast and axilla. Since the lungs, liver, bone, and contralateral breast are the commonest sites of metastases, they must be evaluated. Although metastasis to the brain is seen, it is uncommon in the absence of symptoms.

116. The answer is D. [*Chapter 12 II A 2 c*] Carcinoid tumors are commonest in the periappendiceal region and then in the small bowel. Prognosis is related to the presence of metastases, and the risk of metastases rises with increased tumor size. However, regardless of the presence of liver metastases, an obstructing bowel lesion should be resected, as it may also ulcerate, bleed, or perforate if only bypassed. Small bowel carcinoid tumors have a 30% incidence of multicentricity, and a thorough search of the entire small bowel is needed. Carcinoid tumors arise in the enterochromaffin cells, which are found throughout the bowel mucosa. They have no known association with Meckel's diverticulum. Incidental appendectomies are not usually indicated. Massive liver metastases may cause the *carcinoid,* not carcinoma, syndrome.

117. The answer is B. [*Chapter 2 V B 1, 2 b*] The inguinal canal is the communication between the internal and external rings. The anterior wall of the canal is formed by the external oblique aponeurosis. The posterior wall (floor) of the canal is formed by the transversalis fascia and aponeurosis. Within the floor of the canal is Hesselbach's triangle, which is formed laterally by the inferior epigastric artery, inferiorly by the inguinal ligament, and superomedially by the transversalis fascia and portions of the rectus sheath. An indirect inguinal hernia passes through the internal ring (i.e., laterally to the inferior epigastric vessels) and down the inguinal canal. A direct inguinal hernia occurs in the floor of the inguinal canal at Hesselbach's triangle (i.e., medially to the inferior epigastric vessels) due to an acquired weakness of tissue. The inferior epigastric vessels are the anatomic landmarks that separate the indirect and direct hernias.

118. The answer is C. [*Chapter 16 I D 2 d (1), (2), e (1)*] Antithyroid medications are effective in approximately 50% of patients. Since the actions of propylthiouracil and methimazole are similar, a switch from one to the other would not be likely to change the clinical course. Propranolol controls some of the symptoms of hyperthyroidism through its β-adrenergic blockade, but it does nothing to effect T_4 or T_3 production. Therefore, its use alone would not produce remission. ^{131}I would be contraindicated in a woman of childbearing age because of its possible teratogenic effects. Subtotal thyroidectomy would be the therapy of choice for this patient.

119. The answer is D. [*Chapter 28 IV A 1 b (2), (3)*] A mass in the extremity is a common presentation of a bone tumor, and bone tumors warrant thorough, logical workups. A plain film of the involved area will suggest whether the tumor is benign or malignant. Other appropriate studies include CT of the involved area to delineate the anatomic relationships of the mass, a bone scan to identify the extent of the tumor within the bone, and CT of the chest to determine possible metastatic disease.

120. The answer is B. [*Chapter 10 IV B 2*] Hiatal hernia is an anatomic description of the relationship between the diaphragm and the gastroesophageal junction. It can be associated with gastroesophageal reflux, but there are many patients who have hiatal hernias and no reflux. All of the other answers may contribute to the development of esophageal carcinoma. Chronic irritation of the mucosal lining seems to be of significant importance.

121. The answer is C. [*Chapter 14 III G 3 b, c (2)*] Of the choices listed in the question, percutaneous transhepatic cholangiography is the most precise method of visualizing the area of the bile duct at the hepatic duct confluence. The procedure is usually successful when biliary obstruction is present. At the time of the study, a biopsy using a brush or forceps can be performed, establishing the diagnosis. The other invasive procedure that can be helpful is endoscopic retrograde cholangiography.

122. The answer is C. [*Chapter 4 I B 2 b*] Bronchoscopy is most likely to establish the diagnosis in a patient with a cavitary lung lesion. Aspiration of the cavity's contents usually yields necrotic debris and may not yield carcinoma.

123. The answer is C. [*Chapter 16 I D 2 d (1), (2)*] Radioiodine destroys functional thyroid cells through the concentrated effects of radiation on the gland. Iodine blocks the release of thyroid hormone when given in high doses. Propranolol is a β-adrenergic blocker and has no direct effect on T_4 or T_3. Both propylthiouracil and methimazole block the oxidation of iodide to iodine, but only propylthiouracil blocks the peripheral conversion of T_4 to T_3.

124. The answer is D. [*Chapter 6 I G 1 b*] Injury to the heart may result in bleeding into the pericardial sac, which may result in tamponade. This is a true emergency that must be diagnosed and treated promptly. The classic findings are distended neck veins, hypotension, and pulsus paradoxus. The heart sounds are characteristically decreased. If tamponade is suspected, the pericardial sac should be aspirated, which will usually result in a rapid improvement in the patient's blood pressure. Definitive treatment of the underlying cause of tamponade can then be undertaken. If the pulmonary parenchyma were injured, the resulting hemothorax would appear as a unilateral pleural effusion on chest x-ray. This could occur together with, or independent from, a cardiac injury.

125. The answer is E. [*Chapter 1 V A 2, C 2 c (2)*] Hemolytic reactions in the anesthetized patient can be difficult to diagnose. Unexplained generalized bleeding due to disseminated intravascular coagulation is frequently the only manifestation. The treatment of this emergency requires immediately stopping the transfusion, sending the remaining transfusion blood and a fresh sample of the patient's blood for retyping and recrossmatching, and treatment of the hemoglobinuria to prevent renal failure. This consists of initiating a diuresis with fluids and mannitol and alkalinization of the urine with sodium bicarbonate. Allergic reactions typically cause fever, chills, urticaria, and itching and are treated with diphenhydramine. Epinephrine and steroids are reserved for more serious instances of allergic reactions. Febrile reactions are caused by the antigens on white cells and platelets, which do contaminate all units of packed red blood cells.

126. The answer is C. [*Chapter 23 II C*] At most, the risk of cancer in individuals with fibrocystic breast disease is twice that of unaffected women and may be even lower. It is important to remember that benign cysts do not progress to cancer; they arise de novo. In patients with cystic breasts, any malignant lesions must be detected before they become untreatable.

127. The answer is B. [*Chapter 9 IV C 2 b (1)*] Most angiograms are sensitive down to a level of 0.5 ml/min. The ^{99m}Tc radionuclide scan is much more sensitive, detecting to a level of 0.05 ml/min, but it is much less specific in determining the site of bleeding. If bleeding is proceeding at a rate of 50 ml/min, immediate surgery is indicated.

128. The answer is B. [*Chapter 2 II A 3, 4*] Prophylactic antibiotics should be given 1–2 hours preceding surgery and for only 6–24 hours postoperatively for any operation that carries a risk of postoperative wound infection. Longer periods increase the risk of superinfection with resistant organisms. Narrow-spectrum antibiotics aimed at the usual infecting organism for a particular type of operation are the treatment of choice. Broad-spectrum antibiotics often select for resistant organisms, which are then more difficult to treat than the original organism. Prosthesis insertion carries a significant risk of infection, which is very difficult to eradicate and may result in loss of life or limb. Many studies have demonstrated the usefulness of prophylactic antibiotics in prosthetic surgery. However, most prosthetic infections cannot be sterilized with antibiotics and, thus, require removal of the prosthesis.

129. The answer is C. [*Chapter 5 VI B 1 a*] Squamous cell carcinoma is the commonest tumor of the trachea, and regional lymph node spread is common. Adenoid cystic carcinoma is the second commonest primary tracheal neoplasm and is quite malignant, being characterized by extensive submucosal lymphatic spread. Carcinoid tumors are rarely found in the trachea, being more commonly located in the main stem or lobar bronchi. Squamous papilloma and mucoepidermoid carcinoma are very rare tumors of the trachea.

130. The answer is D. [*Chapter 16 I F 3 a–f*] ^{99m}Tc and ^{131}I scans of the thyroid help to distinguish functioning from nonfunctioning thyroid nodules; however, although most thyroid malignancies are nonfunctioning, radionuclide scans do not distinguish benign from malignant nonfunctioning thyroid nodules. Thyroid ultrasonography is helpful in distinguishing solid from cystic lesions, but it does not distinguish malignant from benign solid lesions. In the absence of a family history of thyroid malignancy, it is unlikely that a thyrocalcitonin assay will be positive. Fine-needle aspiration will provide cytopathologic material to help in the diagnosis of the thyroid nodule and in deciding on its management. If the cytopathologic findings are those of a benign colloid nodule or adenomatous hyperplasia, then careful clinical observation would be indicated.

131. The answer is A. [*Chapter 23 III D 1, F 1 b*] Haagensen's criteria identify those tumors that are locally advanced with regional disease, which is nonresectable (i.e., internal mammary or supraclavicular nodal involvement) or evidence of dermal lymphatic involvement (edema and erythema). Nipple inversion with eczematoid changes is characteristic of Paget's disease, which is operable.

132. The answer is D. [*Chapter 7 XI A 1–3, B 1 a*] The graft of choice for a femoropopliteal bypass is an autogenous saphenous vein graft. This type of graft is a vein that is transplanted from one part of the body to another for use in bypassing an occlusion in either an artery or vein. An autogenous arterial graft is an artery that is removed from one area of the vascular tree and inserted into another area. Of the vascular allografts—that is, vessels removed from one individual and implanted into another individual—arterial allografts are not used because of a high rate of degeneration, while umbilical vein allografts have shown excellent long-term patency for both lower extremity revascularization and hemodialysis vascular access. Dacron grafts are very successful when used for large-vessel replacements, such as in the aorta or iliac vessels.

133. The answer is E. [*Chapter 14 III F*] The patient probably has a biliary blockage, secondary to either a retained common duct stone or to some mechanical problem related to the surgery or the tube. It is most important to maintain adequate drainage; thus, the T tube should not be clamped or removed. A cholangiogram should be obtained. Decisions about further management will be based on the findings.

134. The answer is C. [*Chapter 7 I B 1 a (2)*] Symptoms of arterial occlusion present distally to the site of the involved vessel. In this case, a patient with a superficial femoral artery occlusion would be expected to present with symptoms of claudication in the calf. By taking a careful history, it is frequently possible to make an educated guess as to where the lesion is.

135. The answer is B. [*Chapter 9 Table 9-1*] Massive upper gastrointestinal bleeding is usually due to a bleeding source proximal to the ligament of Treitz. The cause is most likely to be a posterior duodenal ulcer that is eroding into the gastroduodenal artery. Gastritis, esophagitis, a Mallory-Weiss tear, and esophageal varices are less likely causes of massive upper gastrointestinal bleeding.

136–140. The answers are: 136-B, 137-A, 138-D, 139-C, 140-E. [*Chapter 24 I A 3 b, D 2 a, F 1 b*] Hyperacute rejection is associated with preformed antibody and complement deposition on vascular endothelium. Prior to transplant, the recipient's blood is examined for the presence of cytotoxic antibodies specifically directed against antigens on the donor's T lymphocytes (crossmatch test). A transplant cannot be performed if these antibodies are found.

Kidney transplants are occasionally associated with a period of acute tubular necrosis. This is usually temporary. It results from conditions that occur during obtaining or preserving the kidney and is followed by diuresis and normal renal function.

Antilymphocyte globulin and orthoclone are used in cases of acute rejection when high-dose prednisone fails. Chronic rejection is associated with a slow decline in renal function over months or years. There is no known effective therapy.

Accelerated acute rejection is rapidly evolving, occurs within the first week, and is probably a second-set immune response. Treatment with high-dose prednisone, while generally effective in acute rejection, is associated with a poor success rate in accelerated acute rejection.

141–145. The answers are: 141-D, 142-E, 143-A, 144-C, 145-A. [*Chapter 1 IV C 3 a (1) (b) (iii); V A 1 b, 3–6*] Albumin, which is available in concentrations of 5% and 25%, is obtained by fractionating blood from humans. It is used as a volume expander as are whole blood, packed red blood cells, and fresh frozen plasma; however, the latter three should not be used unless there has been a significant blood loss or loss of clotting factors.

Probably the only indication for the transfusion of whole blood is hypovolemia secondary to acute hemorrhage. Fresh whole blood (not more than 24 hours old) would be ideal for this purpose, since platelets and clotting factors would still be active, and many of the adverse biochemical effects of stored blood would be avoided.

Purified factor VIII concentrations do not contain the von Willebrand factor (factor VIII R:WF) and are, therefore, ineffective for treatment. Cryoprecipitate provides both portions of the factor VIII complex and corrects the bleeding disorder of von Willebrand's disease. In addition to high concentrations of factor VIII, cryoprecipitate contains high concentrations of fibrinogen; thus, it is used appropriately to correct afibrinogenemia.

Fresh frozen plasma contains all of the coagulation factors lacking in banked blood, including factors V and VIII. It is used to replace clotting factors during massive transfusion of packed red cells or to correct factor abnormalities found in conditions such as liver disease or disseminated intravascular coagulation.

146–150. The answers are: 146-C, 147-A, 148-B, 149-D, 150-E. [*Chapter 18 III F 4 c; IV B 4 b; V C; Chapter 19 VIII C 1; XI C 1 d*] Information from an initial history and physical examination can be quite helpful in guiding a workup of a neck mass. Most malignant neck masses are painless and relatively slow-growing. Patients with Hodgkin's disease commonly have fever, night sweats, malaise, anorexia, and weight loss. Hoarseness and cough are common presenting signs of laryngeal carcinoma. Radiation in childhood predisposes patients to an increased risk of benign and malignant thyroid tumors. Atypical mycobacteria rarely affects the lungs and commonly presents with skin involvement over the infected node or gland. Rapid growth, fever, and local inflammation are all signs of an acutely infected neck mass.

151–155. The answers are: 151-C, 152-A, 153-B, 154-E, 155-D. [*Chapter 25 VI B 4 c, C 5 c, D 4 b, E 4 b, F 5 d*] Some testicular tumors have been shown to produce human chorionic gonadotropin and α-fetoprotein. These markers have accurately indicated the presence of microscopic metastases and recurrences. In prostatic carcinoma, serum prostatic acid phosphatase is an early and reliable tumor marker. It has accurately indicated extracapsular extensions, metastases, and recurrences. Renal cell carcinoma can be diagnosed and partially staged by renal arteriography. The tumor is usually indicated by neovascularity with contrast pooling and a vascular blush.

Transitional cell carcinoma of the renal pelvis can be demonstrated by retrograde pyelography. A filling defect seen on excretory urography can be outlined more clearly by the retrograde technique, which can differentiate an obstructing calculus or a neoplasm filling the pelvis of a nonfunctioning kidney. In carcinoma of the bladder, cystoscopy is essential. Bladder endoscopy should be performed in the evaluation of all patients with gross painless hematuria and in the follow-up after treatment of a urothelial neoplasm of the bladder, ureter, or renal pelvis. The mucosal surface of the bladder can be inspected directly, and much greater accuracy in diagnosis can be obtained than with radiologic studies.

156–160. The answers are: 156-E, 157-A, 158-C, 159-B, 160-D. [*Chapter 13 VII B 1–4*] Inflammatory polyps are outgrowths of mucosa in response to inflammation; thus, they are also referred to as pseudopolyps. Hyperplastic polyps are small tumors of no clinical significance and are the commonest polyp found in the adult colon. Juvenile polyps are the commonest type of hamartomatous polyps. Like inflammatory and hyperplastic polyps, juvenile polyps have no malignant potential. Tubular and villous adenomas have certain malignant potential with the villous type having a higher incidence of malignancy overall. Familial polyposis is characterized by more than 100 adenomatous polyps (tubular adenoma) of the colon and rectum.

161–165. The answers are: 161-D, 162-C, 163-E, 164-A, 165-B. [*Chapter 6 II B, D–G*] Both anatomy and physiology are important in congenital cardiac surgery. The key to understanding many congenital cardiac malformations (anatomy) lies in determining the level and direction of the resulting shunt (physiology). With the oxymetric data given, the shunt would be evidenced by the change in oxygen saturation in a particular chamber or chambers. Defects causing a left-to-right shunt would result in an increase in oxygen saturation in right-sided chambers. This increase, or step up, in oxygen saturation occurs in the right atrium with an atrial septal defect, in the right ventricle with a ventricular septal defect, and in the pulmonary artery with a patent ductus arteriosus. Defects causing a right-to-left shunt, such as tetralogy of Fallot, would result in cyanosis, manifested by low oxygen saturations in all right-sided chambers, as well as a decrease in oxygen saturation in the left ventricle and aorta. Transposition of the great arteries results in two nearly independent parallel circuits, one recycling unsaturated blood to the periphery, and the other recycling saturated blood to the lungs.

166–170. The answers are: 166-A, 167-B, 168-E, 169-D, 170-C. [*Chapter 17 I B 1 d, 3 b, C 2 a (2); II C 2 a, D 1 a*] Multiple endocrine adenomatosis (MEA) syndromes are characteristic patterns of endocrine hyperfunction, which are inherited as autosomal dominant traits. In all MEA syndromes, the affected endocrine glands develop either hyperplasia, adenoma, or carcinoma.

MEA type I, or Wermer's syndrome, chiefly involves the parathyroid glands, pancreatic islet cells, and the pituitary gland. Hyperparathyroidism is present in 90% of patients, pancreatic tumors occur in 80%, and pituitary tumors occur in 65%. Most patients present with symptoms of peptic ulceration related to the pancreatic gastrinoma (Zollinger-Ellison syndrome) or with symptoms related to the pituitary tumor (e.g., acromegaly, galactorrhea, and Cushing's syndrome). The hyperparathyroidism usually is asymptomatic, evidenced only by an increased serum calcium level.

MEA type II, or Sipple's syndrome, involves medullary thyroid carcinoma (in all patients), pheochromocytoma (in 40% of patients), and parathyroid hyperplasia (in 60% of patients). Medullary thyroid carcinoma often is preceded by nonmalignant hyperplasia of the parafollicular C cells. An elevated serum thyrocalcitonin level is diagnostic. In the premalignant state, infusion of calcium and pentagastrin may be needed to demonstrate the abnormal thyrocalcitonemia.

MEA type III, or mucosal neuroma syndrome, is considered a variant of MEA type II, sharing with it the development of medullary thyroid carcinoma and pheochromocytoma. Patients with MEA type III are distinguished, however, by their characteristically distorted body habitus.

Pancreatic gastrinoma, or Zollinger-Ellison syndrome, is characterized by oversecretion of gastrin, most commonly due to a non-beta islet cell tumor. The excess gastrin stimulates hypersecretion of gastric acid, which ultimately results in peptic ulceration. Abdominal pain secondary to peptic ulceration occurs in 90% of patients. Diarrhea also is common.

Pancreatic cholera is believed to be caused by hypersecretion of vasoactive intestinal peptide due to a pancreatic non-beta islet cell tumor. The syndrome sometimes is referred to as WDHA syndrome for its severe watery diarrhea, hypokalemia, and achlorhydria.

171–175. The answers are: 171-C, 172-D, 173-E, 174-B, 175-D. [*Chapter 11 II A 5, B 2 c, C 3; III A 2, B 1*] Stress ulcers occur in patients undergoing severe stress—from sepsis, severe trauma, burns, and so forth—which causes ischemia of the gastric mucosa and consequent ulceration. Gastric atrophy occurs in chronic (atrophic) gastritis and increases the risk of gastric cancer. (There is no evidence that persons with simple gastric ulcer have a higher incidence of cancer.) Prepyloric ulcers can obstruct the gastric outlet, causing gastric distention, crampy pain, and nausea. Several factors are known to increase the incidence of duodenal ulcer; these include not only understandable factors, such as aspirin or caffeine ingestion, but also the blood type O. Parietal cell antibodies are associated with the less common of the two types of chronic gastritis, type B, which is also associated with vitamin B_{12} malabsorption.

176–180. The answers are: 176-A, 177-C, 178-B, 179-A, 180-A. [*Chapter 16 IV B 4, C 3 b (1)*] Complete thymectomy is the operation of choice for benign and malignant tumors of the thymus gland. Radiation therapy may be beneficial for malignant thymomas, which are nonresectable or which cannot be completely removed. Chemotherapy has not been useful for these neoplasms.

Complete thymectomy appears to be the treatment of choice for all patients with myasthenia gravis except those with purely ocular disease who do just as well with medical therapy (anticholinesterases). The effect of thymectomy on patients with myasthenia gravis and a thymic tumor is less predictable but still advised. Partial thymectomy has no role in the treatment of thymic tumors or myasthenia gravis, except with malignant thymomas when the organ cannot be completely excised safely.

Index